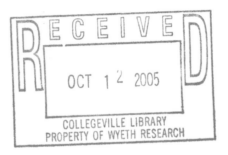

Pharmaceutical Stress Testing

DRUGS AND THE PHARMACEUTICAL SCIENCES

DRUGS AND THE PHARMACEUTICAL SCIENCES

A Series of Textbooks and Monographs

1. Pharmacokinetics, *Milo Gibaldi and Donald Perrier*
2. Good Manufacturing Practices for Pharmaceuticals: A Plan for Total Quality Control, *Sidney H. Willig, Murray M. Tuckerman, and William S. Hitchings IV*
3. Microencapsulation, *edited by J. R. Nixon*
4. Drug Metabolism: Chemical and Biochemical Aspects, *Bernard Testa and Peter Jenner*
5. New Drugs: Discovery and Development, *edited by Alan A. Rubin*
6. Sustained and Controlled Release Drug Delivery Systems, *edited by Joseph R. Robinson*
7. Modern Pharmaceutics, *edited by Gilbert S. Banker and Christopher T. Rhodes*
8. Prescription Drugs in Short Supply: Case Histories, *Michael A. Schwartz*
9. Activated Charcoal: Antidotal and Other Medical Uses, *David O. Cooney*
10. Concepts in Drug Metabolism (in two parts), *edited by Peter Jenner and Bernard Testa*
11. Pharmaceutical Analysis: Modern Methods (in two parts), *edited by James W. Munson*
12. Techniques of Solubilization of Drugs, *edited by Samuel H. Yalkowsky*
13. Orphan Drugs, *edited by Fred E. Karch*
14. Novel Drug Delivery Systems: Fundamentals, Developmental Concepts, Biomedical Assessments, *Yie W. Chien*
15. Pharmacokinetics: Second Edition, Revised and Expanded, *Milo Gibaldi and Donald Perrier*
16. Good Manufacturing Practices for Pharmaceuticals: A Plan for Total Quality Control, Second Edition, Revised and Expanded, *Sidney H. Willig, Murray M. Tuckerman, and William S. Hitchings IV*
17. Formulation of Veterinary Dosage Forms, *edited by Jack Blodinger*
18. Dermatological Formulations: Percutaneous Absorption, *Brian W. Barry*
19. The Clinical Research Process in the Pharmaceutical Industry, *edited by Gary M. Matoren*
20. Microencapsulation and Related Drug Processes, *Patrick B. Deasy*
21. Drugs and Nutrients: The Interactive Effects, *edited by Daphne A. Roe and T. Colin Campbell*
22. Biotechnology of Industrial Antibiotics, *Erick J. Vandamme*
23. Pharmaceutical Process Validation, *edited by Bernard T. Loftus and Robert A. Nash*

24. Anticancer and Interferon Agents: Synthesis and Properties, *edited by Raphael M. Ottenbrite and George B. Butler*
25. Pharmaceutical Statistics: Practical and Clinical Applications, *Sanford Bolton*
26. Drug Dynamics for Analytical, Clinical, and Biological Chemists, *Benjamin J. Gudzinowicz, Burrows T. Younkin, Jr., and Michael J. Gudzinowicz*
27. Modern Analysis of Antibiotics, *edited by Adjoran Aszalos*
28. Solubility and Related Properties, *Kenneth C. James*
29. Controlled Drug Delivery: Fundamentals and Applications, Second Edition, Revised and Expanded, *edited by Joseph R. Robinson and Vincent H. Lee*
30. New Drug Approval Process: Clinical and Regulatory Management, *edited by Richard A. Guarino*
31. Transdermal Controlled Systemic Medications, *edited by Yie W. Chien*
32. Drug Delivery Devices: Fundamentals and Applications, *edited by Praveen Tyle*
33. Pharmacokinetics: Regulatory • Industrial • Academic Perspectives, *edited by Peter G. Welling and Francis L. S. Tse*
34. Clinical Drug Trials and Tribulations, *edited by Allen E. Cato*
35. Transdermal Drug Delivery: Developmental Issues and Research Initiatives, *edited by Jonathan Hadgraft and Richard H. Guy*
36. Aqueous Polymeric Coatings for Pharmaceutical Dosage Forms, *edited by James W. McGinity*
37. Pharmaceutical Pelletization Technology, *edited by Isaac Ghebre-Sellassie*
38. Good Laboratory Practice Regulations, *edited by Allen F. Hirsch*
39. Nasal Systemic Drug Delivery, *Yie W. Chien, Kenneth S. E. Su, and Shyi-Feu Chang*
40. Modern Pharmaceutics: Second Edition, Revised and Expanded, *edited by Gilbert S. Banker and Christopher T. Rhodes*
41. Specialized Drug Delivery Systems: Manufacturing and Production Technology, *edited by Praveen Tyle*
42. Topical Drug Delivery Formulations, *edited by David W. Osborne and Anton H. Amann*
43. Drug Stability: Principles and Practices, *Jens T. Carstensen*
44. Pharmaceutical Statistics: Practical and Clinical Applications, Second Edition, Revised and Expanded, *Sanford Bolton*
45. Biodegradable Polymers as Drug Delivery Systems, *edited by Mark Chasin and Robert Langer*
46. Preclinical Drug Disposition: A Laboratory Handbook, *Francis L. S. Tse and James J. Jaffe*

47. HPLC in the Pharmaceutical Industry, *edited by Godwin W. Fong and Stanley K. Lam*
48. Pharmaceutical Bioequivalence, *edited by Peter G. Welling, Francis L. S. Tse, and Shrikant V. Dinghe*
49. Pharmaceutical Dissolution Testing, *Umesh V. Banakar*
50. Novel Drug Delivery Systems: Second Edition, Revised and Expanded, *Yie W. Chien*
51. Managing the Clinical Drug Development Process, *David M. Cocchetto and Ronald V. Nardi*
52. Good Manufacturing Practices for Pharmaceuticals: A Plan for Total Quality Control, Third Edition, *edited by Sidney H. Willig and James R. Stoker*
53. Prodrugs: Topical and Ocular Drug Delivery, *edited by Kenneth B. Sloan*
54. Pharmaceutical Inhalation Aerosol Technology, *edited by Anthony J. Hickey*
55. Radiopharmaceuticals: Chemistry and Pharmacology, *edited by Adrian D. Nunn*
56. New Drug Approval Process: Second Edition, Revised and Expanded, *edited by Richard A. Guarino*
57. Pharmaceutical Process Validation: Second Edition, Revised and Expanded, *edited by Ira R. Berry and Robert A. Nash*
58. Ophthalmic Drug Delivery Systems, *edited by Ashim K. Mitra*
59. Pharmaceutical Skin Penetration Enhancement, *edited by Kenneth A. Walters and Jonathan Hadgraft*
60. Colonic Drug Absorption and Metabolism, *edited by Peter R. Bieck*
61. Pharmaceutical Particulate Carriers: Therapeutic Applications, *edited by Alain Rolland*
62. Drug Permeation Enhancement: Theory and Applications, *edited by Dean S. Hsieh*
63. Glycopeptide Antibiotics, *edited by Ramakrishnan Nagarajan*
64. Achieving Sterility in Medical and Pharmaceutical Products, *Nigel A. Halls*
65. Multiparticulate Oral Drug Delivery, *edited by Isaac Ghebre-Sellassie*
66. Colloidal Drug Delivery Systems, *edited by Jörg Kreuter*
67. Pharmacokinetics: Regulatory • Industrial • Academic Perspectives, Second Edition, *edited by Peter G. Welling and Francis L. S. Tse*
68. Drug Stability: Principles and Practices, Second Edition, Revised and Expanded, *Jens T. Carstensen*
69. Good Laboratory Practice Regulations: Second Edition, Revised and Expanded, *edited by Sandy Weinberg*
70. Physical Characterization of Pharmaceutical Solids, *edited by Harry G. Brittain*

71. Pharmaceutical Powder Compaction Technology, *edited by Göran Alderborn and Christer Nyström*
72. Modern Pharmaceutics: Third Edition, Revised and Expanded, *edited by Gilbert S. Banker and Christopher T. Rhodes*
73. Microencapsulation: Methods and Industrial Applications, *edited by Simon Benita*
74. Oral Mucosal Drug Delivery, *edited by Michael J. Rathbone*
75. Clinical Research in Pharmaceutical Development, *edited by Barry Bleidt and Michael Montagne*
76. The Drug Development Process: Increasing Efficiency and Cost Effectiveness, *edited by Peter G. Welling, Louis Lasagna, and Umesh V. Banakar*
77. Microparticulate Systems for the Delivery of Proteins and Vaccines, *edited by Smadar Cohen and Howard Bernstein*
78. Good Manufacturing Practices for Pharmaceuticals: A Plan for Total Quality Control, Fourth Edition, Revised and Expanded, *Sidney H. Willig and James R. Stoker*
79. Aqueous Polymeric Coatings for Pharmaceutical Dosage Forms: Second Edition, Revised and Expanded, *edited by James W. McGinity*
80. Pharmaceutical Statistics: Practical and Clinical Applications, Third Edition, *Sanford Bolton*
81. Handbook of Pharmaceutical Granulation Technology, *edited by Dilip M. Parikh*
82. Biotechnology of Antibiotics: Second Edition, Revised and Expanded, *edited by William R. Strohl*
83. Mechanisms of Transdermal Drug Delivery, *edited by Russell O. Potts and Richard H. Guy*
84. Pharmaceutical Enzymes, *edited by Albert Lauwers and Simon Scharpé*
85. Development of Biopharmaceutical Parenteral Dosage Forms, *edited by John A. Bontempo*
86. Pharmaceutical Project Management, *edited by Tony Kennedy*
87. Drug Products for Clinical Trials: An International Guide to Formulation • Production • Quality Control, *edited by Donald C. Monkhouse and Christopher T. Rhodes*
88. Development and Formulation of Veterinary Dosage Forms: Second Edition, Revised and Expanded, *edited by Gregory E. Hardee and J. Desmond Baggot*
89. Receptor-Based Drug Design, *edited by Paul Leff*
90. Automation and Validation of Information in Pharmaceutical Processing, *edited by Joseph F. deSpautz*
91. Dermal Absorption and Toxicity Assessment, *edited by Michael S. Roberts and Kenneth A. Walters*

92. Pharmaceutical Experimental Design, *Gareth A. Lewis, Didier Mathieu, and Roger Phan-Tan-Luu*
93. Preparing for FDA Pre-Approval Inspections, *edited by Martin D. Hynes III*
94. Pharmaceutical Excipients: Characterization by IR, Raman, and NMR Spectroscopy, *David E. Bugay and W. Paul Findlay*
95. Polymorphism in Pharmaceutical Solids, *edited by Harry G. Brittain*
96. Freeze-Drying/Lyophilization of Pharmaceutical and Biological Products, *edited by Louis Rey and Joan C. May*
97. Percutaneous Absorption: Drugs–Cosmetics–Mechanisms–Methodology, Third Edition, Revised and Expanded, *edited by Robert L. Bronaugh and Howard I. Maibach*
98. Bioadhesive Drug Delivery Systems: Fundamentals, Novel Approaches, and Development, *edited by Edith Mathiowitz, Donald E. Chickering III, and Claus-Michael Lehr*
99. Protein Formulation and Delivery, *edited by Eugene J. McNally*
100. New Drug Approval Process: Third Edition, The Global Challenge, *edited by Richard A. Guarino*
101. Peptide and Protein Drug Analysis, *edited by Ronald E. Reid*
102. Transport Processes in Pharmaceutical Systems, *edited by Gordon L. Amidon, Ping I. Lee, and Elizabeth M. Topp*
103. Excipient Toxicity and Safety, *edited by Myra L. Weiner and Lois A. Kotkoskie*
104. The Clinical Audit in Pharmaceutical Development, *edited by Michael R. Hamrell*
105. Pharmaceutical Emulsions and Suspensions, *edited by Francoise Nielloud and Gilberte Marti-Mestres*
106. Oral Drug Absorption: Prediction and Assessment, *edited by Jennifer B. Dressman and Hans Lennernäs*
107. Drug Stability: Principles and Practices, Third Edition, Revised and Expanded, *edited by Jens T. Carstensen and C. T. Rhodes*
108. Containment in the Pharmaceutical Industry, *edited by James P. Wood*
109. Good Manufacturing Practices for Pharmaceuticals: A Plan for Total Quality Control from Manufacturer to Consumer, Fifth Edition, Revised and Expanded, *Sidney H. Willig*
110. Advanced Pharmaceutical Solids, *Jens T. Carstensen*
111. Endotoxins: Pyrogens, LAL Testing, and Depyrogenation, Second Edition, Revised and Expanded, *Kevin L. Williams*
112. Pharmaceutical Process Engineering, *Anthony J. Hickey and David Ganderton*
113. Pharmacogenomics, *edited by Werner Kalow, Urs A. Meyer, and Rachel F. Tyndale*
114. Handbook of Drug Screening, *edited by Ramakrishna Seethala and Prabhavathi B. Fernandes*

115. Drug Targeting Technology: Physical • Chemical • Biological Methods, *edited by Hans Schreier*

116. Drug–Drug Interactions, *edited by A. David Rodrigues*

117. Handbook of Pharmaceutical Analysis, *edited by Lena Ohannesian and Anthony J. Streeter*

118. Pharmaceutical Process Scale-Up, *edited by Michael Levin*

119. Dermatological and Transdermal Formulations, *edited by Kenneth A. Walters*

120. Clinical Drug Trials and Tribulations: Second Edition, Revised and Expanded, *edited by Allen Cato, Lynda Sutton, and Allen Cato III*

121. Modern Pharmaceutics: Fourth Edition, Revised and Expanded, *edited by Gilbert S. Banker and Christopher T. Rhodes*

122. Surfactants and Polymers in Drug Delivery, *Martin Malmsten*

123. Transdermal Drug Delivery: Second Edition, Revised and Expanded, *edited by Richard H. Guy and Jonathan Hadgraft*

124. Good Laboratory Practice Regulations: Second Edition, Revised and Expanded, *edited by Sandy Weinberg*

125. Parenteral Quality Control: Sterility, Pyrogen, Particulate, and Package Integrity Testing: Third Edition, Revised and Expanded, *Michael J. Akers, Daniel S. Larrimore, and Dana Morton Guazzo*

126. Modified-Release Drug Delivery Technology, *edited by Michael J. Rathbone, Jonathan Hadgraft, and Michael S. Roberts*

127. Simulation for Designing Clinical Trials: A Pharmacokinetic-Pharmacodynamic Modeling Perspective, *edited by Hui C. Kimko and Stephen B. Duffull*

128. Affinity Capillary Electrophoresis in Pharmaceutics and Biopharmaceutics, *edited by Reinhard H. H. Neubert and Hans-Hermann Rüttinger*

129. Pharmaceutical Process Validation: An International Third Edition, Revised and Expanded, *edited by Robert A. Nash and Alfred H. Wachter*

130. Ophthalmic Drug Delivery Systems: Second Edition, Revised and Expanded, *edited by Ashim K. Mitra*

131. Pharmaceutical Gene Delivery Systems, *edited by Alain Rolland and Sean M. Sullivan*

132. Biomarkers in Clinical Drug Development, *edited by John C. Bloom and Robert A. Dean*

133. Pharmaceutical Extrusion Technology, *edited by Isaac Ghebre-Sellassie and Charles Martin*

134. Pharmaceutical Inhalation Aerosol Technology: Second Edition, Revised and Expanded, *edited by Anthony J. Hickey*

135. Pharmaceutical Statistics: Practical and Clinical Applications, Fourth Edition, *Sanford Bolton and Charles Bon*

136. Compliance Handbook for Pharmaceuticals, Medical Devices, and Biologics, *edited by Carmen Medina*

137. Freeze-Drying/Lyophilization of Pharmaceutical and Biological Products: Second Edition, Revised and Expanded, *edited by Louis Rey and Joan C. May*

138. Supercritical Fluid Technology for Drug Product Development, *edited by Peter York, Uday B. Kompella, and Boris Y. Shekunov*

139. New Drug Approval Process: Fourth Edition, Accelerating Global Registrations, *edited by Richard A. Guarino*

140. Microbial Contamination Control in Parenteral Manufacturing, *edited by Kevin L. Williams*

141. New Drug Development: Regulatory Paradigms for Clinical Pharmacology and Biopharmaceutics, *edited by Chandrahas G. Sahajwalla*

142. Microbial Contamination Control in the Pharmaceutical Industry, *edited by Luis Jimenez*

143. Generic Drug Product Development: Solid Oral Dosage Forms, *edited by Leon Shargel and Izzy Kanfer*

144. Introduction to the Pharmaceutical Regulatory Process, *edited by Ira R. Berry*

145. Drug Delivery to the Oral Cavity: Molecules to Market, *edited by Tapash K. Ghosh and William R. Pfister*

146. Good Design Practices for GMP Pharmaceutical Facilities, *edited by Andrew Signore and Terry Jacobs*

147. Drug Products for Clinical Trials, Second Edition, *edited by Donald Monkhouse, Charles Carney, and Jim Clark*

148. Polymeric Drug Delivery Systems, *edited by Glen S. Kwon*

149. Injectable Dispersed Systems: Formulation, Processing, and Performance, *edited by Diane J. Burgess*

150. Laboratory Auditing For Quality and Regulatory Compliance, *edited by Donald Singer, Raluca-Ioana Stefan, and Jacobus van Staden*

151. Active Pharmaceutical Ingredients: Development, Manufacturing, and Regulation, *edited by Stanley H. Nusim*

152. Preclinical Drug Development, *edited by Mark C. Rogge and David Taft*

153. Pharmaceutical Stress Testing: Predicting Drug Degradation, *edited by Steven W. Baertschi*

154. Handbook of Pharmaceutical Granulation Technology: Second Edition, *edited by Dilip M. Parikh*

Pharmaceutical Stress Testing

Predicting Drug Degradation

edited by

Steven W. Baertschi

Eli Lilly and Company

Indianapolis, Indiana, U.S.A.

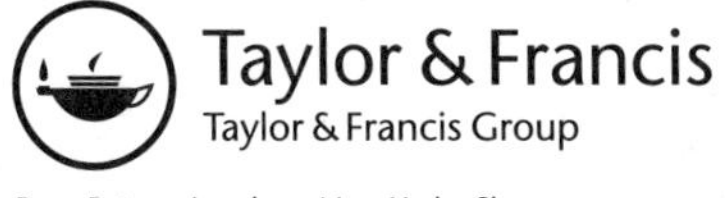

Boca Raton London New York Singapore

Published in 2005 by
Taylor & Francis Group
6000 Broken Sound Parkway NW, Suite 300
Boca Raton, FL 33487-2742

Printed in the United States of America on acid-free paper
10 9 8 7 6 5 4 3 2 1

International Standard Book Number-10: 0-8247-4021-1 (Hardcover)
International Standard Book Number-13: 978-0-8247-4021-4 (Hardcover)

Library of Congress Cataloging-in-Publication Data

Catalog record is available from the Library of Congress

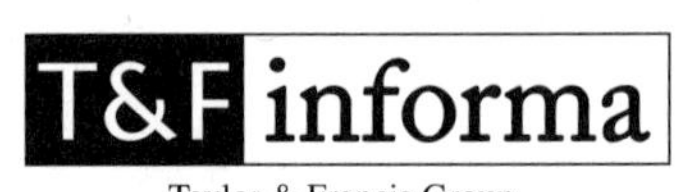

Taylor & Francis Group
is the Academic Division of T&F Informa plc.

Visit the Taylor & Francis Web site at
http://www.taylorandfrancis.com

Preface

Stress testing has long been recognized as an important part of the drug development process. Recent efforts by the International Conference on Harmonization (ICH) with regard to impurities and photostability have brought an increased regulatory scrutiny of impurities, requiring identification and toxicological qualification at very low levels. Coupled with the fact that the pharmaceutical industry is making major efforts to reduce the time it takes to get products to market, the potential for stability and impurity "surprises" that affect the development timeline has increased dramatically.

Stress testing is the main tool that is used to predict stability problems, develop analytical methods, and identify degradation products/pathways. Since there are no detailed regulatory guidelines that direct how stress testing is to be done, nor has there ever been a text/reference book on the subject, stress testing has evolved into an artful science that is highly dependent on the experience of the company or the individuals directing the studies. This book provides readers with a single source reference that benchmarks the current best practices of experienced pharmaceutical scientists/researchers. Questions like "How hot, how long, what conditions are appropriate?" and topics such as mass balance, photostability, oxidative susceptibility, and the chemistry of drug degradation are addressed in an objective, detailed scientific manner, with ample references to relevant guidances and the scientific literature.

Compiling a book to be used as a scientific reference for the topic of pharmaceutical stress testing was a daunting task. Stress testing, as it relates to traditional small molecule pharmaceuticals, is very broad and scientifically complex. Thus, this book seeks to be a practical and scientific guide which will, hopefully, stimulate new ideas and further development of the science.

This undertaking is done with some trepidation, since I realize that discussion of this topic could lead to attempts to formalize or standardize (i.e., regulatory standardization) an area of pharmaceutical science that relies on scientific expertise and flexibility. Each new drug compound, formulation, route of administration, delivery device, etc. has the potential to present unique challenges and unanticipated problems, and should be approached with such a mindset. The pharmaceutical researcher must be free to design and develop new ways to predict and measure stability-related issues through stress testing. Nonetheless, it is hoped that this book will provide a useful and practical scientific guide that is a welcome addition to the library of many pharmaceutical scientists. I am confident that the "artful science" of stress testing will evolve beyond what is represented in this book as other scientists further the science and fill in topics that are poorly covered or missing.

I am indebted to my co-workers, especially Patrick J. Jansen and W. Kimmer Smith for helping to develop our strategies for stress testing over the last decade. I am grateful to Jerry R. Draper, Lindsay N. Maxwell, Bradley M. Campbell, and Michael A. Vance for all their stress testing work over the last several years and the numerous scientists at Eli Lilly and Company who have helped me develop this area through their collaborations. I am grateful to Eli Lilly and Company for allowing me to focus on an area of pharmaceutical science for an extended period of time and for supporting me in my efforts to assemble a book devoted to the topic of stress testing. But most of all I am in debt to my family, especially my wife, Cheryl, for graciously putting up with the "stress" resulting from the effort required to complete this book.

Steven W. Baertschi

Contents

Contributors

Angelo Albini Dipartimento di Chimica Organica, Università di Pavia, Pavia, Italy

Karen M. Alsante Pfizer Global Research & Development, Analytical Research & Development, Groton, Connecticut, U.S.A.

Amy S. Antipas Pfizer Global Research & Development, Groton, Connecticut, U.S.A.

Steven W. Baertschi Eli Lilly and Company, Lilly Research Laboratories, Lilly Corporate Center, Indianapolis, Indiana, U.S.A.

Giovanni Boccardi Discovery Analytics, Discovery Research, Sanofi–Aventis, Milano, Italy

Donald B. Boyd Department of Chemistry, Indiana University–Purdue University at Indianapolis (IUPUI), Indianapolis, Indiana, U.S.A.

Graham Buckton The School of Pharmacy, University of London, London, U.K.

Elisa Fasani Dipartimento di Chimica Organica, Università di Pavia, Pavia, Italy

Simon Gaisford The School of Pharmacy, University of London, London, U.K.

Patrick J. Jansen Eli Lilly and Company, Lilly Research Laboratories, Lilly Corporate Center, Indianapolis, Indiana, U.S.A.

Margaret S. Landis Pfizer Global Research & Development, Groton, Connecticut, U.S.A.

Larry A. Larew Eli Lilly and Company, Lilly Research Laboratories, Lilly Corporate Center, Indianapolis, Indiana, U.S.A.

Steven L. Nail Pharmaceutical Sciences R&D, Eli Lilly and Company, Indianapolis, Indiana, U.S.A.

Mark A. Nussbaum Chemistry Department, Hillsdale College, Hillsdale, Michigan, U.S.A.

Bernard A. Olsen Eli Lilly and Company, Lilly Research Laboratories, Lafayette, Indiana, U.S.A.

Dan W. Reynolds GlaxoSmithKline, Chemical Development, Research Triangle Park, North Carolina, U.S.A.

W. Kimmer Smith Eli Lilly and Company, Lilly Research Laboratories, Lilly Corporate Center, Indianapolis, Indiana, U.S.A.

1

Introduction

Steven W. Baertschi

Eli Lilly and Company, Lilly Research Laboratories, Lilly Corporate Center, Indianapolis, Indiana, U.S.A.

Dan W. Reynolds

GlaxoSmithKline, Chemical Development, Research Triangle Park, North Carolina, U.S.A.

I. GENERAL INFORMATION/BACKGROUND

Stress testing has long been recognized as an important part of the drug development process. Recent efforts by the International Conference on Harmonization (ICH) with regard to impurities (1–4) and stability (5–7) have brought an increased regulatory scrutiny of impurities, requiring identification and toxicological qualification at very low levels. Coupled with efforts by the pharmaceutical industry to reduce the time and cost that it takes to get products to market, the potential for stability and impurity "surprises" that affect the development timeline has increased dramatically. Efforts to improve and streamline processes related to early identification of potential impurity problems are important to the goal of providing new, safe medicines, faster (8).

Stress testing is the main tool that is used to predict stability problems, develop analytical methods, and identify degradation products and pathways. Since there are no detailed regulatory guidelines that describe how to carry out stress testing studies (nor has there ever been a textbook or reference book devoted to the subject), stress testing has evolved into an "artful science" that is highly dependent on the experience of the company and of the individuals directing the studies. Questions, such as "How hot?," "How long?," "How much humidity?," "What pH values should be used?," "What reagents/conditions for oxidative studies should be used?," are faced by every pharmaceutical investigator. As will be described in more detail in the section on "Historical context," this has led to a tremendous variation in stress testing approaches and conditions. A recent article about stress testing (or forced degradation) was even entitled "The Gray Area," in reference to the vagueness of the current guidelines (9).

This book is an attempt to provide a practical and scientific guide for the pharmaceutical scientist to help in designing, executing, and interpreting stress testing studies for traditional small molecule (typically synthetically prepared) drug substances. While the primary emphasis is on the chemical aspects of stress testing, some physical aspects have also been addressed (see, for example, Chapters 9 and 11). While this book is not designed for biologicals, peptides, etc., some of the principles and strategies may be generally applicable. On the formulated product side, the focus of this book is on traditional solid oral dosage forms, although some consideration is given to other dosage forms. Detailed consideration of alternate drug delivery systems (e.g., metered-dose inhalers, transdermal patches, dermal creams, etc.) is beyond the scope of this book.

II. DEFINITIONS/TERMS

It is important to have a clear definition of terms to facilitate the discussion. In the context of pharmaceuticals, "stress testing" is historically a somewhat vague and undefined term, often used interchangeably with the term "accelerated stability." A 1980 article by Pope (10) defined accelerated stability testing as "the validated method or methods by which product stability may be predicted by storage of the product under conditions that accelerate change in a defined and predictable manner." The term "validated" was intended to emphasize that the change occurring under the accelerated conditions must be demonstrated to correlate with normal long-term storage. The United States FDA definition of "accelerated testing" (11) in the February 1987 guideline states that "The term "accelerated testing" is often used synonymously with "stress testing." This usage is understandable in that the term stress testing is used in many industries to describe testing intended to measure how a system functions when subjected to "an applied force or system of forces (12)." More recently, the ICH introduced an important distinction between the two terms in the context of pharmaceutical stability. The ICH defined "accelerated testing" (13) as:

> Studies designed to increase the rate of chemical degradation or physical change of an active drug substance or drug product using exaggerated storage conditions as part of the formal, definitive,

> storage program. These data, in addition to long-term stability studies, may also be used to assess longer-term chemical effects at non-accelerated conditions and to evaluate the impact of short-term excursions outside the label storage conditions such as might occur during shipping. Results from accelerated testing studies are not always predictive of physical changes.

An important aspect of this definition is that the studies are part of the "formal, definitive, storage program." In contrast, ICH, in "Annex 1, Glossary and Information" of the revised stability guideline (6) defined stress testing (drug substance) as:

> Studies undertaken to elucidate the intrinsic stability of the drug substance. Such testing is part of the development strategy and is normally carried out under more severe conditions than those used for accelerated testing.

A more detailed description of stress testing is provided near the beginning of the ICH Stability guideline, under the "Drug Substance" heading:

> Stress testing of the drug substance can help identify the likely degradation products, which can in turn help establish the degradation pathways and the intrinsic stability of the molecule and validate the stability indicating power of the analytical procedures used. The nature of the stress testing will depend on the individual drug substance and the type of drug product involved.
>
> Stress testing is likely to be carried out on a single batch of the drug substance. It should include the effect of temperatures (in 10°C increments (e.g., 50°C, 60°C, etc.) above that for accelerated testing), humidity (e.g., 75% RH or greater) where appropriate, oxidation, and photolysis on the drug substance. The testing should also evaluate the susceptibility of the drug substance to hydrolysis across a wide range of pH values when in solution or suspension. Photostability testing should be an integral part of stress testing. The standard conditions for photostability testing are described in ICH Q1B.
>
> Examining degradation products under stress conditions is useful in establishing degradation pathways and developing and validating suitable analytical procedures. However, it may not be necessary to examine specifically for certain degradation products if it has been demonstrated that they are not formed under accelerated or long term storage conditions.

> Results from these studies will form an integral part of the information provided to regulatory authorities.

The description of stress testing was slightly modified in the revised stability guideline from the original description in ICH Q1A (5). The original Q1A description contained this additional paragraph:

> Stress testing is conducted to provide data on forced decomposition products and decomposition mechanisms for the drug substance. The severe conditions that may be encountered during distribution can be covered by stress testing of definitive batches of drug substance.

The ICH definition of stress testing for the drug *product* is shown below (7):

> Studies undertaken to assess the effect of severe conditions on the drug product. Such studies include photostability testing (see ICH Q1B) and specific testing on certain products (e.g., metered dose inhalers, creams, emulsions, refrigerated aqueous liquid products).

From the ICH definition, it is clear that there is now a [regulatory] differentiation between "accelerated testing" and "stress testing." Stress testing is distinguished by both the severity of the conditions and the focus or intent of the results. Stress testing, which is also often referred to as "forced degradation," is an investigation of the "intrinsic stability" characteristics of the molecule, providing the foundation for developing and validating analytical methods and for developing stable formulations. Stress testing studies are intended to *discover* stability issues, and are therefore *predictive* in nature. Stress testing studies are not a part of the "validated" formal stability program. Rather, pharmaceutical stress testing is a research investigation requiring scientific expertise and judgment. These concepts have ramifications for the design and execution of stress testing studies, which will be explored in more detail later.

III. HISTORICAL CONTEXT

As discussed above, the terms stress testing and accelerated [stability] testing were often used interchangeably in the pharmaceutical industry. Usually these topics were discussed as part of an overall discussion of drug stability and/or prediction of shelf life (14), although in some cases the focus was on degradation pathways or chemical reactivity/stabilization (15). In a classic article by Kennon (16), the effect of increasing temperature (from room temperature to 85°C) on the rates of degradation of pharmaceutical products was discussed in the context of predicting shelf life of pharmaceuticals. This article provided the basis for many articles that followed. For example, the articles by Yang and Roy (17) and Witthaus (18) were extensions of Kennon's original work. Their work led Joel Davis of the FDA to propose what has become known as the "Joel Davis Rule," i.e., 3 months at 40°C/75% relative humidity is roughly equivalent to 24 months at room temperature (25°C) (19). Interestingly, Carstensen has pointed out that prior to the "Joel Davis Rule," the historical "rule-of-thumb" had been that 5 weeks of storage at 42°C is equivalent to two years of storage at room temperature (20). This rule had been derived from work done in 1948 on the stability of vitamin A and it assumes the same activation energy as found for vitamin A. Many other important contributions have been made over the years with regard to kinetic evaluations of drug stability from an "accelerated stability" viewpoint, but a comprehensive review of the literature related to the kinetics of degradation is not the focus here.

It is interesting to consider some of the conditions that have historically been employed in the stress testing of pharmaceuticals, documented both in the "Analytical Profiles of Drug Substances" (21) and by Singh and Bakshi (22). Acidic stress conditions can be found to vary from 0.1 N HCl at 40°C for 1 week (with "negligible degradation") (23), to 0.1 N HCl at 65°C for 21 days (71.6% degradation) (22), to 0.1 N HCl at 105°C for 2 months (with "considerable degradation"), to 4 N HCl under refluxing conditions for 2 days (66% degradation) (24), to 6.5 N HCl at 108°C for 24 hr (50% degradation), to concentrated HCl at room temperature (56.5% degradation) (25). Similar elevated temperatures, times, and base strength have been employed for basic stress conditions. For example, conditions can be found to vary from 0.1 N NaOH at 40°C for 1 week (with negligible degradation) (23), to 0.1 N NaOH at 65°C for 21 days (with 100% degradation) (22), to 0.1 N NaOH under refluxing conditions for 2 days (68% degradation) (24), to 1 N NaOH under boiling conditions for 3 days (7.2% degradation) (26), to 5 N NaOH under refluxing conditions for 4 hr (100% degradation) (27). In terms of oxidative degradation studies, hydrogen peroxide has been employed at strengths from 0.3% to 30% (28). Studies were often conducted at elevated temperatures, e.g., 37°C for 6 hr [3% hydrogen peroxide, 60% degradation (29)], 50°C for 72 hr (3% hydrogen peroxide, 6.6% degradation), and even refluxing conditions for 30 min (3% hydrogen peroxide, extensive degradation) (27) or 6 hr (10% hydrogen peroxide, no significant degradation) (30).

As these examples illustrate, historically there has been tremendous variation in the conditions employed in acid/base and oxidative stress testing studies. There has also been tremendous variation in defining the appropriate "endpoint" of the stress testing studies, i.e., what length of time (and temperature) or amount of degradation is sufficient to end the stress exposure.

Perhaps the most dramatic variability in stress testing conditions is observed in the photostressing of drugs (31), where the lamps and exposures range from short wavelength Hg arc lamps (254 nm, UVC range) to fluorescent light to "artificial light" to halogen lamps to xenon lamps. The variability of photoexposure during pharmaceutical photostability studies has also been documented by surveys of the pharmaceutical industry (32–34).

From the information provided above, it is apparent that stress-testing conditions have varied greatly from compound to compound and from investigator to investigator. Extremely harsh conditions have been commonly used in the past to ensure degradation, even if the conditions far exceeded plausible exposures.

More recently, several articles relevant to stress testing have appeared in the pharmaceutical literature. A paper by Singh and Bakshi (22) in 2000 provides the most thorough collection of references to various degradation studies of drug products, documenting the diversity of conditions and approaches to stress testing. This paper attempts to provide a classification system (Extremely labile, Very labile, Labile, Stable) based on a defined systematic approach. It is not clear from the article on what basis (scientific or otherwise) the classification system was devised; however, the paper does define "endpoints" to stressing (albeit, fairly harsh endpoints), allowing for the conclusion that a particular compound may be regarded as "stable" under a certain set of conditions.

In 1992 (and again in 1994), Boccardi provided some needed guidance on oxidative stress testing by asserting that most pharmaceutical oxidative degradation was the result of autoxidation and that hydrogen peroxide was not a very good reagent to mimic autoxidation processes (35,36). Boccardi was the first to describe the use of radical initiators such as azobisisobutyronitrile (AIBN) for oxidative pharmaceutical stress testing, and he provided a simple procedure with mild conditions he termed "The AIBN Test." In 1996, Baertschi (37) presented and discussed an approach to stress testing that had defined limits of harshness and exposure time. In 1998, Weiser (38), in discussing the role of stress testing in analytical method development, suggested a set of conditions for performing stress testing that was arguably milder than many of the historical studies cited above. In 2001, Alsante et al. (39) provided a guide to stress testing studies that suggested defined limits to the stress conditions. For example, for acidic and basic stressing, Alsante suggested conditions of 1 N HCl and 1 N NaOH for a maximum of 1 week at room temperature. In 2002, the views of the Pharmaceutical Research and Manufacturer's Association (PhRMA) were summarized in an article on forced degradation studies published in Pharmaceutical Technology (40). The PhRMA article did not discuss specifics of conditions of stress, but rather focused more on what kinds of stress testing should be performed for drug substances and products and on the regulatory requirements.

Recent publications on the topic of stress testing/forced degradation studies reveal that there is still a tremendous variability in the conditions employed. A few examples will be discussed here, although this discussion is not intended to be an exhaustive review of the literature.

A degradation study of haloperidol utilized 1 M HCl and 1 M NaOH (refluxed for 5 hr), and 30% hydrogen peroxide (70°C for 5 hr) for the most stressful conditions of the study (41). These conditions appear to have been chosen to enable production of known degradation products (six degradation products shown) to facilitate HPLC method validation efforts. A degradation study of ibuprofen produced 13 degradation products, several of which had never before been detected (42). In this study, oxidative studies were carried out utilizing potassium permanganate (0.05 M) at room temperature up to 16 hr in 0.5 M NaOH; up to 33% hydrogen peroxide at room temperature for 22 hr; and potassium dichromate (0.1 N) at room temperature up to 14 days in 0.5 M HCl. Solid-state studies utilized 50°C up to 8 months and 100°C up to 16 hr to detect volatile degradation products. An NMR study of the aqueous degradation of isophosphoramide mustard was conducted in buffered aqueous solutions in the pH range of 1–13 (43). The degradation of sumatriptan in 0.1 N HCl, 0.1 N NaOH, and in 3% hydrogen peroxide was studied using LC/MS and LC/MS/MS (44). The solutions were heated at 90°C for 30 min to 9 hr. Photostability was assessed by exposure to UV irradiation at 254 nm for 24 hr (no indication of irradiation intensity). A study of the major oxidative degradation products of SCH56592 was conducted by exposure of the drug substance in the solid state to 150°C for 12 days with identification of the major products using LC-MS and LC-NMR (45). Singh et al. (46) describe stress degradation studies of ornidazole and prazosin, terazosin, and doxazosin (47) under conditions designed to be in "alignment" with the ICH Stability guideline (Q1AR). In the case of ornidazole, significant degradation was seen under acidic conditions of 0.1 M HCl to 5 M HCl at 80°C for 12–72 hr, although no degradation products were detected (presumably because of degradation to non-chromophoric products). Studies under basic conditions of 0.1 M NaOH at both 80°C and 40°C revealed complete degradation at time zero. Milder studies were then conducted at pH 8 and 40°C. Oxidative studies involved 3% and 30% hydrogen peroxide at room temperature for 24 and 48 hr, with losses of 8% and 53% of the parent, respectively. Photodegradation studies utilized Option 2 of the ICH photostability guideline (7) with exposures up to 30 days at 7000 lux (over 5 million lux-hr exposure). Similar conditions were employed for prazosin, terazosin, and doxazosin.

In these recent examples of stress testing studies, it is apparent that there is still a great diversity of conditions employed to induce degradation, although the diversity is arguably less than was observed prior to publication of the ICH guidances. This continued diversity of approach could be interpreted in a couple of ways. One interpretation is that stress-testing studies are inherently a research undertaking, and therefore flexibility and scientific judgment are required, leading to diverse conditions and approaches.

Another interpretation is that there is (appropriately or inappropriately) very little guidance (either regulatory or in the scientific literature) on the specifics of the conditions or appropriate endpoints of pharmaceutical stress testing. We assert that both interpretations are valid. Therefore, the goal of this book is to provide additional scientific guidance to the researcher to enable sound, practical, and reasonably consistent approaches to pharmaceutical stress testing.

IV. REGULATORY CONTEXT

The guidance does not explicitly require stress testing be performed or reported at the Phase 1–2 IND stages although it is encouraged to facilitate selection of stability indicating methods (48). Experience has shown, however, that regulatory authorities may still ask questions concerning results from stress testing as early as a Phase 1 IND, especially where potentially toxic degradation products are possible. The guidance does require stress testing for the Phase 3 IND for drug substances and suggests these studies be conducted on drug products. At Phase 3, the guidance strongly suggests, but does not always require, that degradation products detected above the ICH identification thresholds during formal stability trials should be identified. For an NDA, the guidance requires a summary of drug substance and drug product stress studies including elucidation of degradation pathways, demonstration of the stability indicating nature of analytical methods, and identification of significant degradation products (49). Stressing the drug substance under hydrolytic, oxidative, photolytic, and thermolytic conditions in solution and the solid state is required. The design of drug product studies is formulation dependent and is left to the discretion of the applicant.

Although not necessarily directly related to stress testing, the guidance also requires demonstration and/or a summary of an investigation of mass balance (6) in degraded samples from formal stability trials, an assessment of the drug's stereochemical stability (50), and distinguishing drug related and non-drug-related degradation products (4). However, these issues can often be addressed in stress studies fulfilling both scientific need and regulatory requirements. The predictive nature of well-conducted stress studies can forewarn of potential problems in these areas early-on facilitating appropriate and efficient changes in the development strategy if required.

The guidance suggests the analytical assumptions made when determining mass balance should be explained in the registration application (4). Failure to demonstrate mass balance may be acceptable provided a thorough investigation has been conducted to understand the chemistry of the molecule (5). Examining mass balance in stressed samples can reveal the need for better analytical methodology from the start.

The guidance recommends treating chiral impurities as though they were achiral impurities with the caveat that the ICH identification and qualification thresholds may not apply for analytical reasons (50). Experimental demonstration that stereoisomers of the drug substance and its degradation products do not form during stress studies can obviate the need for testing for these potential impurities during formal stability trials. Experience has shown that merely arguing a particular chiral center is unlikely to invert on strictly theoretical grounds is unacceptable to the FDA.

Differentiation between drug-related and non-drug-related degradation products can be achieved with stress studies of the drug substance, drug product, and placebo. These studies should allow discrimination between synthetic process impurities, excipients, degradation products derived from excipients alone and drug-related degradation products including drug-excipient combinations.

The guidance suggests the potential for reactions between active ingredients in combination products should be investigated (49). For a triple combination tablet formulation, the FDA suggested stressing the three actives together under conditions usually applied to a single drug substance. These studies were conducted and reported in the NDA.

The guidance specifies identification thresholds for degradation products observed in formal stability samples of the drug substance and product that depend upon the dosage (1–4). Consideration for not identifying degradation products which are detected at the threshold levels is given for degradation products which are unstable (4). In those cases, a summary of the efforts to isolate and identify the unstable degradation product may suffice.

REFERENCES

1. International Conference on Harmonisation, Impurities in New Drug Substances, Q3A, January, 1996.
2. International Conference on Harmonisation, Impurities in New Drug Substances, Draft, Q3A(R), February, 2002.
3. International Conference on Harmonisation, Impurities in New Drug Products, Q3B, November, 1996.
4. International Conference on Harmonisation, Impurities in New Drug Products, Draft, Q3B(R), October, 1999.
5. International Conference on Harmonisation, Stability Testing of New Drug Substances and Products, Q1A, September, 1994.
6. International Conference on Harmonisation, Stability Testing of New Drug Substances and Products, Q1A(R2), February, 2003.
7. International Conference on Harmonisation, Stability Testing: Photostability Testing of New Drug Substances and Products, Q1B, November, 1996.
8. Görög S. New safe medicines faster: the role of analytical chemistry. Trends Anal Chem 2000; 22:7–8.
9. Dubin CH. The Gray Area. Pharmaceutical Formulation and Quality, Dec/Jan, 2003; 22–29.

10. Pope DG. Accelerated stability testing for prediction of drug product stability. Drug and Cosmet. Ind., Part 1, 54–62, November, 1980 and Part 2, 48–116, December 1980.
11. Guideline for Submitting Documentation for the Stability of Human Drugs and Biologics. Center for Drugs and Biologics, United States FDA, Department of Health and Human Services, Rockville, MD, February, 1987, p. 2.
12. The American Heritage® Dictionary of the English Language. 4th ed. Copyright© 2000 by Houghton Mifflin Company. Boston, MA: Houghton Miffin Company.
13. Reference ICH-Q1A, September 1994. (For drugs to be stored at room temperature, i.e., 25°C, accelerated testing is defined as 40°C/75% relative humidity. For other storage conditions accelerated testing is to be carried out at 15°C above the long-term storage temperature.)
14a. Kulschreshtha HK. Use of kinetic methods in storage stability studies on drugs and pharmaceuticals. Defence Sci J 1976; 26(4):189–204.
14b. Witthaus G. In: Breimer DD, Speiser P, eds. Accelerated Storage Tests: Predictive Value, Topics in Pharmaceutical Sciences. Elsevier, North-Holland Biomedical Press, 1981:275–290.
14c. Carstensen JT. In: Swarbrick JT, ed. Drug Stability. Principles and Practices. 2nd ed. New York: Marcel Dekker, 1995.
15a. Schou SA. Decomposition of pharmaceutical preparations due to chemical changes. Am J Hosp Pharm March 1960; 17:153–161.
15b. Stewart PJ, Tucker IG. Prediction of drug stability. Part 1. Mechanism of drug degradation and basic rate laws. Aust J Hosp Pharm 1984; 14:165–170.
15c. Stewart PJ, Tucker IG. Prediction of drug stability. Part 2. Hydrolysis. Aust J Hosp Pharm 1985; 15(1):11–16.
15d. Stewart PJ, Tucker IG. Prediction of drug stability. Part 3. Oxidation and photolytic degradation. Aust J Hosp Pharm 1985; 15(2):111–117.
16. Kennon LJ. Pharm Sci 1964; 53(7):815–818.
17. Yang W-H, Roy SB. Projection of tentative expiry date from one-point accelerated stability testing. Drug Dev Ind Pharm 1980; 6(6):591–604.
18. Witthaus G. Breimer DD, Speiser P, eds. Accelerated Storage Tests: Predictive Value, Topics in Pharmaceutical Sciences. Elsevier, North-Holland Biomedical Press, 1981:275–290.
19. Davis JS. Criteria for Accelerated Stability Testing, presented at the FDA/ASQC Seminar, March 11, Chicago, IL, 1991.
20. Carstensen JT. Drug Stability: Principles and Practices 2nd. ed. In: Swarbrick JT New York: Marcel Dekker, 1995:3–4.
21. Florey K, Brittain HG, eds. Analytical Profiles of Drug Substances. Vol. 1–25. New York: Academic Press, 1972–1998.
22. Singh S, Bakshi M. Guidance on conduct of stress tests to determine inherent stability of drugs. Pharma Technol Online April, 2000, 1–14.
23. Bridle JH, Brimble MT. A stability indicating method for dipyridamole. Drug Dev Ind Pharm 1993; 19:371–381.
24. Padmanabhan G, Becue I, Smith JB. Cloquinol. In: Florey K, ed. Analytical Profiles of Drug Substances. Vol. 18. New York: Academic Press, 1989:76–77.

25. Gröningsson K, Lindgren J-E, Lundbeg E, Sandberg R, Wahlén A. Lidocaine base and hydrochloride. In: Florey K, ed. Analytical Profiles of Drug Substances. Vol.14. New York: Academic Press. 1985:226–227.
26. Lagu AL, Young R, McGonigle E, Lane PA. High performance liquid chromatographic determination of suprofen in drug substance and capsules. J Pharm Sci 1982; 71(1):85–88.
27. Muhtadi FJ. Analytical profile of morphine. In: Florey K, ed. Analytical Profiles of Drug Substances. Vol. 17. New York: Academic Press, 1988:309.
28. Maron N, Wright G. Application of photodiode array UV detection in the development of stability-indicating LC methods: determination of mefenamic acid. J Pharm Biomed Anal 1990; 8:101–105.
29. Nassar MN, Chen T, Reff MJ, Agharkar SN. Didanosine. In: Brittain HG, ed. Analytical Profiles of Drug Substances and Excipients. Vol. 22. New York: Academic Press, 1993:216–219.
30. Johnson BM, Chang P-TL. Sertraline hydrochloride. In: Brittain HG, ed. Analytical Profiles of Drug Substances and Excipients. Vol. 24. New York: Academic Press, 1996:484.
31. See Table V in Singh S, Bakshi M. Guidance on conduct of stress tests to determine inherent stability of drugs. Pharma Technol Online April, 2000; 1–14.
32. Anderson NH, Johnston D, McLelland MA, Munden P. Photostability testing of drug substances and drug products in UK pharmaceutical laboratories. J Pharm Biomed Anal 1991; 9(6):443.
33. Thoma K. Survey of twenty German manufacturers (1995). In: Tønnesen H, ed. Photostability of Drugs and Drug Formulations. London: Taylor & Francis, 1996:136–137.
34a. Thatcher SR, Mansfield RK, Miller RB, Davis CW, Baertschi, SW. Pharmaceutical photostability: a technical and practical interpretation of the ICH guideline and its application to pharmaceutical stability: Part I, Pharmaceutical Technology, March 2001; 25(3):98–110.
34b. Thatcher SR, Mansfield RK, Miller RB, Davis CW, Baertschi SW. Pharmaceutical photostability: a technical and practical interpretation of the ICH guideline and its application to pharmaceutical stability: Part II, Pharmaceutical Technology, April 2001; 25(4):50–62.
35. Boccardi G, Deleuze C, Gachon M, Palmisano G, Vergnaud JP. J Pharm Sci 1992; 81(2):183–185.
36. Boccardi G. Il Farmaco 1994; 49(6):431–435.
37. Baertschi SW. The Role of Stress Testing in Pharmaceutical Product Development, presented at the American Association of Pharmaceutical Scientists Midwest Regional Meeting, Chicago, IL, May 20, 1996.
38. Weiser WE. Developing analytical methods for stability testing. Pharma Technol 1998:20–29.
39. Alsante KM, Friedmann RC, Hatajik TD, Lohr LL, Sharp TR, Snyder KD, Szczesny EJ. Degradation and impurity analysis for pharmaceutical drug candidates. In: Ahuja S, Scypinski S, eds. Handbook of Modern Pharmaceutical Analysis. Vol. 3. Separation Science and Technology. Academic Press, 2001: 85–172.

40. Reynolds DW, Facchine KL, Mullaney JF, Alsante KM, Hatajik TD, Motto MG. Available guidance and best practices for conducting forced degradation studies. Pharma Technol February 2002; 26(2).
41. Trabelsi H, Bouabdallah S, Bouzouita K, Safta F. Determination and degradation study of haloperidol by high performance liquid chromatography. Pharm Biomed Anal 2002; 29:649–657.
42. Caviglioli G, Valeria P, Brunella P, Sergio C, Attilia A, Gaetano B. Identification of degradation products of Ibuprofen arising from oxidative and thermal treatments. J Pharm Biomed Anal 2002; 30:499–509.
43. Breil S, Martino R, Gilard V, Malet-Martino M, Niemeyer U. Identification of new aqueous chemical degradation products of isophosphoramide mustard. J Pharm Biomed Anal 2001; 25:669–678.
44. Xu X, Bartlett MG, Stewart JT. Determination of degradation products of sumatriptan. J Pharm Biomed Anal 2001; 26:367–377.
45. Feng W, Liu H, Chen G, Malchow R, Bennett F, Lin E, Pramanik B, Chan T-M. Structural characterization of the oxidative degradation products of an antifungal agent SCH56592 by LC-NMR and LC-MS. J Pharm Biomed Anal 2001; 25:545–557.
46. Bakshi M, Singh B, Singh A, Singh S. The ICH guidance in practice: stress degradation studies on ornidazole and development of a validated stability-indicating assay. J Pharm Biomed Anal 2001; 26:891–897.
47. Ojha T, Bakshi M, Chakraborti AK, Singh S. The ICH guidance in practice: stress decomposition studies on three piperazinyl quinazoline adrenergic receptor-blocking agents and comparison of their degradation behavior. J Pharm Biomed Anal 2003; 31:775–783.
48. FDA: Guidance for Industry: INDs for Phase 2 and 3 Studies; Chemistry, Manufacturing, and Controls Information (Issued May 2003).
49. Submitting Documentation for the Stability of Human Drugs and Biologics (CDER, Issued February, 1987).
50. International Conference on Harmonisation; Guidance on Q6A Specifications: Test Procedures and Acceptance Criteria for New Drug Substances and New Drug Products: Chemical Substances. December, 2000.

2

Stress Testing: A Predictive Tool

Steven W. Baertschi and Patrick J. Jansen

Eli Lilly and Company, Lilly Research Laboratories, Lilly Corporate Center, Indianapolis, Indiana, U.S.A.

I. INTRODUCTION

As described in Chapter 1, stress testing is the main tool that is used to predict stability-related problems, develop analytical methods, and identify degradation products and pathways. Stability-related issues can affect many areas, including the following:

- Analytical methods development
- Formulation and package development
- Appropriate storage conditions and shelf-life determination
- Safety/toxicological concerns
- Manufacturing/processing parameters
- Absorption, distribution, metabolism, and excretion (ADME) studies
- Environmental assessment

It is worth discussing briefly each of these stability-related areas.

A. Analytical Methods Development

In order to assess the stability of a compound, one needs an appropriate method. The development of stability-indicating analytical method, particularly an impurity method, is a "chicken and egg" type of problem. That is, how does one develop an impurity method to detect degradation products when one does not know what the degradation products are? Stress-testing studies can help to address this dilemma. Stressing the parent compound under particular stress conditions can generate samples containing degradation products. These samples can then be used to develop suitable analytical procedures. It is important to note that the degradation products generated in the stressed samples can be classified as "potential" degradation products that may or may not be formed under relevant storage conditions. It is also important to note that not all relevant degradation products may form under the stress conditions. Both accelerated and long-term testing studies are used to determine which of the potential degradation products actually form under normal storage conditions and are, therefore, relevant degradation products. The strategy for developing a stability-indicating method is described in detail in Chapter 4.

B. Formulation and Packaging Development

The knowledge gained from stress testing is useful for formulation and packaging development. Well-designed stress-testing studies can determine the susceptibility of a compound to hydrolysis, oxidation, photochemical degradation, and thermal degradation. This information is then taken into consideration when developing the formulation and determining the appropriate packaging. For example, if stress-testing studies indicate that a compound is rapidly degraded in acid, then consideration might be given to developing an enteric-coated formulation that protects the compound from rapid degradation in the stomach. Similarly, if a compound is sensitive to hydrolysis, packaging that protects from water vapor transmission from the outside of the package to the inside of the package may be helpful to ensure long-term storage stability. Other degradation mechanisms (e.g., oxidative degradation or photodegradation) can also be prevented or minimized by the use of appropriate packaging and/or formulation. Knowledge of potential drug–excipient interactions is also critical to developing the best formulation.

C. Appropriate Storage Conditions and Shelf-Life Determination

Determining appropriate storage conditions for a drug substance or product requires knowledge of the conditions that induce degradation and the degradation mechanisms. Most of this information can be obtained from stress-testing studies combined with accelerated stability testing. Accurate shelf-life predictions, however, are best made with data from formal long-term stability studies.

D. Safety/Toxicological Concerns

If stress-testing studies indicate the formation of (a) known toxic compound(s), steps can be taken early on to inhibit the formation of the toxic compound(s) and to develop sensitive analytical methods to accurately detect and quantify. Stress-testing studies can also facilitate preparation/isolation of a degradation product for toxicological evaluation when synthetic preparation is not feasible.

E. Manufacturing/Processing Parameters

Degradation can also occur during manufacturing or processing steps. Knowledge of what conditions lead to degradation of the parent compound can help to design appropriate controls/conditions during manufacturing/processing. For example, if a compound is susceptible to degradation at low pH, then either the manufacturing steps under low pH conditions can be avoided or the time and/or temperature can be more carefully controlled to minimize the degradation. It is not uncommon to observe degradation during formulation processing, for example, wet granulation, milling, etc. An understanding of the degradation that may occur during the formulation processing steps can help in choosing conditions to ensure maximum stability of the drug substance (e.g., oxidative susceptibility may lead to the use of processing in an inert-gas atmosphere).

F. ADME Studies

ADME characteristics of a drug are extensively studied prior to marketing. These studies typically involve identification of the major metabolites, a process that can be difficult owing to the complex matrix (living organism) and often very low levels. Occasionally, degradation products detected in stress-testing studies are also metabolites. In these cases, it is usually easier to generate larger quantities of the metabolite for characterization using the stress condition rather than isolate it from the living organism. It is also possible that nonenzymatic degradation can occur in vivo, and therefore an understanding of what degradation pathways might be relevant under physiological conditions can be important to understanding the ADME of a new drug.

G. Environmental Assessment

The environmental assessment deals with the fate of the drug in the environment. The information gained from stress testing can be useful for designing and interpreting environmental studies, as the degradation of the drug in the environment will often be similar to degradation observed during stress-testing studies.

II. PREDICTIVE VERSUS DEFINITIVE

It is important to remember that stress testing is *predictive* in nature (as opposed to *definitive*). That is, the degradation products formed under stress conditions may or may not be relevant to the actual storage conditions of the drug substance and/or to the degradation chemistry of the drug product. This reality is reflected in the ICH definition of stress testing, where it is stated:

> Examining degradation products under stress conditions is useful in establishing degradation pathways and developing and validating suitable analytical methods. However, such examination may not be necessary for certain degradation products if it has been demonstrated that they are not formed under accelerated or long term storage conditions (from Ref. 1.)

Therefore, the degradation products formed during stress testing can be thought of as "potential" degradation products. Ideally, stress conditions should result in the formation of all potential degradation products. The "significant" or "relevant" degradation products that occur during long-term storage or shipping (as revealed by accelerated testing and long-term stability studies) should thus be a subset of the "potential" degradation products. This concept is illustrated in Figure 1. The overall strategy of stress testing is, therefore, to predict *potential* issues related to stability of the molecule—either as the drug substance alone or as a formulated product. This strategy is outlined in Figure 2.

As shown in Figure 2, the overall strategy is similar for both drug substance and product. The strategy begins with stress testing of the drug substance using discriminating or "screening" methods (2). Such methods should be capable of separating and detecting a broad range of degradation products and can be used for degradation and impurity investigations. In practice, RP-HPLC with UV detection is by far the most common analytical technique currently used for the detection of impurities. A discriminating RP-HPLC method utilizing a broad gradient elution is recommended for covering a wide polarity range. Other separation techniques or detection modes may be employed, but the key concept is to develop and use methodology that will maximize separation and provide the most universal detection. The screening method can be developed/optimized by analysis of partially degraded samples and the use of standard method development procedures and tools (3). The analysis of stressed samples should reveal the "potential" degradation products formed under the various stress conditions. Accelerated testing and analytical evaluation using the same broad screening method can determine the "significant" degradation products. Methods designed to separate and detect only the significant degradation products (i.e., those that form at significant levels under accelerated and long-term storage conditions) can then be developed and optimized. Such methods, which have been referred to elsewhere as "focused" methods (2), are designed for regulatory registration in the marketing application and use in quality control laboratories for product release and stability.

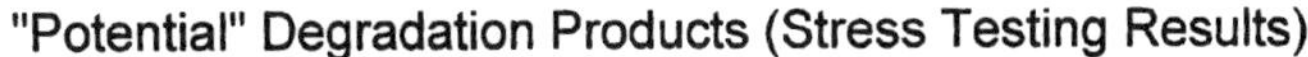

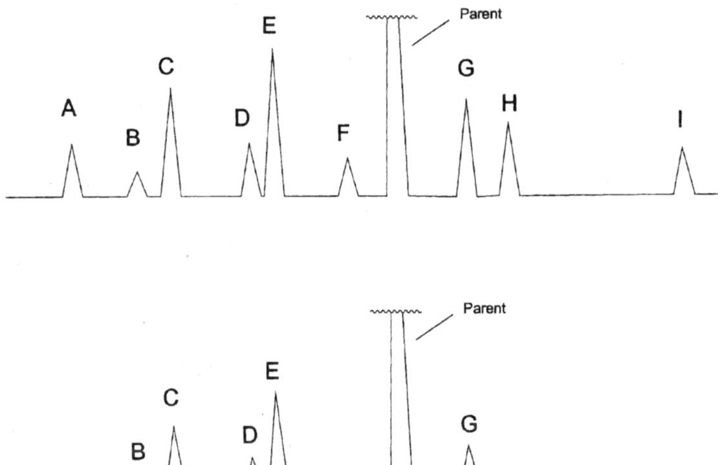

Figure 1 Cartoon illustration of hypothetical chromatograms from stress testing (upper) and accelerated or long-term stability studies. Peaks A–I represent all the degradation products from stress-testing studies under various stress conditions and are therefore classified as "potential" degradation products. Peaks B–E and G represent the products that form at significant levels during formal stability studies and are therefore classified as the "actual" or "relevant" degradation products.

The information gathered during stress testing of the drug substance is used to guide the formulation of the drug product. As described in detail in Chapter 13, drug-excipient compatibility studies (4–7) can be performed to determine whether or not individual excipients, excipient blends, or trial formulations have any significant adverse interactions with the parent drug. A broad screening method such as that developed for drug substance stress testing should be used for the analytical evaluation of such studies. As discussed in Chapter 11, microcalorimetric techniques may also be useful for the analysis of drug–excipient interactions (8–11). Once a suitable formulation has been developed, stress-testing studies can be performed on the formulation and any resulting degradation products can be compared to the degradation products formed during stress-testing studies of the drug substance alone. In an analogous manner to the strategy for the drug substance, the "significant" degradation products can be determined via accelerated and long-term stability studies, and focused methods can be developed for regulatory registration and use in quality control laboratories for product release and stability.

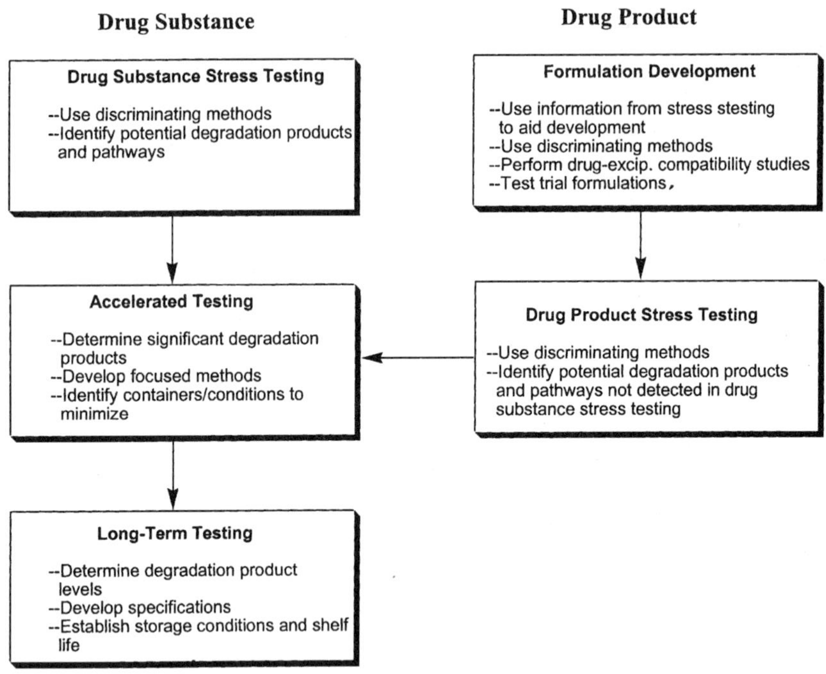

Figure 2 Overall strategy for the prediction, identification, and control of stability-related issues.

The key to the strategy outlined earlier is to have well-designed stress-testing studies that form all potential degradation products. As discussed in Section II, ICH defines stress testing as an investigation of the "intrinsic stability" characteristics of the molecule. As the term "intrinsic stability" appears to be foundational to the understanding, yet has no clear definition, it is worth discussing. The concept of "intrinsic stability" has four main aspects:

1. Conditions leading to degradation
2. Rates of degradation (Relative or Otherwise)
3. Structures of the major degradation products
4. Pathways of degradation

Once these four areas have been investigated and understood, stability-related issues can be identified or predicted. It is worth considering in more detail the four main aspects of intrinsic stability mentioned earlier.

III. INTRINSIC STABILITY: CONDITIONS LEADING TO DEGRADATION

As described in the PhRMA "Available Guidance and Best Practices" article on forced degradation studies (12), stress testing should include conditions that examine specifically for four main pharmaceutically relevant degradation mechanisms (2): (a) thermolytic, (b) hydrolytic, (c) oxidative, and (d) photolytic. The potential for these degradation pathways should be assessed in both drug substance and formulated product (and/or drug–excipient mixtures). These mechanisms can be assessed in a systematic way by exposure to stress conditions of heat, humidity, photostress (UV and VIS), oxidative conditions, and aqueous conditions across a broad pH range.

A. Thermolytic Degradation

Thermolytic degradation is usually thought of as degradation caused by exposure to temperatures high enough to induce bond breakage, that is, pyrolysis. For the purposes of simplification (although, admittedly, perhaps oversimplification) in the context of drug degradation, we will use the term thermolytic to describe reactions that are driven by heat or temperature. Thus, any degradation mechanism that is enhanced at elevated temperatures can be considered a "thermolytic pathway." The following list of degradation pathways, while not an exhaustive list, can be thought of as thermolytic pathways: hydrolysis/dehydration, isomerization/epimerization, decarboxylation, rearrangements and some kinds of polymerization reactions. Note that hydrolytic reactions are actually a subset of thermolytic pathways using this construct. In addition, note that oxidative and photolytic reactions are not included in this list (as they are not primarily driven by temperature) but are discussed separately in more detail (see below). The ICH Stability guideline suggests studying "… the effect of temperatures in 10°C increments above the accelerated temperature test condition (e.g., 50°C, 60°C, etc.)… ." It is not clear why the guideline suggests 10°C increments, but it may be related to the importance of understanding whether or not any degradation (in the solid state) mechanisms change as a result of increasing temperature. Studies with such temperature increases would be useful for constructing Arrhenius plots to allow prediction of degradation in the solid state rates at different temperatures; however, for many pharmaceutical small molecule drug substances, it would take several months of storage at the elevated temperatures to induce enough degradation to provide meaningful kinetic data from which to construct such plots.

As discussed in Chapter 1 (Sections III and IV), the kinetics of drug degradation has been the topic of numerous books and articles. The Arrhenius relationship is probably the most commonly used expression for evaluating the relationship between rates of reaction and temperature for a given order of reaction (For a more thorough treatment of the Arrhenius equation and prediction of chemical stability, see Ref. 13). If the decomposition of a drug obeys the Arrhenius relationship [i.e., $k = A \exp(-E_a/RT)$, where k is the degree of rate constant, A is the "pre-exponential factor" or "frequency factor" (i.e., the frequency of collisions among reactants irrespective of energy), R is the universal gas constant, and T is the temperature in degrees in Kelvin], it is possible to estimate the effect of temperature on the degradation rate of a compound, providing the "energy of activation" (E_a) is known (14).

Connors et al. (15) assert that most drug substances have energies of activation (E_as) of 12–24 kcal/mol, although E_as > 24 kcal/mol are not uncommon (16). In 1964, Kennon (17) compiled the activation energies for decomposition of a number of drug compounds and found the average to be 19.8 kcal/mol. Davis (18), a retired FDA reviewer, has asserted that 20 kcal/mol is a "quite conservative" estimate for the average E_a of decomposition of drug compounds. The "Joel Davis Rule", an historical rule-of-thumb that has been commonly used in the pharmaceutical industry, states that acceptable results from 3-month stability testing of a drug product at 37–40°C can be used to project a tentative expiry date of 2 years from the date of manufacture. Yang and Roy (19) have shown that this rule-of-thumb is valid only if the E_a is >25.8 kcal/mol (19). The PhRMA "Available Guidance and Best Practices" on forced degradation provides estimates of the effects of elevated temperature based on a very conservative assumption of 12 kcal/mol (12). Waterman (20) has asserted that the relative humidity under which a solid drug product is stored is a critical variable when attempting to use the Arrhenius relationship. Waterman showed evidence that degradation rates of formulated products (with pathways involving hydrolytic or oxidative degradation) often hold to the Arrhenius relationship if the relative humidity is held constant at the different elevated temperatures. Further research in this area may provide significant improvements in the predictability of solid state drug degradation rates from stress testing and accelerated stability studies.

Table 1 shows rates of degradation relative to 25 °C assuming energies of activation of 12, 15, and 20 kcal/mol assuming that the degradation kinetics follows Arrhenius kinetics. Table 2 shows the increase in rate for each 10°C increase in temperature for the same 12, 15, and 20 kcal/mol energies of activation. Tables 1 and 2 can be used to estimate the effect of stress temperatures on the rate of a degradation reaction for a particular E_a. It is apparent from Tables 1 and 2 that the increase in reaction rate is dependent on the E_a, and that a low energy of activation (e.g., 12 kcal/mol) results in a less-dramatic increase in reaction rate as temperature is increased.

The PhRMA guidance and Alsante et al. (21) have recommended a conservative approach of assuming that for every 10°C increase in temperature the reaction rate approximately doubles. This is approximately equivalent to assuming an E_a of 12 kcal/mol.

Using the information provided in Tables 1 and 2, it is straightforward to calculate the effect of temperature on the degradation rate to enable

Table 1 Rates of Degradation (Relative to 25°C) Assuming Arrhenius Kinetics and Energies of Activation (E_a) of 12, 15, and 20 kcal/mol

Temperature (°C)	Relative rate assume E_a=12 kcal/mol	Relative rate assume E_a = 15 kcal/mol	Relative rate assume E_a = 20 kcal/mol
25	1	1	1
30	1.39	1.52	1.75
40	2.62	3.37	5.05
50	4.78	7.10	13.65
60	8.36	14.33	34.79
70	14.20	27.74	83.98

prediction/estimation of degradation rates at lower temperatures (e.g., room temperature) for different energies of activation. For example, if one assumes an activation energy of 12 kcal/mol, stressing at 70°C for 1 week would be roughly the same as 100 days at 25°C (14.2 × 7 days = 99.4 days). Similarly, assuming an activation energy of 20 kcal/mol and stressing for one week at 70°C would be roughly the same as 588 days at 25°C (83.98 × 7 days = 587.86 days).

It should be noted here that solid-state reactions often proceed in an "autocatalytic" pathway (similar to oxidative degradation kinetics) involving an induction period (lag), followed by a period of rapidly increasing degradation and then a slowing down of the degradation rate as the drug is consumed (22,23). Thus, solid-state reaction kinetics will often follow an "S"-shaped curve when degradation vs. time is plotted. This kind of reaction kinetics is often more pronounced in formulated solid oral dosage forms (for reasons which will not be discussed here). It is reasonable to question whether or not Arrhenius kinetics will hold if the solid-state degradation is autocatalytic. Arrhenius kinetics is typically observed in the

Table 2 Relative Increase in Rates of Degradation as Temperature is Increased, Assuming Arrhenius Kinetics and Energies of Activation (E_a) of 12, 15, and 20 kcal/mol

Temperature (°C)	Increase in Rate of Reaction (E_a = 12 kcal/mol)	Increase in Rate of Reaction (E_a =15 kcal/mol)	Increase in Rate of Reaction (E_a = 20 kcal/mol)
25–30	1.39	1.52	1.75
30–40	1.88	2.22	2.89
40–50	1.82	2.11	2.71
50–60	1.75	2.02	2.55
60–70	1.70	1.94	2.41

degradation of solid pharmaceutical products (within temperature ranges discussed in what follows) presumably because most solid-state degradation studies involve only modest amounts of degradation (e.g., $\leq 5\%$) and are therefore typically operating in the "induction" or "lag" period of the solid-state degradation. If solid-state degradation studies are carried out to higher levels of degradation (e.g., >10–30% degradation), it is likely that degradation rate prediction via Arrhenius kinetics would not be feasible. For an in depth discussion of the applicability of Arrhenius kinetics to pharmaceutical degradation see Waterman (20).

Note that the above information assumes that the decomposition follows the same pathways at all the temperatures. This assumption will not be true for all compounds, but for the majority of small molecule drug compounds, it is our experience that the degradation pathways will usually be the same up to ~70°C. Precedence can be found in regulatory guidelines and in the scientific literature for using temperatures up to 50°C (4), 60°C (1), and even 80°C (25) and 85°C (17,26) for stress testing and "accelerated stability" studies. However, the references to stressing at 80°C and 85 °C suggest that such high temperatures are optional and may lead to different decomposition pathways for some compounds. One example of changes in degradation mechanism above 80°C is the case of SB-243213 (27). In this case, stress studies at room temperature up to 80°C showed the same degradation profile. In contrast, stressing at 100°C showed a large number of new degradants not observed at lower temperatures. Another example of changes in degradation mechanism as a function of temperature can be seen in the case of cefaclor.

Cefaclor is an oral cephalosporin antibiotic whose degradation pathways have been studied extensively (28). As shown by Dorman et al. (28), the degradation profile of cefaclor after storage at 85°C is significantly different than the profile observed upon storage at room temperature or at 40°C. Olsen et al. (29) have shown that the degradation pathways of cefaclor at room temperature do not change as the temperature is increased to ~ 70 °C (see also Fig. 2 of Chapter 8). Somewhere between 70°C and 85 °C, different degradation pathways begin to occur, illustrating that there is a risk of introducing nonrelevant degradation pathways, as stressing temperatures of drug substances and products are increased.

It is noteworthy that *oxidative* reaction rates, whether in solid state or in solution, may not be readily predicted using just thermal stress. For this reason, oxidative degradation is broken out into a separate category (see the section on Oxidative Degradation for more discussion).

In conclusion, on the basis of evaluation of the literature and kinetic considerations in conjunction with our stress-testing experience over the last 15 years, temperatures of up to 70°C (at high and low humidities) should provide a rapid, reasonably predictive assessment of the solid-state degradation pathways and relative stabilities of most drug substances at lower temperatures. A time period of 1 to 2 months under these stress conditions is recommended.

B. Hydrolytic Degradation

Drug degradation that involves reaction with water is called hydrolysis. Stewart and Tucker (30) have asserted that hydrolysis and oxidation are the two most common mechanisms of drug degradation. The experience of the authors and extensive reviews of drug degradation literature are consistent with their assertion. Given that water is present at significant levels in many drugs (e.g., hydrates), in many excipients, and even at normal atmospheric conditions it is not surprising that hydrolysis is a common degradation problem. Because hydrolysis is such a common reaction, it has been described in detail elsewhere and, therefore, will not be extensively dealt with in this chapter. Rather, just a few of the more important aspects will be discussed, with relevant literature references given to facilitate further study.

Stewart and Tucker assert that hydrolysis is affected by pH, buffer salts, ionic strength, solvent, and other additives such as complexing agents, surfactants, and excipients, and each of these factors is discussed in some detail. Waterman et al. (31) provide a comprehensive treatment of hydrolysis as it relates to pharmaceuticals, with thorough discussions of mechanisms, formulation considerations, pH, ionic strength, buffers, solid-state considerations, hydrolysis of lyophiles, liquid dosage forms, packaging, etc.

Hydrolysis reactions are typically acid or base catalyzed. Acidic, neutral, and basic conditions should therefore be employed in order to induce potential hydrolytic reactions. This is especially important when the compound being tested has (an) ionizable functional group(s) and can exist in different ionization states under relevant aqueous conditions. It is particularly important to be sure to test hydrolysis at unique protonation states, unless there are a large number of ionizable functional groups as is often the case with peptides and proteins. In cases such as these, a practical approach is to simply expose the sample to a wide pH range in defined increments (e.g., 1 pH unit). A pH range of 1 (e.g., 0.1 M HC1) to 13 (e.g., 0.1 M NaOH) has been used by a number of major pharmaceutical companies (32) for the most acidic and most basic extremes of aqueous stress testing. As discussed in the section on Historical and Regulatory Context mentioned in Chapter 1, more acidic (e.g., $pH < 1$) and basic (e.g., $pH > 13$) conditions can and have been employed. These unusually acidic or basic conditions may simply speed up acid or base-catalyzed hydrolysis, but there is an increased risk of inducing unrealistic degradation pathways (e.g., from protonation of sites with very low pKs that can alter the site(s) of hydrolytic attack).

One problem that is often faced in designing hydrolytic stress tests is compound solubility. Many small molecule drugs are not soluble in water at the concentrations typically used for analytical evaluation (i.e., 0.1–1 mg/mL) across the entire pH range (32). Thus, either a slurry/suspension must be used to examine the hydrolytic stability of a compound or a cosolvent must be added to facilitate dissolution under the conditions of low solubility. The two most commonly used cosolvents are acetonitrile and methanol (32). Because methanol has the potential of participating in the degradation chemistry (e.g., acting as a nucleophile to react with electrophilic sites or intermediates in the degradation pathways), it should be used with caution (especially under acidic conditions) if the compound being tested contains a carboxylic acid, ester, or amide as these groups may react with methanol. Acetonitrile is generally regarded as an inert solvent and is typically preferable to methanol in hydrolytic stress-testing studies (32). It should be recognized, however, that acetonitrile is not completely inert and can participate in the degradation reactions leading to artifactual degradation results. For example, acetonitrile is known to contribute to base-catalyzed epoxidation reactions in the presence of peroxides (33). Acetonitrile will also degrade, in the presence of base (e.g., pH 13) and/or acid (e.g., pH 1) under elevated temperatures, to detectable levels of acetamide and/or acetic acid, which can show up as early eluting peaks (when monitoring at low wavelengths) on RP-HPLC. The size of the HPLC peaks from these two products is relatively small, and the use of stressed blank solutions (solvent system without drug stressed under the same conditions) permits ready identification of these peaks. In acidic acetonitrile/water solutions, tertiary alcohols can undergo a Ritter reaction to form amides (see Chapter 3). In the presence of radicals [e.g., generated during prolonged sonication as part of the analytical workup or in the presence of free radical initiators such as 2, 2-azo*bis*isobutyronitrile (AIBN)], acetonitrile can be oxidized to small amounts of formyl cyanide that will readily react with nucleophiles (such as amines), resulting in a "formylation" reaction (Fig. 3). Nonetheless, most of these side reactions of acetonitrile are relatively minor and acetonitrile remains the most frequently used cosolvent for hydrolysis studies. Other cosolvents that have been recommended for hydrolytic stress-testing studies (34) are shown in Table 3.

It is worth discussing the potential effects of cosolvents on the degradation rates and pathways. It is often thought that the apparent hydrolytic degradation rate of a drug will be increased by the use of a cosolvent to facilitate dissolution, and while this is often true, it is also often *not* true. (In our experience, roughly 25–40% of the time the observed degradation rate in aqueous conditions will be slower with the addition of a cosolvent such as ACN when compared with an aqueous slurry/suspension.) The overall hydrolytic degradation rate will depend on the specific mechanism(s) involved in the degradation pathway(s). The degradation reactions and rates

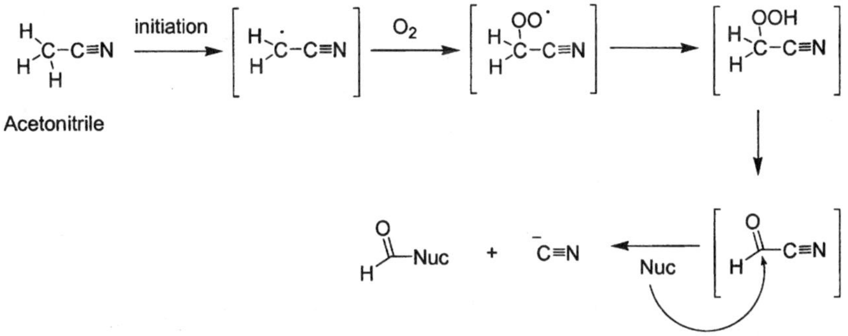

Figure 3 Potential side reaction of acetonitrile in the presence of radicals.

involved will depend on a variety of factors such as the dielectric constant, solvent polarity, ionic strength, whether or not the solvent is protic or aprotic, the surface energy (i.e., of the solid–liquid interface in a slurry/suspension), etc. (35–37). For example, a degradation reaction involving acid-catalyzed hydrolysis with a cationic intermediate or a polarized transition state will be facilitated by a solvent with a high dielectric constant, and the addition of a cosolvent that reduces the effective dielectric constant will reduce the rate of such a reaction. Solvation of a compound in an aqueous cosolvent mixture may involve formation of a "solvent cage" of the more nonpolar solvent around the compound, potentially leading to some protection from hydrolysis. Solvent composition can also affect tautomeric states of molecules (38,39), which in turn can affect both degradation rates and pathways. The effective pH of an aqueous solution will also change upon addition of a cosolvent (40), which can both affect the degradation rate and change the degradation pathway(s) (e.g., by facilitating different protonation states).

The use of elevated temperature is appropriate (though not required) for aqueous solution stress-testing studies. As discussed in Section III. A, elevated temperatures up to 70°C should accelerate the hydrolytic degradation

Table 3 Organic Cosolvents that have been Used for Stress-Testing Studies

Acidic pH	Neutral pH	Basic pH
Acetonitrile[a]	Acetonitrile[a]	Acetonitrile[a]
DMSO	NMP	DMSO
Acetic Acid		Glyme[a]
Propionic Acid		Diglyme
		p-Dioxane

[a]Volatile solvent: may evaporate at higer temperatures.

processes in a meaningful way. Higher temperatures can be used, but the risk of non-Arrhenius behavior increases significantly as temperature is increased further. Tables 1 and 2 can be used to help predict degradation rates at different temperatures, with the assumptions of Arrhenius behavior and specific activation energies.

In conclusion, we assert that testing of the hydrolytic susceptibility of a drug substance should involve exposure to acidic, neutral, and basic conditions in the pH range of 1–13, preferably under 100% aqueous conditions. When solubility is low, the use of an inert water miscible cosolvent (e.g., acetonitrile) is appropriate, but it should be recognized that the presence of a cosolvent may either speed up or slow down the hydrolysis, and there is a possibility that degradation pathways could also change in the presence of a cosolvent. Therefore, it may be useful to stress the compound as a slurry in 100% aqueous conditions in addition to stressing in the presence of a cosolvent. Elevated temperatures with an upper limit of 70°C are recommended for accelerating the hydrolytic reactions. The longest recommended time period for stressing at the highest temperature is 2 weeks, although longer times can certainly be used if desired.

C. Oxidative Degradation

As mentioned in Section III.B, oxidative reactions are one of the two most common mechanisms of drug degradation. Oxidative drug degradation reactions are typically autoxidative, that is the reaction is radical initiated. Radical-initiated reactions start with an initiation phase involving the formation of radicals (this step is rate-limiting), followed by a propagation phase and eventually a termination phase. Thus, the reaction kinetics will often follow an "S"-shaped curve when degradation vs. time is plotted (22,23,41) and will not follow Arrhenius kinetics. In the solid state, it is not clear whether or not oxidative degradation reactions have significant propagation phases. It has been recently suggested that autoxidative degradation reactions in solid oral dosage forms do not have significant propagation phases (presumably due to lack of mobility), and therefore, observed deviations from Arrhenius kinetics may be from (a) different cause(s) (42). The picture is further complicated by the complex nature of oxidative reactions, where oxidative intermediates are often thermally unstable and may decompose via alternate pathways at elevated temperatures (43). Increases in temperature, therefore, may not lead to predictable changes in degradation rates, and the observed oxidative rates and pathways may be different than those observed at lower temperatures. In solution, oxidative rates and pathways may be dependent on the dissolved oxygen concentration. Thus, the reaction rate in solution may actually be *reduced* at higher temperatures because of the decrease in oxygen content of the solvent. This may be partially overcome by bubbling oxygen or air through the solution while heating or by storing the solution under oxygen in an airtight vessel with high pressure (at least a few atmospheres). Regardless, the degradation kinetics will likely not follow Arrhenius kinetics, and therefore short-term stress studies may not accurately predict long-term stability. Instead, the susceptibility to oxidative degradation can be studied in solution using a radical initiator (e.g., AIBN, 40°C, up to 1 week) and exposure to hydrogen peroxide (e.g., 0.3% hydrogen peroxide, up to 1 week at room temperature, in the dark) in separate studies. As both of these oxidative susceptibility studies are in solution, it may be useful to control the pH such that all relevant protonation states of the drug are tested. For example, if the compound being tested contained one ionizable functional group (e.g., an amine) with a p*K* of 7, the oxidative tests could be carried out 1 pH unit above and below. It should be noted here that room temperature storage is sufficient for the hydrogen peroxide test. The use of higher temperatures (e.g., >30°C) with hydrogen peroxide should be done with caution because the O–O bond is a weak bond that will readily cleave at elevated temperatures to form hydroxyl radicals, a much harsher oxidative reagent. The use of transition metals [e.g., copper (II) and iron (III) at ~1–5 mM, 1–3 days] is also recommended for evaluation of oxidative susceptibility. For a more thorough discussion on oxidative degradation and stress testing, see Refs. 20, 43–45 and Chapter 7.

D. Photolytic Degradation

Photolytic degradation (as it applies to pharmaceutical stability) is the degradation that results from exposure to ultraviolet or visible light in the wavelength range of approximately 300–800 nm. Exposure to radiation at wavelengths <300 nm is not needed because a pharmaceutical compound would not experience such exposure during its life cycle. The "first law" of photochemistry [Grotthus (1817) and Draper (1843)] states, "only radiation that is absorbed by a molecule can be effective in producing chemical changes in the molecule." Thus, in order for photolytic degradation to occur, radiation must be absorbed—either by the drug substance or by the formulation. Photodegradation rates are therefore directly dependent on the amount of incident radiation and on the amount of radiation that is absorbed by the compound or the formulation. It is important to remember that a compound may undergo photolytic degradation even if it does not itself absorb radiation in the UVA or visible region. This can only happen if there is some additional agent in the formulation, intentionally or adventitiously present, that facilitates absorption. Reed et al. (46) have documented a classic example of this phenomenon, describing a phenyl ether-based drug substance that exhibited photodegradation with both UVA and visible light exposure even though the drug molecule itself did not absorb at wavelengths >300 nm. In this case, the presence of low levels of iron (III) was found to chelate with carboxylates present in the formulation (citrate), leading to a complex that absorbed in the UVA and visible regions. The proposed mechanism for photodegradation was the formation of hydroxyl radicals (via the photo-Fenton reaction), which caused oxidative degradation of the drug.

It is important to remember that the ICH photostability guideline (Q1B) refers to both forced degradation studies (stress testing) and confirmatory testing. As confirmatory photostability testing is designed to be a part of the definitive, formal stability testing, it can be thought of as being analogous to an accelerated stability study. Thus, the minimum recommended exposure outlined in Q1B (i.e., 1.2 million lux-hr visible and 200 W-hr/m^2 UVA) is not the exposure recommended for forced degradation studies. In fact, there is no mention of recommended exposures for forced degradation studies and the design is left open. A member of the original ICH Photostability Expert Working Group recommended an exposure of three to five times the minimum ICH confirmatory exposure for forced degradation studies (47). Interestingly, early versions of the guideline (during Step 1 of the ICH process) suggested that forced degradation studies should use exposures in the range of five to 10 times the confirmatory exposure recommendations. A photoexposure in the range of three to 10 times the confirmatory exposure seems a reasonable amount of photostress for forced degradation studies, remembering that photodegradation of the compound being studied beyond 20–30% would not be necessary or desired.

It should be remembered that photodegradation products formed under stress conditions (i.e., "potential" photodegradation products) may not always be observed under confirmatory conditions. Such differences may be exacerbated by the use of different photon sources [i.e., ICH Option 1 vs. Option 2 (48)] for stress testing and confirmatory studies, and therefore it may be prudent to use the same source for both studies to avoid confusion.

Evaluation of the propensity of a drug substance (or formulation) to undergo photodegradation should be guided by the ICH QIB guidance document on photostability testing (48). As this topic has been covered extensively elsewhere (49–53), including Chapter 10 in this book, it will not be discussed in detail here.

IV. INTRINSIC STABILITY: RATES OF DEGRADATION

A critical part of evaluation of "intrinsic stability" is the apparent rate of degradation under various conditions that lead to degradation. A rigorous evaluation of the kinetics of degradation is generally not the focus of stress-testing studies, but useful information can be gained by kinetic evaluation. For example, relative rates of degradation at different pH conditions allows an assessment of which pH conditions will provide the most (or least) stable environment for a compound. Such information is useful for evaluation of analytical sample preparation conditions (e.g., the sample solvent for analytical assay) and is critical to some liquid formulations where stability must be maximized in order to achieve acceptable shelf life. It can also be applicable in designing stable solid-state formulations. For example, if a compound is known to show instability under basic conditions, basic excipients that may cause an alkaline microenvironment in a formulation may be wisely avoided. Kinetics of degradation obtained from stress testing may also reveal the order of a reaction, whether or not a solid-state degradation is catalyzed by humidity or if the reaction is autocatalytic. Such information can be very useful in designing stability studies and interpreting early time point results. Kinetics of solid-state reactions have been thoroughly discussed elsewhere (For reviews of pharmaceutical kinetics see Ref. 54.) and will not be discussed further here.

In addition to following the kinetics of the disappearance of the parent compound, it can be very important in developing an understanding of the degradation pathways to follow the rates of formation of the different degradation products. Examination of the degradation profile from early time points (e.g., 0–5% degradation) can reveal which products are the primary or first formed products and which are secondary. This can be especially important, as it is not uncommon for the degradation profiles observed during real-time stability studies to contain a mixture of both primary and secondary degradation products.

V. INTRINSIC STABILITY: STRUCTURES OF THE MAJOR DEGRADATION PRODUCTS

Knowledge of the structures of the major degradation products of a drug compound is a prerequisite to understanding the degradation pathways. Understanding the degradation pathways allows an assessment to be made of the sites in the compound that are susceptible to degradation under the different conditions. Such information is essential to an understanding of the "intrinsic stability" characteristics of a drug compound. The critical issue is, then, what are the "major" degradation products that need to be identified.

There appear to be two major schools of thought on this issue. One school asserts structure elucidation need only occur for those degradation products that are formed (in either the drug substance or the product) under long-term storage or accelerated testing stability studies at levels approaching or exceeding the ICH impurity threshold levels established in the relevant impurity guidelines (55,56). Using this line of thinking, major degradation products that occur during stress testing do not need to be identified unless they are also formed at significant levels during the shelf life of the product under long-term storage conditions (or possibly after 6 months storage under accelerated stability conditions, i.e., 40°C/75% relative humidity). Such an approach relies on the results of the analytical testing strategies and methods to resolve, detect, and accurately quantify the degradation products so that the major degradation products can be discerned. Assumptions have to be made regarding the response factors of the unknown degradants, the resolution from the parent compound, and the elution of the degradants from the column (assuming HPLC is the analytical technique). This strategy can be termed a "technique-oriented approach" (2) because it relies on the analytical technique to provide comprehensive and accurate results. The technique-oriented approach is strengthened by use of additional analytical techniques (different HPLC columns and conditions, alternative separation techniques, different detectors, etc.). There are significant advantages to this approach, as there is a significant cost in resources and time to determine response factors and to elucidate chemical structures. Examination of part of the ICH definition of stress testing seems to support this approach:

> However, it may not be necessary to examine specifically for certain degradation products if it has been demonstrated that they are not formed under accelerated or long term storage conditions.

Examining the sentence preceding the foregoing quote, however, reveals the context:

> Examining degradation products [under stress conditions] is useful in [establishing degradation pathways] and developing and validating suitable analytical methods.

One cannot establish a degradation pathway merely by identification of the *conditions* that lead to the degradation and noting the peaks that are observed in a chromatogram. Identification of a pathway involves both the conditions of degradation and the structures involved. Another problem with the technique-oriented approach is the reality that current analytical separation and detection technologies are not ideal in that they cannot ensure resolution and quantification of unknown degradation products. When using HPLC with UV detection, the response factors of degradation products (relative to the parent compound) can be vastly different or even zero (e.g., nonchromophoric degradation products may not be detected with UV detectors at wavelengths >200 nm). In addition, as the degradation products are unknown (with unknown polarity, solubility, and volatility characteristics), it cannot be known whether the degradation products will resolve from the parent, will elute from the column, or will even be amenable to the analytical technique. (For more discussion on this topic, see Chapters 4 and 6). Nonetheless, it can be argued that as long as the analytical method(s) result(s) in *detection* of degradation products (i.e., peaks in an HPLC–UV chromatogram), there are no clear regulatory requirements for structure elucidation of degradation products observed only during stress testing.

The other school of thought can be described as following a chemistry-guided approach (2). The chemistry-guided approach relies on scientific evaluation of the *chemistry* to guide the interpretation of the data and the selection of appropriate analytical techniques. An essential part of the chemistry-guided approach is developing an understanding of the structures of the major degradation products observed by the analytical method, which in turn allows an evaluation of the pathways, leading eventually to a rational assessment of the completeness of the investigation, and the appropriateness of the analytical methodology.

An example of the use of the chemistry-guided approach can be seen in the case of LY297802 (Fig. 4) (2), described in Chapter 6. In this example, degradation was observed upon exposure of a solution of the drug substance to cool white fluorescent light with no analytically observed (HPLC with UV detection) increases in degradation products. Additional analysis using another technique, LC/MS, revealed no additional information. Close examination of the container in which the degradation occurred, however, revealed a faintly observable insoluble film. The insoluble film was collected and analyzed by electron ionization (El)-MS, revealing that the major component of the material was elemental sulfur (S_8). This finding revealed that the photodegradation involved decomposition of the chromophoric part of the molecule (the thiadiazole ring). Because attempts to detect these non-chromophoric degradation products by LC/MS were unfruitful, consideration was given to the possibility of the formation of volatile degradation products (which might not be detected by LC/MS). Analysis by GC/FID (and subsequently EI–MS) led to the identification of the other, previously undetected degradation products (i.e., *n*-butyl thiocyanate and the quinuclidine nitrile species, Figure 4). This example serves to illustrate how the identification of a just a single degradation product (elemental sulfur in this case) can guide the analytical approaches used for a particular compound (chemistry-guided approach).

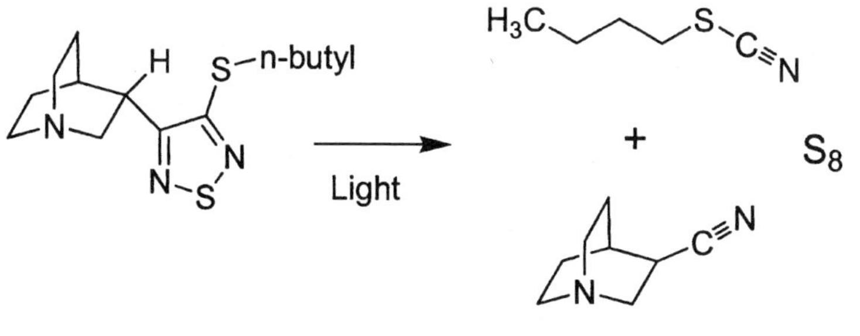

Figure 4 Structure of LY297802 and major photodegradation products.

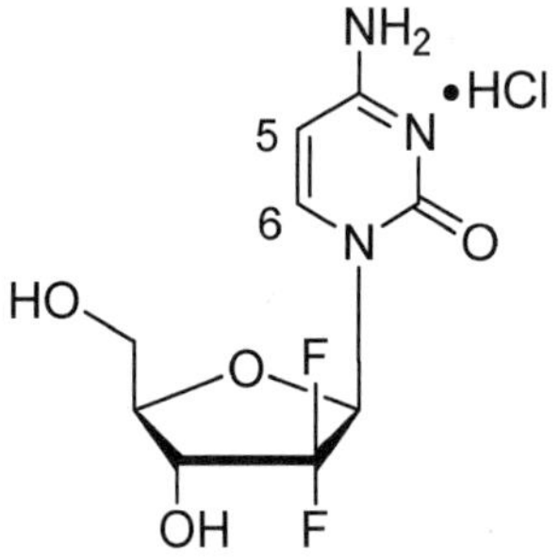

Figure 5 Structure of gemcitabine hydrochloride.

Another example of using the chemistry-guided approach is illustrated with the β-difluoronucleoside, gemcitabine hydrochloride (2′-deoxy-2′,2′-difluorocytidine, Figure 5) (57). Gemcitabine hydrochloride is currently marketed as a lyophilized powder; however, there was an interest in developing a solution formulation. Therefore, a study was designed to generate the data needed to construct an Arrhenius plot to enable prediction of degradation rates of solutions of gemcitabine at proposed storage conditions. The study solutions were also monitored for impurities resulting from the degradation of gemcitabine in order to compare the degradation profile of the investigational formulation to that of the marketed formulation.

During the course of the investigation, a significant mass balance issue was detected. Solutions of gemcitabine that exhibited a significant loss of the parent showed only a very minor increase in impurities. (Refer to Table 4 for selected results illustrating the mass balance issue and to Figure 6 for an HPLC chromatogram obtained on a solution thermally stressed at 70°C for 2 days.) Examination of the HPLC chromatogram (Fig. 6) indicates that the only significant impurity detected was the β-uridine analog (Fig. 7), a known degradation product of gemcitabine. The levels of the β-uridine analog were

Table 4 HPLC Results Obtained on Thermally Stressed Solutions of Gemcitabine Hydrochloride

Condition	Gemcitabine assay (% Initial)	Related substances (%)	Mass balance (%)	Relative Mass Balance deficit[a](%)
70°C/2 days	82.5	4.89	87.4	61.2
55°C/7 days	85.9	3.49	89.4	67.1
40°C/28 days	91.4	1.86	93.3	72.2
30°C/56 days	94.3	1.12	95.4	75.7

[a]See chapter 6 for a discussion of "relative mass balance deficit"

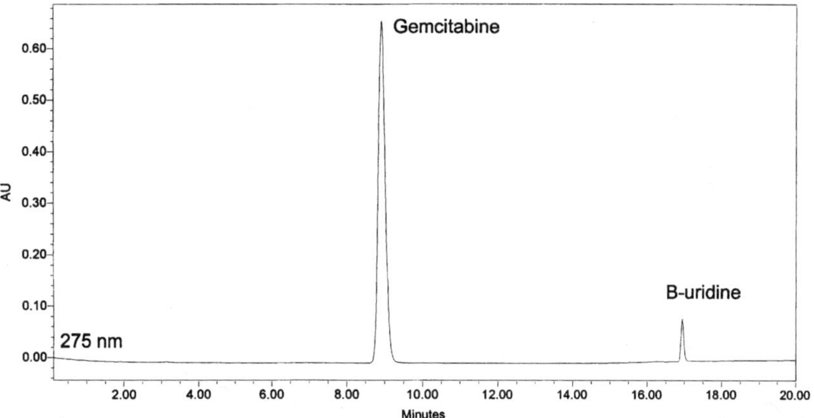

Figure 6 HPLC chromatogram obtained on a solution of gemcitabine hydrochloride in pH 3.2 acetate buffer stressed at 70°C for 2 days.

not high enough to account for the loss of the parent, indicating the formation of other degradation products that were not being detected.

A survey of the literature revealed a significant amount of information published on the degradation of cytidine, a structurally related nucleoside. Several papers (58) suggest a mechanism for deamination of cytidine to uridine that involves intermediates in which a nucleophile has been added to position 6 of the cytosine moiety resulting in loss of the 5, 6 double bond. If the analogous chemistry were to occur with gemcitabine, the intermediates formed would likely have a significantly different UV spectrum than gemcitabine and might not be detected at the wavelength used in the HPLC method (275 nm). The wavelength was therefore changed to 205 nm and the stressed sample was re-examined. The chromatogram is shown in Figure 8. At 205 nm, two additional impurities were detected. While isolating the two impurities for spectroscopic characterization (using a preparative HPLC

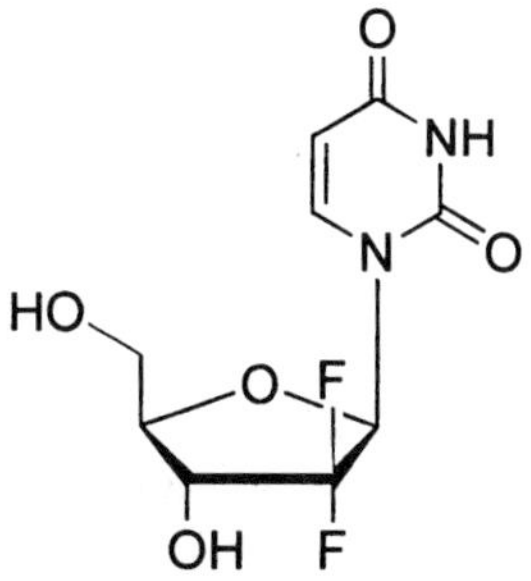

Figure 7 Structure of the β-uridine analog of gemcitabine.

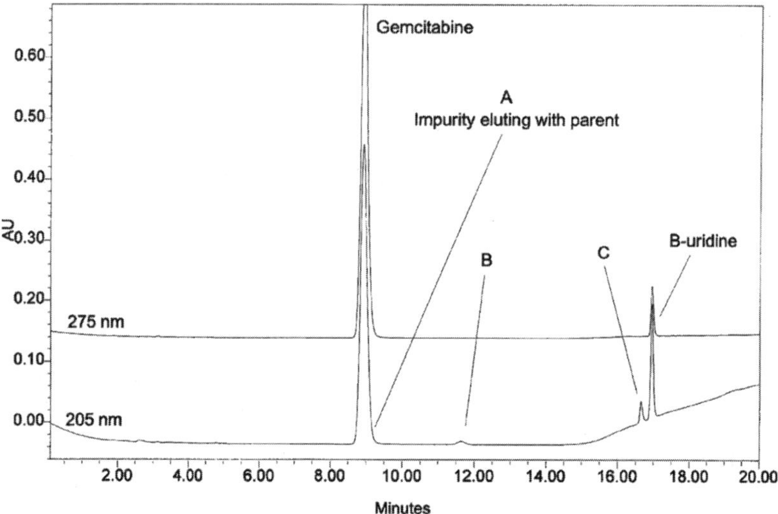

Figure 8 HPLC chromatograms obtained on a gemcitabine hydrochloride in pH 3.2 acetate buffer stressed at 70°C for 2 days.

column with a different mobile phase and gradient), a third impurity was discovered. This third impurity was found to coelute with the parent gemcitabine peak on the analytical HPLC method. Isolation, structural characterization, and degradation studies of the three additional impurities confirmed that they were intermediates in the formation of the β-uridine analog. The structures and proposed mechanism are given in Sch. 1.

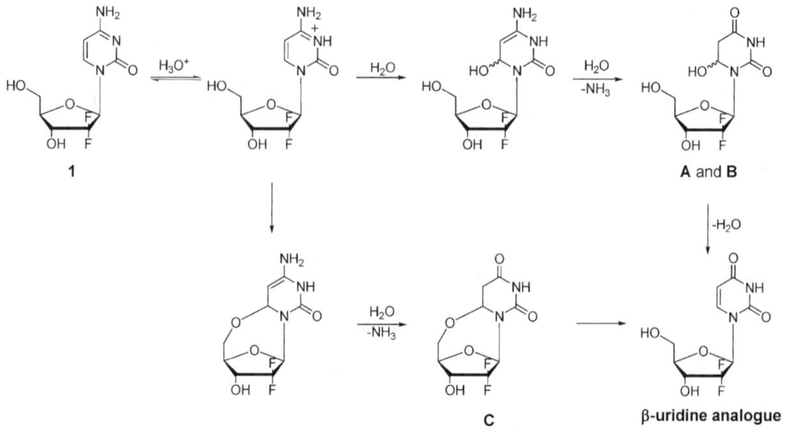

Scheme 1 Proposed deamination mechanism of gemcitabine in acidic aqueous solution.

Structural information of stress-induced degradation products can also be used to assess the potential for formation of toxic degradation products. Both ICH guidelines on impurities (drug substance and drug product) specifically address the issue of potential toxic impurities:

> However, analytical procedures should be developed for those potential impurities that are expected to be unusually potent, producing toxic or pharmacological effects at a level not more than the identification threshold. (From Refs. 55 and 56.)

Determining the structures of the major degradation products can reveal whether or not a known carcinogen or toxic compound is or might possibly be formed. When the structure(s) are novel, one cannot know for sure whether or not the compound will be unusually potent or toxic from the structure alone. Nonetheless, certain functional groups are often regarded as potentially toxic, and scientists in the field of toxicology routinely evaluate compounds for toxicological potential on the basis of structure.

Determining structures of degradation products arising during stress testing can also be useful for preclinical discovery efforts during structure–activity relationship investigations. An understanding of the parts of the molecule that are labile or susceptible to degradation can help in the design of less reactive, more stable analogs. The development of a stable formulation is also aided by an understanding of the reactive parts of the drug molecule. Drug-excipient compatibility studies (which are a form of stress testing) often lead to new, unknown degradation products. The rational development of a stable formulation is greatly aided by a chemical understanding of the reactions leading to degradation. See Chapter 13 for a thorough discussion of drug-excipient compatibility studies.

Elucidation of the structures of degradation products is typically a collaborative research undertaking that involves analytical, organic, and physical chemistry knowledge combined with spectroscopic information. It is not possible to define a precise process for the determination of an unknown degradation product, but common approaches are apparent in the modern laboratory as evidenced by the literature. Once a degradation product has been targeted for structure elucidation, a decision is made as to whether or not to begin spectroscopic characterization of the unknown in a mixture or after isolation and purification. Although the UV spectrum of the unknown can be obtained via HPLC with photodiode array UV detection, the first piece of spectroscopic information that is often sought is the molecular weight. HPLC/MS (especially with electrospray or atmospheric pressure chemical ionization in either the negative or the positive ion mode) is commonly used in the pharmaceutical industry to obtain molecular weight information. Often times, the MS information (i.e., molecular weight and fragmentation information) can provide enough information to allow proposal of a likely structure (59). Accurate mass MS can be especially useful in that it not only provides the molecular weight, but can also provide the molecular formula (60). Knowledge of organic chemistry and the conditions that led to the formation of the unknown are critical to making plausible structural proposals. When a structure is proposed, often times the proposal can be tested by comparison to "authentic standards" (i.e., if the compound has already been prepared via efforts of the synthetic organic chemists or if such a compound can easily be synthetically prepared). If the chromatographic retention and MS information (or, alternatively, the UV spectrum) of the unknown match the authentic standard, it is usually regarded as sufficient evidence to establish the structure. Alternatively, when the structure proposal involves a novel structure that is not available or readily prepared synthetically, further characterization is needed and consideration is given to isolation and purification. HPLC/NMR, while expensive and technologically demanding, is maturing as a technique and is now used in some laboratories as an alternative to isolation and purification (61,62). Nonetheless, HPLC/NMR is still generally used for situations where the unknowns are difficult to isolate and purify or when samples amounts are limited (63,64).

Isolation and purification of unknowns can be accomplished by a variety of techniques (e.g., preparative HPLC or TLC, flash chromatography, extraction, etc.) (65). Preparative HPLC, RP or NP, is probably the most widely used technique in the pharmaceutical industry for purification of milligram to gram quantities of low-level impurities. Once an unknown is isolated, spectroscopic characterization by MS and NMR is usually sufficient to unambiguously assign structures. UV, IR, and/or Raman are often used to identify specific chromophores or functional groups. Spectroscopic characterization of unknown impurities leading to structure elucidation is a process that has been discussed extensively elsewhere (66–68) and need not be reproduced here.

In summary, we advocate a chemistry-guided approach to developing an understanding of the intrinsic stability characteristics of a pharmaceutical compound. Acquiring structural information of the degradation products observed during stress testing facilitates such an approach.

VI. INTRINSIC STABILITY: PATHWAYS OF DEGRADATION

As defined by ICH and by the earlier discusion, stress testing is useful to "help identify the likely degradation products, which can in turn help establish the degradation pathways and the intrinsic stability of the molecule and validate the stability indicating power of the analytical procedures used." Establishing the pathways of degradation is critical, therefore, to developing an understanding of the intrinsic stability of the molecule, and degradation pathway information provides a scientific foundation for the validation of the stability indicating power of the analytical methodology.

The determination of degradation product structures (discussed earlier) provides the critical information needed to allow proposal (and testing) of plausible degradation pathways. The importance of this approach is seen in the example of LY297802 (discussed in Sec. XI). The example of LY297802 shows the importance of determining degradation product structures in order to understand the degradation pathways. Another example can be found in the case of duloxetine hydrochloride.

Duloxetine hydrochloride is a compound that is unstable under acidic conditions (69), degrading to four main compounds (70). The structures of the degradation products were determined and are shown in Figure 9. The structures revealed that the aryl ether linkage of duloxetine is acid labile, from which degradation pathways could be proposed. The structures and proposed pathways do not implicate other nonobserved degradation products, as was the case for both LY297802 and gemcitabine hydrochloride (see the earlier section). Thus, the structures and pathways help to provide assurance that the major degradation products are being resolved and detected. The critical step in the degradation pathways is the formation of a cationic intermediate (Fig. 10). The proposal of the cationic intermediate is important for a few reasons. First, it shows that there is one primary acid-labile site in the molecule. Second, it allows for an understanding of the instability; that is, it becomes apparent that the stability of the cationic intermediate is likely a major contributor to the acid instability of duloxetine. Such information can be important in designing ways to stabilize the compound, for example, liquid formulations using solvents with a low dielectric constant or solid formulations with excipients and packaging that minimize

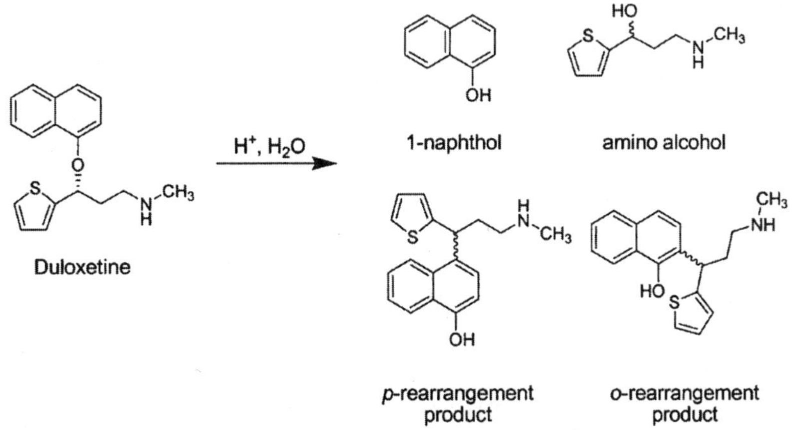

Figure 9 The structures of duloxetine and the four main acidic hydrolysis products.

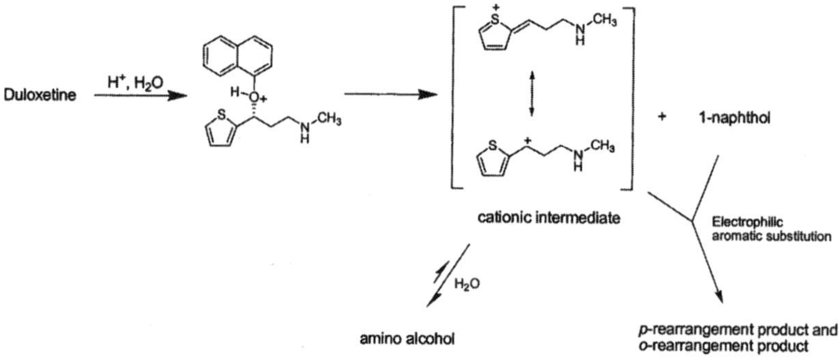

Figure 10 Proposed acid-catalyzed degradation pathways for duloxetine.

the levels of moisture. Degradation pathway information can also be useful for new drug discovery efforts involving modifications to the chemical structure in order to reduce the ability of the adjacent aromatic group (e.g., the thiophene) to delocalize and stabilize the cation. The ability of thiophene to stabilize the charge is due, in large part, to the location of sulfur atom in relation to the site of attachment of the alkyl side chain.

Stress-testing studies should also be conducted on the formulated drug product because drugs can and often do degrade differently in the presence of excipients. One such example is duloxetine hydrochloride, the molecule discussed in the preceding paragraph. Because duloxetine is unstable in solution at pH values <2.5, enteric polymer-coated formulations were developed to prevent its acid degradation in the stomach and to provide for subsequent rapid disintegration and release in the small intestine (69). A

	HPMCAS	HPMCP
R =	H	CH_3
	CH_3	$CH_2CH(OH)CH_3$
	$COCH_3$	COC_6H_4COOH
	$COCH_2CH_2COOH$	
	$CH_2CH(OH)CH_3$	
	$CH_2CH(OCOCH_3)CH_3$	
	$CH_2CH(OCOCH_2CH_2COOH)CH_3$	

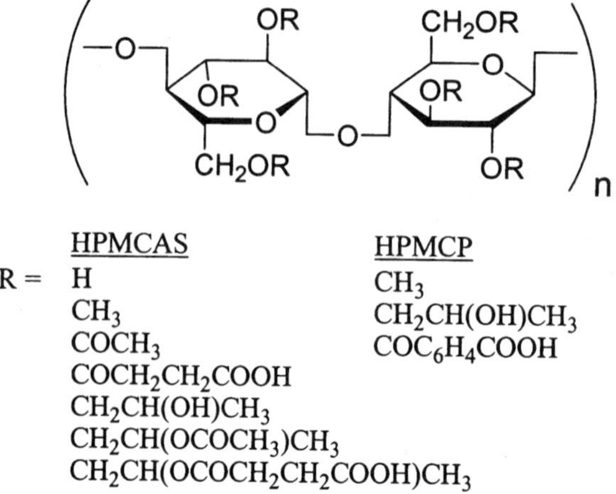

Figure 11 Structures of enteric polymers HPMCAS and HPMCP.

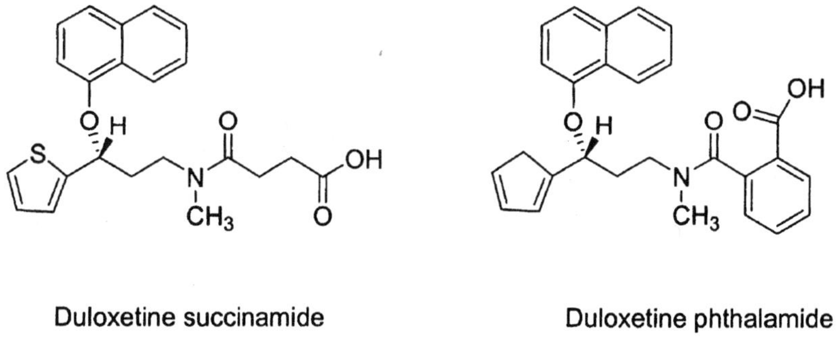

Duloxetine succinamide

Duloxetine phthalamide

Figure 12 Structures of duloxetine succinamide and duloxetine phthalamide, the major impurities resulting from interaction between duloxetine and the enteric coatings HPMCAS and HPMCP during stress testing or long-term stability studies.

tablet formulation coated with the enteric polymer hydroxypropyl methylcellulose phthalate (HPMCP) was originally developed, but a formulation consisting of pellets coated with the enteric polymer hydroxypropyl methylcellulose acetate succinate (HPMCAS) contained in a capsule was the desired market formulation. The structures of the enteric polymers are given in Figure 11.

During stress testing (60°C for 14 days) of the HPMCAS-coated pellet formulation, an unknown impurity eluting after duloxetine was detected by HPLC. This impurity was also detected at significant levels in stability samples stored at either 30°C/60% relative humidity or at 40°C/75% relative humidity. Subsequent analysis of stability samples of HPMCP-coated tablets indicated the presence of a different impurity that also eluted after duloxetine. Structural characterization of these impurities indicated that the impurity formed in the HPMCAS-coated pellets was a duloxetine succinamide and that the impurity formed in the HPMCP-coated tablets was a duloxetine phthalamide (see Fig. 12 for structures). These impurities are the result of an interaction of duloxetine with the enteric polymers. The formation of the duloxetine succinamide in the commercial formulation was minimized by increasing the thickness of the barrier layer that separates duloxetine from the enteric coating. In this case, early stress testing of the formulation uncovered a significant degradation problem that was easily corrected by making a relatively minor change in the formulation. Without knowledge of the structure of the impurity and its origin, it would have been difficult to minimize its formation.

VII. INTERPRETATION OF THE RESULTS OF STRESS TESTING

One of the more interesting and challenging aspects of stress testing involves interpreting the results of stress testing such that the data becomes meaningful to the development process. For example, what levels of instability are indicative of problems for analytical handling, manufacturing/processing, formulation, patient "in use," and storage and distribution? Can stress-testing results be easily interpreted to conclude whether or not a compound will have high-, medium-, or low-stability concerns for the development process? These questions are difficult as there are no (as yet) scientifically derived criteria for predicting the "developability" of a new drug entity. Such interpretive criteria would be very useful for the pharmaceutical development process.

Attempts have been made to use stress-testing results to classify compounds as extremely labile, very labile, labile, and stable (71). The basis for this classification system was the personal experience of the authors. In this section we will attempt to outline and discuss some of the factors that need to be considered when attempting to interpret the results of stress testing, and to provide references to other resources. It is our opinion that insufficient information has been gathered to provide a definitive classification system.

Interpretation of stress-testing results has several different facets. An obvious consideration is the degradation rate under a particular condition. The rates of degradation are critically important for determination of shelf life (although stress-testing results should not be used for shelf-life determination) and for handling considerations during manufacturing, formulation, and analysis. In addition to the kinetic interpretation, it is important to understand what the stress-testing results indicate about mechanism of degradation (e.g., from the structures of degradation products and the degradation pathways involved). Such information is important in designing the appropriate degradation-control strategies (2) (e.g., developing a stable formulation, appropriate packaging and storage conditions, and relevant analytical methodologies).

A. Solid State

There are three main stress conditions evaluated during stress testing in the solid state: temperature, humidity, and photostability. The stress of elevated temperature is perhaps the stress condition that lends itself most directly to predictive interpretation. This assumes, of course, that Arrhenius kinetics is observed within the range of long-term storage temperature to the stressed temperature(s). Assuming Arrhenius kinetics and reasonable energies of activation, predictions can be made to relate the amount of degradation and increases of individual degradation products at the stress temperature to the long-term storage temperature. This topic is discussed in detail in Sec. IX.A.

The solid-state stress of elevated humidity provides information related to the need for protection from exposure to high or low humidity. Such information is generally considered to be only semiquantitative in nature, that is, whether or not the stability of the compound is best at high or low humidity. Quantitative correlations (e.g., is there a critical relative humidity threshold?) are difficult and would require additional experiments (e.g., statistically designed experiments).

The solid-state stress of exposure to light (i.e., ultraviolet and visible radiation) is guided by the ICH guideline on photostability (48). The ICH guideline is primarily directed toward *confirmatory* photostability testing, which outlines photoexposure levels for the purpose of identifying potential photostability problems that may be encountered during storage and distribution of the marketed product. Most of these types of problems can be addressed by modifications of packaging, labeling, and/or formulation (with some associated expense). Very little guidance is given to interpretation of photostress studies (which the guideline refers to as "forced degradation testing") in relation to the development process:

> The forced degradation studies should be designed to provide suitable information to develop and validate test methods for the confirmatory studies. These test methods should be capable of resolving and detecting photolytic degradants that appear during the confirmatory studies. When evaluating the results of these studies, it is important to recognize that they form part of the stress testing and are not therefore designed to establish qualitative or quantitative limits for change. (from Ref. 48.)

Thus, photostressing studies are primarily useful for developing an understanding of the photochemistry of the drug and for developing appropriate analytical methodologies. See Chaper 10 for further discussion of this topic.

One possible use of photostability/photostressing studies is assessment of the potential for problems in manufacturing and analytical handling. It has been recommended by EFPIA that 100,000 lux-hr is a reasonable amount of light exposure to determine whether or not special precautions should be considered during manufacture (47). This level of light exposure should also provide a reasonable estimation of problems that might be encountered during analytical and formulation development. Of course, the potential for exposure to UV light may also need to be assessed depending on the lighting conditions of the analytical laboratories and the manufacturing facility. The best way to assess the potential light exposure would be to make actual measurements in the actual laboratories and manufacturing facilities.

B. Solution: Acid/Base Stress-Testing Results

These results will indicate whether or not the drug molecule has a particular instability in aqueous conditions as a function of pH. An approximate pH profile can sometimes be constructed from the data, but caution should be exercised because it is not uncommon for a drug compound to be relatively insoluble in some pH ranges, and some samples may require cosolvents in order to achieve dissolution. If precise information on either kinetics or the precise pH range of maximum stability is desired (e.g., for a compound that will have a liquid formulation), further studies in which the solvents, the ionic strength, the buffer type, and the concentration are carefully controlled should be conducted.

Stress testing information can be relevant for ADME concerns. Critical evaluation of the pH 1–2 degradation rate data can help assess the potential need for enteric coating of drugs to be administered orally. The pH of gastric fluid (worst case) can be roughly simulated using 0.1 N HCl (pH 1). While transit times in the stomach are highly variable (dependent on variables such as %liquids/solids ingested, amount ingested, fasting level), most literature values fall within the time of 30 min to 4 hr (72). Assuming a worst case transit time (4 hr exposure to the acidic environment in the stomach), it seems reasonable to *consider* the potential need for an enteric-coated formulation if a loss of potency of ~10–20% or greater is observed after 4 hr at 40°C in 0.1 N HCl; assuming first-order kinetics of degradation, this degradation rate would correspond to a half-life of ~26 hr. Consideration of the potential need for enteric coating would involve many factors. For example, do the acidic degradation products raise questions of safety or efficacy? How rapid is the absorption? What is the half-life of the compound in the body? What are the pharmacological needs for efficacy of the parent? These questions need to be addressed on a case-by-case basis in an interdisciplinary manner (e.g., scientists from ADME, pharmacokinetics, analytical, formulations, and medical/clinical areas).

Evaluation of solution stability under neutral to moderately basic (e.g., pH 6–9) can help in assessing the potential for nonenzymatic breakdown of the compound under physiologically relevant conditions (e.g., pH 7.5). Such information can be useful not only for metabolism studies, but also for pharmacokinetic concerns (i.e., understanding how long a compound might remain intact in vivo) and what degradation products might form under such conditions. Thus, for example, if a compound degrades at pH 7.5 at a rate significantly faster than the half-life of the compound, the nonenzymatically formed degradation products will likely contribute to the metabolic profile of the compound.

Evaluation of degradation rates under different pH conditions also provides needed information related to analytical concerns. For example, how much degradation might occur during the analytical workup under specific pH conditions. Can samples be prepared and held at room temperature for a specified length of time without appreciable degradation? Do samples need to be refrigerated in order to maintain stability during analysis? Answers to these questions are fairly straightforward if the analytical constraints are defined.

For additional discussion on this subject, see Sec. III.B.

C. Solution: Oxidative Stress-Testing Results

It can be difficult to translate oxidative stress-testing results into accurate predictions of the susceptibility of a compound to oxidation. This is partially because oxidative mechanisms can be quite diverse and complex and oxidative degradation often does not follow typical Arrhenius kinetic models. For a more indepth discussion of this subject, see Chapter 7.

In Chapter 7, Boccardi suggests that the two most relevant tests for prediction of oxidative susceptibility of a drug compound involves the use of radical initiators (such as AIBN) for testing susceptibility to autoxidation and the use of dilute hydrogen peroxide for testing susceptibility to oxidation by peroxides (e.g., from excipients). Boccardi asserts that, assuming a test involving use of AIBN in an equimolar basis with the drug, after 48 hr at 40°C, compounds that are sensitive to autoxidation will likely be degraded $> 10\%$ whereas compounds that are relatively stable to autoxidation will likely be degraded no more than a few percent. Harmon (73) has recently developed an oxidative susceptibility stress test for ranking of compounds with respect to their potential for oxidizing in typical oral dosage formulations. The predictability of this promising new system remains to be documented in the literature with examples. A scientifically sound approach to quantitative assessment of the oxidative susceptibility of Pharmaceuticals would be a valuable contribution to the future of pharmaceutical development.

In the case of hydrogen peroxide, it is difficult to associate a percent degradation with a classification of oxidizability. If there are amines present in the molecule, especially tertiary amines, oxidation is usually rapid if the amine is uncharged (e.g., the free base). A protonated cationic amine is protected and the oxidation rate will be greatly reduced. In general, however, it is the experience of the authors that if a 0.3% solution of hydrogen peroxide induces $<5\%$ degradation in 24 hr at room temperature, the compound is not particularly sensitive to peroxides and will likely not require special considerations for development. Alternatively, an $\sim 20\%$ or more degradation in 24 hr may indicate a particularly sensitive compound that could require special efforts in the formulation and/or storage conditions to ensure oxidative stability.

VIII. SUMMARY

Stress testing is an important tool for the prediction of stability-related problems. The results of stress testing can be useful to many areas of pharmaceutical research and development beyond the obvious areas of analytical, formulation, and packaging development. Well-designed stress-testing studies can lead to a thorough understanding of the intrinsic stability characteristics of the drug molecule. We advocate a chemistry-guided approach to stress-testing, where structures of the major degradation products are determined and degradation pathways are proposed and tested. The quantitative interpretation of stress testing results is an underdeveloped area for which additional research is needed.

REFERENCES

1. Stability testing of new drug substances and products. International Conference on Harmonisation, QlA(R2), February 2003.
2. Olsen BA, Baertschi SW. Strategies for investigation and control of process-related and degradation-related impurities in Pharmaceuticals. In: Ahuja S, Alsante KM, eds. Handbook of Isolation and Characterization of Impurities in Pharmaceuticals, Volume 5 of Separation Science and Technology. San Diego, CA: Academic Press, 2003.
3. Snyder LR, Glajch JL, Kirkland JJ. Practical HPLC Method Development. New York: John Wiley and Sons, 1988.
4. Monkhouse DC, Maderich A. Whither compatibility testing? Drug Dev Ind Pharm 1989; 15(13):2115–2130.
5. Serajuddin ATM, Thakur AB, Ghoshal RN, Fakes MG, Ranadive SA, Morris KR, Varia SA. Selection of solid dosage form composition through drug–excipient compatibility testing. J Pharm Sci 1999; 88(7):696–704.
6. Crowley P, Martini L. Drug–excipient interactions. Pharm Technol Europe (March) 2001; 13(3):26–28, 30–32, 34.
7. Akers MJ. Excipient–drug interactions in parenteral formulations. J Pharm Sci 2002; 91(11):2293–2300.
8. Selzer T, Radau M, Kreuter J. The use of isothermal heat conduction microcalorimetry to evaluate drug stability in tablets. Int J Pharm 1999; 184:199–206.
9. Wissing S, Craig DQM, Barker SA, Moore WD. An investigation into the use of stepwise isothermal high sensitivity DSC as a means of detecting drug–excipient incompatibility. Int J Pharm 2000; 199:141–150.
10. Schmitt EA, Peck K, Yang S, Geoffroy J-M. Rapid, practical and predictive excipient compatibility screening using isothermal microcalorimetry. Thermochim Acta 2001; 380:175–183.
11. McDaid FM, Barker SA, Fitzpatrick S, Petts CR, Craig DQM. Further investigations into the use of high sensitivity differential scanning calorimetry as a means of predicting drug–excipient interactions. Int J Pharm 2003; 252:235–240.
12. Reynolds DW, Facchine KL, Mullaney JF, Alsante KM, Hatajik TD, Motto MG. Available guidance and best practices for conducting forced degradation studies. Pharm Technol (February) 2002; 26(2): 48–54.
13. Dieter K. In: Grimm W, Thoma K, Krummen K, eds. Stability testing in the EC, Japan, and the USA: Scientific and Regulatory Requirements. Chapter 4. Stuttgart: Wissenschaftliche Verlagsgesellschaft mbH Stuttgart, 1993.
14. Jerussi RA. Stability testing and generics. J cGMP Compliance 1999; 3(4): 28–32.

15. Connors KA, Amidon GL, Stella VL. Chemical Stability of Pharmaceutical: A Handbook for Pharmacistss. 2nd ed. New York: Wiley and Sons, 1986:19 and reference 3.
16. Connors KA. Chemical Kinetics: The Study of Reaction Rates in Solution. New York: VCH Publishers, 1990:191; Table 5–1.
17. Kennon LJ. Use of models in determining chemical pharmaceutical stability. J Pharm Sci 1964; 53(7):815–818.
18a. Davis JS. The dating game. Proprietary Assocation's Twelfth Manufacturing Controls Seminar, New Jersey, Oct 5–6. 1978.
18b. Davis JS. Criteria for accelerated stability testing. FDA/ASQC Seminar, Chicago, IL, March 11, 1991.
19. Yang W-H, Roy SB. Projection of tentative expiry date from one-point accelerated stability testing. Drug Dev Ind Pharm 1980; 6(6):591–604.
20. Waterman KC, Adami RC, Accelerated aging: Prediction of chemical stability of pharmaceuticals. Int J pharm 2005; 293: 101–125.
21. Alsante KM, Friedmann RC, Hatajik TD, Lohr LL, Sharp TR, Snyder KD, Szczesny EJ. Degradation and impurity analysis for pharmaceutical drug candidates. In: Ahuja S, Scypinski S, eds. Handbook of Modern Pharmaceutical Analysis, Volume 3 of Separation Science and Technology. San Diego, CA: Academic Press, 2001:85–172.
22. Connors KA, Amidon GL, Stella VJ. Solid state chemical decomposition. In: Chemical Stability of Pharmaceuticals: A Handbook for Pharmacists. 2nd ed. Chapter 6. New York: John Wiley and Sons, 1986:116–119.
23. Monkhouse DC, Campen LV. Solid state reactions—theoretical and experimental aspects. Drug Dev Ind Pharm 1984; 10(8&9):1175–1276.
24. Pope DG. Accelerated stability testing for prediction of drug product stability. Drug Cosmet Ind (December) 1980; 48–116.
25. Grimm VW. Stabilitätsprüfung pharmazeutischer Zubereitungen. Pharm Ind 1975; 37(10):815–825.
26. Witthaus G. Accelerated storage tests: predictive value. In: Breimer DD, Speiser P, eds. Topics in Pharmaceutical Sciences. Amsterdam, The Netherlands: Elsevier/North-Holland Biomedical Press, 1981:275–290.
27. Sims JL, Carreira JA, Carrier DJ, Crabtree SR, Easton L, Hancock SA, Simcox SR. A new approach to accelerated drug–excipient compatibility testing. Pharm Dev Technol 2003; 8(2):119–126.
28a. Baertschi SW, Dorman DE, Occolowitz JL, Spangle LA, Collins MW, Bashore FN, Lorenz LJ. Isolation and characterization of degradation products arising from aqueous degradation of cefaclor. J Pharm Sci 1997; 86(5): 526–539.
28b. Dorman DE, Lorenz LJ, Occolowitz JL, Spangle LA, Collins MW, Bashore FN, Baertschi SW. Isolation and structure elucidation of the major degradation products of cefaclor in the solid state. J Pharm Sci 1997; 86(5):540–549.
29. Olsen BA, Perry FM, Snorek SV, Lewellen PL. Accelerated conditions for stability assessment of bulk and formulated cefaclor monohydrate. Pharm Dev Technol 1997; 2(4):303–312.
30. Stewart PJ, Tucker IG. Prediction of drug stability. Part 2. Hydrolysis. Aust J Hosp Pharm 1985; 15(1):11–16.

31. Waterman KC, Adami RC, Antipas AS, Arenson DR, Carrier R, Hong J, Landis MS, Lombardo F, Shah JC, Shalaev E, Smith SW, Wang H. Hydrolysis in pharmaceutical formulations. Pharm Dev Tech 2002; 7(2): 113–146.
32. Alsante KM, Martin L, Baertschi SW. A stress testing benchmarking study. Pharm Technol (February) 2003; 27(2):60–72.
33a. Payne GB, Deming PH, Williams PH. Reactions of hydrogen peroxide. VII. Alkali-catalyzed epoxidation and oxidation using nitrile as co-reactant. J Org Chem 1961; 26:659–663.
33b. Laus G. Kinetics of acetonitrile-assisted oxidation of tertiary amines by hydrogen peroxide. J Chem Soc Perkins Trans 2001; 2:864–868.
34. Reynolds DW. Available regulatory guidance and best practices for conducting forced degradation studies. Forced Degradation Studies: Best Practices for the Pharmaceutical Industry. Institute for International Research, Princeton, NJ, Feb 24–25, 2004.
35. Stewart PJ, Tucker IG. Prediction of drug stability. Part 2. Hydrolysis. Aust J Hosp Pharm 1985; 15(1):11–16.
36a. Dawber J Graham. Relationship between solvatochromic solvent polarity and various thermodynamic and kinetic data in mixed solvent systems. J Chem Soc Faraday Trans 1990; 86(2):287–291.
36b. Alfassi ZB, Padmaja S, Neta P, Huie RE. Solvent effects on the rate of reaction of $Cl_2(dot)^-$ and $SO_4(dot)^-$ radicals with unsaturated alcohols. Int J Chem Kinet 1993; 25:151–159.
36c. Manege LC, Ueda T, Hojo M, Fujio M. Concentrated salt effects on the rates of solvolyses involving carbocations as reaction intermediates in acetone–water mixed solvents. J Chem Soc Perkin Trans 1998; 2:1961–1965.
36d. Osamu Ito, Hisanori Watanabe. Effect of preferential solvation on reactivity of a free radical in binary solvent systems. J Chem Soc Faraday Trans 1994; 90(4): 571–574.
37a. LePree JM, Connors KA. Solvent effects on chemical processes. 11. Solvent effects on the kinetics of decarboxylative dechlorination of *N*-chloro amino acids in binary aqueous-organic solvents. J Pharm Sci 1996; 85(6): 560–566.
37b. Skwierczynski RD, Connors KA. Solvent effects on chemical processes. 8. Demethylation kinetics of aspartame in binary aqueous-organic solvents. J Pharm Sci 1994; 82(12):1690–1696.
37c. Calmon J-P, Canavy J-L. Solvent effects on the kinetics of alkaline hydrolysis of dimethylacetylacetone. Part 1. Influence of alcohol–water mixtures. J Chem Soc Perkin II 1972; 8:706–710.
38. Bates RG. Medium effects and pH in nonaqueous solvents. In: Solute–Solvent Interact 1969: Coetzee J. F, ed. Marcel Dekker, New York, 45–96.
39. Watarai H, Suzuki N. Keto-enol tautomerization rates of acetylacetone in mixed aqueous media. J Inorg Nucl Chem 1974; 36:1815–1829. Great Britain: Pergamon Press.
40a. Castells CB, Rafols C, Roses M, Bosch E. Effect of temperature on pH measurements and acid–base equilibria in methanol–water mixtures. J Chromatogr A 2003; 1002(1–2):41–53.

40b. Canals I, Portal JA, Bosch E, Roses M. Retention of ionizable compounds on HPLC. 4. Mobile-phase pH measurement in methanol/water. Anal Chem 2000; 72(8):1802–1809.

40c. Espinosa S, Bosch E, Roses M. Retention of ionizable compounds in high-performance liquid chromatography. IX. Modeling retention in reversed-phase liquid chromatography as a function of pH and solvent composition with acetonitrile-water mobile phases. J Chromatogr A 2002; 947(1):47–58.

41. Johnson DM, Gu LC. Autoxidation and antioxidants. In: Swarbrick J, Boylan JC, eds. Encyclopedia of Pharmaceutical Technology. Vol. 1. New York: Marcel Dekker, 1988:425–429.

42. Munson E, Schoenich C. Oxidation reactions in the solid state: mechanisms and comparison to solution chemistry. Oxidative Degradation and Stabilization Conference. Institute for International Research, Princeton, NJ, July 20–21, 2004.

43. Boccardi G. Autoxidation of drugs: prediction of degradation impurities from results of reaction with radical chain initiators. Il Farmaco 1994; 49(16): 431–435.

44. Hovorka SW, Schöneich C. Oxidative degradation of Pharmaceuticals: theory, mechanisms, and inhibition. J Pharm Sci 2001; 90(3):253–269.

45. Waterman KC, Adami RC, Alsante KM, Jinyang H, Landis MS, Lombardo F, Roberts CJ. Stabilization of pharmaceuticals to oxidative degradation. Pharm Dev Technol 2002; 7(1):1–32.

46. Reed RA, Harmon P, Manas D, Wasylaschuk W, Galli C, Biddell R, Bergquist PA, Hunke W, Templeton AC, Ip D. The role of excipients and package components in the photostability of liquid formulations. J Pharm Sci Technol 2003; 57(5):351–368.

47. Anderson NH. Photostability testing: design and interpretation of tests on drug substances and dosage forms. In: Tønnesen HH, ed. Photostability of Drugs and Drug Formulations. Great Britain: Taylor & Francis, 1996:307.

48. Stability testing: photostability testing of new drug substances and products. International Conference on Harmonisation, Q1B, Nov 1996.

49a. Thatcher SR, Mansfield RK, Miller RB, Davis CW, Baertschi SW. Pharmaceutical photostability: a technical and practical interpretation of the ICH guideline and its application to pharmaceutical stability: Part I. Pharm Technol March 2001; 25(3):98–110.

49b. Thatcher SR, Mansfield RK, Miller RB, Davis CW, Baertschi SW. Pharmaceutical photostability: a technical and practical interpretation of the ICH guideline and its application to pharmaceutical stability: part II. Pharm Technol April 2001; 25(4):50–62.

50a. Tønnesen HH, ed. The Photostability of Drugs and Drug formulations. Great Britain: Taylor & Francis, 1996.

50b. Tønnesen HH, ed. The Photostability of Drugs and Drug formulations. 2nd ed. Boca Raton, Florida: CRC Press LLC, 2004.

51. Piechocki J, ed. Pharmaceutical Photostability and Stabilization Technology. New York: Marcel Dekker. In preparation.

52. Albini A, Fasani E. Drugs: Photochemistry and Photostability. Royal Society of Chemistry, 1998.

53. Tønnesen HH. Photodecomposition of drugs. Encyclopedia of Pharmaceutical Technology. New York: Marcel Dekker 2002:2197–2203.
54a. Connors KA. In: Chemical Kinetics: The Study of Reaction Rates in Solution. New York: VCH Publishers, 1990.
54b. Carstensen JT. Drug Stability: Principles and Practices. 2nd ed. New York: Marcel Dekker, 1995.
55. Impurities in new drug substances. International Conference on Harmonisation, Q3A(R), Feb 2003.
56. Impurities in new drug products. International Conference on Harmonisation, Q3B(R), Feb 2003.
57. Jansen PJ, Akers MJ, Amos RM, Baertschi SW, Cooke GG, Dorman DE, Kemp CAJ, Maple SR, McCune KA. The degradation of the anti-tumor agent gemcitabine hydrochloride in an acidic aqueous solution at pH 3.2 and identification of degradation products. J Pharm Sci 2000; 89(7):885–891.
58a. Wechter WJ, Kelly RC. The mechanism of the deamination of cytidine. Collect Czech Chem Commun 1970; 35:1991–2002.
58b. Notari RE, Witiak DT, DeYoung JL, Lin AJ. Comparative kinetics of cytosine nucleosides. Influences of a 6-methyl substituent on degradation rates and pathways in aqueous buffers. J Med Chem 1972; 15:1207–1214.
59. Wu Y. The use of liquid chromatography–mass spectrometry for the identification of drug degradation products in pharmaceutical formulations. Biomed Chromatogr 2000; 14:384–396.
60. Winger BE, Kemp CAJ. Characterization of pharmaceutical compounds and related substances by using HPLC FTICR–MS and tandem mass spectrometry. Am Pharm Rev 2001; 4(2):55–63.
61. Wilson ID, Griffiths L, Lindon JD, Nicholson JK. HPLC/NMR and related hyphenated NMR methods. In: Görög S, ed. Identification and Determination of Impurities in Drugs. New York: Elsevier, 2000:299–322.
62. Peng SX. Hyphenated HPLC–NMR and its applications in drug discovery. Biomed Chromatogr 2000; 14:430–441.
63. Sharman GJ, Jones IC. Critical investigation of coupled liquid chromatography–NMR spectroscopy in pharmaceutical impurity identification. Magn Reson Chem 2003; 41:448–454.
64. Cummings PG, Offen P, Olsen MA, Kennedy-Gabb S, Zuber G. LC/MS, LC/NMR, FTIR: an integrated approach to impurity identification in pharmaceutical development formulation. Am Pharm Rev 2003; 6(3):88, 90, 92.
65a. Gorman PM, Jiang H. Isolation methods I: thin-layer chromatography. In: Ahuja S, Alsante KM, eds. Handbook of isolation and characterization of impurities in Pharmaceuticals, Separation Science and Technology, v. 5. Chapter 9. New York: Academic Press, 2003.
65b. Guinn M, Bates R, Hritzko B, Shanklin T, Wilcox G, Guhan S. Isolation methods II: Column Chromatography. In: Ahuja S, Alsante KM, eds. Handbook of Isolation and Characterization of Impurities in Pharmaceuticals, Separation Science and Technology, v. 5. Chapter 10. New York: Academic Press, 2003.
66. Tollsten L. HPLC/MS for drug impurity identification. In: Görög S, ed. Identification and Determination of Impurities in Drugs. New York: Elsevier, 2000:266–297.

67a. Burinsky DJ, Wang F. Mass spectral characterization. In: Ahuja S, Alsante KM, eds. Handbook of Isolation and Characterization of Impurities in Pharmaceuticals, Separation Science and Technology, v. 5. Chapter 11. New York: Academic Press, 2003.
67b. Lohr LL, Jensen AJ, Sharp TR. NMR characterization of impurities. In: Ahuja S, Alsante KM, eds. Handbook of Isolation and Characterization of Impurities in Pharmaceuticals, Separation Science and Technology, v. 5. Chapter 12. New York: Academic Press, 2003.
67c. Feinberg TN. Hyphenated characterization techniques. In: Ahuja S, Alsante KM, eds. Handbook of Isolation and Characterization of Impurities in Pharmaceuticals, Separation Science and Technology, v. 5. Chapter 13. New York: Academic Press, 2003.
67d. Alsante KM, Hatajik TD, Lohr LL, Santafianos D, Sharp TR. Solving impurity/degradation problems: case studies. In: Ahuja S, Alsante KM, eds. Handbook of Isolation and Characterization of Impurities in Pharmaceuticals, Separation Science and Technology, v. 5. Chapter 13. New York: Academic Press, 2003.
68. Görög S. New safe medicines faster: the role of analytical chemistry. Trends Anal Chem 2003; 22:7–8.
69. Jansen PJ, Oren PL, Kemp CA, Maple SR, Baertschi SW. Characterization of impurities formed by interaction of duloxetine HC1 with enteric polymers hydroxypropyl methylcellulose acetate succinate (HPMCAS) and hydroxypropyl methylcellulose phthalate (HPMCP). J Pharm Sci 1998; 87(1):81–85.
70. Bopp RJ, Breau AP, Faulkinbury TJ, Heath PC, Miller C, Stephan EA, Weigel LO, Wong DT. The rearrangement of duloxetine under mineral acid conditions. 206th National American Chemical Society Meeting, San Diego, CA; Mar 13, 1993; ORGN 111.
71. Singh S, Bakshi M. Guidance on conduct of stress tests to determine inherent stability of drugs. Pharm Technol Online (April)2000; 1–14.
72. Dressman JB. Comparison of Canine and human gastointestinal physiology. Pharm Res 1986; 3(3):123–131.
73. Harmon PA. Development of a peroxy radical mediated oxidative stressing system for predicting general oxidative sensitivity in solid dosage forms. Forced Degradation Studies: Best Practices for the Pharmaceutical Industry. Institute for International Research, Princeton, NJ, Feb 24–25, 2004.

3

Stress Testing: The Chemistry of Drug Degradation

Steven W. Baertschi
Eli Lilly and Company, Lilly Research Laboratories, Lilly Corporate Center, Indianapolis, Indiana, U.S.A.

Karen M. Alsante
Pfizer Global Research & Development, Analytical Research & Development, Groton, Connecticut, U.S.A.

I. INTRODUCTION

In this chapter, we will examine the major mechanisms of chemical decomposition of pharmaceuticals in the context of common functional groups. The major mechanisms of chemical decomposition of pharmaceuticals include hydrolysis/dehydration, oxidation, isomerization/epimerization, decarboxylation, rearrangements, dimerization/polymerization, and photolysis and transformation products involving reaction with excipients/salt forms. In order to develop an understanding of the chemistry of such reactions, a basic knowledge of organic chemistry is needed. Providing such a background is not the purpose of this book, and therefore the reader may find it useful to consult more advanced organic chemistry textbooks and literature references. A good general organic chemistry reference is given by March (1). Stewart and Tucker (2) have provided excellent references for consideration of drug degradation mechanisms. An in-depth discussion of the various mechanisms is beyond the scope of this chapter, but some discussion is warranted.

The mechanisms of hydrolysis/dehydration, isomerization/epimerization, decarboxylation, rearrangements and some kinds of polymerization reactions can be generalized into a condition that has been called "thermolytic" (3); these reactions are generally sensitive to temperature and can be accelerated by elevating the temperature under various conditions in the solid state (low and high humidity) and in solutions and/or slurries. *Hydrolytic* reactions (which are also "thermolytic" in nature) can be accelerated both by exposure to elevated temperature as well as by exposure to a broad pH range. *Oxidative* degradation of pharmaceuticals is generally the result of autoxidation, the rate of which usually will not be accelerated by temperature in a predictable manner, but rather by the formation of radicals (via initiators such as transition metals, low levels of peroxides, or molecular oxygen). Many polymerization reactions are the result of radical-initiated processes. *Photolytic* reactions are [obviously] caused by the absorption of photons from exposure to various sources of light (e.g., sunlight, metal halide lamps, fluorescent lamps, or other indoor lighting sources), and therefore these reactions can be induced by exposure to photolysis sources emitting in the 290–800 nm region. More detailed discussions of the design of stress-testing studies to evaluate these major degradation pathways (i.e., thermolytic, hydrolytic, oxidative, and photolytic) can be found in other chapters in this book (Chapters 2, 4, 7, and 10).

II. DEGRADATION OF COMMON FUNCTIONAL GROUPS

The degradation chemistry of a variety of common functional groups, organized by functionality, is discussed in this chapter. Some discussion of photolytic chemistry of functional groups is provided, but for a more thorough discussion of photochemistry, see Chapter 10. This list of functional groups is not intended to be exhaustive, nor is the discussion intended to be comprehensive, as there exist volumes of reference books on the chemistries associated with various functional groups and heterocycles. For example, "The Chemistry of Functional Groups" series was founded by Professor Saul Patai (1918–1998) and in 38 years has published more than 120 volumes covering all aspects of organic chemistry (4). The discussion in the present chapter is intended to provide a quick and practical reference to the degradation chemistry of some of the more common functional groups found in the structures of common active pharmaceutical ingredients (APIs).

A. Carbonyl Chemistry

1. Esters, Lactones

Esters are subject to general acid or base-catalyzed hydrolysis to form a carboxylic acid and an alcohol. Both are equilibrium reactions and readily occur when equilibrium is shifted to the right. Base-catalyzed hydrolysis

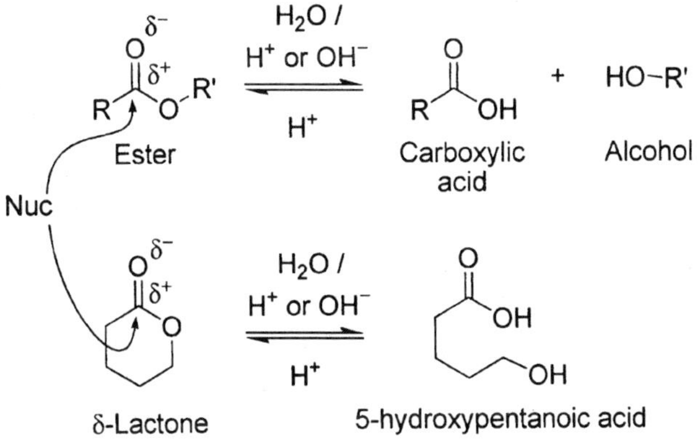

Figure 1 Hydrolysis of esters and lactones.

(saponification) of esters is fast with the more powerful attacking -OH nucleophile yielding the salt of the acid. Acid-catalyzed ester hydrolysis is slower. Acids catalyze the reaction by making the carbonyl carbon more electropositive (by protonation of the carbonyl oxygen) and therefore more susceptible to nucleophilic attack. Lactones are simply cyclic esters, and are therefore subject to the same acid/base hydrolysis chemistry as an ester (Fig. 1).

The carbonyl carbon of these moieties is electrophilic, and therefore nucleophilic reactions are likely to occur via nucleophilic attack on the carbonyl carbon. In highly aqueous systems, the nucleophile is usually water. In the case of lactones, the smaller the lactone ring, the higher the ring strain, and therefore the more susceptible to hydrolysis (rate of hydrolysis of $\beta > \gamma > \delta$). For a more thorough discussion of acid/base hydrolysis, see Stewart and Tucker (2) and March (5). Esters and lactones are not particularly susceptible to oxidation.

A classic example of ester hydrolysis is demonstrated with aspirin. Aspirin hydrolyzes under acidic and basic conditions to yield acetic and salicylic acid (Fig. 2) (6). Aspirin easily hydrolyzes because it is an activated ester (i.e., the leaving group, carboxylate anion, can readily stabilize the anionic charge). An additional API example that undergoes ester hydrolysis is cyclandelate (7).

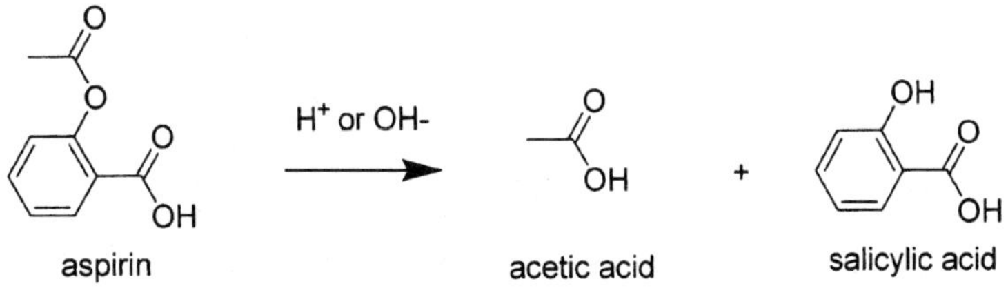

Figure 2 Hydrolysis of aspirin to acetic and salicylic acid.

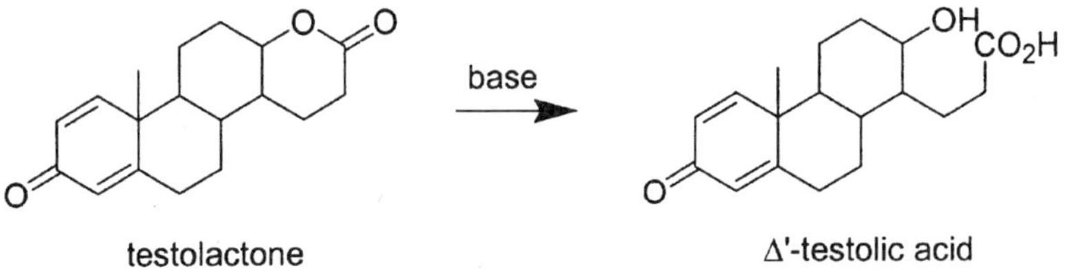

testolactone

base

Δ'-testolic acid

Figure 3 Testolactone degradation.

The API testolactone will undergo ring opening of the lactone to Δ′-testolic acid in strongly alkaline solution (Fig. 3) (8).

An additional example of lactone hydrolysis includes the API lovastatin (9). In addition to lactone cleavage reactions, lactone formation can also occur as in the case of the API cephalosporin cefuroxime sodium (Fig. 4) (10).

2. Amides, Lactams

Amides are subject to acid or base-catalyzed hydrolysis to form a carboxylic acid and an amine (Fig. 5). Amides are more stable than their corresponding esters since -NHR is a poorer leaving group than -OR for esters. Therefore, water alone is not sufficient to hydrolyze most amides at a significant rate. Prolonged heating is also required even with acidic or basic catalysts. However, in pharamaceutical degradation studies, where we are not monitoring for stoichiometric chemistry, the hydrolysis of amides is often observed at levels of concern at room temperature conditions during the shelf life of many products. Thiol amides are much more readily hydrolyzed than are amides. The rate of hydrolysis of thiol esters, esters, and amides (thiol esters > esters > amides) is a reflection the pK_a of the conjugate acid of the leaving group. The greater the tendency of the conjugate acid of the leaving group to ionize to the anion (i.e., the lower the pK_a), the better the leaving group and the faster the hydrolysis (5). Lactams, imides, cylic imides, and hydrazines also undergo this reaction. Amides and lactams are not particularly susceptible to oxidation.

Acetominophen is a classic example of an API that readily undergoes amide hydrolysis. Acetominophen undergoes acid and base-catalyzed hydrolysis to yield *p*-aminophenol and acetic acid (Fig. 6) (11).

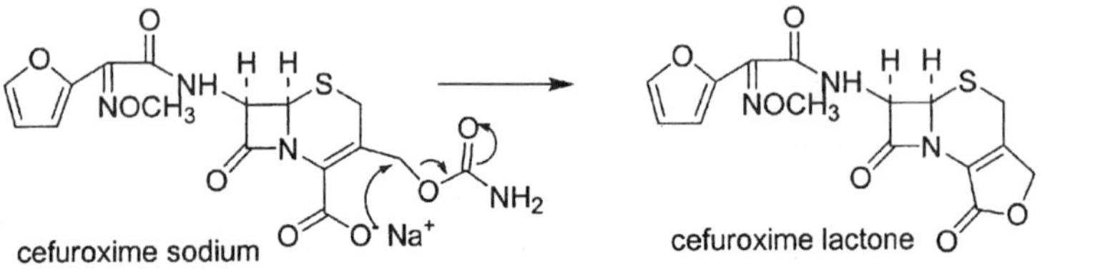

cefuroxime sodium

cefuroxime lactone

Figure 4 Cefuroxime sodium lactone formation.

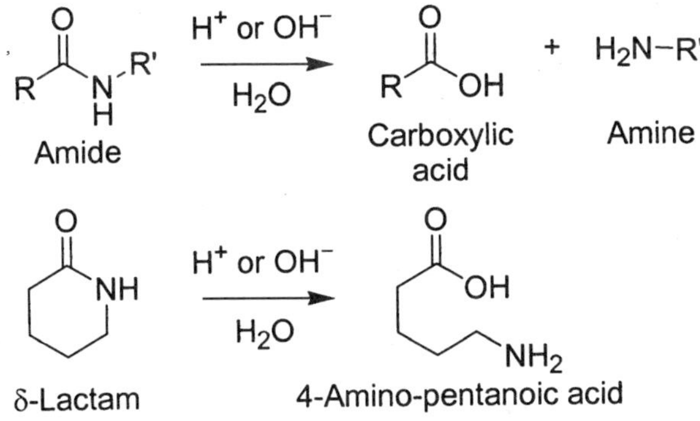

Figure 5 Hydrolysis of amides and lactams.

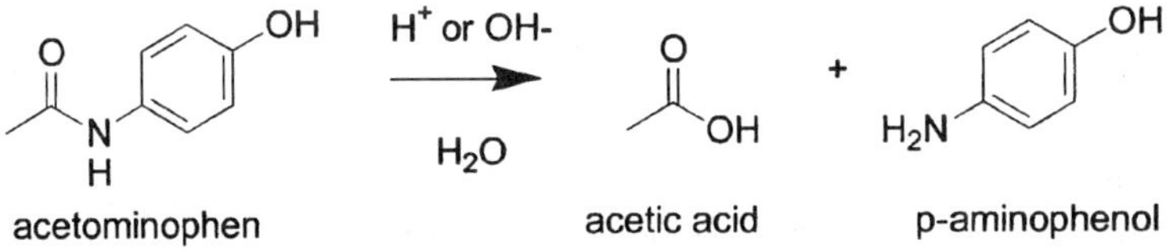

Figure 6 Acid and base-catalyzed hydrolysis of acetominophen.

Other API amide hydrolysis examples include chloramphenicol (12), indomethacin under alkaline conditions (13), lidocaine (14), azintamide (15), terazosin (16), flutamide (17), oxazepam, and chlordiazepoxide (18). Lidocaine does not readily hydrolyze in aqueous solution under thermal or basic conditions (Fig. 7) (19). The enhanced stability is due to the steric hindrance of the two *o*-methyl groups. Hydrolysis does occur more readily in acidic conditions rather than basic conditions presumably because the rate-limiting step, protonation of the carbonyl, is not affected by the steric hindrance of the *o*-methyl.

Other APIs have shown lactam formation. In the case of baclofen, formation of the corresponding lactam is observed at 50°C (Fig. 8) (20).

A subset of lactams is the β-lactam functionality, the chemistry of which has been studied extensively. *The β-lactam functionality has been thoroughly studied because the biological activity of the β-lactam antibiotics (e.g., penicillins, cephalosporins, etc.) is the result of the presence of the β-lactam moiety (Fig. 9). The electrophilic carbonyl of the β-lactam reacts with certain "penicillin binding proteins" found in bacteria to form a covalent bond (ester-linked) with the protein (23,24). The protein is thereby inactivated, bacterial cell wall

* For specific examples of articles dealing with β-lactam degradation chemistry see Ref. 21. For general information on the chemistry of β-lactams see Ref. 22.

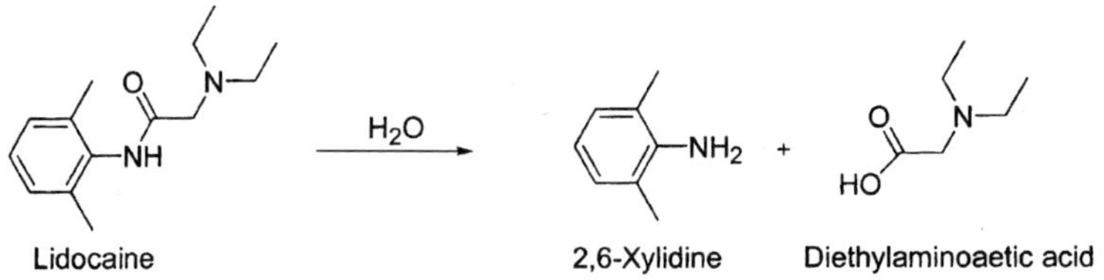

Lidocaine $\xrightarrow{H_2O}$ 2,6-Xylidine + Diethylaminoaetic acid

Figure 7 Lidocaine API amide hydrolysis under acidic conditions.

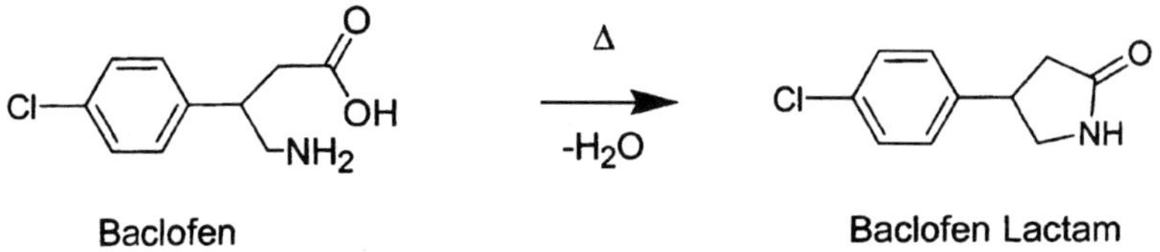

Baclofen $\xrightarrow[-H_2O]{\Delta}$ Baclofen Lactam

Figure 8 Degradation of baclofen to form the baclofen lactam.

synthesis is inhibited, and growing bacteria cells are induced to undergo lysis. It is noteworthy that when a β-lactam undergoes hydrolysis, the initially formed product (Fig. 9, R"=OH) is generally not stable and undergoes further degradation to other products.

The electrophilic carbonyl of the β-lactam can also result in degradation by polymerization (25) as shown in the polymerization of ampicillin

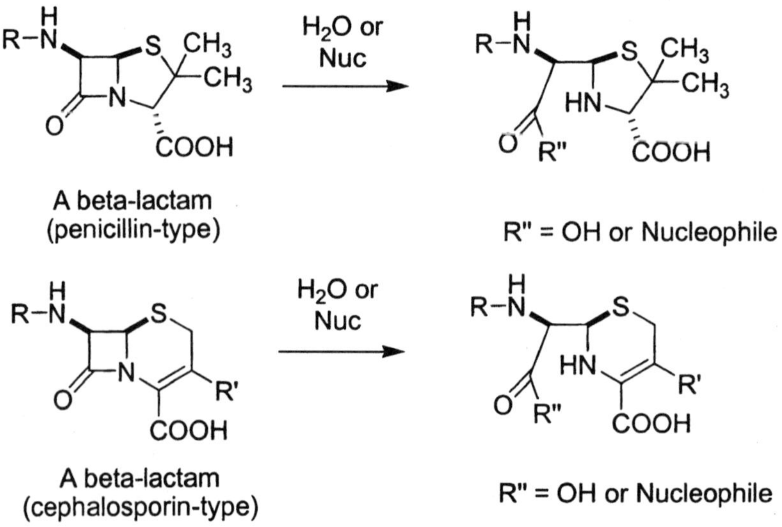

A beta-lactam (penicillin-type) $\xrightarrow{H_2O \text{ or Nuc}}$ R" = OH or Nucleophile

A beta-lactam (cephalosporin-type) $\xrightarrow{H_2O \text{ or Nuc}}$ R" = OH or Nucleophile

Figure 9 The highly electrophilic carbonyl carbon of β -lactam antibiotics reacts readily with nucleophiles.

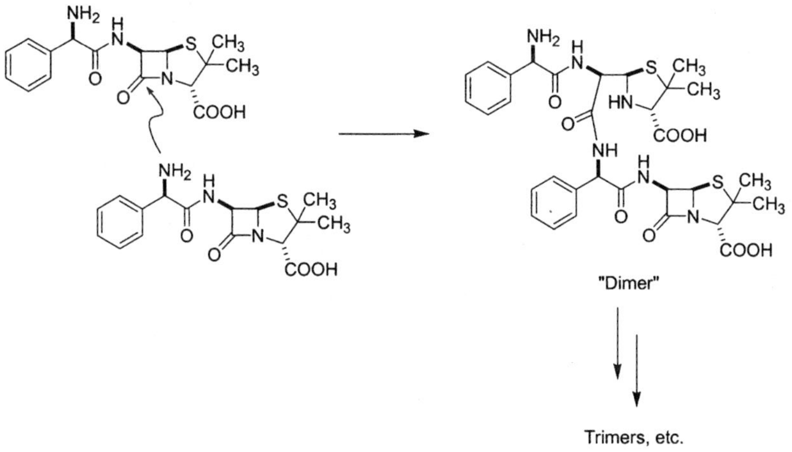

Figure 10 Polymerization of the β-lactam antibiotic ampicillin.

(26) in Figure 10, although not all polymerization reactions of β-lactams occur directly from a nucleophilic attack on the β-lactam (see for example, ceftazidime (27)). In general, the polymerization of β-lactams occurs as is shown in Figure 10. The β-lactam is not particularly susceptible to oxidation, but the sulfur atom in these antibiotics is susceptible to oxidation to the sulfoxide and sulfone (for more information on sulfoxide/sulfone chemistry, see the section on Sulfonyl chemistry).

β-Lactam containing APIs are susceptible to lactam hydrolysis as observed with the β-lactam antiobiotic penicillin G (18). Amoxicillin degradation is typical of penicillin hydrolysis reactions. Under basic conditions, amoxicillin decomposes by ring opening of the lactam ring to penicilloic acid, which ultimately loses CO_2 and forms penilloic acid (28). A general scheme for penicillin degradation is available in *Analytical Profiles of Drug Substances* (29).

3. Carbamic Esters

Carbamic esters also hydrolyze by ester/amide carbonyl chemistry (described above) to the corresponding carbamic acid followed by carbamic acid decarboxylation (Fig. 11). Carbamic esters are not particularly susceptible to oxidation.

Example APIs containing carbamic ester functional groups with the potential for hydrolysis are loratadine (Fig. 12) and pipazetate (18).

4. Imides

Imides can hydrolyze to give a mixture of products resulting from nucleophilic attack of water on either carbonyl carbon, as shown in Figure 13. In the case of cyclic imides, such as maleimide, an intramolecular cyclization reaction can

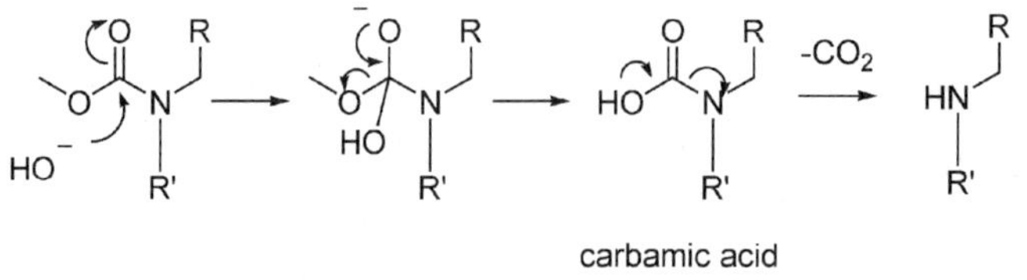
-CO2
HO
carbamic acid

Figure 11 Carbamic ester hydrolysis.

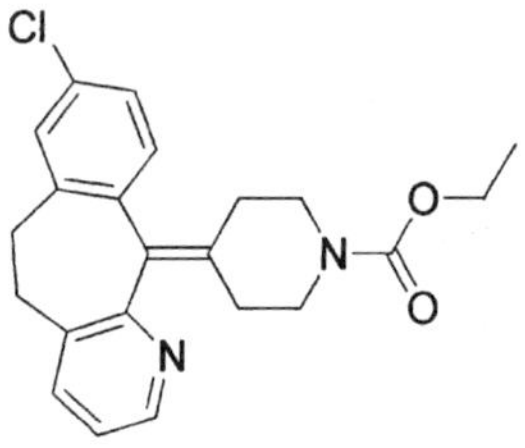

Figure 12 Carbamic ester containing API, loratadine.

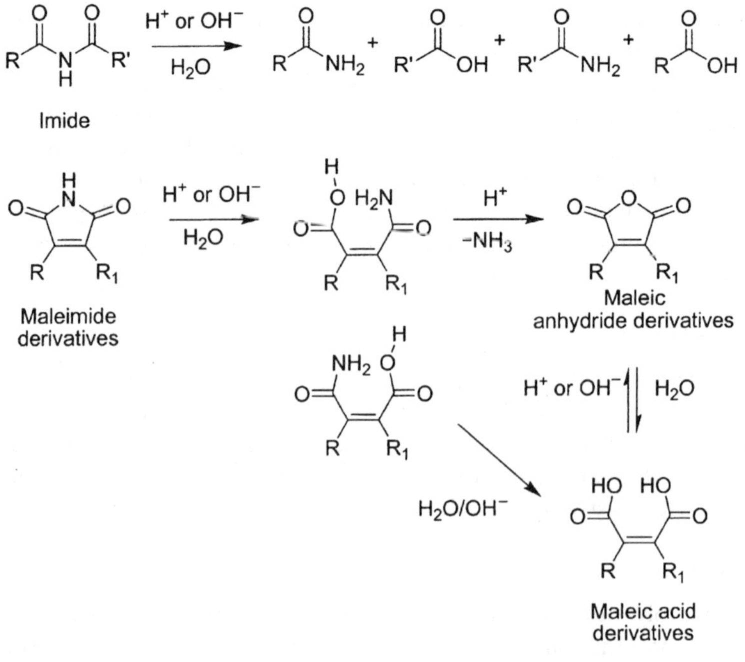
Imide
H+ or OH−
H2O
Maleimide derivatives
H+
-NH3
Maleic anhydride derivatives
H2O/OH−
Maleic acid derivatives

Figure 13 Hydrolysis of imides.

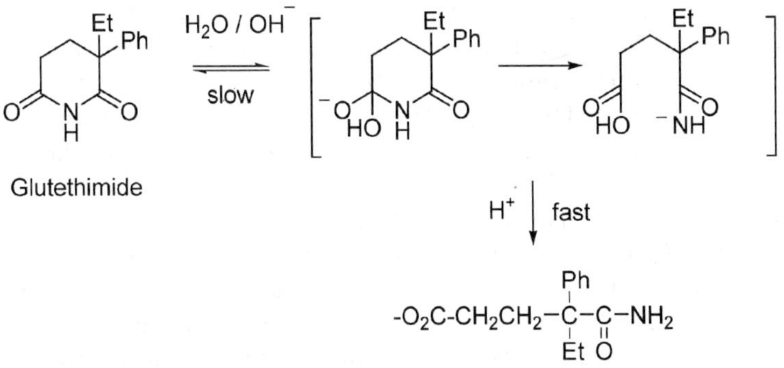

Figure 14 Mechanism of glutethimide hydrolysis.

occur subsequent to the ring-opening hydrolysis, leading to the release of ammonia and the formation of maleic anhydride. Alternatively, the ring-opened product can hydrolyze further without ring closure to form maleic acid.

An example of imide hydrolysis occurs with the cyclic imide-containing API glutethimide (Fig. 14). The mechanism proposed involves direct attack by a hydroxyl ion on the unhindered carbonyl followed by ring cleavage (30).

Additionally, imide hydrolytic decomposition is observed with the API phenobarbital in alkaline solution to produce α-ethylbenzeneacetic acid and urea (Fig. 15) (31).

5. Carboxylic Acids

Carboxylic acids *typically* have pK_a's in the range of ~2–5.5 (although some can be significantly outside this range, depending on the nature of the substituents) (32) and it is therefore helpful to consider the ionization state of the group when evaluating the chemistry. Below the pK_a, the group is protonated and therefore the carbonyl carbon is more electrophilic. The car-

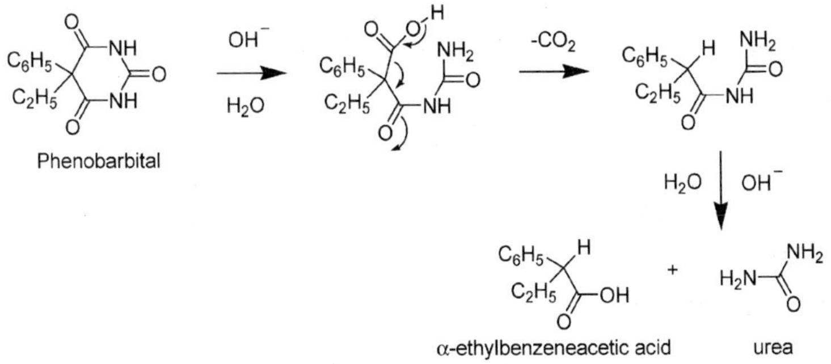

Figure 15 Imide hydrolysis of phenobarbital in basic conditions.

bonyl can undergo nucleophilic attack to form esters, amides, thioesters, etc. In the case of attack by an alcohol, the reaction product is an ester, and the reaction is called an esterification reaction (Fig. 16). This can occur as an artifact reaction when acid/base hydrolysis reactions are performed using an alcohol co-solvent system such as methanol. Esters of the API parent compound can also be observed as process-related impurities, especially when alcohol solvents are used in the recrystallization step.

Above the pK_a, the carboxylate is anionic and the charge is resonance stabilized; the group is therefore less electrophilic and does not have a good leaving group. Therefore, reactions with nucleophiles are significantly suppressed when compared to the protonated form. Carboxylic acids are not prone to oxidative degradation.

Some carboxylic acids can decarboxylate under the right conditions (33). For example, if the carboxylic acid is β to a keto group, acid or base-catalyzed decarboxylation can occur as shown in Figure 17.

As an example, the API moxalactam disodium undergoes decarboxylation at the benzylic site to form decarboxylated moxalactam in the solid state (Fig. 18) (34).

Decarboxylation of the API diflunisal occurs under thermal conditions. Diflunisal contains a β-hydroxyl group. Tautomerization to the β-keto form permits a decarboxylation reaction to occur, eventually leading to a dimerization reaction to form diflunisal descarboxydiflunisal ester (Fig. 19) (35). Other API decarboxylation examples include norfloxacin (36) and terazosin (37).

An example excipient that is reactive with APIs containing carboxylic acids is polyvinyl alcohol. Polyvinyl alcohol containing secondary hydroxyl

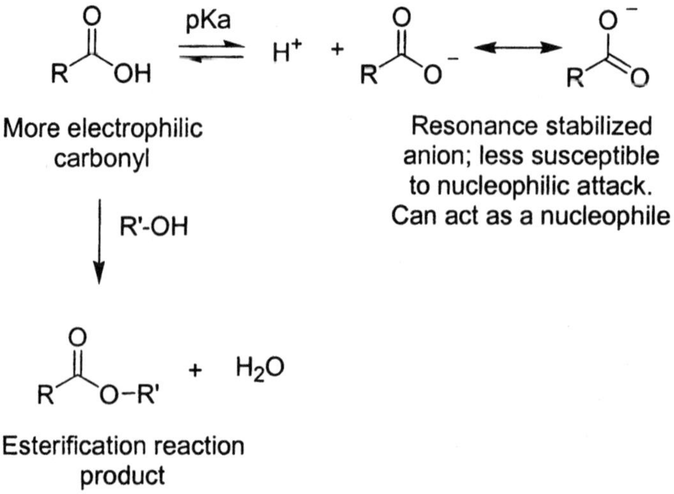

Figure 16 Chemistry of carboxylic acids.

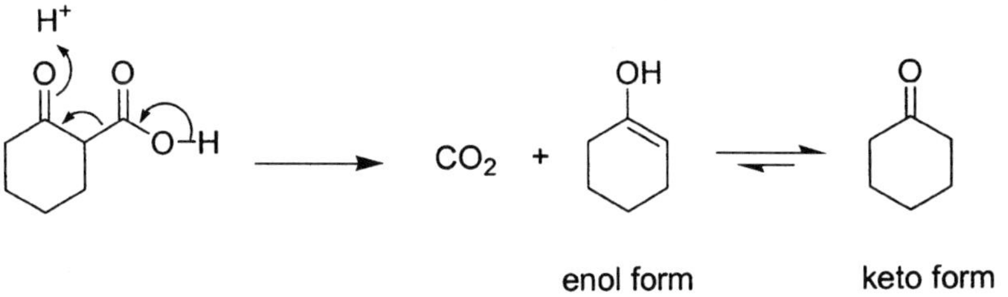

H^+

CO_2 +

enol form

keto form

Figure 17 Decarboxylation of a β-keto carboxylic acid.

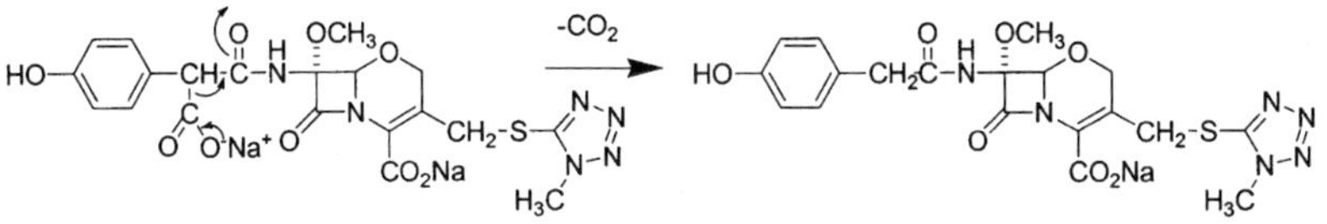

$-CO_2$

Figure 18 Moxalactam disodium decarboxylation.

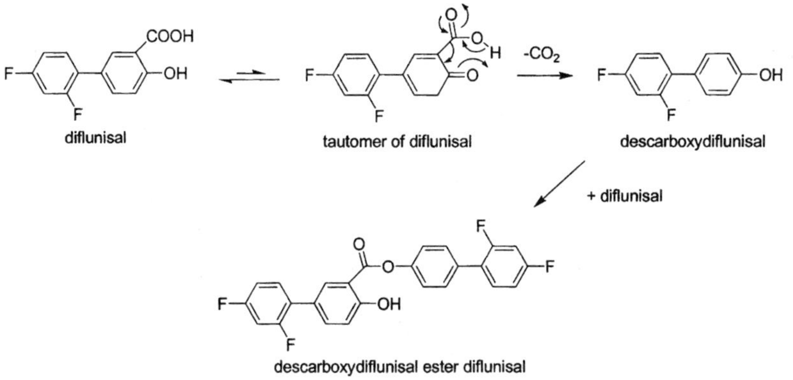

diflunisal

tautomer of diflunisal

descarboxydiflunisal

+ diflunisal

descarboxydiflunisal ester diflunisal

Figure 19 Diflunsal decarboxylation and dimer ester formation.

groups is susceptible to esterification reactions (38). Other excipient sources of hydroxyls that react with APIs containing carboxylic acids are carbohydrates/sugars such as lactose, mannitol, sucrose, β-cyclodextrins, and polyethylene glycols.

6. Ketones, Aldehydes

Ketones and aldehydes have electrophilic carbonyls that significantly contribute to the chemistry of these functional groups. In general, aldehydes tend to be more electrophilic and will often exist in aqueous solutions in hydrated form as a gem-diol (Fig. 20). This is an important consideration when attempting to characterize by NMR an unknown that may contain an

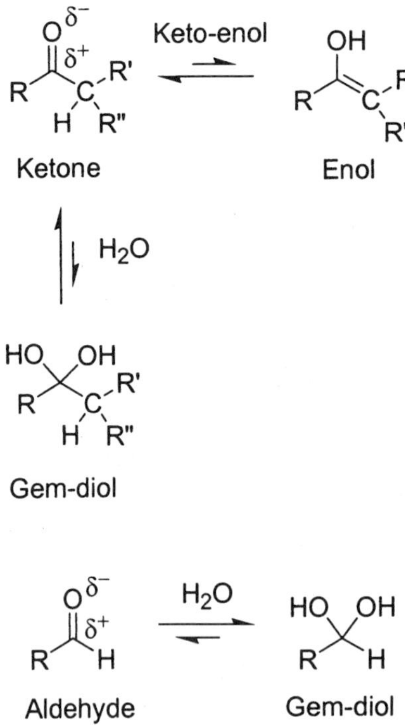

Figure 20 Chemistry of ketones and aldehydes.

aldehyde, since in D_2O the aldehyde might exist predominantly as a gem-diol but in organic solvents such as $CDCl_3$ the aldehydic form will likely predominate. Isolated ketones may also readily react with water to form a gem-diol, although generally to a much lesser extent (39). Ketones (and aldehydes) will undergo a rapid tautomerization (catalyzed by either acid or base) known as the keto-enol tautomerism if there is a hydrogen atom on the carbon alpha to the carbonyl (see Fig. 20). Thus, chiral centers adjacent to the carbonyl of ketones and aldehydes are often (but not always) readily epimerized via this tautomerization.

Because of their significant electrophilic character, aldehydes are often unstable and will react with nucleophiles. For example, a common reaction of aldehydes is the formation of a hemiaminal with amines. If the amine is a primary amine, the hemiaminal can dehydrate to form an imine as shown in Figure 21. The reaction of aldehydes with primary and secondary amines is a well-studied reaction pathway because it is a common reaction pathway of reducing sugars and amino acids, and this reaction pathway is known as the Maillard reaction (40). In the case of amino acids and sugars, this reaction leads to discoloration, or "browning." This reaction will be discussed in greater detail in the Amines–Maillard Reaction section.

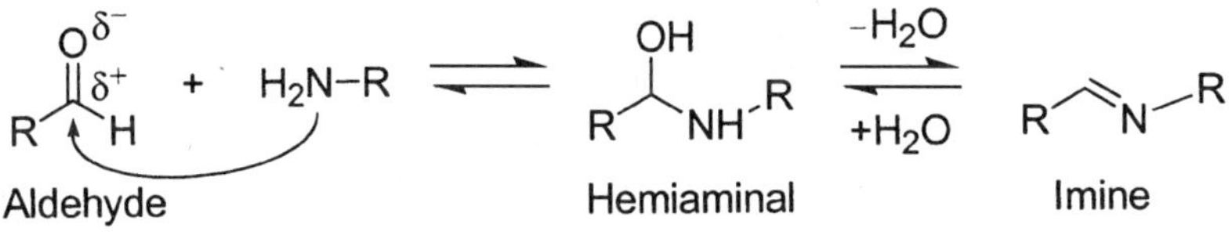

Figure 21 Reaction of aldehydes with amines.

Aldehydes are susceptible to oxidation to the corresponding carboxylic acid, but ketones are generally not oxidized under pharmaceutically relevant conditions. When ketones are conjugated with one or more double bonds, as in the case of an α,β-unsaturated ketone (also called an "enone"), the carbonyl is less electrophilic but is still susceptible to nucleophilic attack at either the carbonyl carbon (1,2-addition) or at the β-carbon (1,4-addition, or "Michael addition") (Fig. 22).

The carbon alpha to the carbonyl of aldehydes and ketones can act as a nucleophile in reactions with other electrophilic compounds or intermolecularly with itself. The nucleophilic character is imparted via the keto-enol tautomerism. A classic example of this reactivity is seen in the aldol condensation (41), as shown in Figure 23. Note that the aldol condensation is potentially reversible (retro-aldol), and compounds containing a carbonyl with a hydroxyl at the β-position will often undergo the retro-aldol reaction. The aldol condensation reaction is catalyzed by both acids and bases. Aldol products undergo a reversible dehydration reaction (Fig. 23) that is acid or base catalyzed. The dehydration proceeds through an enol intermediate to form the α,β-unsaturated carbonyl containing compound.

The API haloperidol was found to be incompatible with 5-(hydroxymethyl)-2-furfuraldehyde, an impurity (resulting from degradation of lactose) in anhydrous lactose, and an adduct transformation product is formed (Fig. 24) (42).

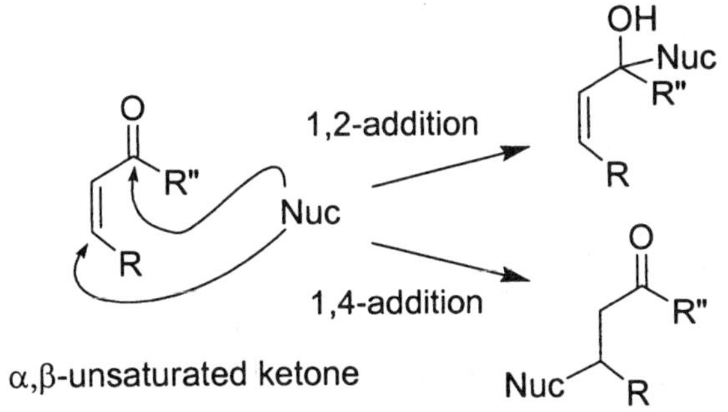

Figure 22 Reactions of α,β-unsaturated ketones with nucleophiles.

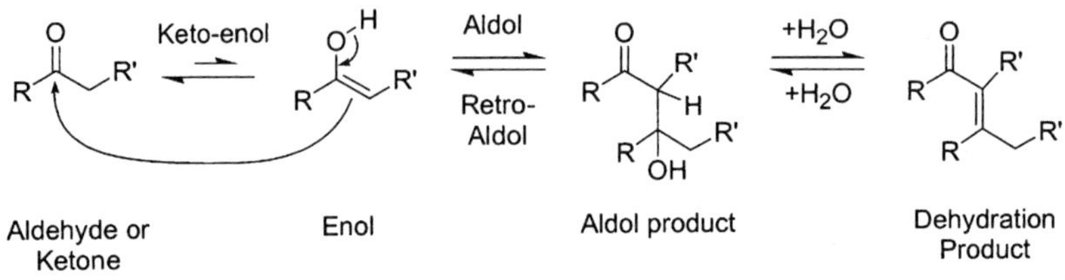

Figure 23 "Aldol" condensation and dehydration reaction.

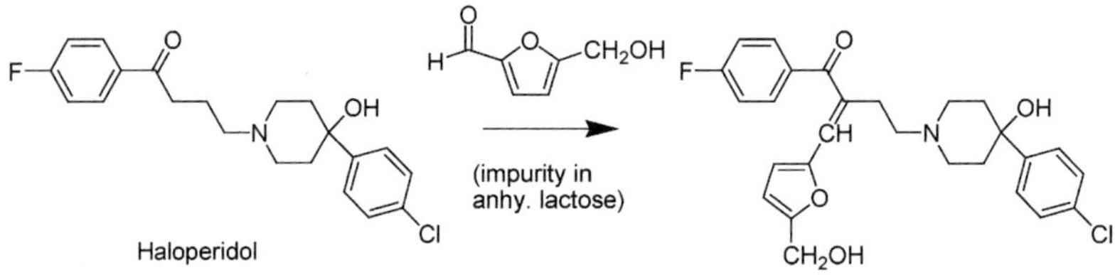

Figure 24 Haloperidol adduct transformation product resulting from reaction with an impurity in anhydrous lactose .

Aldehydes and ketone derivatives that absorb light at wavelengths greater than approx. 300 nm are known to be photolabile (Fig. 25) (43). The lowest lying excited state, typically an n-π^* transition, behaves as an electrophilic radical. Common reactions of aldehydes and ketones in their photoexcited states include reduction via intermolecular hydrogen abstraction and fragmentation either via α cleavage (Norrish Type I) or via intramolecular γ-hydrogen atom abstraction followed by C_α–C_β cleavage (Norrish Type II).

7. Acetals/Ketals

Hemi-acetal and hemi-ketal functional groups (Fig. 26) are very susceptible to base-catalyzed hydrolysis and are also susceptible to acid catalyzed hydrolysis. In contrast, acetals and ketals are extremely resistant to hydrolysis by base. For acetals and ketals, only acid-catalyzed hydrolysis occurs

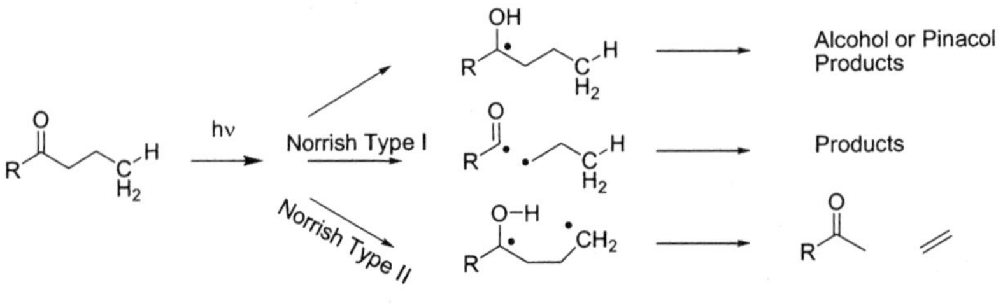

Figure 25 Aldehyde/ketone photochemistry.

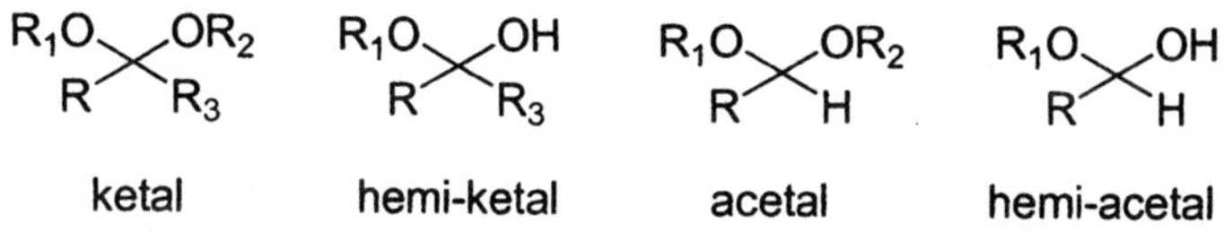

R_1O, OR_2, R, R_3 — ketal; R_1O, OH, R, R_3 — hemi-ketal; R_1O, OR_2, R, H — acetal; R_1O, OH, R, H — hemi-acetal

Figure 26 Basic structures of ketals, hemi-ketals, acetals, and hemi-acetals.

$$RCH(OR')_2 \underset{}{\overset{H^+}{\rightleftharpoons}} RCH(\overset{+}{H}OR')(OR') \underset{}{\overset{\text{slow}, -R'OH}{\rightleftharpoons}} R\overset{+}{C}H\text{-}OR' \overset{+H_2O}{\rightleftharpoons} RCH(\overset{+}{O}H_2)\text{-}OR' \overset{-H^+}{\rightleftharpoons}$$

Acetal

$$RCH(OH)\text{-}OR' \overset{H^+}{\rightleftharpoons} RCH(OH)\text{-}\overset{+}{O}R'H \overset{-R'OH}{\rightleftharpoons} R\overset{+}{C}H\text{-}OH \overset{-H^+}{\rightleftharpoons} RCH{=}O$$

Hemi-acetal

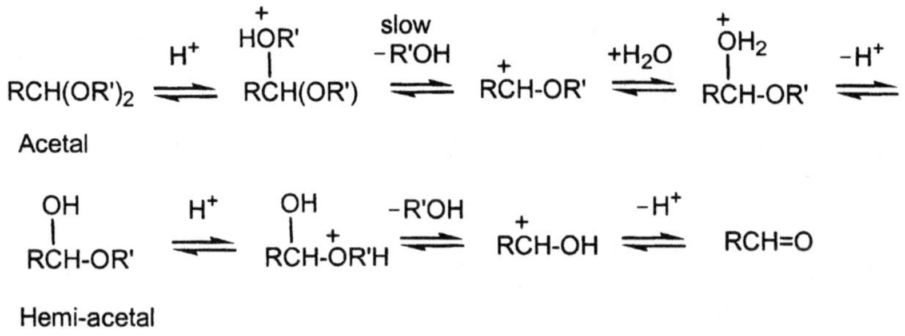

Figure 27 Acid-catalyzed (S_N1) hydrolysis mechanism of acetals and hemiacetals.

(18). The acid-catalyzed reaction proceeds by an S_N1 mechanism as shown in Figure 27.

Triamcinolone acetonide contains a cyclic ketal group that can be readily cleaved by a variety of organic acids (Fig. 28) (44).

B. Nitrogen-Containing Functional Groups

1. Nitriles

Nitriles are susceptible to hydrolysis via nucleophilic attack of water on the electropositive carbon atom, especially under strongly acidic and basic conditions (Fig. 29). Nitriles hydrolyze to imidic acids, which tautomerize to amides. Amides can be hydrolyzed further to carboxylic acids, although much more slowly. Nitriles are susceptible to oxidation by peroxides under mildly basic conditions (e.g., pH 7.5–8) as has been documented in the case

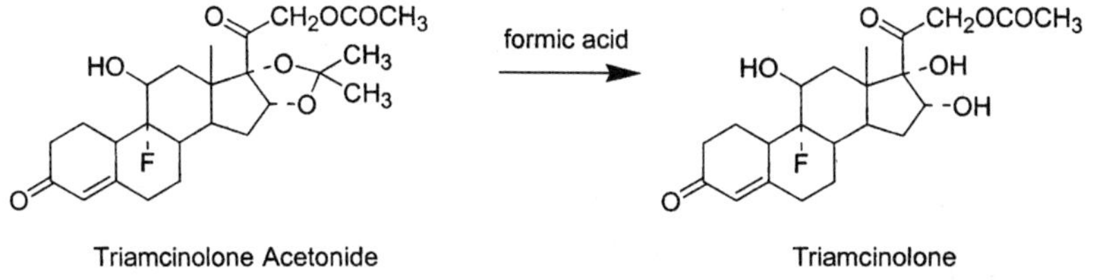

Triamcinolone Acetonide —formic acid→ Triamcinolone

Figure 28 Triamcinolone acetonide ketal hydrolysis under acidic conditions.

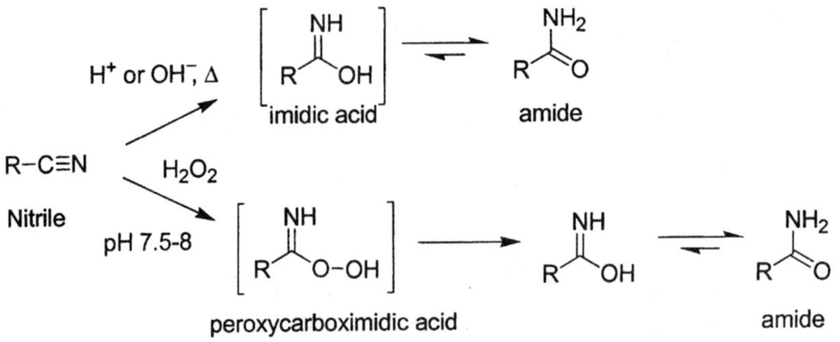

Figure 29 Hydrolysis and oxidation of nitriles.

of acetonitrile (45,46). The nitrile adds peroxide to form an unstable peroxycarboximidic acid. This unstable intermediate is a reactive oxidizing species and can oxidize other species present while being concomitantly reduced to the amide (Fig. 29).

Acid hydrolysis of the nitrile in the API cimetidine leads to the corresponding amide which then undergoes further degradation through loss of the $CONH_2$ moiety via a pathway that is analogous to a β-keto acid decarboxylation (Fig. 30) (47).

If the carbon alpha to the nitrile contains a proton, the potential exists for radical-initiated oxidation, leading to oxidative degradation. Such

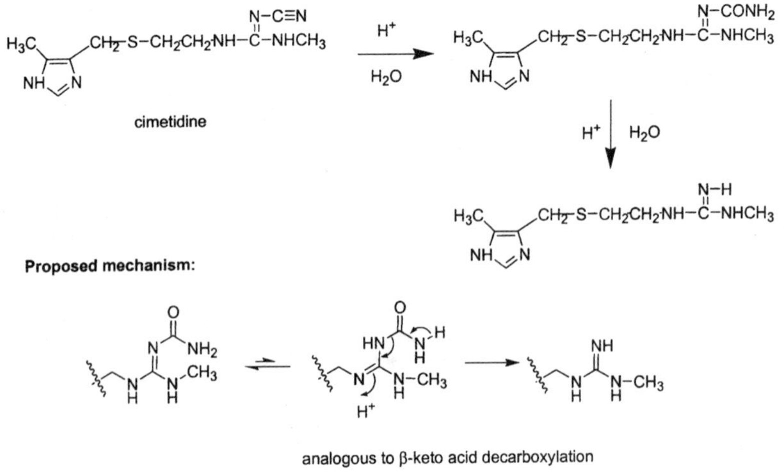

Figure 30 Hydrolysis of the nitrile in cimetidine leads to an unstable compound that undergoes further degradation.

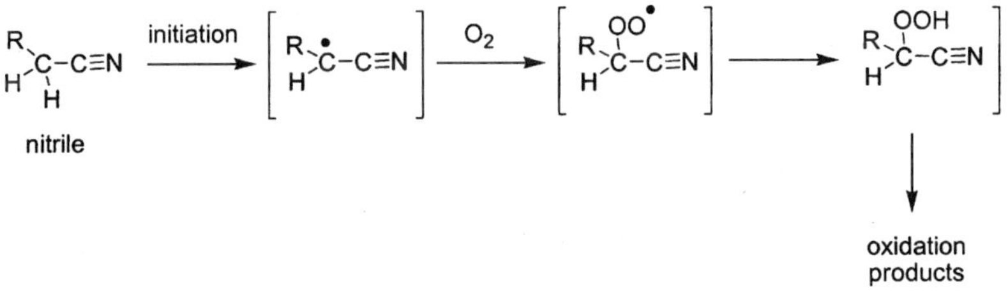

Figure 31 Potential autoxidation degradation pathway of nitriles.

reactivity has been observed for acetonitrile (Fig. 31) (48,49), in spite of the fact that acetonitrile is generally regarded as an inert solvent.

The API diphenoxylate hydrochloride undergoes degradation under acidic conditions with peroxide to hydrolyze the tertiary amine to a hydroxyl followed by hydrolysis of the nitrile to the amide. Further degradation occurs by ring closure as the hydroxyl group adds to the amide group (Fig. 32) (50).

2. Amines

Amines are a very common functional group in pharmaceuticals and are prone to a variety of degradation reactions. Amines can be primary, secondary, or tertiary, aryl, or alkyl. The protonation state of amines is critical to an understanding of the degradation chemistry. Most primary, secondary, and tertiary alkyl amines have pK_a's in the range of 7.5–11.5. Aryl amines tend to be much less basic and have pK_a's in the range of 3–6 (e.g., pK_a of aniline is 4.6). When amines are unprotonated (i.e., in the neutral "free base" form), they are nucleophilic, more easily oxidized, and more volatile. Primary and secondary amines are nucleophilic and will react readily with electrophiles such as aldehydes (as present in reducing sugars) to undergo the first steps of the Maillard reaction (Fig. 43). Amines will also react with trace levels of formaldehyde (or other aldehyde impurities adventitiously present) to form hemiaminals with the potential for dehydration to imines and cross-linking with other amines or nucleophiles as shown in Figure 33. Such

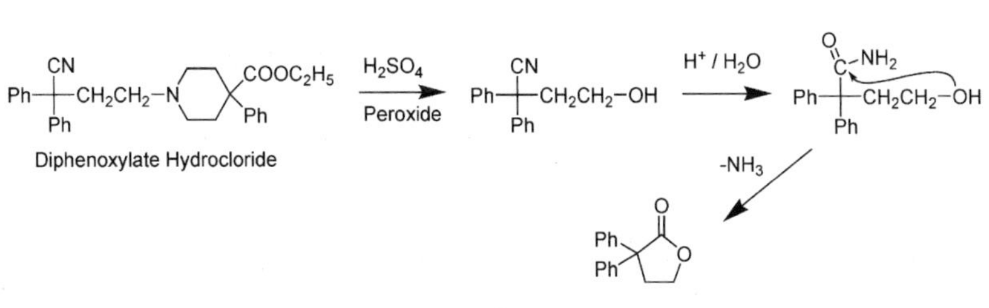

Figure 32 Degradation of the nitrile-containing API diphenoxylate hydrochloride under acidic conditions in the presence of peroxide.

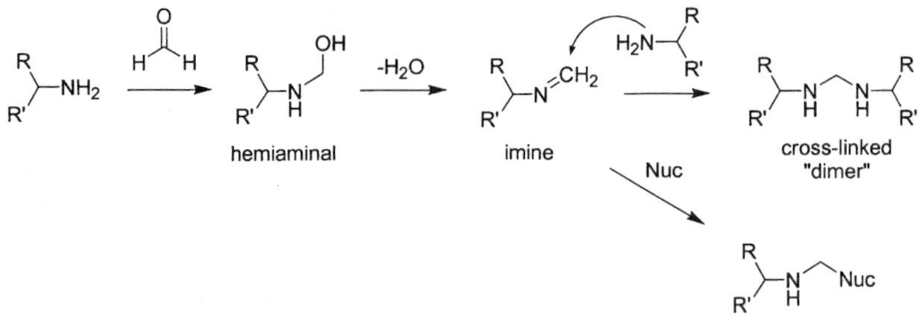

Figure 33 Reaction of an amine with formaldehyde.

reactions of amines with formaldehyde have been documented in the literature and should be considered as possible degradation pathways (51,52). This chemistry is commonly observed with drug product degradation. Polymeric excipients (such as polyethylene glycol and polysorbates) are a common source of formaldehyde from breakdown of the polymeric chain (53).

Tertiary amines are known for their propensity to oxidize to the amine oxide (N-oxide) during long-term storage (54) (Fig. 34). A classic example of

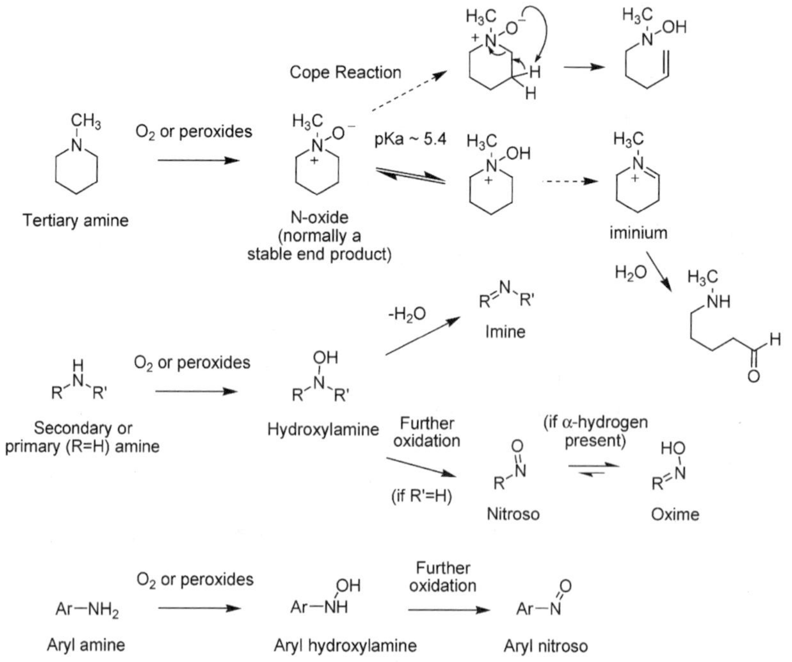

Figure 34 Oxidative reactions of amines. Formation of N-oxides from oxidation of tertiary amines and formation of hydroxylamines from oxidation of primary and secondary amines.

the oxidation of a tertiary amine to form an N-oxide is the case of raloxifene hydrochloride (54a). The tertiary amine of raloxifene hydrochloride is protonated and the formation of the N-oxide was not observed to a significant extent during stress testing studies or upon long-term or accelerated storage of the API. Surprisingly, the product (tablet formulation) showed a propensity to form the N-oxide degradation product upon long-term storage (Fig. 35). It was concluded from an extensive investigation that the N-oxide formation was the result of residual peroxide in the povidone binder and crospovidone disintegrant present in the tablet formulation.

Tertiary amine oxides are generally thought to be relatively stable end products of oxidative degradation, but some amine oxides readily degrade further to other products. Amine oxides are known to degrade via a pathway (Fig. 34) known as the Cope reaction (55) (not to be confused with the Cope rearrangement), although this reaction typically requires exposure to high temperatures (e.g., 100–150°C). In this case, the amine oxide cleaves to form an alkene and a hydroxylamine. Another degradation pathway of tertiary amine oxides occurs via protonation of the oxygen and dehydration to the iminium ion, which can react further with water to hydrolyze to a hemiaminal and further degrade to an aldehyde and a secondary amine (Fig. 34). This pathway is illustrated by Zhao et al. (56) in their work with a morpholine acetal substance P antagonist (Fig. 36).

Oxidation of secondary or primary amines (although in our experience not a common degradation pathway for solid dosage forms) results in the formation of hydroxylamines. Hydroxylamines may not always be observed or may be difficult to isolate. Dehydration to the imine (along with further hydrolysis) should be considered possible if hydroxylamines are formed. For primary amines, further oxidation to the nitroso can occur, but the nitroso can tautomerize to the oxime (if there is an α-hydrogen present). Protonation of amines to the cationic form greatly reduces their oxidation rate, but oxidative degradation of tertiary amines may still present problems for long-term storage or formulation, as was observed in the case of

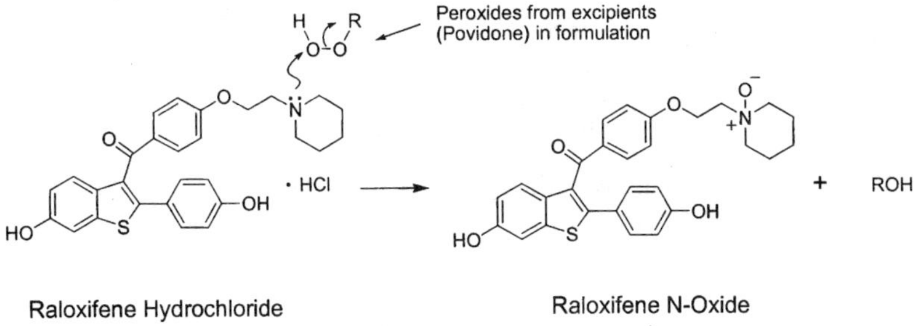

Peroxides from excipients (Povidone) in formulation

Raloxifene Hydrochloride · HCl → Raloxifene N-Oxide + ROH

Figure 35 Excipient-induced (povidone and crospovidone) oxidation of a tertiary amine (raloxifene hydrochloride).

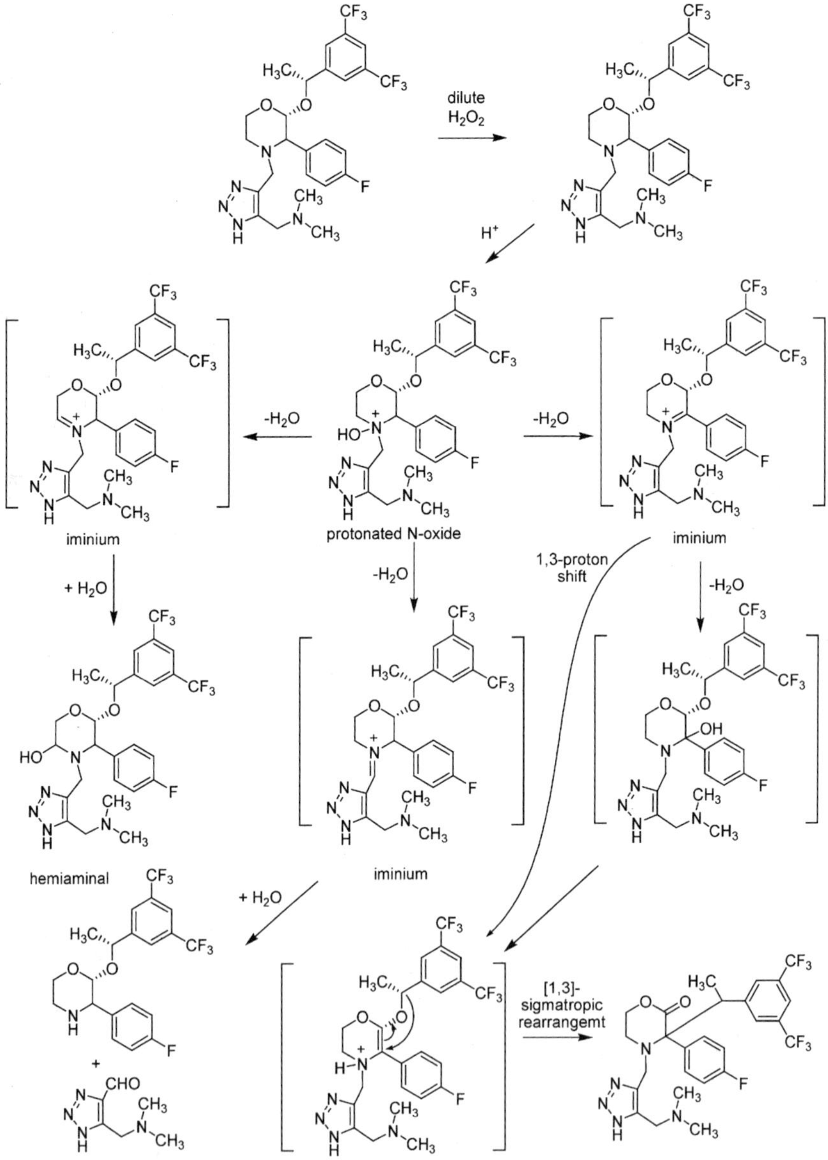

Figure 36 Proposed degradation pathways for an amine oxide degradation product. The counterion (chloride) is not shown for simplicity.

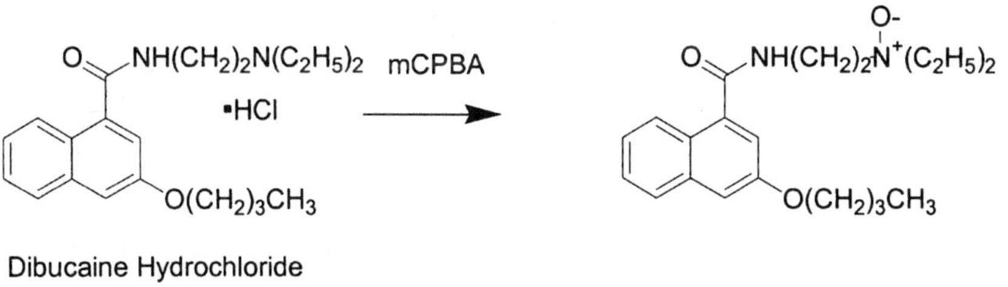

Figure 37 Dibucaine hydrochloride N-oxide formation.

raloxifene hydrochloride (54). Oxidation of aryl amines leads to aryl hydroxylamines, which are susceptible to further oxidation to aryl nitroso compounds.

Heteroaromatic amines can oxidize to the corresponding N-oxide, which are typically stable enough to be isolated and detected as degradation products. The N-oxide functionality typically increases the reactivity of the aromatic ring. For example, the N-oxide functionality in pyridine N-oxide facilitates both electrophilic and nucleophilic substitution at the alpha and gamma positions (57).

Aliphatic amines are subject to simple hydrolysis to the resulting hydroxyl compound or elimination to form a double bond. In either case, ammonia is released from the API.

Using oxidation conditions of *m*-chloroperbenzoic acid, the API dibucaine can be easily oxidized to its N-oxide analog (Fig. 37) (58). An additional example includes the API flavoxate hydrochloride, which degrades to the corresponding N-oxide in 3% aqueous hydrogen peroxide (59).

Dealkylation is also a common degradation reaction for amines (Fig. 38). As shown in the mechanistic scheme, dealkylation involves oxidation of the amine by peroxide followed by decomposition (dehydration) of the hydroxylamine to the corresponding imine. Water attack on the imine occurs to yield the corresponding primary amine and aldehyde.

An example of a tertiary amine dealkylation via oxidative degradation is seen with diphenoxylate hydrochloride (Fig. 32). An example of a secondary amine dealkylation via oxidative degradation, the API brinzolamide undergoes a dealkylation reaction converting the secondary amine to a primary amine in the presence of heat, light (neutral pH), and peroxide

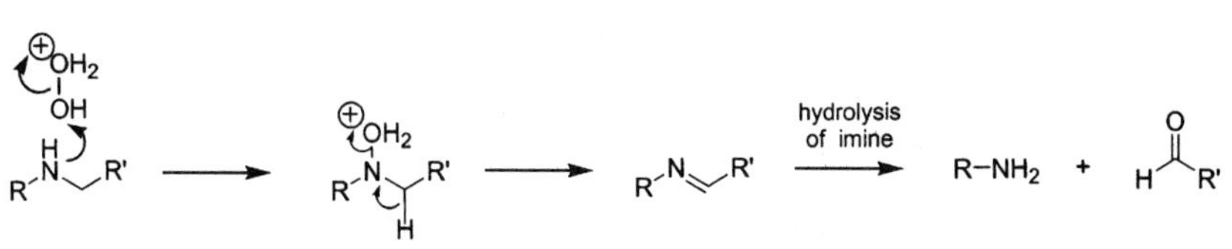

Figure 38 Proposed mechanism of amine dealkylation.

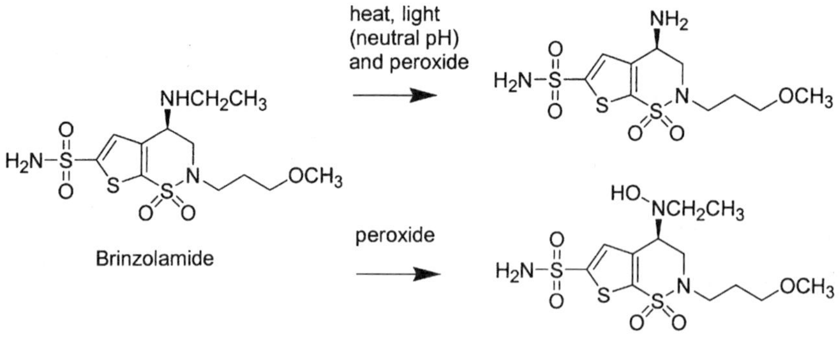

Figure 39 Brinzolamide oxidative degradation leading to N-dealkylation.

(Fig. 39). In the presence of peroxide, brinzolamide also undergoes conversion to the corresponding hydroxylamine (60).

In the presence of light, dorsolamide hydrochloride also undergoes amine dealkylation from a secondary to a primary amine, which presumably occurs via oxidation to the hydroxylamine, dehydration to the imine, and subsequent hydrolysis to form the primary amine (Fig. 40) (61).

The API bumetanide reacts under acidic conditions to the convert the secondary amine into the corresponding primary amine (Fig. 41) (62). The mechanism is analogous to the Hofmann–Martius reaction resulting in the debutylated amine and *n*-butyl chloride (the chloride presumably comes from HCl) (63).

3. Amines–Reaction with Formaldehyde and Other Aldehydes

Formaldehyde, along with other short-chain aldehydes such as acetaldehyde, is a low molecular weight, volatile, reactive contaminant that can be present at low levels from a variety of sources (e.g., excipients such as polyethylene oxide, polyethylene glycol (64,65), or from carbohydrate degradation (66), solvent contamination (51), packaging materials (52), etc.). Formaldehyde is known to react with amines (Fig. 33) to form a reactive N-hydroxymethyl compound (a hemiaminal) that can further react with other nucleophiles. Reaction of formaldehyde with amino acids (67) can cause

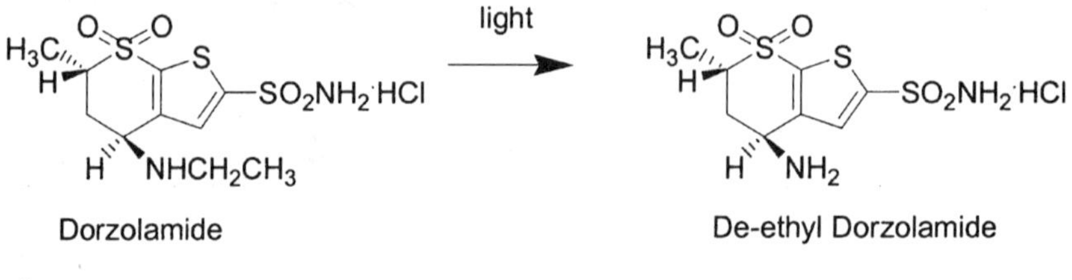

Figure 40 Dorzolamide photodegradation leads to N-dealkylation.

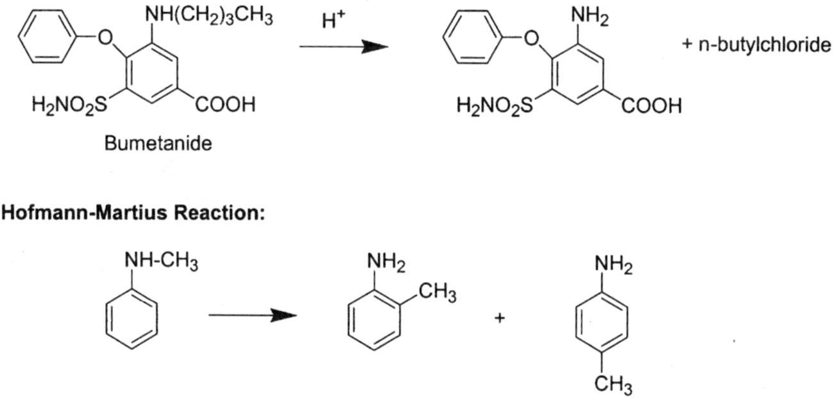

Figure 41 Bumetanide degradation under acidic conditions.

cross-linking of amino groups in gelatin to form an insoluble protein (68), which can inhibit dissolution of gelatin capsules (69). Because of its ubiquitous nature and propensity to react with pharmaceutical products (70), it has been suggested that exposure of APIs to formaldehyde should be considered for inclusion into routine "preformulation screens" (71). In addition, reaction of amines with formic acid can occur to yield N-formyl adducts.

The importance of and potential for reaction of APIs with aldehydes is illustrated by the L-tryptophan impurities incident. In 1989, a link between an outbreak of eosinophilia–myalgia syndrome (EMS) and the use of L-tryptophan as an over-the-counter dietary supplement was made. The outbreak of EMS resulted in more than 36 deaths and greater than 1500 serious illnesses (72). The L-tryptophan linked to this outbreak was manufactured by a single firm in Japan, and low levels of impurities present in lots manufactured by this firm have been postulated as the agents responsible for this toxic reaction, In particular, the impurity 1,1′-ethylidenebis(L-tryptophan), also known as EBT, was identified as a possible causal agent (73,74). This impurity is the reaction product of acetaldehyde and two molecules of L-tryptophan during the synthesis (Fig. 42). A definitive correlation of EMS with EBT or other impurities present in the L-tryptophan supplement was not made, however, possibly because of the difficulty of establishing an accurate animal model for the disease and the uncertainties in extrapolating such results to humans. Regardless, this significant tragedy has served to underscore the importance of developing an understanding of the potential impurities present from either processing or degradation.

4. Amines–The Maillard Reaction

The Maillard reaction, first described by Louis Maillard in 1912 (40), is not a single reaction but rather a collection of complex reactions between some

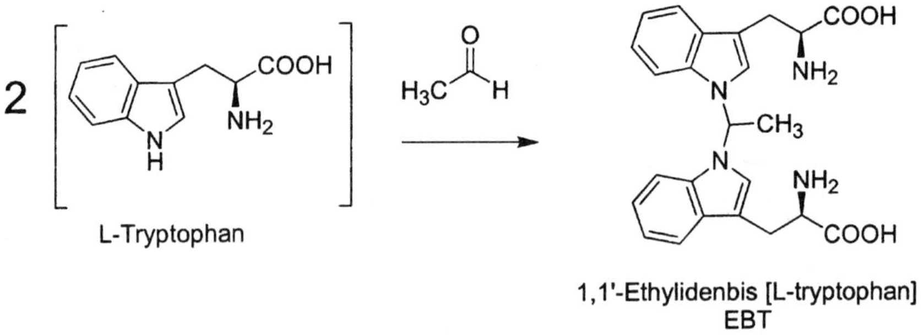

2 L-Tryptophan H_3C–CHO → 1,1'-Ethylidenbis [L-tryptophan] EBT

Figure 42 Reaction of L-tryptophan with acetaldehyde to form EBT.

amines and reducing sugars, resulting in the production of brown pigments (75). This reaction is sometimes known as the "Maillard browning reaction," and has been extensively studied and reviewed (40,76). The article by Wirth et al. (40) is an excellent starting point for understanding the chemistry of this degradation pathway and its relevance to pharmaceuticals. The Maillard reaction is classically represented by considering the reaction of a primary amine with a reducing sugar in its aldehydic form. The chemistry of the Maillard reaction is represented in Figure 43. The initial steps show that the anomeric carbon of a reducing sugar (e.g., lactose) is susceptible to nucleophilic attack by amines, which, upon loss of OH^-, gives rise to an unstable iminium ion. This iminium ion species can lose a proton and tautomerize to form an α-amino ketone that is known as the "Amadori rearrangement product" (ARP) (77).

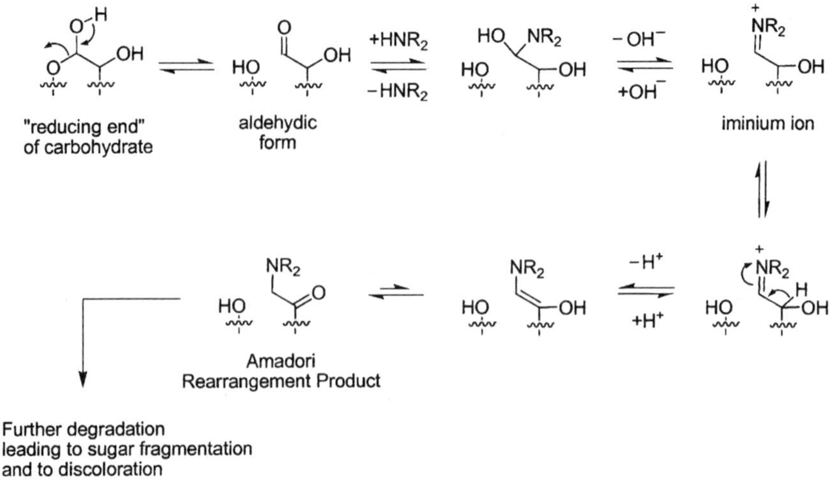

"reducing end" of carbohydrate ⇌ aldehydic form ⇌ (+HNR_2 / −HNR_2) ⇌ (−OH^- / +OH^-) iminium ion ⇌ (−H^+ / +H^+) ⇌ Amadori Rearrangement Product → Further degradation leading to sugar fragmentation and to discoloration

Figure 43 Initial steps of the Maillard browning reaction involving an Amadori rearrangement stable intermediate.

A lesser-known degradation reaction of amines is the propensity to undergo formylation upon extended storage in formulations with carbohydrates, especially reducing sugars such as lactose. This has been described by Wirth et al. (40a) in a study of the reaction of fluoxetine hydrochloride with lactose (Fig. 44).

The ARP is an important intermediate in the Maillard reaction. Under pharmaceutically relevant storage conditions, the ARP can accumulate as an impurity to significant levels as was described in the cases of fluoxetine hydrochloride (40a) and pregabalin (78). As shown in Figure 44, in the case of fluoxetine–lactose formulations, the glycosylamine is also observed as a significant degradation product. It should be noted that although the structure of the fluoxetine–lactose ARP is shown as acyclic, it will exist in solution as a mixture of pyranose and furanose forms, both of which are diastereomeric (79). Thus, the ARP may be observed chromatographically as several peaks, possibly interconverting on-column. In addition to the glycosylamine and ARP degradation products, another significant product identified by Wirth et al. was N-formyl-fluoxetine. The degradation pathway leading to the N-formyl product was not clearly delineated, but must be the result of reaction of the secondary amine with a small fragment of the lactose skeleton. Glyoxal was proposed as a possible formylating agent that could result from the degradation of ARP. Regardless of the precise mechanism of formation, N-formylation should be considered as a possible degradation pathway for formulations of amine-containing APIs with reducing (e.g., lactose) and possibly non-reducing (e.g., microcrystalline cellulose) carbohydrate excipients.

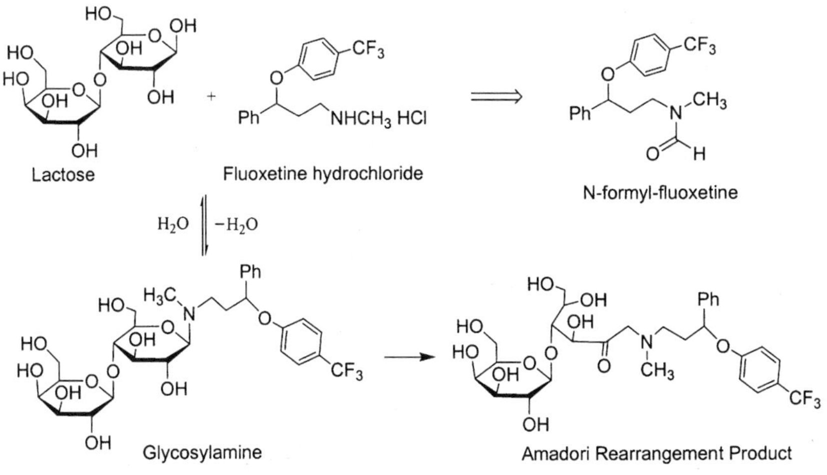

Lactose + Fluoxetine hydrochloride ⟹ N-formyl-fluoxetine

H_2O ⇅ $-H_2O$

Glycosylamine ⟶ Amadori Rearrangement Product

Figure 44 Maillard reaction of lactose and fluoxetine HC1 yielding major degradants glycosylamine, Amadori rearrangement product, and N-formyl fluoxetine.

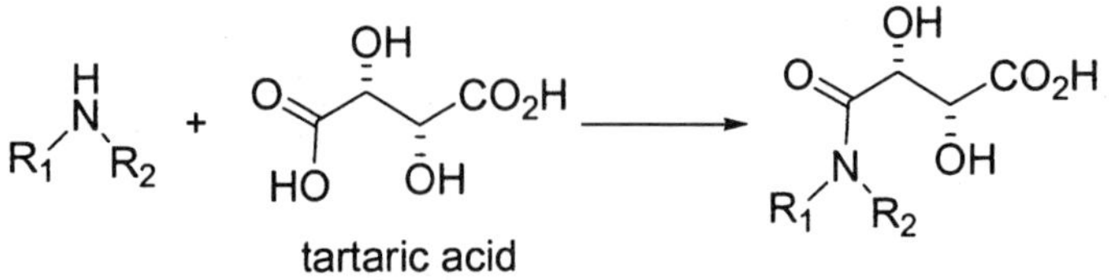

Figure 45 Amine reaction with tartaric acid.

The Maillard reaction is more susceptible with amorphous lactose than with crystalline lactose; therefore, this reaction is expected to be more of a concern for spray-dried material (80). Since the reaction is acid/base catalyzed, it is ideal to maintain a neutral pH environment with lactose-based products.

5. Amines–Reaction with Salts and Excipients Containing Carboxylic Acids

Amines are particularly prone to reaction with excipients and salt counterions, as shown in Figure 45 for tartaric acid. The potential for a reaction with magnesium stearate or stearic acid is particularly of concern with an API containing a primary amine. In the case of norfloxacin, formation of a stearoyl derivative was observed in tablets containing magnesium stearate after prolonged storage at 60°C (Fig. 46) (81).

The potential for reaction of a primary amine salt with its counterion is exemplified by seproxetine maleate (82). In formulations with pregelatinized starch, after storage at 25°C and 40°C for 3 months, a 1,4-Michael addition adduct was formed between the primary amine of seproxetine and maleate (Fig. 47). In formulations containing talc, after similar storage, an amide linkage was formed (1,2-addition adduct). While these reactions were not specifically excipient-induced (i.e., the same reactions can occur without the presence of excipients), it is still of interest from a formulation viewpoint since the excipients catalyzed the reactions. It is noteworthy that these reactions were greatly suppressed when using the fumarate salt (the *trans* configuration of maleate).

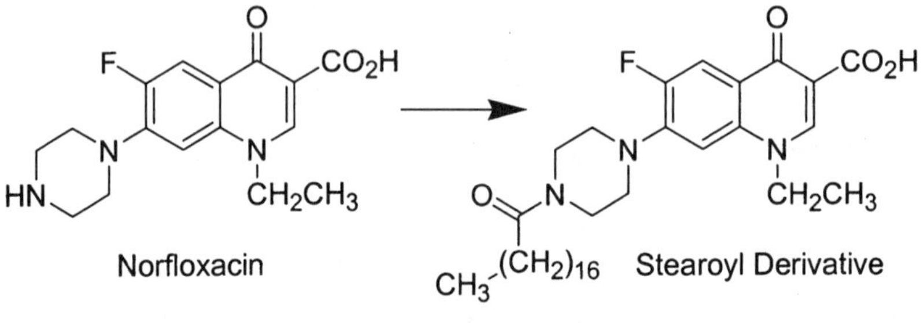

Figure 46 Norfloxain reaction with magnesium stearate.

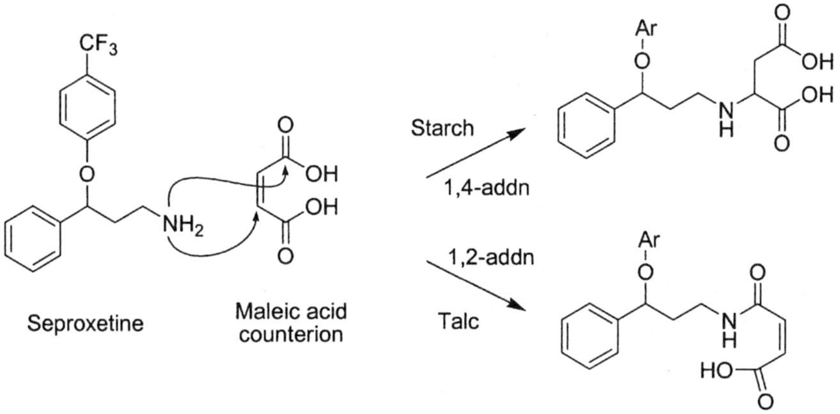

Figure 47 Reaction of a primary amine with its maleate counterion in stressed formulations.

6. Amines–Reaction with Formulation Components

Amines containing APIs have also been known to react with other formulation components such as flavoring agents and even enteric coating constituents. An example of the reaction of a primary amine with a flavoring agent is illustrated in Figure 48 (83). In this example, the API was formulated in a ready-to-use liquid, oil-based formulation, and vanillin was one of the

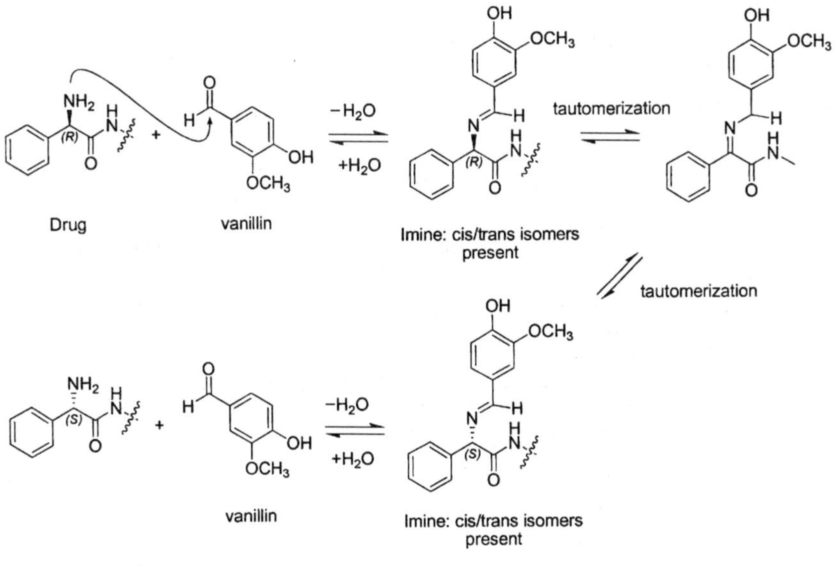

Figure 48 Aldehydes plus amines: reaction of API with flavoring agent.

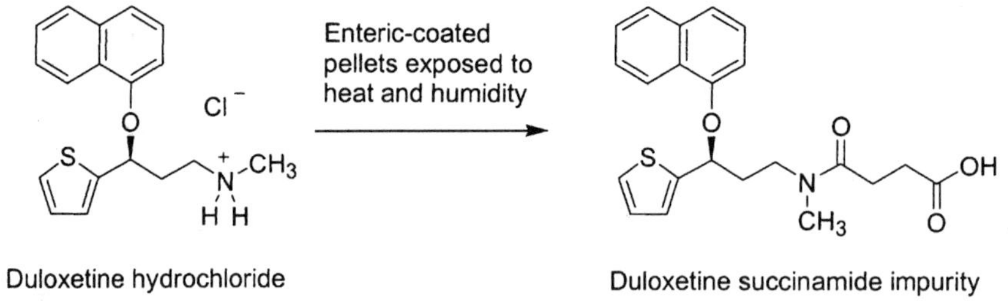

Enteric-coated pellets exposed to heat and humidity

Duloxetine hydrochloride

Duloxetine succinamide impurity

Figure 49 Structures of duloxetine hydrochloride and a low level impurity formed upon aging of enteric-coated pellets.

flavoring components. Upon long-term storage, low levels of new impurities were observed, several of which appeared to be unstable and difficult to isolate. It was determined that the degradation-related impurities were the result of the reaction of the primary amine with the aldehydic functionality of vanillin, leading to cis/trans imines, and also to inversion of the chiral center.

Another example of an amine reacting with a formulation component is found in the case of duloxetine hydrochloride (84). This example, which is also discussed in Chapter 2, is summarized in Figures 49 and 50. In this example, the secondary amine of duloxetine hydrochloride reacted with the enteric coating polymer hydroxypropyl methylcellulose acetate succinate (HPMCAS) to form a succinamide degradation product. This reaction occurred under both stress conditions (60°C for 14 days) and during formal stability studies (30°C/60% relative humidity and 40°C/75% relative

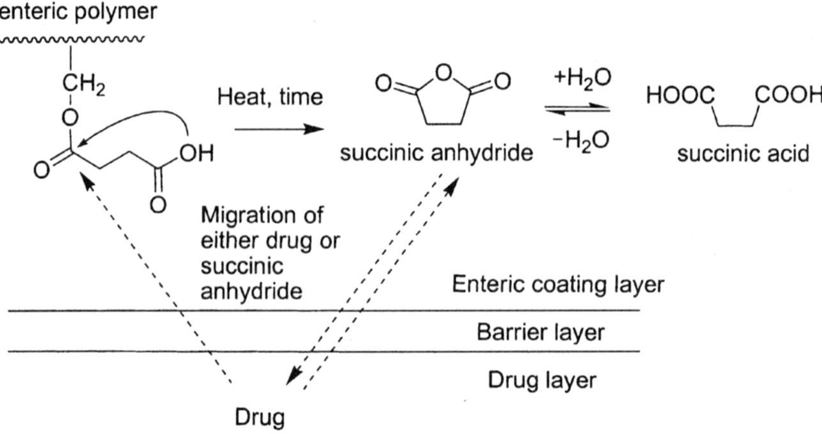

Figure 50 Proposed pathways for the interaction of duloxetine hydrochloride with HPMCAS to form duloxetine succinamide.

humidity). The reaction is especially interesting in that there was a physical separation (different physical layers) of the API from the HPMCAS enteric polymer. Since it was concluded from spiking experiments that duloxetine hydrochloride did not react with free succinic acid present in the enteric polymer layer, an alternate pathway was proposed. It was postulated that the degradation product was forming either via migration of duloxetine hydrochloride to facilitate intimate contact with the polymer, or by degradation of the polymer to form succinic anhydride, which could migrate to the API layer of the formulation (Fig. 50). The degradation reaction was minimized by increasing the size of the barrier layer between the API and enteric polymer layers.

Yet another example of an amine reacting with a formulation component is that of meropenem (85). Meropenem is a secondary amine containing drug substance that is formulated as a blend of crystalline drug and sodium carbonate. It was determined that meropenem exists partially as a covalent, carbon dioxide adduct (a carbamate) in both the solid powder and in the reconstituted solution for injection. Under acidic conditions, the carbamate protonates and the resulting carbamic acid derivative rapidly loses carbon dioxide to regenerate the parent drug. The overall degradation reaction is represented in Figure 51.

7. Imines

Imines readily hydrolyze under basic or acidic conditions. Figure 52 shows the acid-catalyzed hydrolysis of imines. When developing methods to detect imines, it is often necessary to use neutral pH conditions to optimize the stability of the imine. An example of imine formation and hydrolysis is found in the degradation chemistry of the API sertraline hydrochloride (Fig. 53) (86).

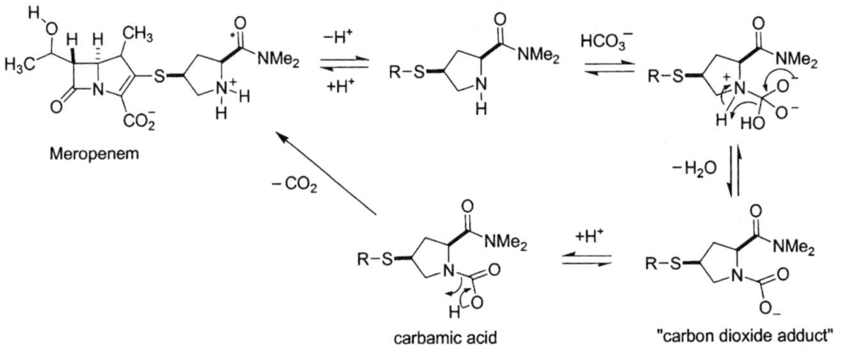

Figure 51 Meropenem, a secondary amine, reacts with sodium carbonate to form a carbon dioxide adduct.

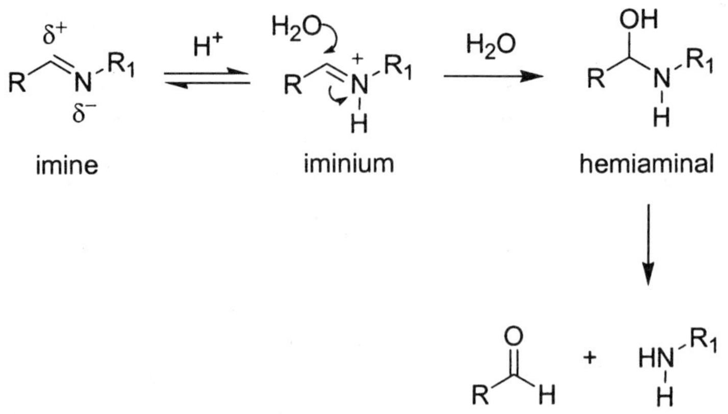

Figure 52 Imine hydrolysis.

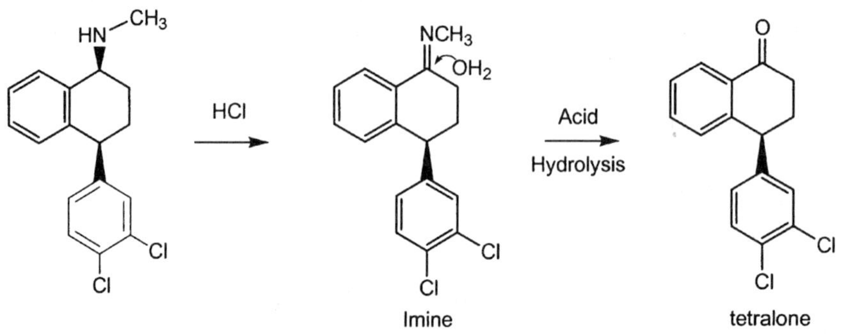

Figure 53 The secondary amine of sertraline hydrochloride is oxidized to an imine and then hydrolyed to a ketone under acidic conditions.

Other API examples include methaqualone (87) and terbutaline sulfate in which the amine converts to an imine followed by imine hydrolysis (88). In the case of diazepam under acidic aqueous conditions, the imine undergoes hydrolysis to the corresponding benzophenone (Fig. 54) (89).

In the case of xylometazoline hydrochloride, imine hydrolysis chemistry occurs to open the 4,5-dihydro-lH-imidazole ring (Fig. 55) (90). Similar degradation chemistry is observed for the following APIs: flurazepam hydrochloride (91), clorazepate dipotassium (92), clonazepam (93), methaqualone (94), chlordiazepoxide, and oxazepam (18).

8. Hydrazines

Hydrazines $[(R)_2\text{-N-N-}(R)_2]$ do not readily hydrolyze. Procarbazine hydrochloride, which contains a hydrazine moiety, undergoes oxidation by atmospheric oxygen in the presence of moisture or in aqueous solution to form

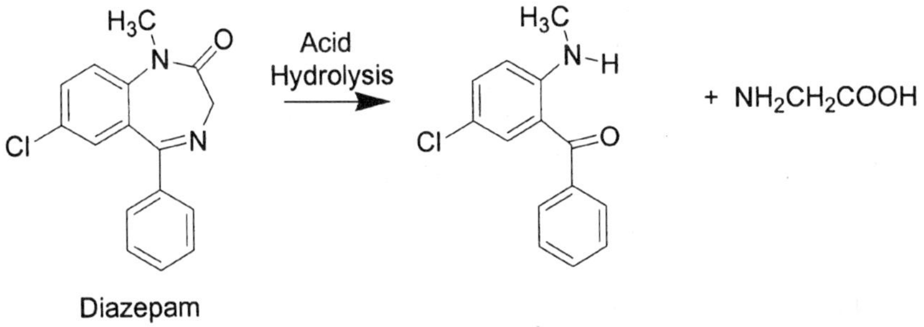

Diazepam

Figure 54 Diazepam acid hydrolysis. Both the imine and the lactam undergo hydrolysis to yield a benzophenone derivative.

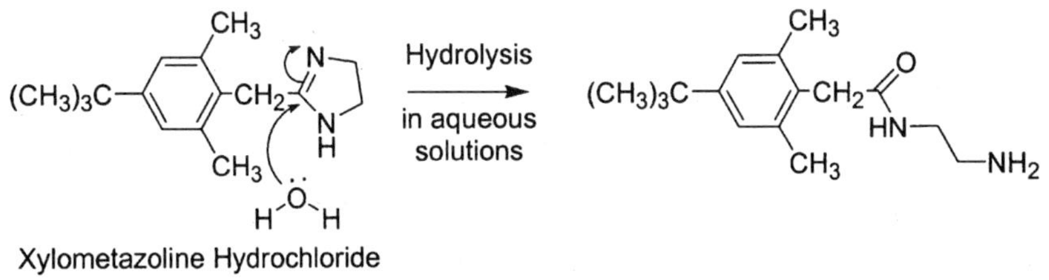

Xylometazoline Hydrochloride

Figure 55 The imine of xylometazoline undergoes ring opening hydrolysis.

the diazene and hydrazone compounds shown in Figure 56. The hydrazone undergoes further decomposition in the presence water to form the resulting aldehyde and hydrazine (analogous to imine degradation chemistry) (95).

9. Enamines

Enamines are susceptible to acid-catalyzed hydrolysis (last step of the Stork enamine reaction) (96). Under acidic conditions, examines protonate to form the tautomeric iminium ion, which undergoes hydrolysis to the ketone as shown in Figure 57. The iminium ion undergoes hydrolysis quite readily since there is a contributing resonance form with a positive charge on the carbon (97).

Enamines are susceptible to photoreactivity with singlet oxygen (singlet oxygen is formed through the photosensitization of ground state molecular oxygen) as shown in Figure 58.

The API nizatidine contains an enamine functionality (Fig. 59). Degradation of the enamine functionality under acid and basic conditions yields the subsequent amine. After irradiation with a mercury lamp in an aqueous solution, nizatidine degraded to the corresponding urea compound from the addition of water to the nitro-substituted enamine followed by cleavage (consistent with the enamine photochemistry scheme, Figure 58) (98).

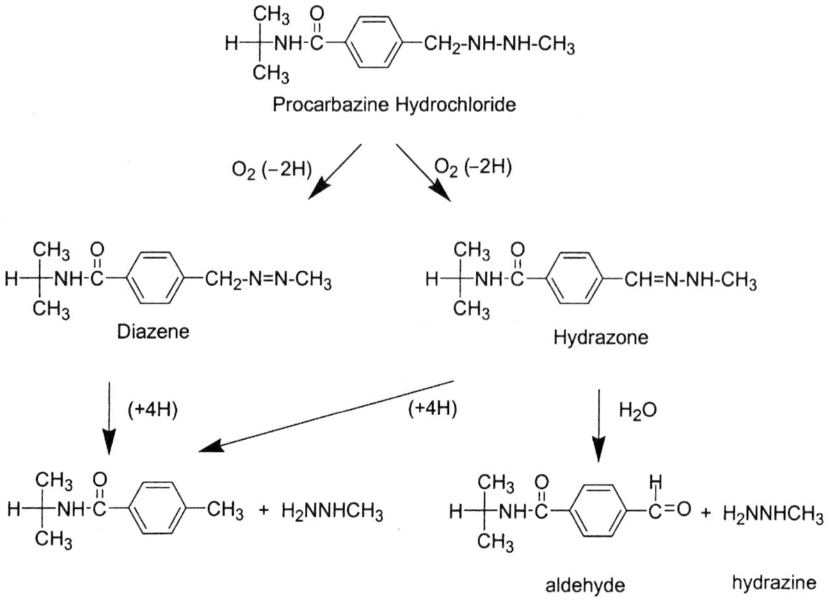

Procarbazine Hydrochloride

Diazene

Hydrazone

aldehyde

hydrazine

Figure 56 Degradation of procarbazine hydrochloride.

enamine

iminium

hemiaminal

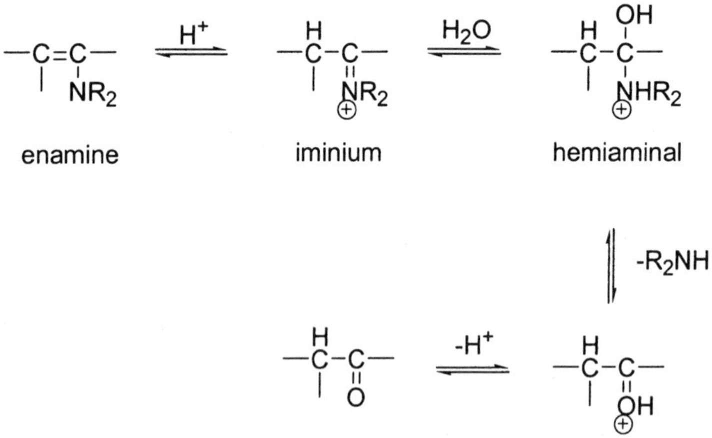

Figure 57 Mechanism of enainine hydrolysis.

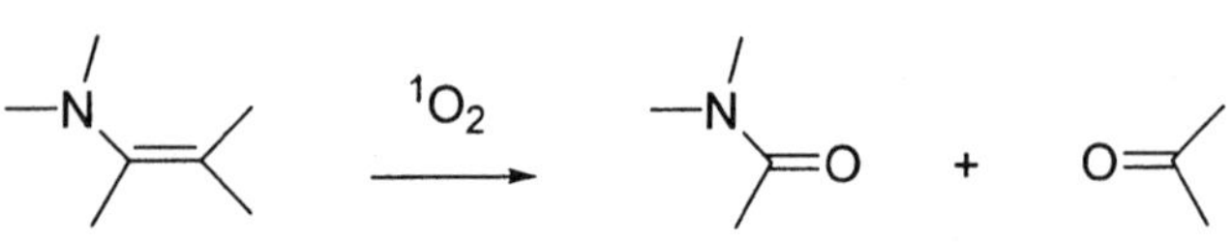

Figure 58 Enamine reaction with singlet oxygen (photochemistry).

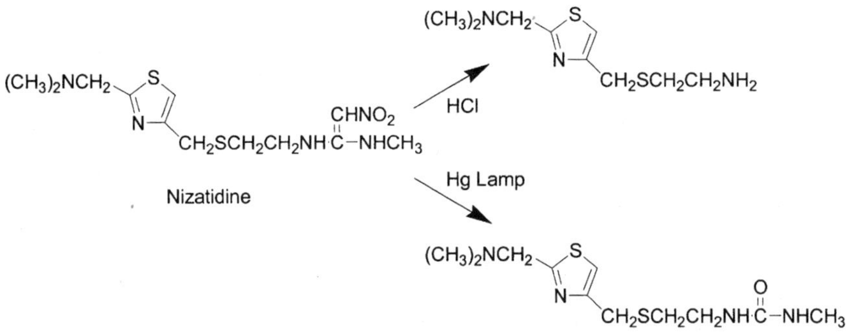

Figure 59 Nizatidine degradation chemistry demonstrates the reactivity of the enamine functionality.

10. Nitro Groups

Certain nitroaromatic groups are susceptible to photochemical reactivity (43). A well-known nitro group degradation reaction occurs for the API nifedipine (Fig. 60). Under ultraviolet as well as visible radiation, the nitro group of nifedipine is rapidly converted to a nitroso compound along with aromatization to a substituted pyridine ring (99). In the presence of molecular oxygen, the nitroso functionality is re-oxidized to the nitro derivative (100).

C. Sulfur-Containing Functional Groups

1. Sulfonamides

Sulfonamides are generally susceptible to acid hydrolysis, but are not readily hydrolyzed under basic conditions (Fig. 61) (101). Primary alcohols react rapidly only with N,N′-disubstituted sulfonamides to yield sulfonic esters. Sulfonamides are not susceptible to oxidation since the sulfur is already oxidized.

Photolysis at 254 nm of arylsulfonamides of aliphatic amines yields the corresponding free amine (102). In the presence of light, the API

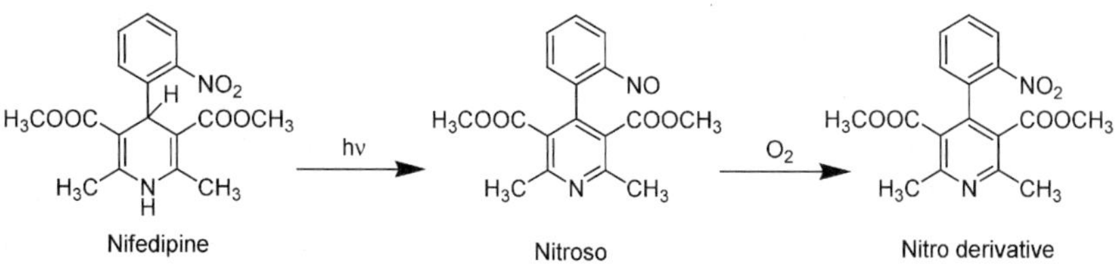

Figure 60 Nifedipine photochemistry.

$$RSO_2NR''_2 + H_2O \xrightarrow{H+} RSO_2OH + NHR''_2$$

$$RSO_2NR''_2 + R'OH \xrightarrow{H+} RSO_2OR' + NHR''_2$$

Figure 61 Sulfonamide degradation chemistry.

brinzolamide in solution undergoes cleavage of the sulfonamide to yield the corresponding des-sulfonamide (Fig. 62) (103).

The API sulfamerazine undergoes hydrolysis on the sulfonamide group to form the products shown in Figure 63 (104). The API sulfamethazine degrades under acidic conditions to produce sulfanilic acid and 2-amino-4,6-dimethyl-pyrimidine (105). Additionally, aryl hydrolysis also occurs to yield the 2-hydroxy-4-methylpyrimidine and sulphanilamide.

2. Sulfonylureas

Sulfonylureas undergo hydrolysis as shown in the mechanistic scheme in Figure 64 (106). Under acid-catalyzed conditions, water addition leads to loss of an amine and formation of a carbamic acid derivative. Acid-catalyzed loss of CO_2 from the carbamic acid derivative yields the corresponding sulfonamide. It was proposed that initial protonation is the rate-determining step in the hydrolysis.

An example of an API containing the sulfonylurea functionality is glibenclamide (Fig. 65) (107). Acid degradation produces the corresponding sulfonamide, amine, and carbon dioxide.

D. Thiols, Ethers, Epoxides, Aziridines

1. Thiols

Thiols can hydrolyze to the corresponding hydroxyl via acid or base catalysis, releasing hydrogen sulfide in the process (Fig. 66). Thiols are ionizable and will typically exist as the anion at pHs higher than 8–9 (pK_a's depend, of course, on the substituents and can vary substantially).

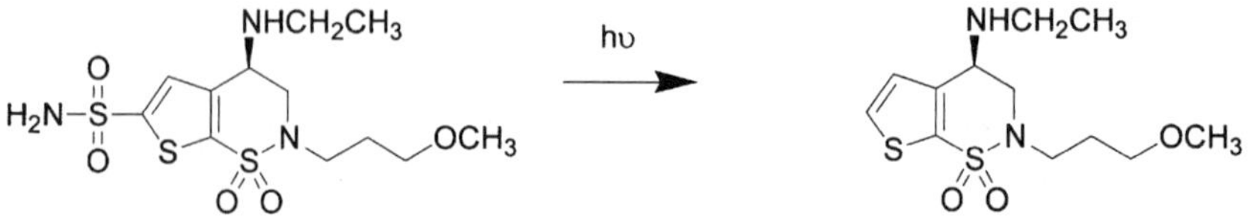

Figure 62 Photodegradation chemistry of the sulfonamide-containing brinzolamide.

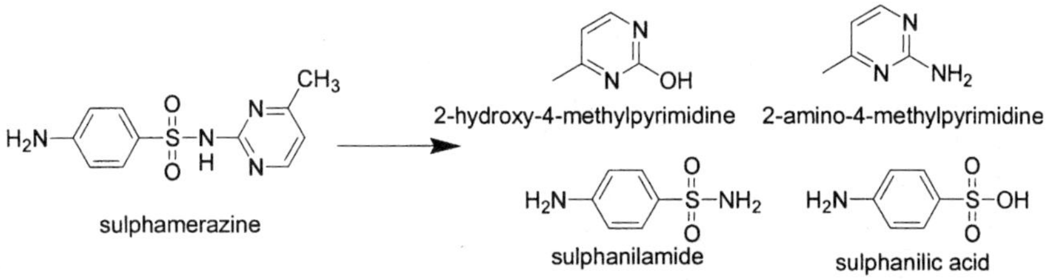

Figure 63 Sulfamerazine degradation chemistry under hydrolytic conditions.

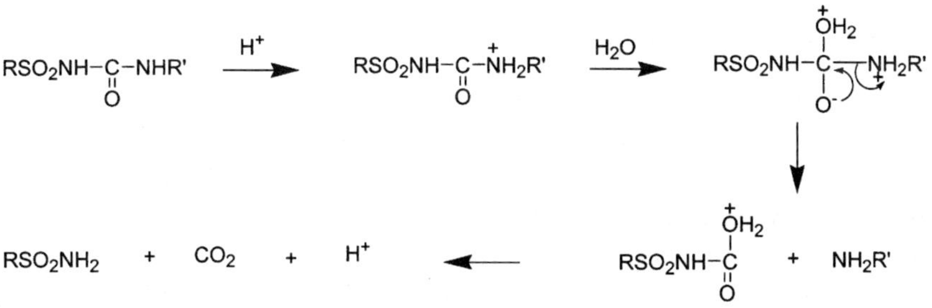

Figure 64 Sulfonylurea hydrolysis chemistry.

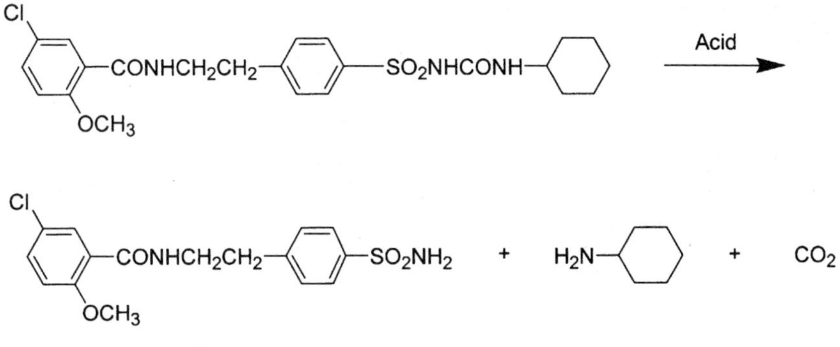

Figure 65 Glibenclamide sulfonylurea hydrolysis chemistry.

$$R\text{-}SH \xrightarrow{H^+/OH^-} R\text{-}OH + H_2S$$

Figure 66 Thiol hydrolysis reaction scheme.

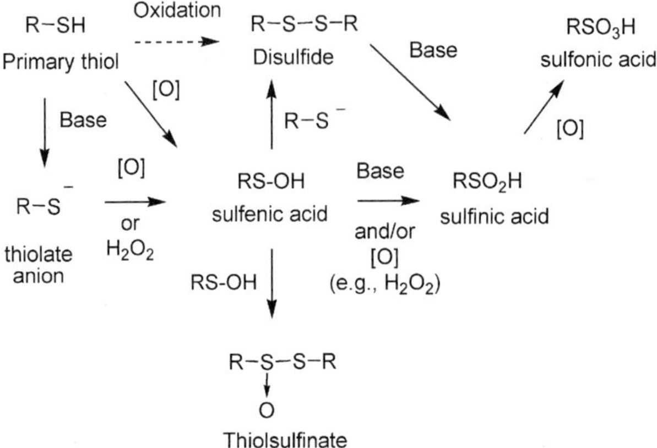

Figure 67 Oxidative degradation pathways of thiols.

Thiols are susceptible to oxidation by peroxides, molecular oxygen, and other oxidizing processes (e.g., radical-catalyzed oxidation) (Fig. 67). Because thiols easily complex with transition metals, it is believed that most thiol autoxidation reactions are metal-catalyzed (108). Autoxidation of thiols is enhanced by deprotonation of the thiol to the thiolate anion. Thiol oxidation commonly leads to disulfides, although further autoxidation to the sulfinic and, ultimately, sulfonic acid can be accomplished under basic conditions. Disulfides can be reduced back to the thiol (e.g., upon addition of a reducing agent such as dithiothreitol). Thiols are nucleophilic and will readily react with available electrophilic sites. For a more thorough discussion, see Hovorka and Schöneich (108) and Luo et al. (200).

2. Ethers, Thioethers

Both ethers and thioethers can be hydolyzed via acid-catalysis to the corresponding alcohol or thiol, respectively, but are reasonably stable to neutral and basic conditions (Fig. 68).

Ether hydrolysis is observed for the API timolol maleate. Under pH 5 aqueous autoclave conditions (120°C), three degradants were isolated.

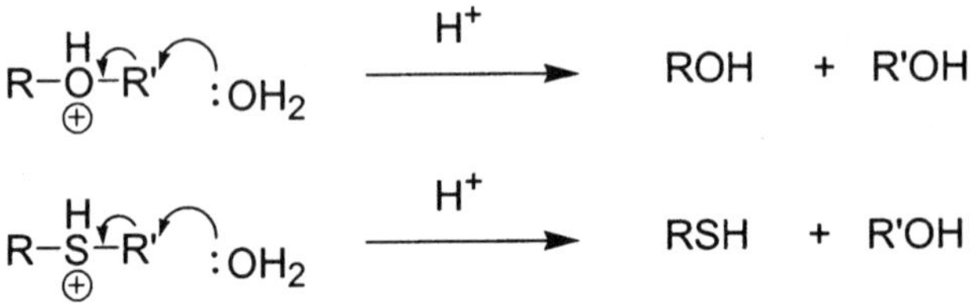

$$R{-}\overset{H}{\underset{\oplus}{O}}{-}R' \quad :OH_2 \xrightarrow{H^+} ROH + R'OH$$

$$R{-}\overset{H}{\underset{\oplus}{S}}{-}R' \quad :OH_2 \xrightarrow{H^+} RSH + R'OH$$

Figure 68 Ether, thioether hydrolysis under acidic conditions.

Figure 69 depicts the degradants and the proposed degradation pathway involving: (1) rearrangement to isotimolol, (2) ether cleavage to form 4-hydroxy-3-morpholino-l,2,5-thiadiazole, and (3) oxidation followed by ether cleavage to form 4-hydroxy-3-morpholino-l,2,5-thiadiazole-l-oxide (109).

Duloxetine hydrochloride is an example of an aryl ether that is particularly unstable to hydrolysis under acidic conditions (84). The acid instability led to the development of an enteric-coated formulation to protect the compound from the acidic environment of the stomach. The reason for the susceptibility to hydrolysis is the stability of the cationic intermediate (Fig. 70), which is stabilized by delocalization into the aromatic thiophene ring. See Chapter 2 for additional discussion of the chemistry of this compound.

Thioether hydrolysis is observed for the API cefamandole nafate under slightly acidic, slightly basic and aqueous photolysis conditions to the resulting thiol and alcohol (Fig. 71) (110).

Additional examples of thioether hydrolysis in solution include the API moxalactam disodium to form thiotetrazole (111). Thioethers are susceptible to oxidation to sulfoxides and sulfones (Fig. 72).

Ethers are susceptible to autoxidation (i.e., radical-initiated oxidation) to form unstable hydroperoxides. These hydroperoxides can decompose through various pathways to yield the corresponding alcohols, carboxylic

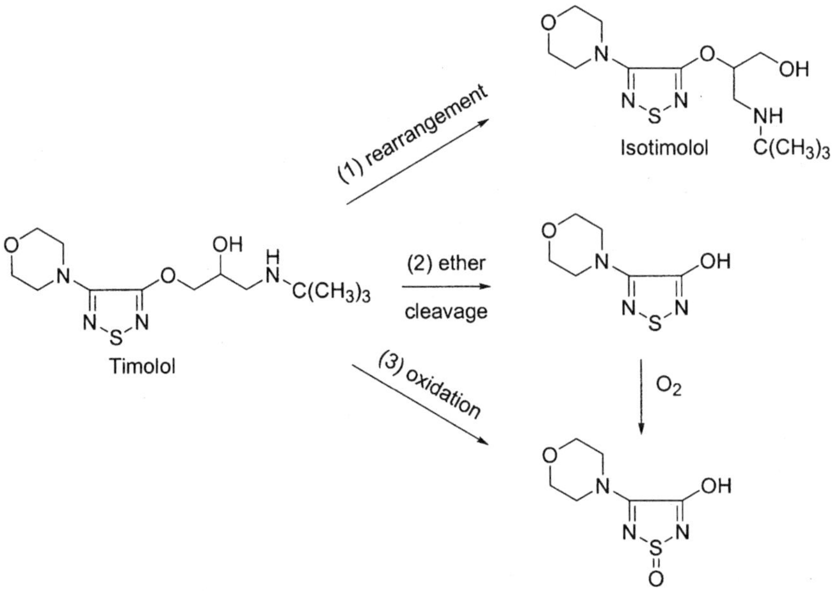

Figure 69 Proposed aqueous solution (aqueous autoclave conditions, 120°C (degradation pathway for timolol maleate.

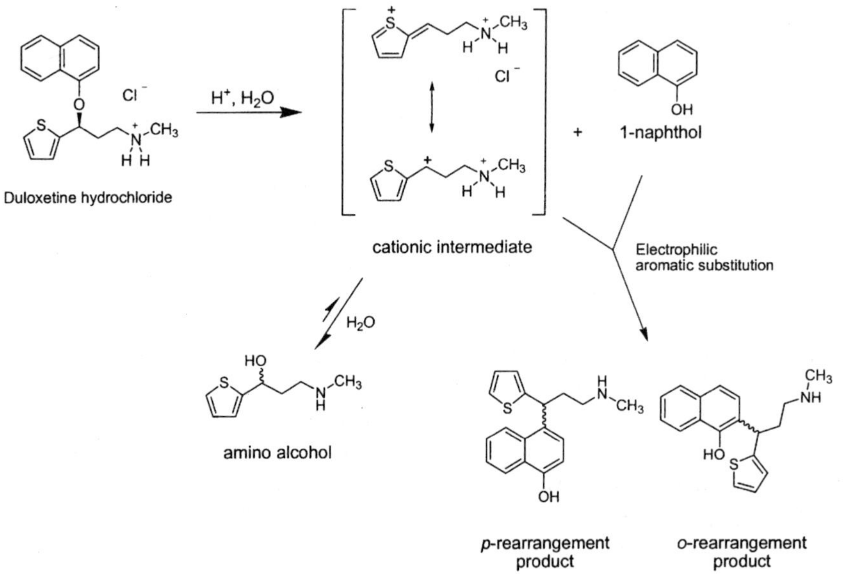

Duloxetine hydrochloride

H^+, H_2O

cationic intermediate

1-naphthol

Electrophilic aromatic substitution

H_2O

amino alcohol

p-rearrangement product

o-rearrangement product

Figure 70 Hydrolysis of the ether linkage of duloxetine hydrochloride under acidic conditions.

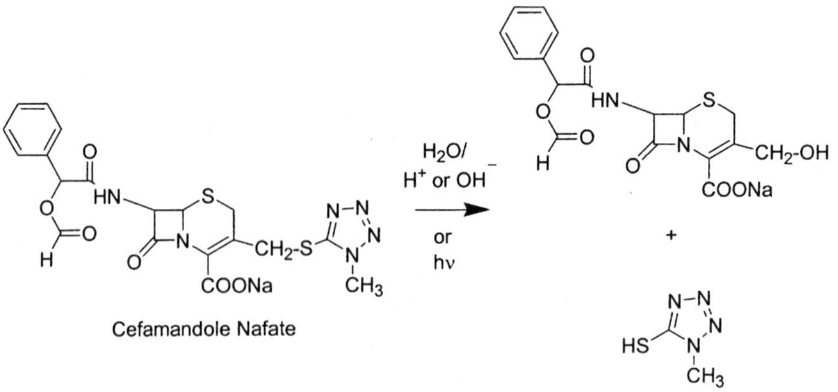

H_2O/ H^+ or OH^- or hν

Cefamandole Nafate

Figure 71 Hydrolysis of the thioether in cefamandole.

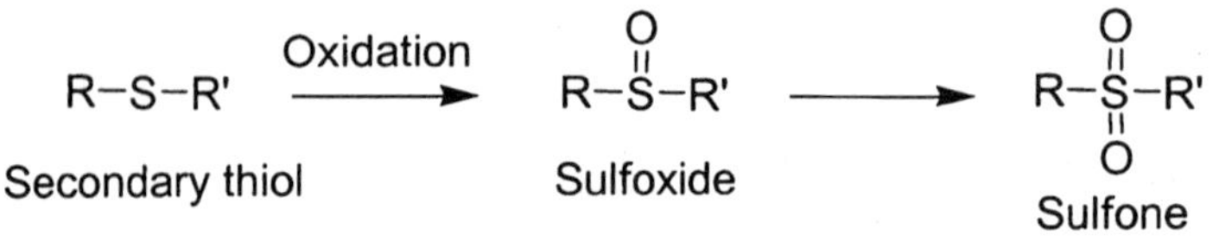

R–S–R' —Oxidation→ R–S(=O)–R' → R–S(=O)(=O)–R'

Secondary thiol Sulfoxide Sulfone

Figure 72 Oxidation of thioethers.

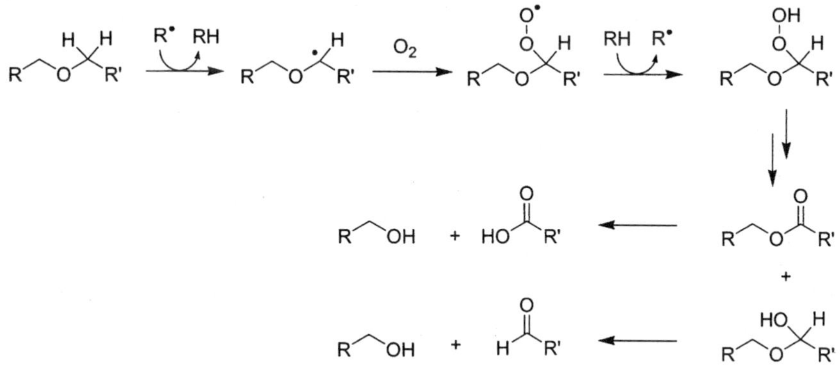

Figure 73 Oxidative degradation of ethers.

acids, and aldehydes (Fig. 73). Ether oxidation can occur at the carbon α to the oxygen. Initiation occurs to generate a radical stabilized by the α-oxygen. Molecular oxygen can then add to the radical at the diffusion-controlled rate followed by hydrogen atom abstraction to yield the corresponding hydroperoxide which can subsequently decompose to the ester and aldehyde secondary degradation products (Fig. 73): Hydrolysis of the ester yields a carboxylic acid and an alcohol.

The API fluphenazine enanthate undergoes oxidation of a secondary aryl thioether to the resulting sulfoxide (Fig. 74) (112).

Additional API examples of thioether to sulfoxide degradation include cimetidine (113), timolol (114), nizatidine (115). The API pergolide mesylate degrades to the corresponding sulfoxide as well as the sulfone (Fig. 75) under light exposures of 3×10^6 lux-hrs or upon aging under long-term storage conditions (116).

The API fenoprofen calcium is a diaryl ether. Degradation of fenoprofen under intense ultraviolet light in solution yields a mixture of isomeric biphenyls via a photo-Fries rearrangement mechanism (Fig. 76) (117).

3. Epoxides

Epoxides are typically very reactive functional groups that are susceptible to nucleophilic attack by water (hydrolysis to form diols) or other

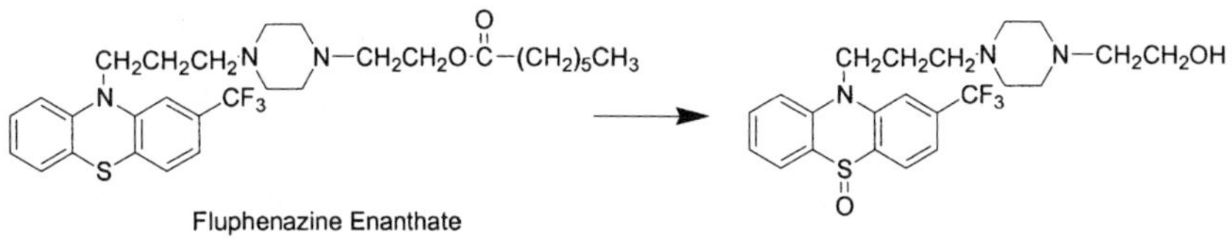

Fluphenazine Enanthate

Figure 74 Oxidation of the thioether of fluphenazine enanthate to the sulfoxide.

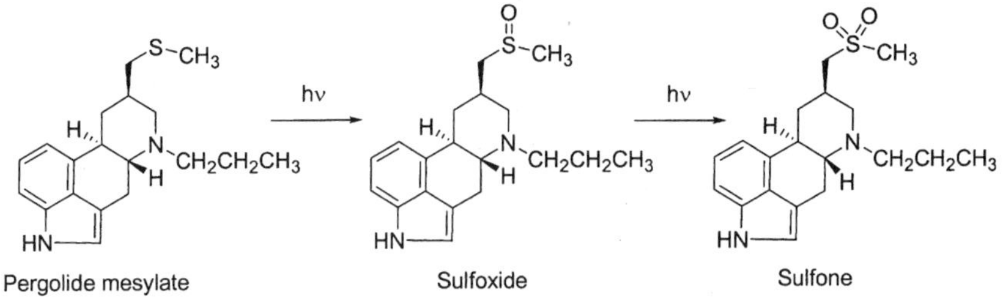

Pergolide mesylate
Sulfoxide
Sulfone

Figure 75 The thioether of pergolide mesylate oxidizes to the sulfoxide and sulfone in the presence of light or during long-term storage.

nucleophiles. The three-membered oxirane ring contains significant strain and the ring opening relieves this strain. Hydrolysis to the diol is catalyzed by both acid (S_N1 mechanism, cationic intermediate) and base (S_N2 mechanism, direct nucleophilic attack). The diol formed from hydrolysis of the

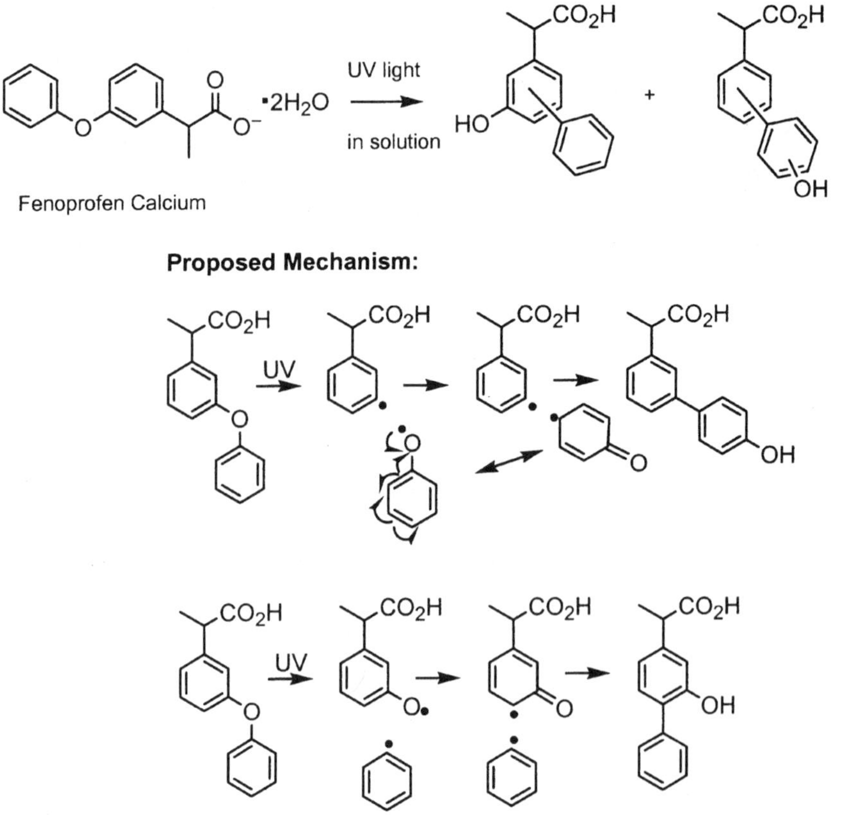

Fenoprofen Calcium

Proposed Mechanism:

Figure 76 Fenoprofen calcium photodegradation and proposed mechanism.

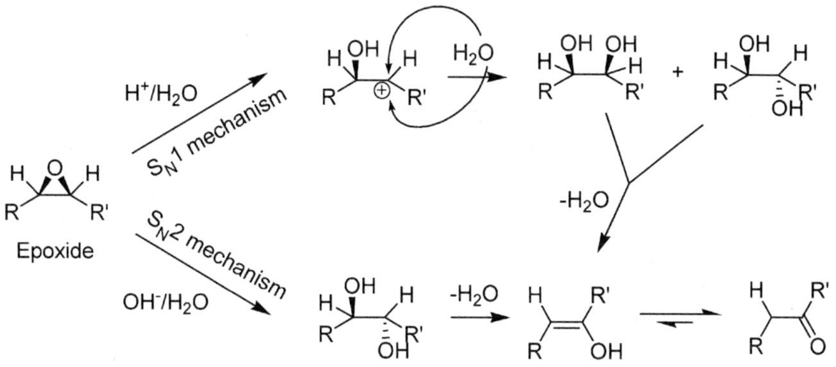

Figure 77 Hydrolysis of an epoxide via acid or base catalysis.

epoxide ring may react further by dehydration and tautomerization to form a ketone, as shown in Figure 77.

4. Aziridines

Aziridines, nitrogen containing three-membered rings, are also subject to ring opening reactions, in the same manner as epoxides. The API mitomycin C contains an aziridine ring. In aqueous acidic solutions, aziridine ring opening occurs with retention of configuration at C2 and water attack at Cl from both faces (S_N1 mechanism) yielding *cis* and *trans*-mitosene (Fig. 78) (119). In basic solutions, the aziridine ring remains intact, with nucleophilic attack on the quinone to hydrolyze the amine, yielding 7-hydroxymitosane.

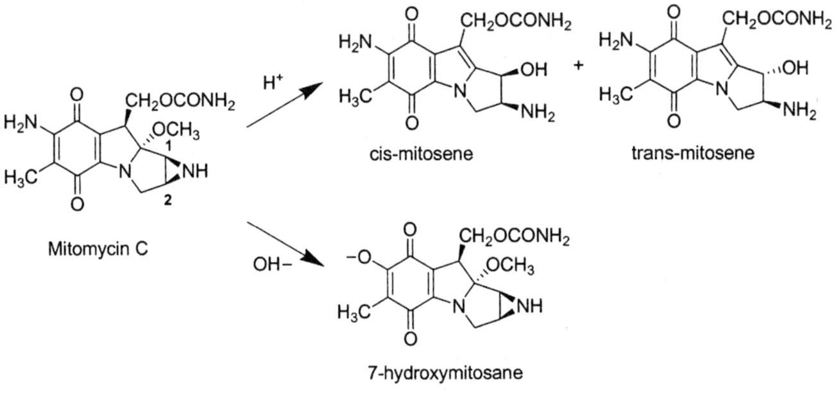

Figure 78 Hydrolysis reactions of Mitomycin C involving acid-catalyzed (S_N1 mechanisms) aziridine ring opening to *cis* and *trans*-mitosene and base-catalyzed, hydrolysis of the amino moiety.

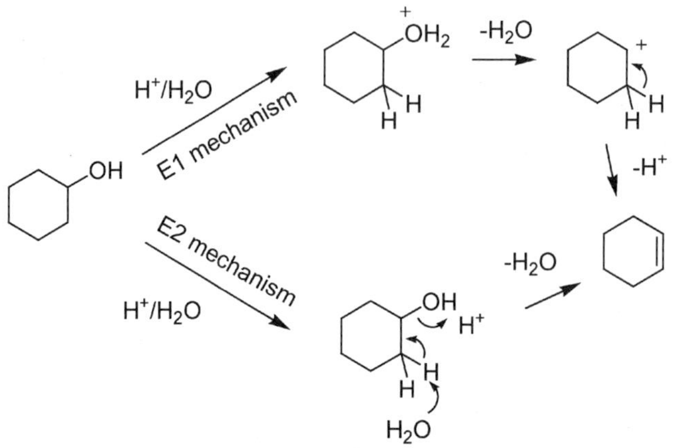

Figure 79 Acid-catalyzed alcohol dehydration.

E. Hydroxyls Groups, Alkyl Halides

1. Hydroxyls

Hydroxyls can act as nucleophiles, although they are less nucleophilic than amines or thiols. Under acidic conditions, hydroxyls can be eliminated in a dehydration reaction (Fig. 79). Elimination reactions can occur as an El reaction (elimination unimolecular) or E2 reaction (elimination bimolecular). The El elimination mechanism proceeds through formation of a carbocation intermediate as the rate-determining step with loss of water whereas the E2 mechanism is second order with the base abstraction of a proton and loss of the leaving group occurring simultaneously (120).

Elimination reaction occurs under acidic conditions for the API vitamin D analog to yield the corresponding major degradation products, E/Z isomers (Fig. 80) (121).

Hydroxyls are not readily ionizable under normal pH conditions (e.g., pH 1–13). Hydroxyls have often been observed to participate in intramole-

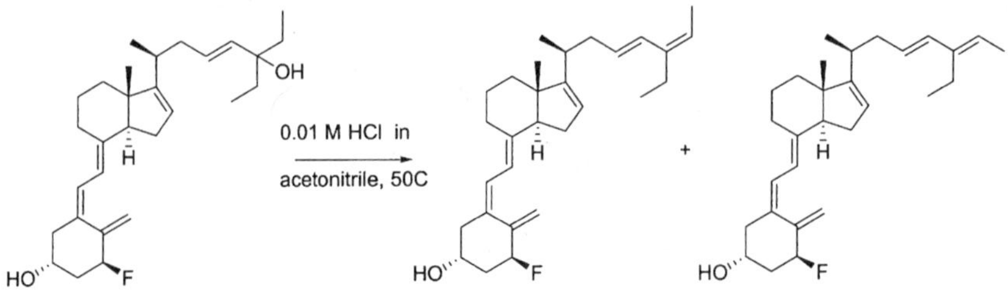

Figure 80 Vitamin D analog degradation under aqueous conditions leads to elimination of the tertiary alcohol.

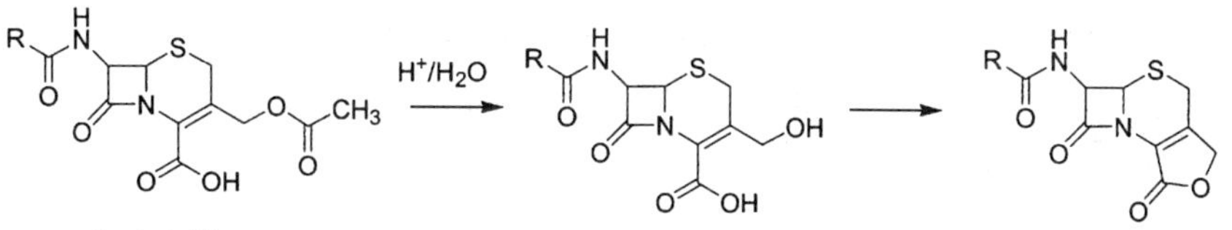

Cephalothin

Figure 81 Lactone formation from intramolecular hydroxyl attack on a carboxylic acid.

cular cyclization reactions to form lactones from carboxylic acids, esters, and thioesters, especially if the lactone formed is a five- or six-membered ring. This kind of degradation reaction is illustrated by degradation studies of the β-lactam antibiotic cephalothin (122) (Fig. 81).

Under oxidative stress conditions, primary and secondary hydroxyls can be oxidized to the corresponding aldehyde and ketone derivatives. Oxidation of a secondary hydroxyl to a ketone (4′-oxolactone) is observed for the API lovastatin (Fig. 82) (123).

Tertiary hydroxyls can undergo several reactions under acidic conditions to form artifacts in degradation experiments. In acidic acetonitrile/water solutions, primary, secondary and tertiary alcohols can undergo a Ritter reaction to form amides (Fig. 83).

It has also been observed that tertiary hydroxyls form chloro artifact compounds under acidic conditions using HCl (Fig. 84).

Ester formation with hydroxyl-containing APIs has been observed for acid salts (e.g., succinic acid, citric acid, formic acid, acetic acid, etc.) as well as excipients (e.g., stearic acid, magnesium stearate). See Figure 85 for an example of the reaction of a hydroxyl group with succinic acid (124).

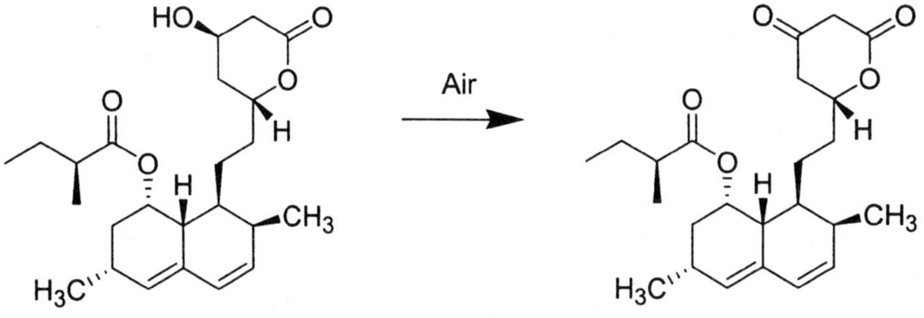

Lovastatin

Oxolactone

Figure 82 Degradation of Lovastatin via oxidation of a secondary hydroxyl to a ketone.

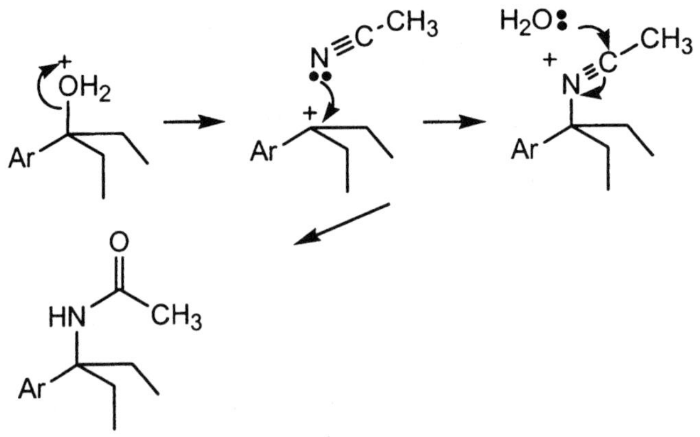

Figure 83 Ritter reaction of tertiary alcohols to form amides under acidic conditions in acetonitrile.

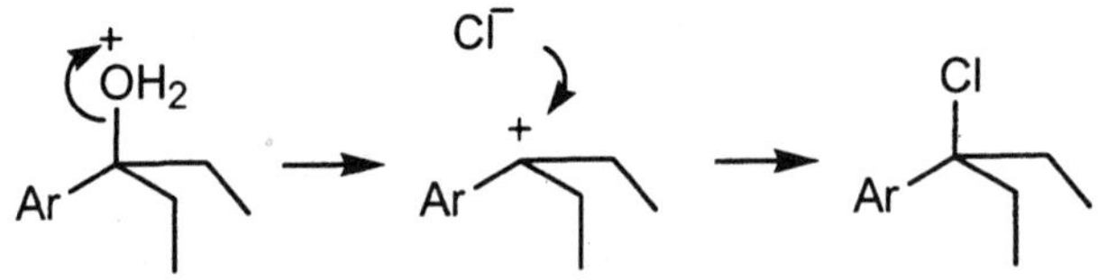

Figure 84 Formation of chloro artifact compounds under acidic (HCl) conditions.

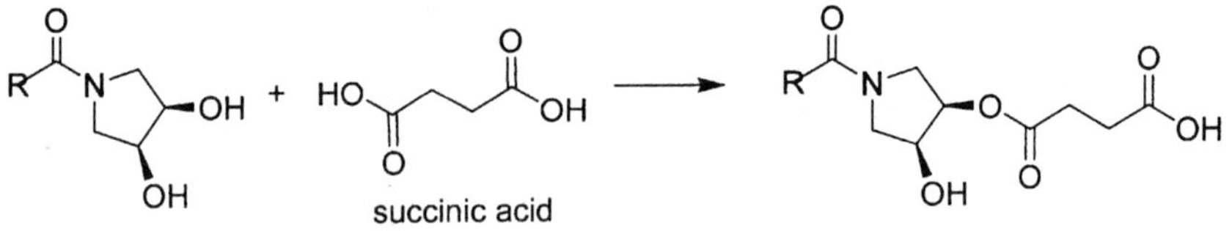

Figure 85 Esterification reaction of a hydroxyl-containing API and its counterion, succinic acid.

2. Phenols

Phenols are known to undergo facile oxidation, and the oxidative chemistry has been studied extensively. For a review, see Ref. 125. The hydroxyl is strongly electron-donating into the phenyl ring, and is the key to the oxidizability of the ring. Abstraction of the proton provides a particularly stable radical that can lead to reaction with molecular oxygen as shown in Figure 86. Deprotonation of the phenol at high pH to the phenolate anion greatly catalyzes the autoxidation process (base-catalyzed autoxidation). The phenolate anion is also an effective nucleophile and can react with electrophilic species at either the oxygen or the *ortho* or *para* positions. Phenolic

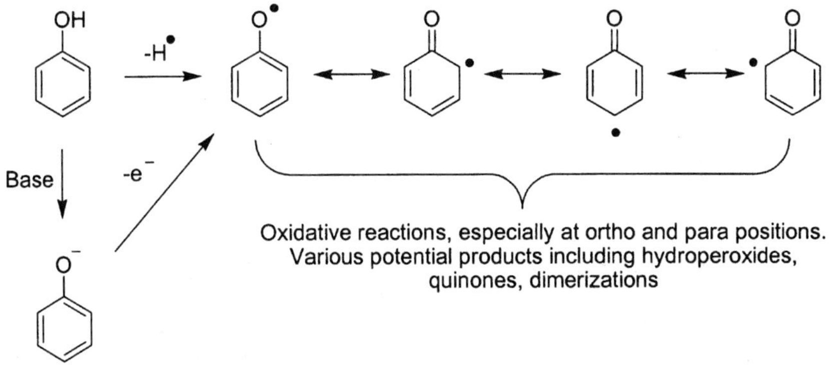

Oxidative reactions, especially at ortho and para positions. Various potential products including hydroperoxides, quinones, dimerizations

Figure 86 Simplified view of oxidative degradation chemistry of phenolic compounds.

compounds have been known to oxidize in the presence of Cu^{2+} or Fe^{3+} ions, especially in the presence of acetonitrile.

The API epinephrine is an *o*-diphenol containing a hydroxyl group in the α-position that is easily oxidized by molecular oxygen (Fig. 87). Oxidation is proposed to occur through the transient formation of epinephrine quinone with subsequent formation of adrenochrome (126). This class of compounds (the adrenergics, including adrenaline and isoprenaline) also undergoes this reaction to the adrenochrome upon irradiation in aqueous solution (127).

A similar oxidation and intramolecular cyclization is observed for the *o*-diphenol levarterenol (128).

3. Alkyl Halides

Alkyl and aryl halides are susceptible to hydrolysis leading to a hydroxyl plus the resulting halo acid (Fig. 88). For alkyl halides, the hydrolysis can occur via S_N1 (cationic intermediate, associated with a racemization if the center is asymmetric), S_N2 (direct nucleophilic attack with inversion of configuration) or by other mechanisms, but a detailed mechanistic discussion is beyond the scope of this chapter.

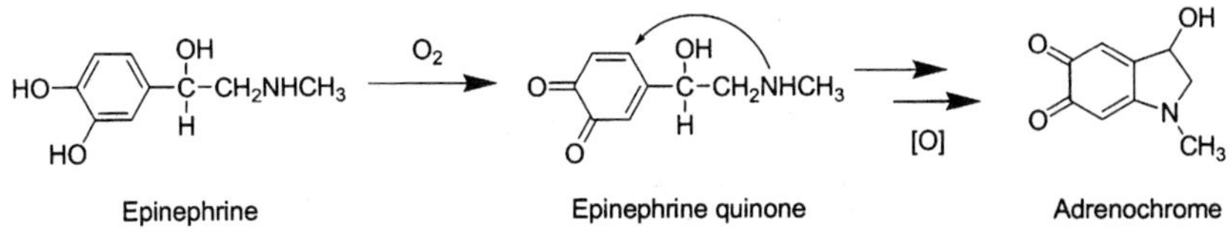

Epinephrine — Epinephrine quinone — Adrenochrome

Figure 87 Oxidation of epinephrine to adrenochrome.

$$RX + H_2O \longrightarrow X^- + ROH_2^+ \xrightarrow{-H^+} ROH + H^+ + X^-$$

$$RX + OH^- \longrightarrow X^- + ROH$$

Figure 88 Alkyl halide hydrolysis (acid and base catalyzed).

The susceptibility of alkyl halides to hydrolysis is a function of the halide (generally, I > Br > Cl > F). In contrast, the rates of aryl halide hydrolysis are generally F > Cl > Br > I. The reversal of the order of rates is because aryl halides hydrolyze via an addition-elimination reaction (March, (129)). The nucleophilic addition step, which is typically the rate-determining step, is facilitated by the strongly electronegative fluorine.

The conformation of an alkyl halide can have a dramatic affect on its susceptibility for elimination. For example, if the halide is oriented anti-periplanar (90° torsion angle) or syn-periplanar (0° torsion angle) to a hydrogen on an adjacent carbon, the elimination of the halo-acid is greatly favored. Hydrolysis of alkyl halides can be dramatically facilitated by the presence of a nitrogen or sulfur attached to the carbon alpha to the halide. This enhancement of solvolysis (e.g., 10–1000 times faster) is the result of intramolecular nucleophilic attack of the sulfur or nitrogen to form a transient cationic three-membered ring (an episulfonium ion in the case of sulfur or an aziridinium ion in the case of a nitrogen) as shown in Figure 89. Such neighboring group assistance requires conformational flexibility in order to form the three-membered ring. The neighboring group assistance

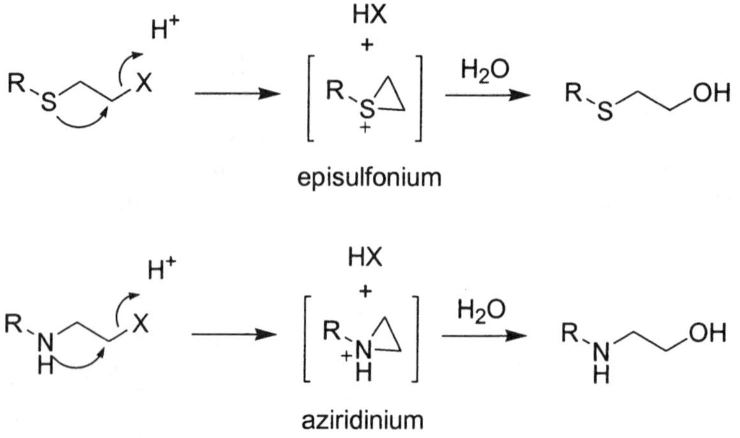

Figure 89 Neighboring sulfur or nitrogen group assistance of solvolysis of alkyl halides.

mechanism consists essentially of two S_N2 substitutions (one intramolecular and one intermolecular) (1).

Hydrolysis of the API melphalan is an example involving nitrogen group assistance of solvolysis of a dialkyl halide to form the dialkyl alcohol (Fig. 90) (130).

Hydrolysis of the dichloroacetamide functionality occurs in aqueous solutions with the API chloramphenicol under basic conditions. A primary route of decomposition for chloramphenicol in aqueous solution involves hydrolysis of the covalent chlorine of the dichloroacetamide functional group (131).

Aryl halides are often susceptible to photochemical degradation. As described in Chapter 10 later in this book, cleavage of the C–X bond occurs with low quantum yield for aryl chlorides (132), higher quantum yields for aryl bromides and iodides (133), and high quantum yields for some aryl fluorides (e.g., fluoroquinolones) (134). Aryl chlorides are photolabile to homolytic and/or heterolytic dechlorination (43). For sertraline hydrochloride, decomposition of the aryl dichloride moiety occurs in solution when exposed to light (ultraviolet and fluorescent conditions). As shown in the following proposed mechanism, the major photochemical decomposition products include mono-chloro- and des-chloro-sertraline via homolytic cleavage (Fig. 91) (86).

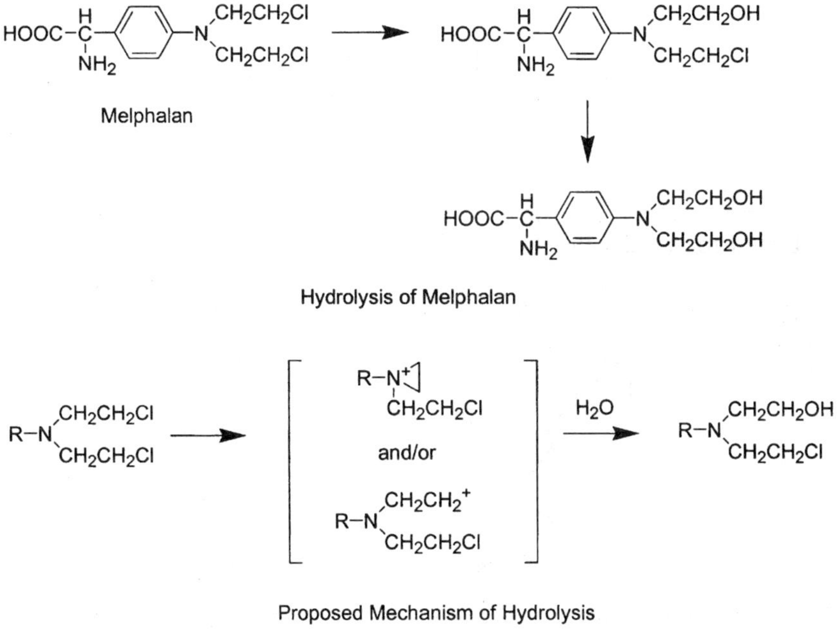

Melphalan

Hydrolysis of Melphalan

Proposed Mechanism of Hydrolysis

Figure 90 Hydrolysis of melphalan and proposed mechanism.

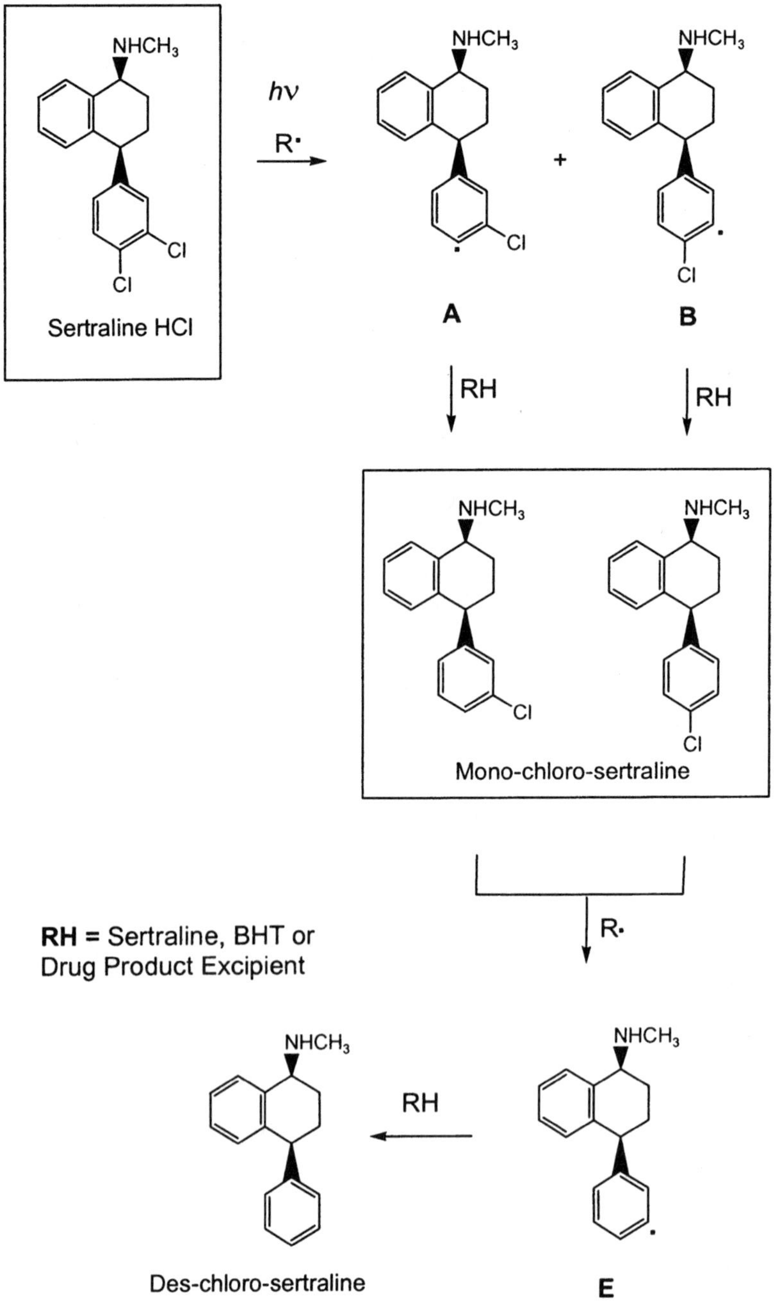

Figure 91 Sertraline HCl photodegradation in solution.

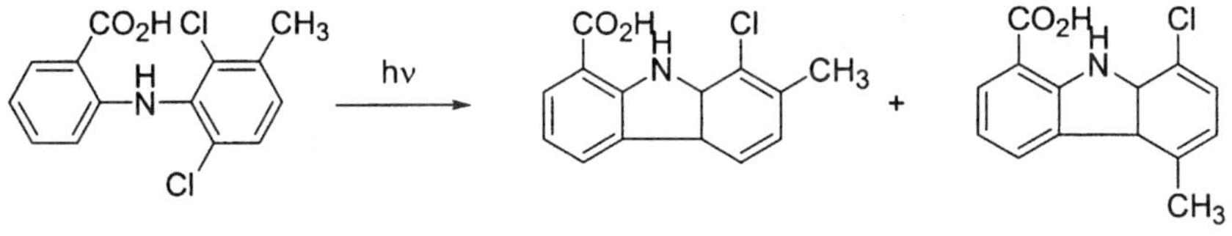

Figure 92 Meclofenamic acid photochemical-induced dechlorination.

Aromatic dechlorination under light is also observed for the API meclofenamic acid (135). Meclofenamic acid undergoes photochemical dechlorination and ring closure to carbazole products (Fig. 92).

The cardiac agent API amiodarone was observed to deiodinate sequentially upon irradiation in deaerated ethanol to yield the mono iodo product and finally the des iodo product (Fig. 93) (136). Formation of aryl radicals during the de-iodination process was supported by a spin-trapping study.

F. Conjugated Double Bond Systems

Conjugated double bond systems are susceptible to autoxidation chemistry. The free radical process of autoxidation consists of a chain sequence involving three distinct types of reactions: initiation, propagation, and termination (Fig. 94) (137). The initiation step involves production of a free radical to begin the chain reaction. Using a radical chain initiator is a valid method of accelerating autoxidation. Radical chain initiating diazenes undergo thermal bond homolysis to yield two radicals and molecular nitrogen. A labile hydrogen atom is then abstracted from the API or excipient by the radicals. Molecular oxygen then reacts with the API or excipient free radical at the diffusion-controlled rate of approximately $10^9\,M^{-1}s^{-1}$, depending on the solvent system. The peroxyl radical formed then abstracts a radical in the rate-determining step.

Termination of the autoxidation chain process occurs as peroxyl radicals couple to yield non-radical products. This reaction takes place through an unstable tetroxide intermediate. Primary and secondary tetroxides decompose rapidly by the Russell termination mechanism to yield three non-radical products via a six-membered cyclic transition state (Fig. 95). The decomposition yields the corresponding alcohol, carbonyl compound, and molecular oxygen (often in the higher energy singlet oxygen state) three

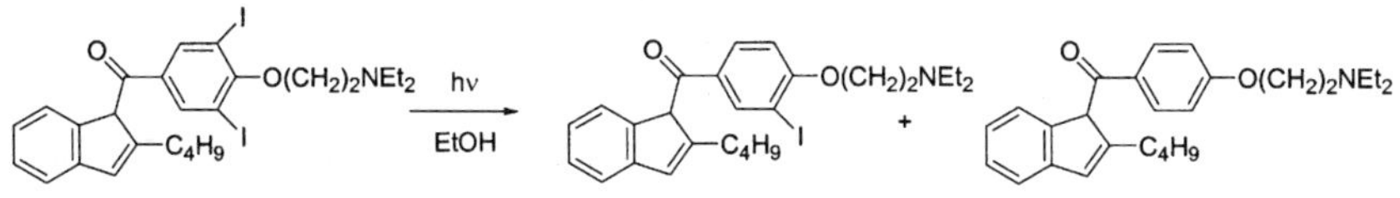

Figure 93 Amiodarone photochemical-induced deiodination.

Initiation:

$$In_2 \longrightarrow 2In\cdot$$

$$In\cdot + RH \longrightarrow InH + R\cdot$$

Propagation:

$$R\cdot + O_2 \longrightarrow ROO\cdot$$

$$ROO\cdot + RH \xrightarrow{kp} R\cdot + ROOH$$

Termination:

$$2ROO\cdot \longrightarrow ROOOOR$$

$$ROOOOR \longrightarrow \text{nonradical products}$$

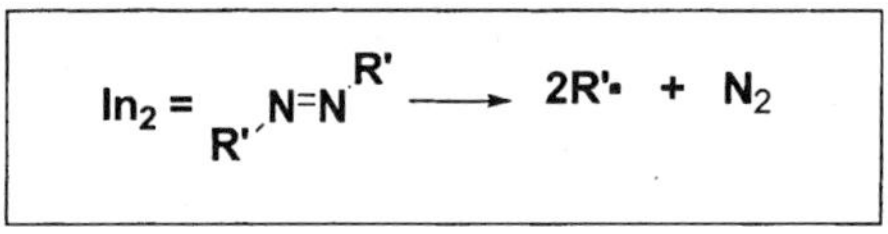

$$In_2 = R'N{=}NR' \longrightarrow 2R'\cdot + N_2$$

Figure 94 Autoxidation chain reaction.

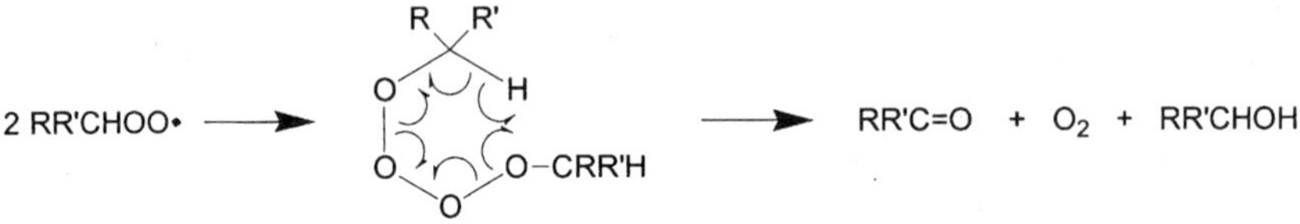

$$2\ RR'CHOO\cdot \longrightarrow [\text{cyclic tetroxide intermediate: } O\text{–}O\text{–}O\text{–}O\text{–CRR'H}, \text{ with } C(R)(R')\text{–H}] \longrightarrow RR'C{=}O + O_2 + RR'CHOH$$

Figure 95 Russell termination mechanism.

non-radical products that terminate the chain process (138). Oxidations can be catalyzed by peroxide-containing excipients (e.g., PEGs, Tween 80/polysorbates, povidone, etc.).

1. Benzyl Groups

Benzyl groups are stable to most conditions but are susceptible to autoxidation as shown in Figure 96. This susceptibility to autoxidation is due to the stability of the benzylic radical formed upon abstraction of a benzylic hydrogen. The benzylic radical (a π delocalized radical) is stabilized by resonance into the phenyl ring. Such resonance delocalization could also be provided by other aryl groups or by extended conjugation (139), and therefore any sp^3 hybridized methine or methylene attached to an aryl group or to a group with extended conjugation provides a favorable site for autoxidation to occur.

If the benzylic site is chiral with a labile hydrogen, epimerization reactions may also occur. As shown in Figure 97, sertraline HC1 API in solution degrades under photo conditions to the trans sertraline product. This is

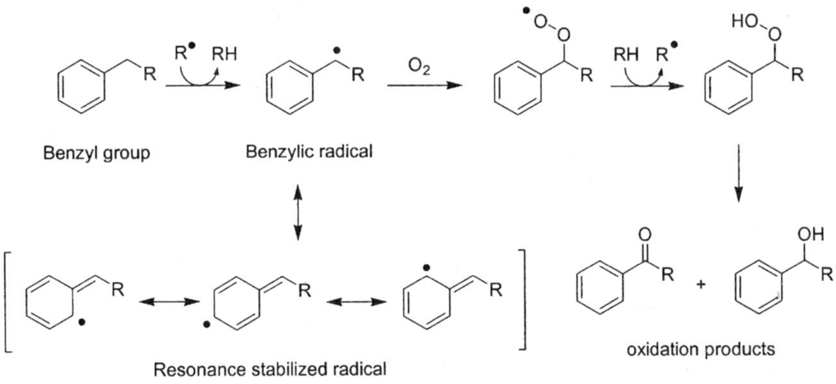

Benzyl group
Benzylic radical
Resonance stabilized radical
oxidation products

Figure 96 Oxidative degradation of benzyl groups.

proposed to form through a dibenzylic radical intermediate. If the degradation chemistry is performed in an aqueous environment, hydroxyl addition to the dibenzylic site can also occur. Additionally, chiral benzylic alcohols are likely to undergo racemization reactions under acidic conditions via a cationic intermediate. Due to the low bond dissociation energy of the benzylic C–H bond and ease of radical formation, another reaction to keep in mind is dimerization of two molecules of the API at the benzylic center.

Benzylic amine containing compounds are particularly susceptible to autoxidation with subsequent hydrolysis; such reaction often occur during stress testing using radical initiators. These compounds readily oxidize to the corresponding imine, which subsequently undergo hydrolysis to the primary amine and aldehyde derivatives.

Imipramine hydrochloride API undergoes oxidation at the benzylic site to form the corresponding benzyl hydroxyl compound (Fig. 98). Subsequent elimination of the hydroxyl occurs to give an extended conjugation in

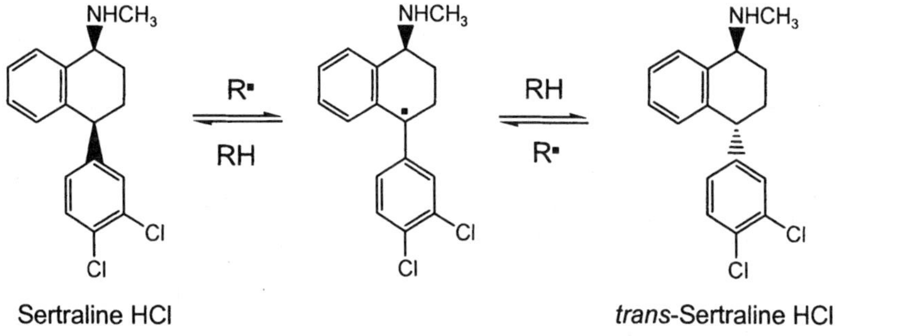

Sertraline HCl
trans-Sertraline HCl

Figure 97 Sertraline HCl API epimerization at dibenzylic position to *trans*-sertraline.

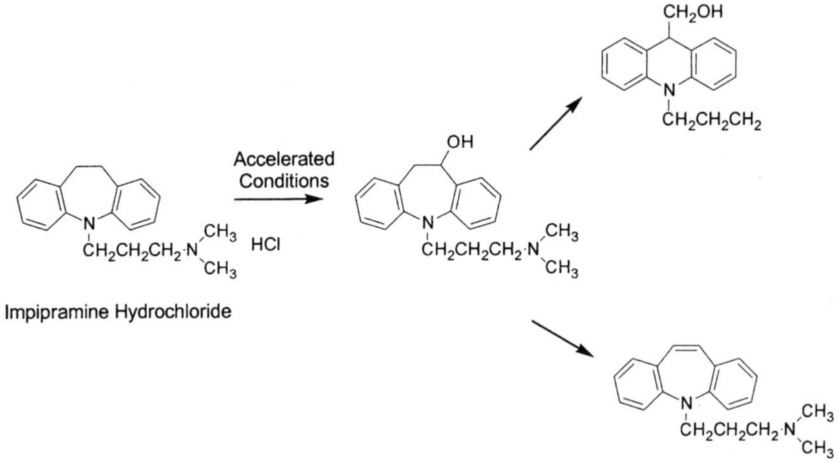

Accelerated Conditions
Impipramine Hydrochloride

Figure 98 Impipramine hydrochloride benzylic oxidation chemistry.

the molecule. By another pathway, the benzyl hydroxyl compound undergoes ring rearrangement from a seven- to a six-membered ring (140).

For the following compound (Fig. 99), the isopropyl benzylic site is oxidized to the corresponding hydroperoxide (141). The hydroperoxide

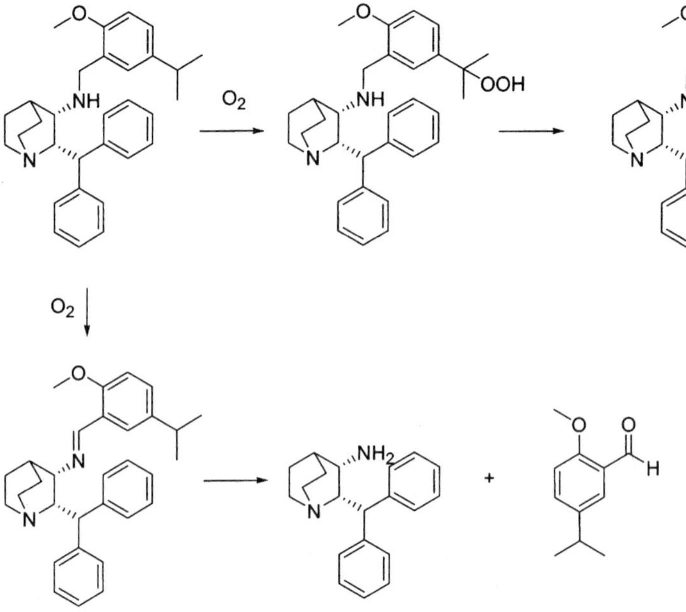

Figure 99 Oxidation degradation pathways for an API candidate.

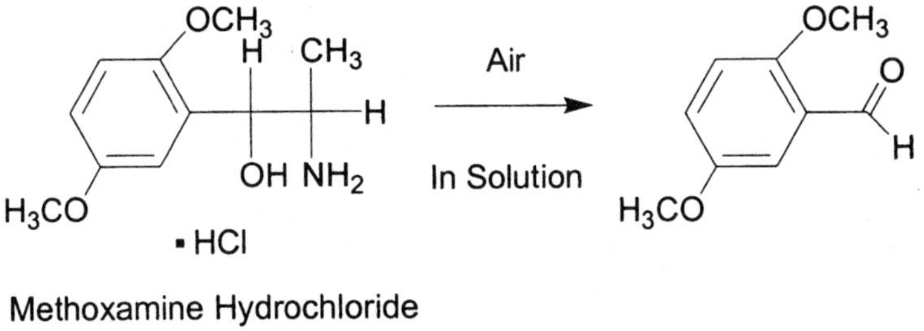

Figure 100 Methoxamine HCl undergoes oxidation at the benzylic position.

undergoes secondary degradation to the corresponding alcohol. Additionally, an imine is formed through a proposed benzylic oxidation step to the hydroperoxide followed by collapse to the imine. The imine undergoes hydrolysis to the corresponding aldehyde and amine.

The API methoxamine hydrochloride, which contains a benzyl hydroxyl, was found to decompose in aqueous solution to the primary degradation product 2,5-dimethoxybenzaldehyde, presumably via a benzylic radical autoxidation pathway (Fig. 100) (142).

The benzyl hydroxyl containing API cyclandelate undergoes oxidation to the corresponding ketone, 3,3,5-trimethylcyclohexyl phenylglyoxalate (143). Low level benzylic oxidation is observed for the API ibuprofen. Oxidation to form the ketone derivatives at both benzylic sites to yield isobutyl acetophenone and 2-(4-isobutyrylphenyl)-propionic acid has been reported (144).

2. Olefins

Olefins can undergo a number of degradation reactions that may be observed during storage and distribution or when subjected to stress-testing conditions. When subjected to peroxides, olefins can undergo epoxidation and dihydroxy addition reactions (Fig. 101). Epoxidation followed by S_N2 reaction with water resulting in anti-hydroxylation can occur by treatment with hydrogen peroxide and formic acid, common excipient impurities in drug product formulations (145).

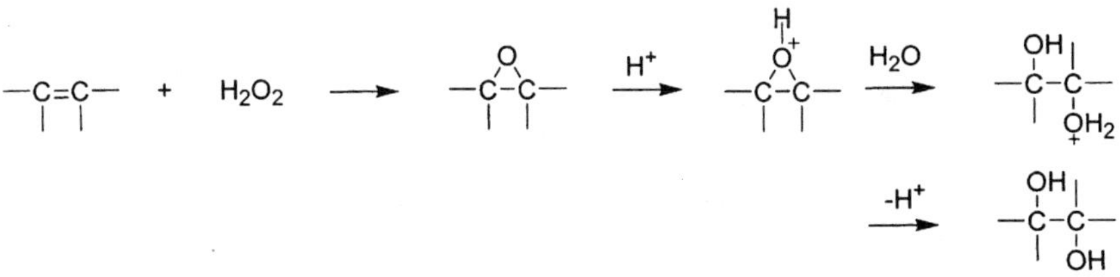

Figure 101 Epoxidation and dihydroxy addition of olefins.

In the case of the API dihydroergocristine methanesulfonate, autoxidation of the olefin moiety yields the corresponding autoxidation products (Fig. 102) (146).

Olefins are susceptible to isomerization. The API ivermectin undergoes isomerization under basic conditions due to the weak acidity of the allylic proton (which is also alpha to a carbonyl) on C2. The two resulting degradants can be derived from the delocalized carbanion formed from dissociation of the proton at C2. Reprotonation at C2 generates the epimeric product and reprotonation at C4 generates the structural isomer (Fig. 103) (147).

The API thiothixene contains an olefin moiety that undergoes photo-induced cleavage to the major decomposition product, the corresponding thioxanthone, through an endoperoxide intermediate (Fig. 104). The proposed mechanism of ketone formation occurs through addition of singlet oxygen to the olefin resulting in a dioxetane intermediate that then collapses to the thioxanthone degradant or by the formation of a charge transfer complex with oxygen forming a hydroperoxide intermediate (148).

For the diene containing API lovastatin, oxidation of the diene to the corresponding epoxide occurs in the presence of air (149).

Olefins are also susceptible to cycloaddition reactions (Fig 105) (150). In particular, some olefin-containing APIs can dimerize with another molecule of API to form a 2+2 cycloaddition product under photo conditions (151). A classic example of such a 2+2 cycloaddition catalyzed by UV radiation is that of the nucleoside thymidine (Fig. 106) (152,153). These reactions are proposed to go through more than one mechanism: concerted, diradical, electron transfer, and radical ion pairs.

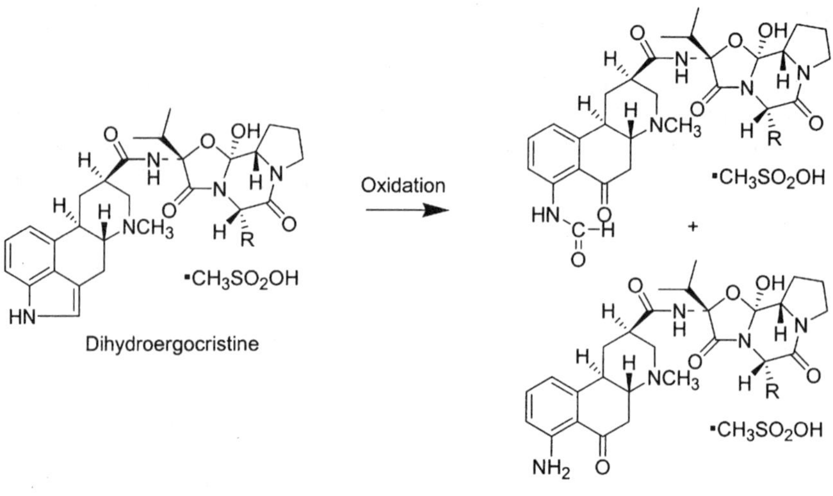

Figure 102 Autoxidation products of dihydroergocristine.

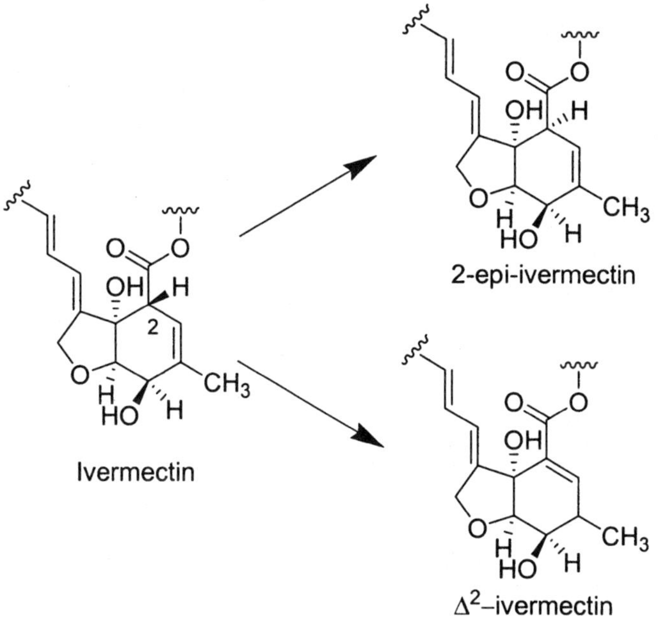

Ivermectin

2-epi-ivermectin

Δ^2–ivermectin

Figure 103 Alkaline hydrolysis products of API ivermectin.

Olefins are also susceptible to photodegradation reactions other than cycloaddition reactions (43). The olefin bond is susceptible to *E(trans)–Z(cis)* isomerization as well as oxidation (Fig. 107) (154). Photochemical *E–Z* isomerization has a major role in photobiological systems and has practical applications in vitamin A and vitamin D industrial processes

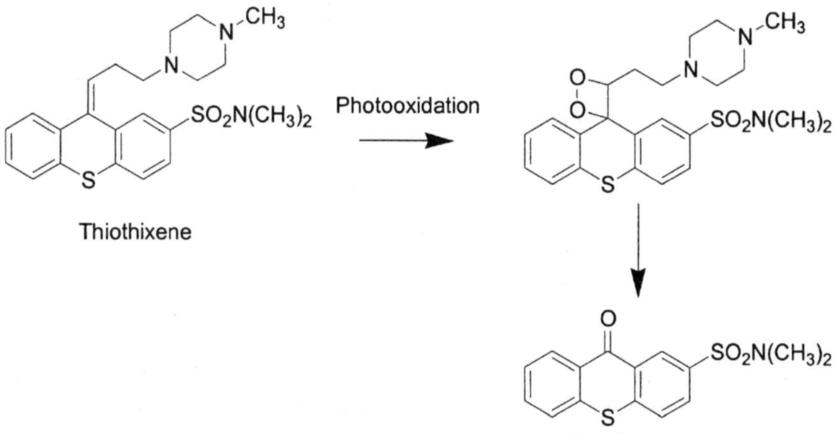

Thiothixene

Photooxidation

Figure 104 Photooxidation of thiothixene.

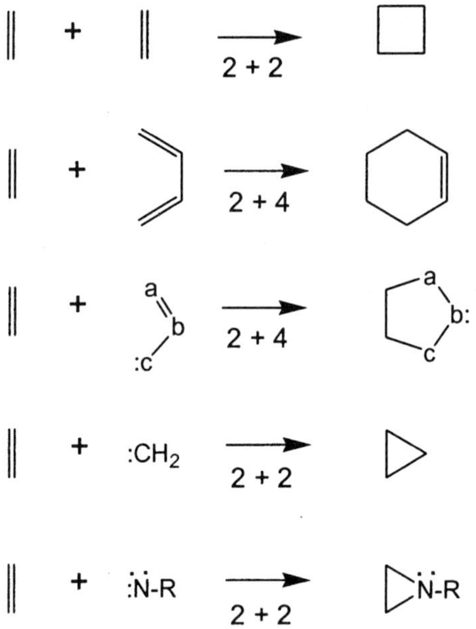

Figure 105 Cycloaddition reactions of olefins.

(155). Photoexcitation of the olefin followed by relaxation of the excited state allows rotation about the olefin yielding a twisted geometry that can produce either ground state *cis* or *trans* product. The sunscreen additive octylmethoxycinnamate undergoes *cis–trans* isomerization with high quantum yield as well as (2+2) cycloaddition reaction yielding a dimeric product (Fig. 108) (156). The *trans*-isomer was found to photoisomerize on irradiation at wavelengths greater than 300 nm. Photodimers were also separated

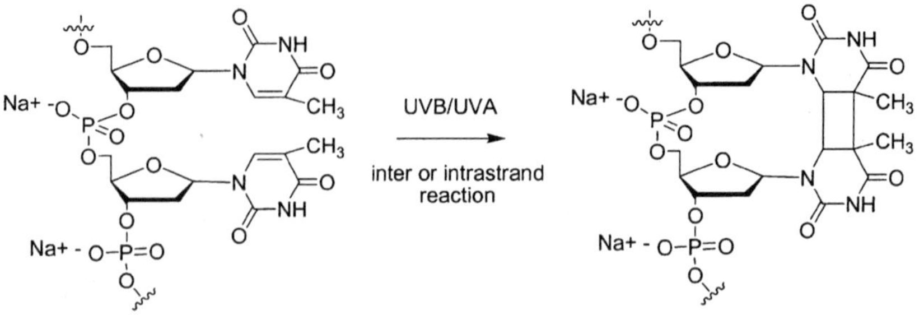

Figure 106 Illustration of thymidine 2+2 photocyclization reaction to form a cyclobutane ring. Note that the reaction can occur between neighboring thymidines on the same DNA strand (intrastrand) or between two different strands to form interstrand cross-links.

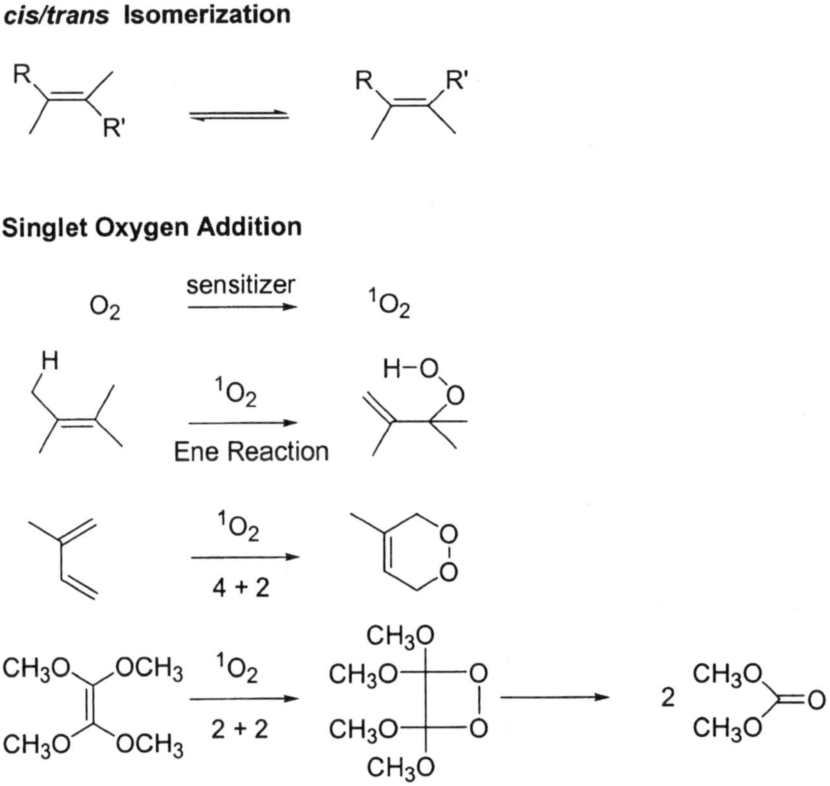

cis/trans **Isomerization**

Singlet Oxygen Addition

$O_2 \xrightarrow{\text{sensitizer}} {}^1O_2$

${}^1O_2$, Ene Reaction

${}^1O_2$, 4 + 2

${}^1O_2$, 2 + 2

Figure 107 Olefin photochemistry.

and identified, and indicate that the sunscreen absorber can undergo (2+2) cycloaddition reactions with itself.

3. Allylic Groups

As mentioned with benzyl groups, an allylic center is also quite susceptible to autoxidation chemistry (Fig. 109). The allylic hydrogen has a weak C–H bond dissociation energy due to the resonance stabilization energy of the resulting allylic radical (157).

4. Fatty Acids

Fatty acids (which are also known as "lipids") consist of a carboxyl function with an aliphatic chain. The aliphatic chain can be either saturated (i.e., no double bonds), monounsaturated (i.e., one double bond), or polyunsaturated (i.e., multiple double bonds). See Figure 110 for examples of fatty acid structures.

Saturated fatty acids (FAs) such as stearic acid are susceptible to degradation reactions typical of those for carboxyl groups. When

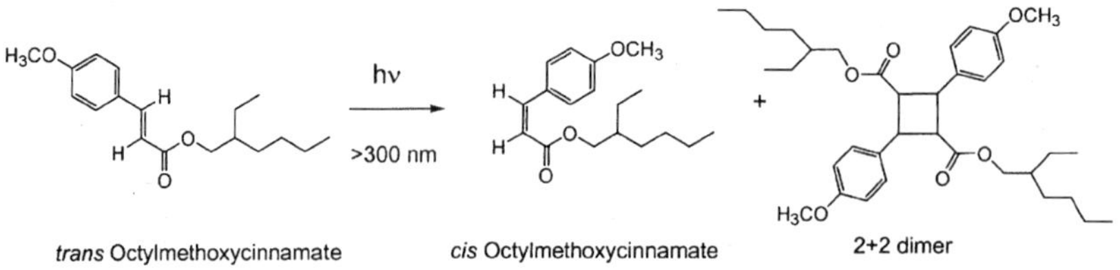

Figure 108 Photochemistry of the sunscreen octylmethoxycinnamate: *trans–cis* Isomerization and dimerization (2+2 cycloaddition).

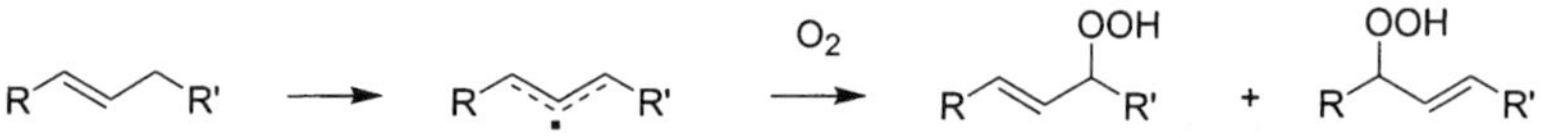

Figure 109 Allyl radical autoxidation mechanism.

protonated, the carboxyl group is electrophilic and can react with nucleophiles such as amines (to form amides) or alcohols (to form esters). When deprotonated, the carboxylate can act as a nucleophile. Saturated FAs are very stable to oxidative conditions. Unsaturated FAs, however, are very susceptible to autoxidation due to the presence of allylic or "doubly allylic" pentadienyl hydrogens that can be abstracted to form a stabilized radical as discussed immediately above (Fig. 94 for a detailed mechanism of the autoxidation chain process). Polyunsaturated FAs such as arachidonic acid contain pentadienyl hydrogens, which are particularly susceptible to hydrogen atom abstraction to form an extended delocalized radical. Such radicals readily form under ordinary atmospheric storage conditions, trapping molecular oxygen and giving rise to hydroperoxides, hydroxyls, aldehydes, endoperoxides, epoxides, and even cyclized prostaglandin-like compounds (as shown in Figure 111 for arachidonic acid).* Autoxidation of arachidonic acid yields six different peroxyl products, and four of these peroxyl radicals can undergo intramolecular cyclization to the dioxolane shown in the figure. The cyclization products can further degrade to multiple products via three main pathways: (1) substitution homolytic intramolecular (SH_i) ; (2) cyclization (k_c) ; and (3) further oxidation (O_2). Autoxidation process following the cyclization pathway have been documented both in vitro and in vivo in the case of arachidonic acid to form so called "isoprostanes" (159–161).

Vitamin E is effective as an antioxidant in arachidonate autoxidation, trapping the kinetic peroxyl radical product before cyclization can occur. Adding vitamin E in arachidonate autoxidation results in reducing radical cyclization products and forming the kinetic product distribution, six simple trans, cis diene hydroperoxides.

* For review articles on mechanisms of autoxidation of polyunsaturated lipids see Ref. 158.

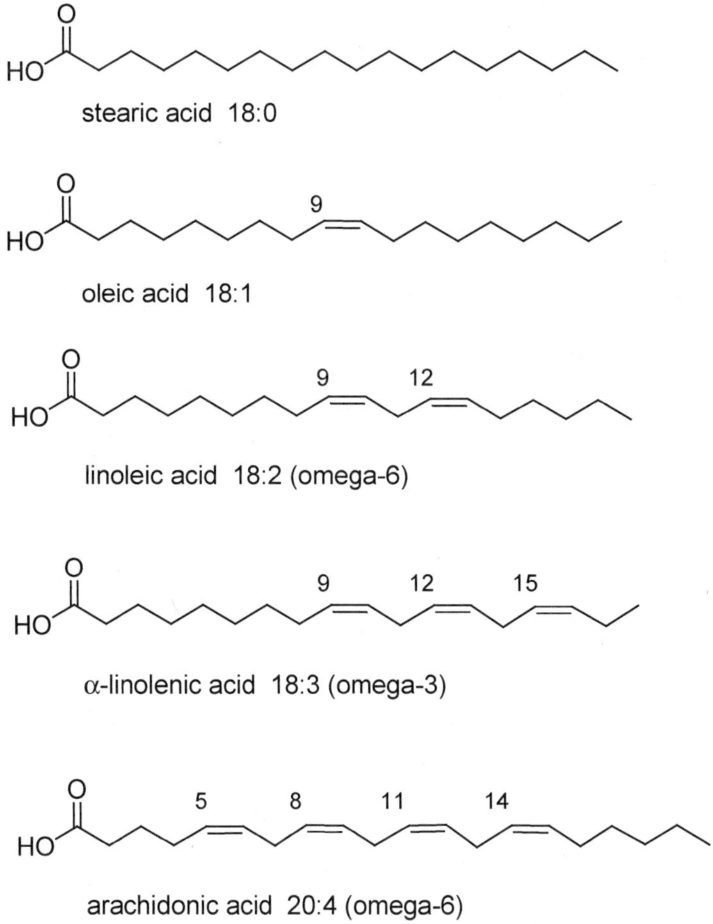
HO
O
stearic acid 18:0
HO
O
9
oleic acid 18:1
HO
O
9
12
linoleic acid 18:2 (omega-6)
HO
O
9
12
15
α-linolenic acid 18:3 (omega-3)
HO
O
5
8
11
14
arachidonic acid 20:4 (omega-6)

Figure 110 Structures of some common fatty acids.

G. Racemization, Isomerization, Ring Transformations, and Dimerization

1. Racemization of Chiral Centers

Racemization of chiral centers often involves a planar intermediate reaction center (e.g., carbon-centered radical, cation, or anion) where the reacting molecule can approach the reaction center either from one side of the planar surface or the other side resulting in either partial or complete racemization of the chiral center.

Epimerization of the API reserpine to 3-isoreserpine occurs readily in strong acid solution but has also been observed in solution using heat and

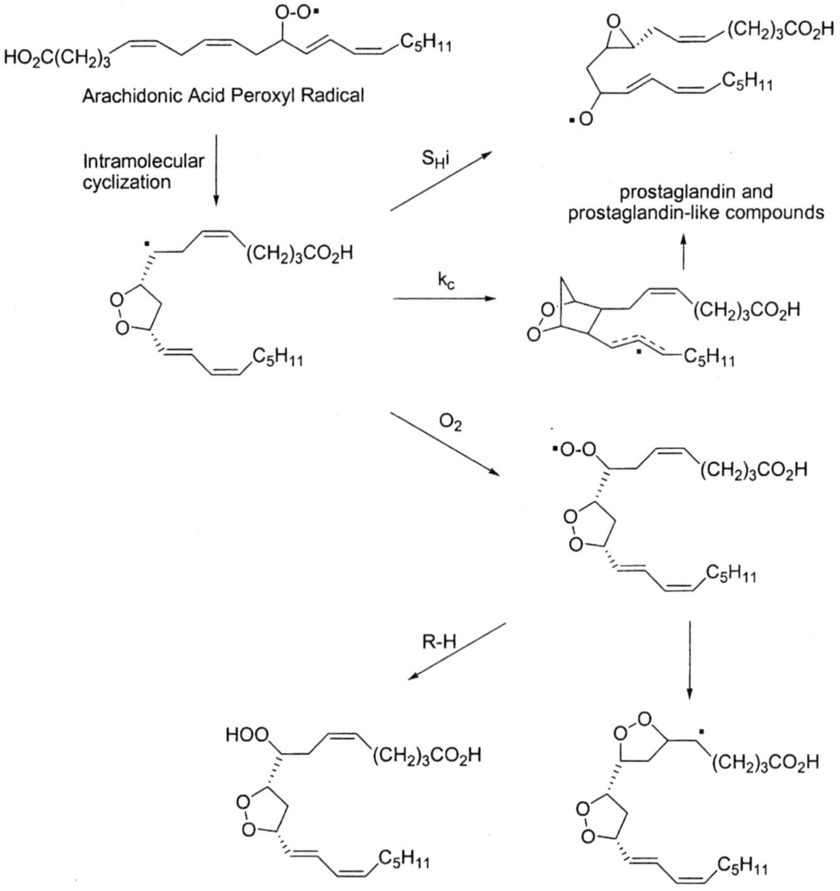

Figure 111 Overview of the complex autoxidation pathways of arachidonic acid.

light conditions (Fig. 112). The epimerization in this example has been shown to be initiated by protonation of C-2 followed by ring opening to yield an intermediate in which C-3 is planar and oriented for efficient ring closure to 3-isoreserpine (162).

Racemization of brinzolamide to the S isomer occurs under heat and light (pH independent) conditions (Fig. 113). This can occur via a radical mechanism from radical formation at the chiral center to form a resonance stabilized planar radical with hydrogen atom addition occurring on both sides of the planar carbon centered-radical to racemize the stereocenter (163).

Epimerization also occurs under basic conditions for the lactone containing API pilocarpine, which has a chiral center α to the carbonyl (Fig. 114) (164).

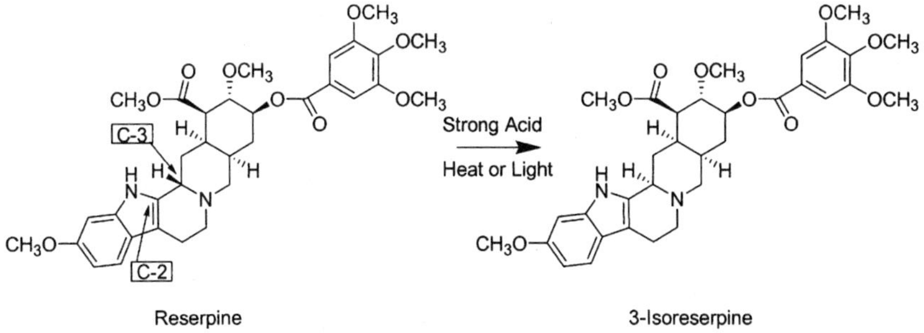

Reserpine → (Strong Acid; Heat or Light) → 3-Isoreserpine

Figure 112 Racemization of reserpine to 3-isoreserpine.

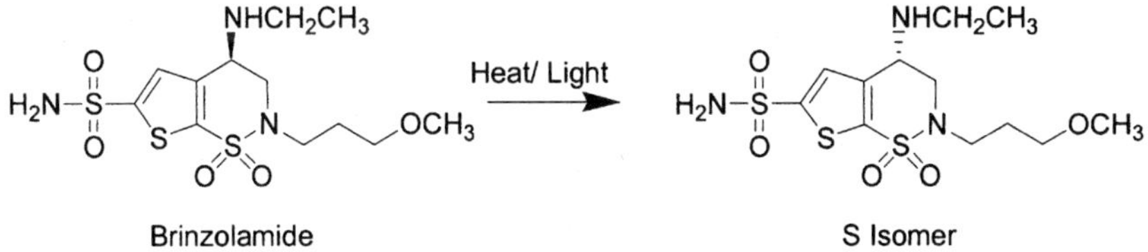

Brinzolamide → (Heat/ Light) → S Isomer

Figure 113 Racemization of brinzolamide.

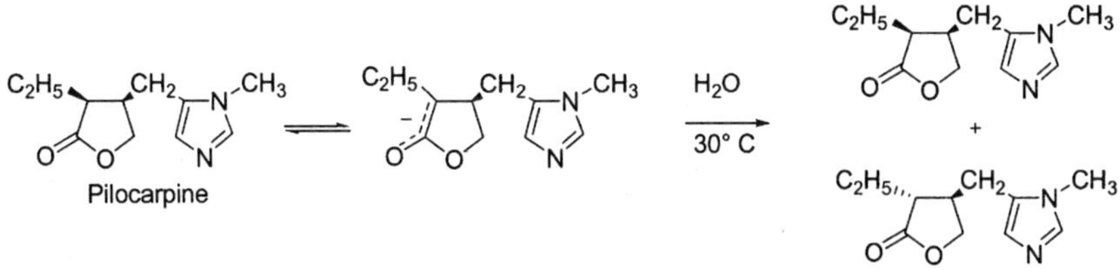

Pilocarpine ⇌ … → (H_2O, 30° C)

Figure 114 Hydrolysis and racemization mechanism of pilocarpine.

2. Ring Transformations

Ring transformations are common in pharmaceuticals. The API lorazepam containing a seven-membered non-aromatic ring can lose a molecule of water and rearrange with the driving force being formation of a six-membered aromatic pyrimidine ring (Fig. 115) (165).

Imidazole and thiazole rings have demonstrated instability under photolysis conditions. For example, the API thiabendazole undergoes cleavage of the thiazole ring to form benzimidazole-2-carboxamide and benzimidazole as well as cleavage of the imidazole ring to form thiazole-4-(*N*-carbomethoxy)-carboxamide (Fig. 116) (106).

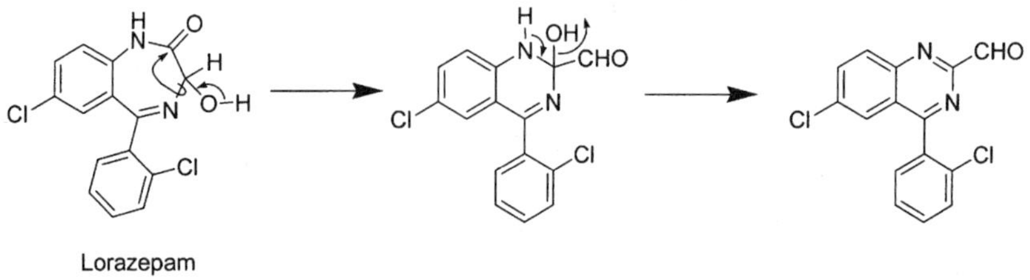

Lorazepam

Figure 115 Lorazepam ring transformation.

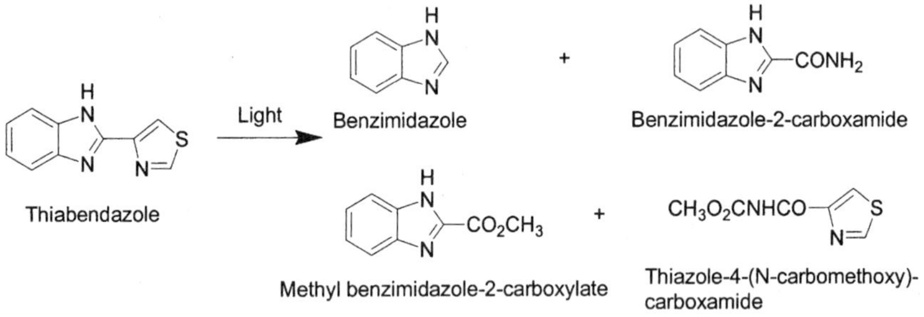

Thiabendazole — Light → Benzimidazole + Benzimidazole-2-carboxamide; Methyl benzimidazole-2-carboxylate + Thiazole-4-(N-carbomethoxy)-carboxamide

Figure 116 Thiabendazole photodegradation.

The API norfloxacin contains a piperazine ring. This undergoes degradation under light conditions in the solution and solid state to form the ring-opened ethylene diamine derivative and amino derivative (Fig. 117). Additional degradants observed in the solid state include the amino and formyl derivatives (167).

The APIs dipivefrin and epinephrine undergo ring formation when subjected to basic conditions to form adrenochrome (Fig. 87) (168).

3. Isomerization Reactions

The API etoposide contains a strained *trans*-γ-lactone ring that undergoes acid and base-catalyzed degradation. Under basic conditions, the degradation

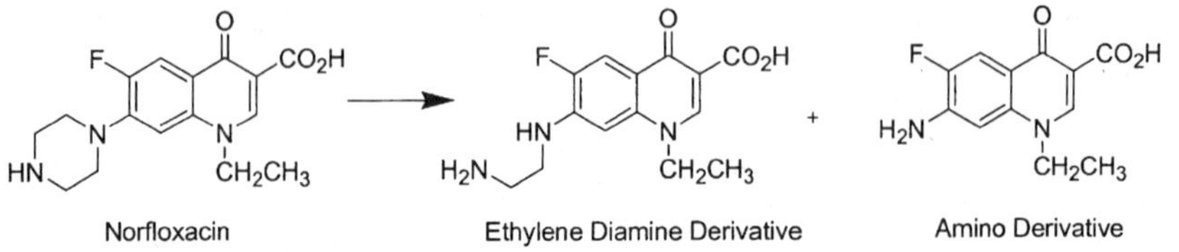

Norfloxacin → Ethylene Diamine Derivative + Amino Derivative

Figure 117 Norfloxacin piperzine ring cleavage to ethylene diamine upon exposure to light.

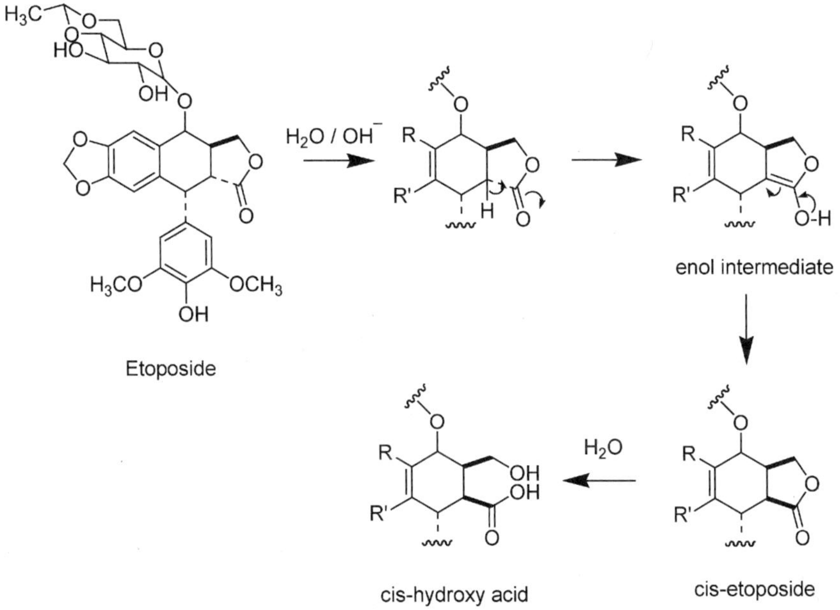

Figure 118 Base-catalyzed epimerization of etoposide.

of etoposide occurs through epimerization of the *trans*-γ-lactone ring to the *cis*-γ-lactone ring through a planar enol intermediate. Secondary degradation of the *cis*-etoposide then occurs to the *cis*-hydroxy acid (Fig. 118) (169).

Cephalosporin antibiotics will undergo isomerization of the double bond from the Δ^3-position to the Δ^2-position (Fig. 119), especially when the 4-carboxyl group is esterified (e.g., to enhance bioavailability) (170). The isomerization reaction is subject to general and specific base catalysis in both directions (171). The reaction also occurs (although at a much slower rate) during either solution or solid-state degradation of non-esterified cephalosporins as in the case of cefaclor (21). In the case of cefaclor, the protonation at C4 occurred stereospecifically to give the 4*S* configuration (proton is β).

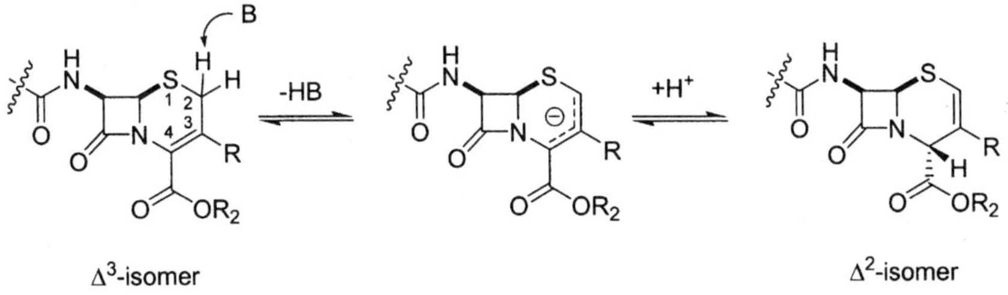

Figure 119 Cephalosporin isomerization of the oleﬂn Δ^3-position to the Δ^2-position.

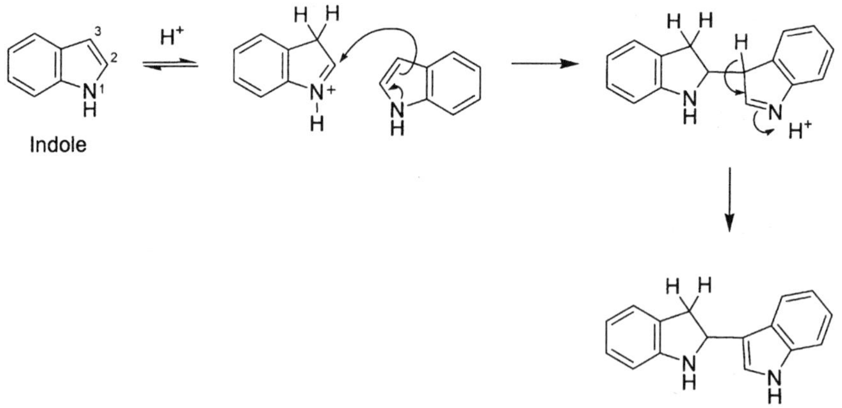

Indole

Figure 120 Dimerization mechanism for indoles under acidic conditions.

4. Dimerization

Many compounds will undergo dimerization reactions: those containing thiols (e.g., disulfide formation) olefins, alcohols, and carboxylic acids (or other carbonyl chemistry e.g., aldol condensation reactions). Indoles have been shown to dimerize under acidic conditions. The dimerization is presumed to occur as shown in Figure 120 via protonation at C3 and nucleophilic attack of a second indole on C2. Phenols have been shown to dimerize under free radical initiated oxidative conditions, usually to ortho phenols. Nalidixic acid API undergoes dimerization under thermolysis conditions to decarboxylate and produce a dimeric structure (Fig. 121) (172).

H. Carbohydrates, Nucleic Acids, Amino Acids

1. Carbohydrates, sugars

A comprehensive or thorough discussion of carbohydrate chemistry is beyond the scope of this chapter. A simple sugar is a straight-chain aldehyde

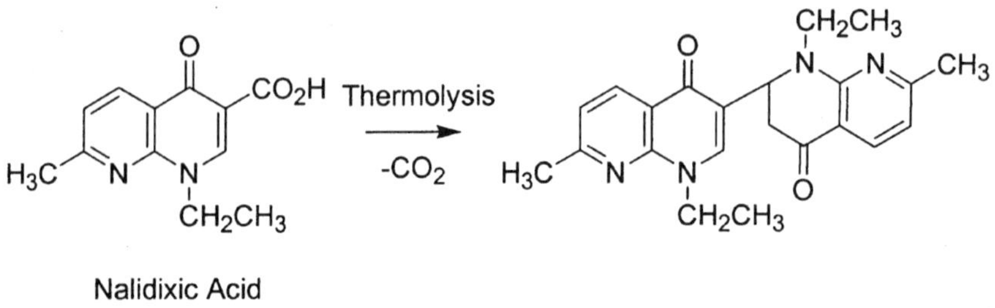

Thermolysis $-CO_2$

Nalidixic Acid

Figure 121 Nalidixic acid decarboxylation and dimerization.

or ketone that has alcohol functional groups on each of the remaining carbons. The aldehyde or ketone functional groups of a simple sugar can interact intramolecularly with a hydroxyl, forming a cyclic hemiacetal, either five- or six-membered rings containing one oxygen, furanose, or pyranose forms, respectively.

In aqueous solution, monosaccharides (containing five or more carbon atoms) occur in ring (or cyclic) forms (173). These molecules are known as pyranoses (six-membered ring) or furanoses (five-membered ring) since they resemble pyran and furan, respectively (as shown in Figure 122 for glucose). The rings form as a result of the aldehyde (or ketone) reacting with a hydroxyl group further along the chain (usually at the penultimate carbon) and forming a hemiacetal (or hemiketal) link. This is a general hemiacetal (hemiketal) reaction where aldehydes (ketones) combine with alcohols.

An extra chiral center is produced at the hemiacetal (or hemiketal) carbon (former carbonyl carbon). The hydroxyl group can be either below (α) or above (β) the plane of the ring structure. Monosaccharides that differ only in the configuration of the groups at the hemiacetal (hemiketal) carbon are known as *anomers.* The hemiacetal (hemiketal) carbon is known as the anomeric carbon (Fig. 122).

Sugars with a free hydroxyl on the anomeric carbon (hemiacetals) are known as reducing sugars because they can open to the aldehydic form and then be readily oxidized to the carboxylic acid. The free anomeric carbon is often called the reducing end. Non-reducing sugars are simple sugars that have an ether linkage of a hydroxyl group present at the anomeric carbon so that the cyclic form cannot readily open to the easily oxidized aldehydic form. Reducing sugars include lactose, fructose, glucose, and maltose. Non-reducing sugars include cellulose, sucrose, trehalose, and mannitol (mannitol is an alditol having all hydroxyl groups and therefore no cyclic/aldehydic forms).

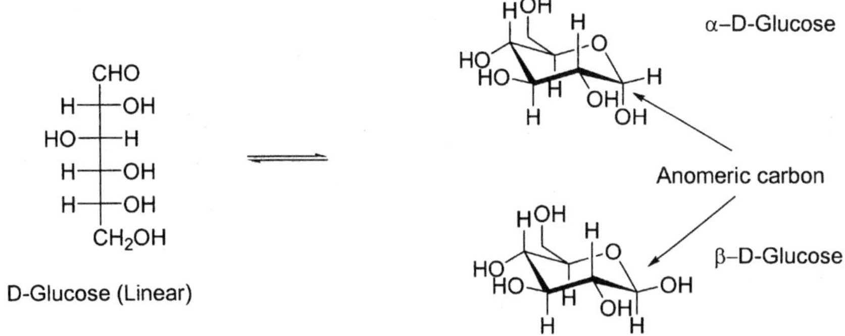

Figure 122 Glucose open chain (aldehydic form) and cyclic pyranose (hemiacetal) form.

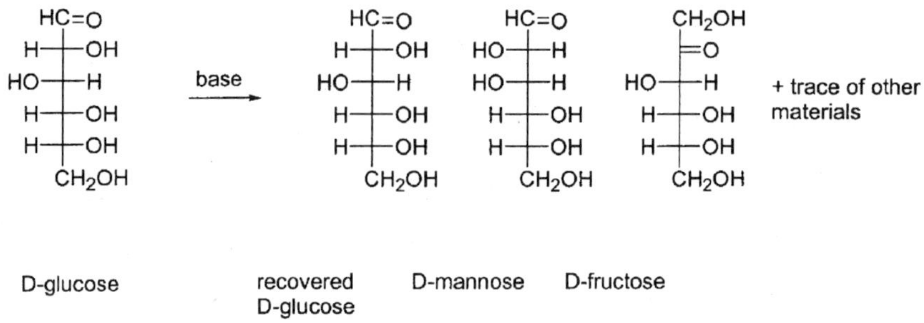

Figure 123 D-Glucose reaction under basic conditions.

In base, aldoses and ketoses rapidly equilibrate to mixtures of sugars (Fig. 123) (174). Most sugars react with alcohols under acidic conditions to yield cyclic acetals (glycosides). Glycoside formation, like acetal formation, is catalyzed by acid and involves cation intermediates (Fig. 124).

An alkyl group located on a carbon alpha to a heteroatom (in the case of sugars, the anomeric carbon) prefers the equatorial position (as expected), but a polar group (such as hydroxyl or -OR) prefers the axial position. This preference is known as the anomeric effect (Fig. 125), and this is the reason for the greater stability of α-glycosides over β-glycosides (175). For example, pyranose sugars substituted with a polar electron-withdrawing group such as halogen or alkoxy at Cl are often more stable when the substituent has an axial orientation rather than an equatorial position (176).

The magnitude of the anomeric effect depends on the substituent with the effect decreasing with increasing dielectric constant of the environment.

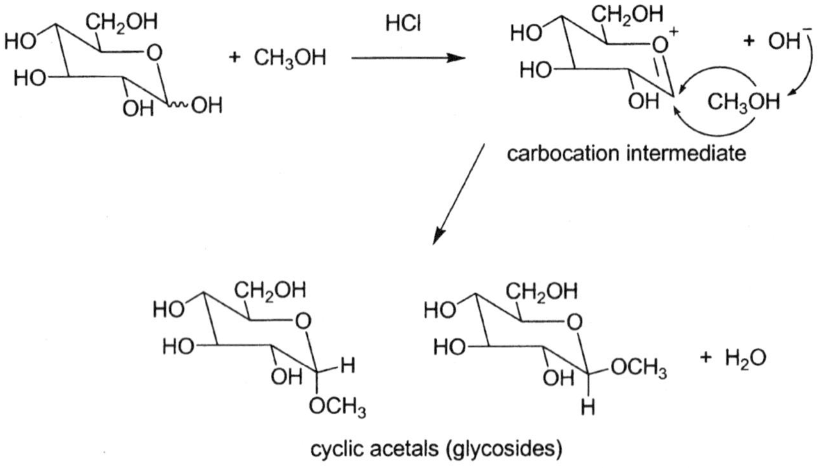

Figure 124 Reaction of sugars with alchols to yield glycosides under acidic conditions.

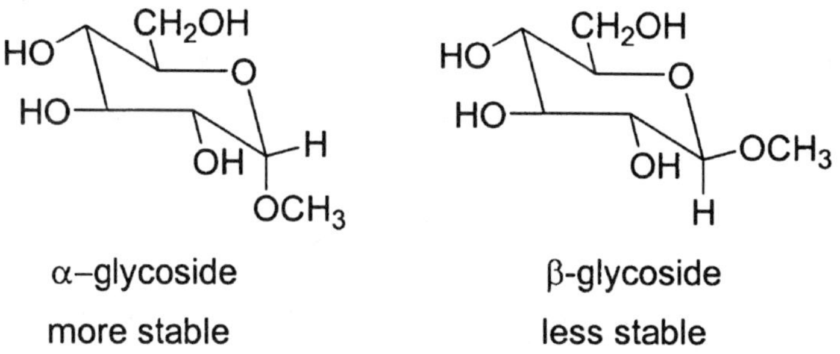

Figure 125 Anomeric effect, stability of α-glycosides over β-glycosides.

In Figure 126, the tri-*O*-acetyl-β-D-xylopyranosyl chloride anomeric effect of the single chlorine drives the equilibrium to favor the conformation with the three acetoxy groups in the axial positions. From a molecular orbital viewpoint, the anomeric effect results from an interaction between the lone pair electrons on the pyran oxygen and the $\sigma*$ orbital associated with the bond to the C2 substituent.

Anomeric center reactivity has been observed for the API lincomycin hydrochloride. Lincomycin HCl contains a carbohydrate portion that undergoes thioglycoside hydrolysis at the carbohydrate anomeric center (Fig. 127) (177).

2. Nucleic Acids

Nucleic acids, similar to peptides and proteins, can possess not only primary structure but also secondary and tertiary structure. For example, oligomeric

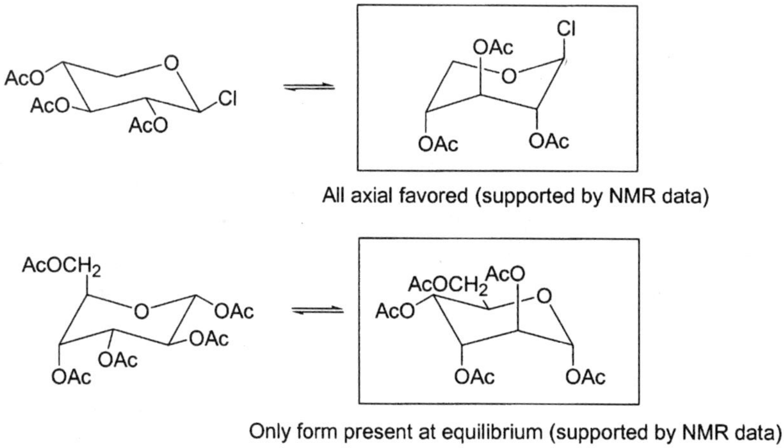

Figure 126 Equilibria in compounds that exhibit the anomeric effect.

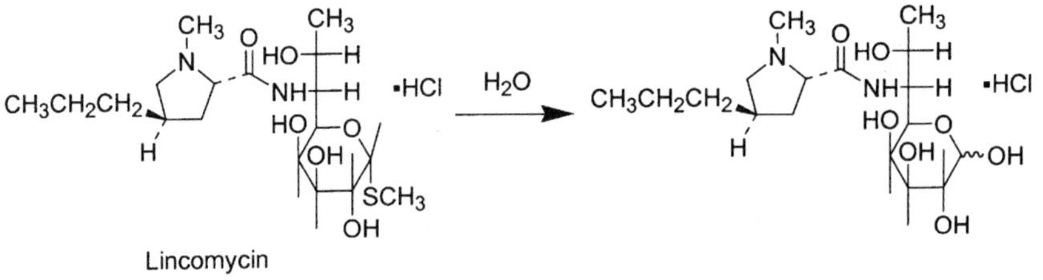

Figure 127 Lincomycin HCl thiogiycoside hydrolysis at the carbohydrate anomeric center.

and polymeric nucleic acid structures can form duplex structures via hydrogen-bonded base pairing. The discussion here will focus only on a few of the major degradation pathways of the primary structure. More extensive reviews of nucleic acid chemistry can be found in the literature (178,179).

While not all drugs that are nucleic acid derivatives are oligomers, for those that are oligomeric, hydrolysis of the phosphodiester bond is one of the prominent degradation pathways. Such degradation leads to a break in the sugar-phosphate backbone as shown in Figure 128 for RNA strands. See Pogocki and Schöenich (179) for an in-depth discussion of this topic.

Depurination, or hydrolysis of the N-glycosidic bond, occurs for both RNA and DNA strands (oligomers/polymers) or analogs (monomers). RNA is much less prone to depurination than DNA as a result of the inductive effect of the 2′-OH group (180). Acid-catalyzed depurination is illustrated in Figure 129.

When R is a strongly electron-withdrawing group, the nucleoside/tide can be significantly stabilized to depurination. Such is the case for gemcita-

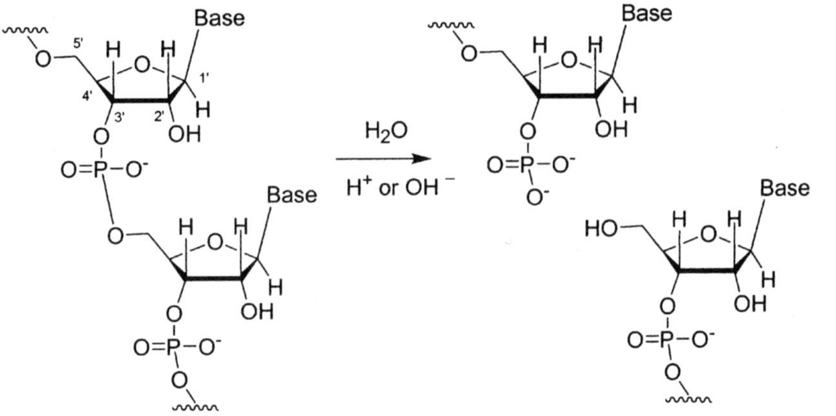

Figure 128 Hydrolysis of the phosphodiester backbond of an RNA strand.

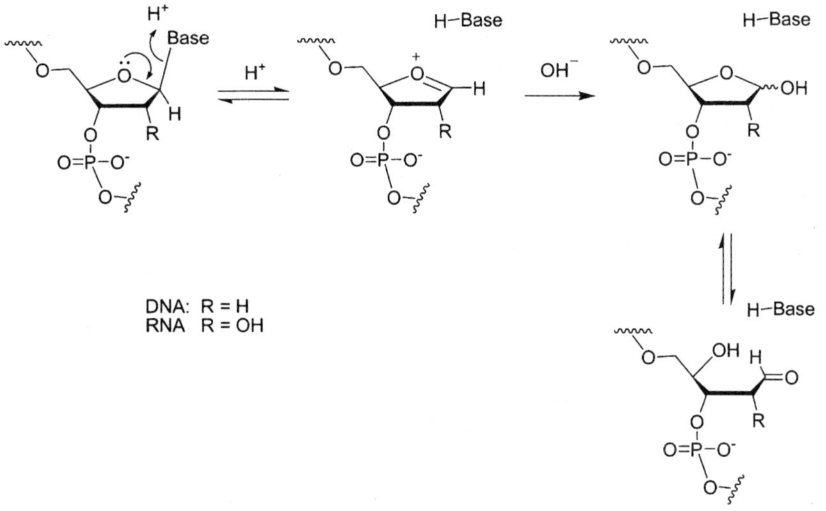

Figure 129 Acid-catalyzed depurination of a nucleic acid.

bine (2′-deoxy-2′,2′-difluorocytidine), a β-difluoronucleoside. The aqueous degradation of gemcitabine under acidic, mildly acidic (pH 3.2), and basic conditions has been studied and the degradation chemistry is shown in Figures 130 and 131 (181). As shown in the figures, depurination does not occur to a measurable extent; rather, nucleophilic attack of the cytidine at C6 (by either water or intramolecular attack by the 5′-hydroxyl) occurs first, leading eventually to deamination. Under basic conditions, a remarkable

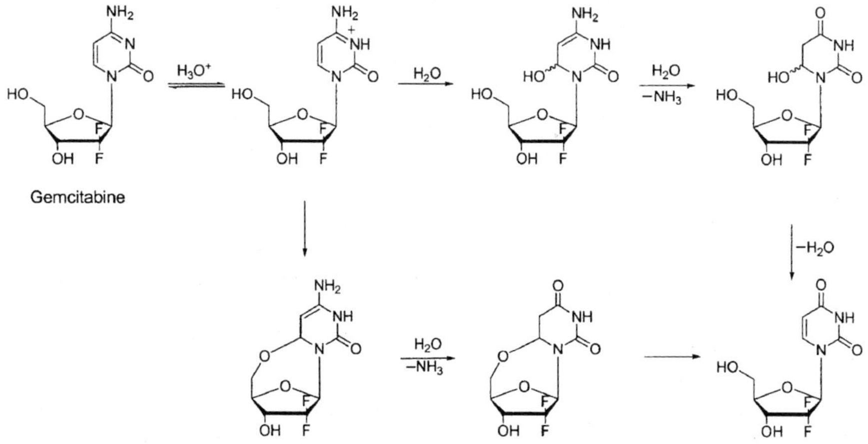

Figure 130 Proposed aqueous acidic degradation pathways of gemcitabine.

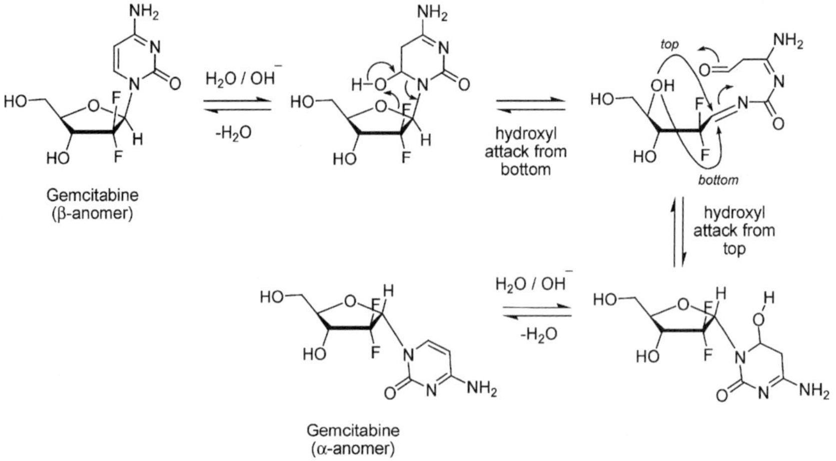

Figure 131 Base-catalyzed degradation of gemcitabine does not induce depurination, but rather anomerization of the base from β to α.

anomerization reaction occurs (shown in Figure 131) illustrating the resistance of the difluoronucleoside to depurination.

Oxidative degradation of nucleic acids has been studied extensively. See the reviews by Pogocki and Schoenich (179) and by Waterman et al. (182) for excellent discussions of this topic.

3. Amino Acids

Protein degradation commonly includes aggregation, deamidation, isomerization, racemization, disulfide bond exchange, hydrolysis, and oxidation (183). Amino acid residues most likely to undergo degradation include asparagines (Asn), aspartic acid (Asp), methionine (Met), cysteine (Cys), glutamine (Gln), histidine (His), lysine (Lys), and serine (Ser). For liquid drug product formulations, the major degradation pathways are hydrolysis, deamidation, and isomerization (184). For lyophilized powder and tablet formulations, the major degradation reactions are similar to the solution formulations, although removal of water through lyophilization results in reduced rates of hydrolysis. In microsphere depot formulations, aggregation and oxidation are the main causes of peptide degradation.

Aggregation. Protein aggregation has two forms: non-covalent (involving the interaction of two or more denatured proteins) and covalent (e.g., disulfide bond formation and/or peptide condensation reactions).

Deamidation, isomerization and racemization. These three reactions are common degradation pathways of proteins and peptides. These reactions are especially prevalent for peptides containing asparagine (Asn) and glutamine (Gln) residues. In the deamidation reaction, the Asn or Gln amide

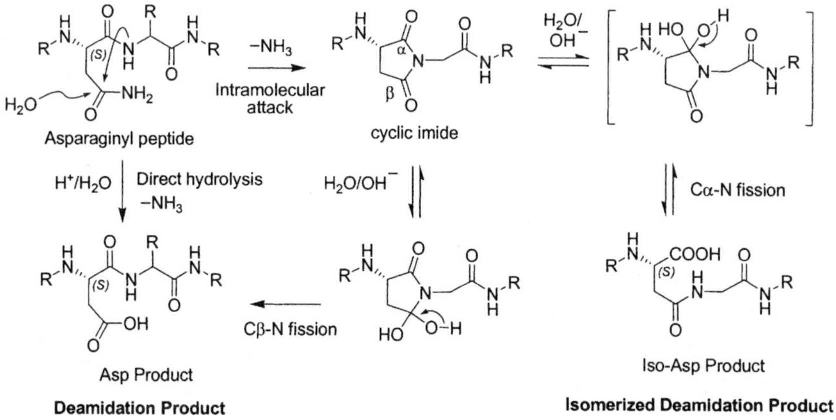

Figure 132 "Deamidation" reactions: asparagine to Asp and IsoAsp.

side chains are hydrolyzed to form a carboxylic acid. During this deamidation process, an isomerization reaction can occur in which the peptide backbone is transferred from the α-carboxyl of the Asn or Gln to the side chain β or γ-carboxyl. Asn–Gly and Asn–Ser are most likely to deamidate. Deamidation is accelerated at alkaline pH conditions through a proposed cyclic imide intermediate. Under acidic conditions, direct deamidation occurs without the cyclic intermediate. In addition to the primary structure, the secondary and tertiary structures also influence the rate of deamidation. Denatured proteins allow increased conformational mobility to form the cyclic intermediate.

These reactions have been extensively described in the literature (185–189). It has been shown that at low pH (e.g., pH < 2), although the cyclic imide does form, the deamidation occurs primarily via direct hydrolysis. When the pH is >5, however, the deamidation occurs exclusively via the cyclic imide. The isoAsp product resulting from deamidation is always formed in a 2- to 4-fold excess compared to the Asp product, although the excess is reduced as the pH rises. The maximum stability toward deamidation is generally in the pH 3–4 range.

In a racemization reaction, the configuration about the α-carbon of the amino acid is inverted. For Asn and Gln amino acids, the racemization is facilitated by enolization of the succinimide, as shown in Figure 133.

Isomerization of aspartyl-X residues can occur via a succinimide intermediate (Fig. 132)*. The isomerized aspartyl residue can be detected by peptide mapping, Edman sequencing, and selective methylation of the iso-Asp peptide using carboxyl methyl transferase enzyme. Succinimide sites

* For isomerization articles see Ref. 190.

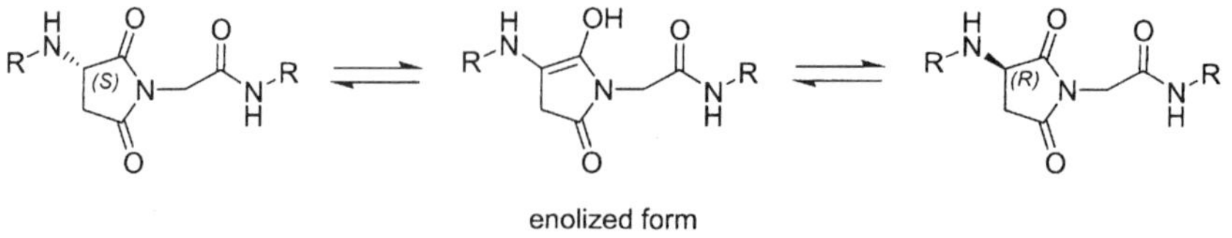

Figure 133 Racemization of an asparagine residue via a cyclic imide intermediate.

in proteins can be detected by basic hydroxylamine cleavage at the succinimide residue and subsequent N-terminal sequencing (192). Peptide bonds of apartyl residues are cleaved under acidic conditions 100 times faster than other peptide bonds with aspartyl–proline peptide bonds, being most labile. Hydrolysis occurs at either the N or C-terminal peptide bonds adjacent to the aspartyl residue. Techniques such as SDS-PAGE and SDS-NGS CE are the most useful to detect peptide bond cleavage fragments.

Disulfide bond exchange. Disulfide linkages are important in determining protein tertiary structure. Disulfide bond formation and/or exchange may occur during metal-catalyzed oxidation of the cysteine residue. This may lead to protein aggregation due to the formation of intermolecular disulfide bonds. In addition to cysteine disulfide bond formation, cysteine is susceptible to oxidation (Fig. 134) (200) (See also discussion on thiol chemistry earlier in this chapter).

Hydrolysis. Peptide bonds of aspartic acid (Asp) residues are cleaved under dilute acidic conditions. Hydrolysis can take place at the N-terminal, the C-terminal, or both terminal peptide bonds adjacent to the Asp residue.

Oxidation. The side chains of cysteine (Cys), histidine (His), methionine (Met), tryptophan (Trp), and tyrosine (Tyr) residues are susceptible to oxidation. Oxidation can result in loss of protein activity. Met is the most reactive residue, oxidizing even with atmospheric oxygen to form Met-sulfoxide, which is frequently observed in proteins (Fig. 135). Additional sources of oxidation include oxidizing agents (peroxides in excipients), metal-catalyzed oxidation and photo-oxidation. Oxidation can be detected

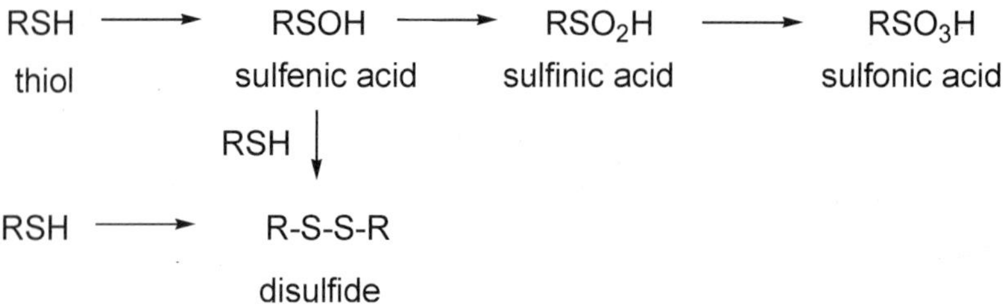

Figure 134 Cysteine oxidation and disulfide bond formation (See also Fig. 67).

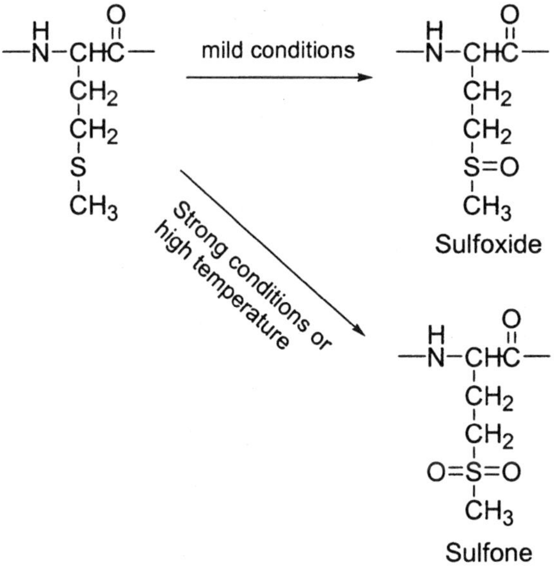

Figure 135 Methionine oxidation.

analytically by reversed phase HPLC and HIC (hydrophobic interaction chromatography). Peptide mapping and mass spectrometry are useful for determination of oxidation sites.

Photodegradation. UV/Vis exposure can induce protein oxidation, aggregation, and backbone cleavage. For example, oxidation has been observed in the histidine residue of human growth hormone (hGH) exposed to photostability conditions (6.7×10^6 lux hours). The proposed oxidation mechanism and product is shown in Figure 136.

Beta-elimination. Beta elimination of cysteine, serine, threonine, lysine, and phenylalanine residues proceed via a carbanion intermediate. This mechanism is influenced by metal ions and favored under basic conditions (190, 191).

Other degradation mechanisms. Additional degradation reactions include N-terminal degradation to form pyroglutamic acid formation (Fig. 137) (193) and N-terminal degradation diketopiperazine formation (Fig. 138) (194).

I. Reactions with Buffer Systems

While buffering systems are ideally considered to be unreactive with pharmaceuticals, buffers are known to enhance certain reactions (buffer catalysis) and there are documented cases of covalent reactions with general chemical compounds and with pharmaceuticals. For example, TRIS [tris

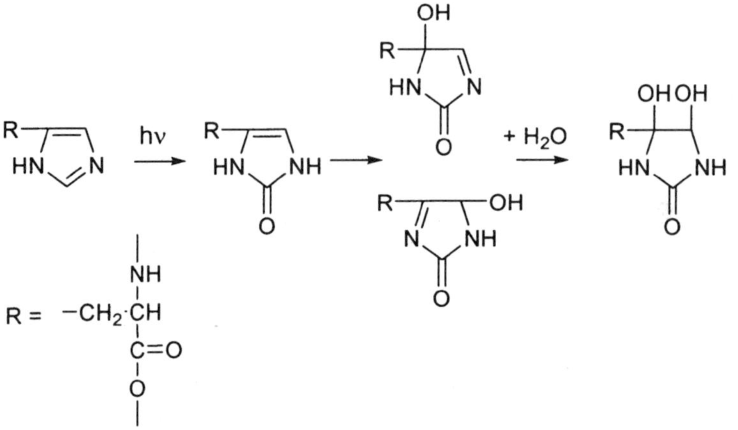

Figure 136 Histidine oxidation in hGH.

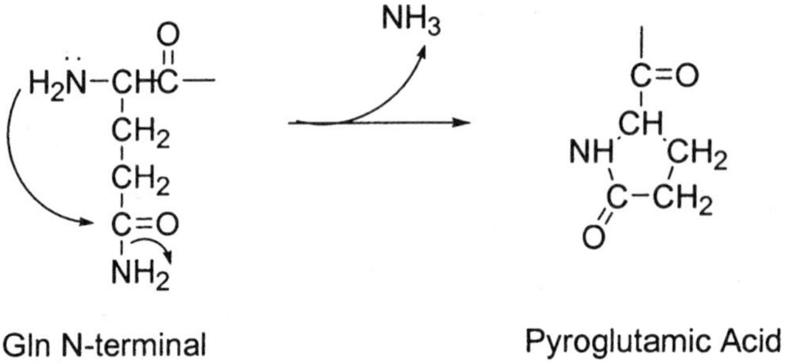

Figure 137 Pyroglutamic acid formation.

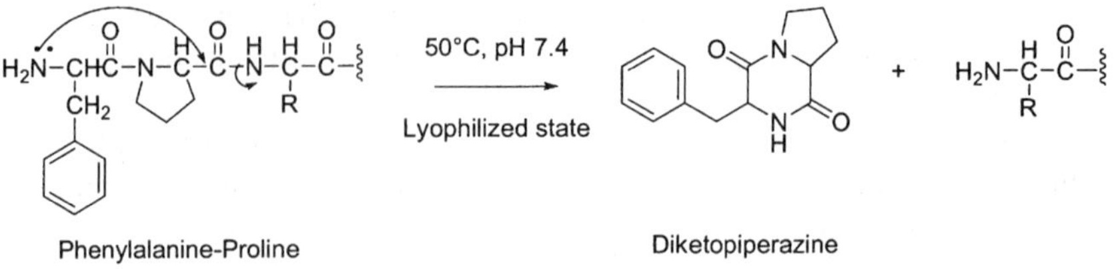

Figure 138 N-Terminal diketopiperazine formation.

(hydroxymethyl) aminomethane] has been shown to react with aldehydes (195,196). An example of covalent reaction with buffers is seen in the case of clerocidin, which has been shown to react with TRIS and with phosphate (197). Clerocidin is a complex microbial terpenoid characterized by the presence of several electrophilic groups—a strained epoxy ring, an α,

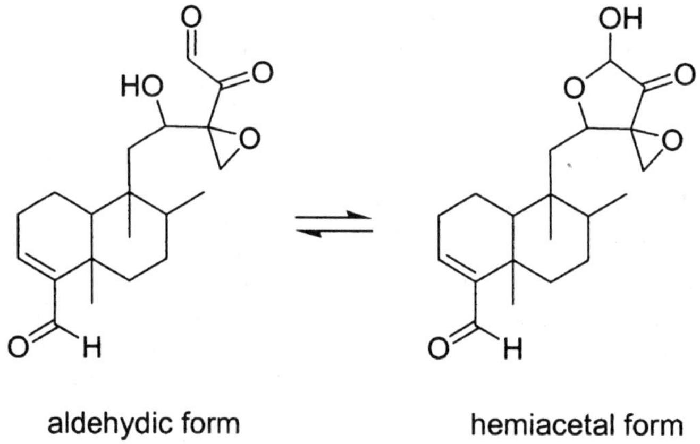

aldehydic form

hemiacetal form

Figure 139 Structure of the two forms of Clerocidin.

β-unsaturated aldehyde, and a second aldehyde functionality that is α to a ketone and is in equilibrium with a cyclic hemiacetal form (Fig. 139). In the presence of phosphate buffer (50 mM, pH 7.4, 37°C), the phosphate anion attacks the epoxy ring of Clerocidin to form two different mono-phosphate adducts (Fig. 140). A second molecule of phosphate can nucleophilically attack the electrophilic ketone to form a relatively unstable bis-adduct. In the presence of TRIS buffer (50 mM, pH 7.4, 37°C), the aldehydic carbon reacts with the nitrogen of TRIS to form an imine, and an intramolecular cyclization reaction then occurs from nucleophilic attack of one of the hydro-

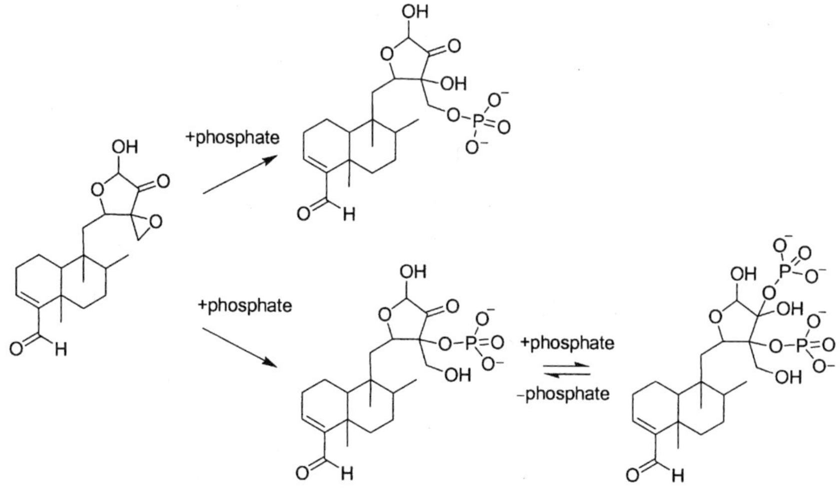

+phosphate

+phosphate

+phosphate

-phosphate

Figure 140 Reaction of Clerocidin with phosphate buffer (pH 7.4).

xyls of TRIS on the ketone of clerocidin to form a hemiacetal (Fig. 141). Opening of the epoxy ring via either attack of water or attack of a second molecule of TRIS results in either a mono-TRIS or a bis-TRIS adduct.

III. COMPUTATIONAL TOOL FOR EVALUATING POTENTIAL DEGRADATION CHEMISTRY–CAMEO

Degradation prediction is extremely useful in understanding potential degradation pathways of a drug compound (see reference for original summary) (198). The computer program CAMEO (Computer Assisted Mechanistic Evaluation of Organic Reactions) has been particularly helpful (199). The analyses cover the following key degradation conditions: basic, acidic, radical, oxidative/reductive, and photochemical as well as mechanistic interpretations of these reactions. The CAMEO prediction results can be used as an initial guide to possible degradants; however, the CAMEO-predicted degradants are not an all inclusive list of every degradation product that will actually be observed in stability studies. In general, the CAMEO

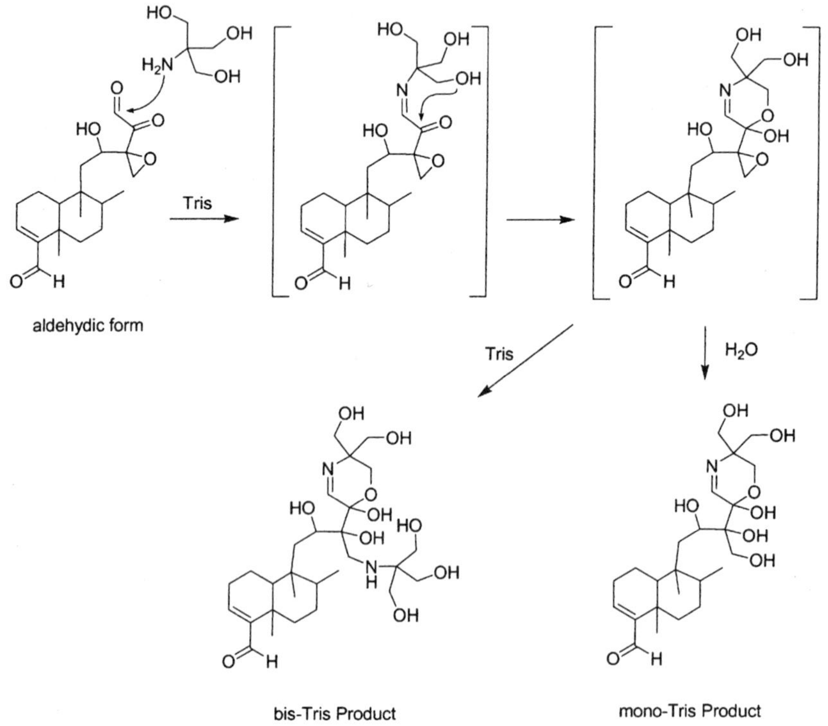

aldehydic form

bis-Tris Product

mono-Tris Product

Figure 141 Reaction of Clerocidin with Tris buffer (pH 7.4).

algorithms have been designed to give product mixtures that often times stop at the primary degradation level. In actual degradation studies, we are not performing stoichiometric chemistry and low-level secondary, ternary, etc. degradants may be observed in actual samples. CAMEO predictions often times overlook these secondary degradants. This is preferable to rules that are too restrictive and reject a key product observed in actual degradation or ICH stability or stress studies. It is also likely that certain products predicted can undergo further decomposition. For example, primary and secondary hydroperoxides typically undergo further radical termination reactions in actual degradation studies to produce non-radical termination products such as ketones and alcohols. Overall, these CAMEO-predicted degradation products assist in degradation characterization studies.

Some functional group transformations that CAMEO is particularly successful at predicting are: amide hydrolysis under basic conditions, hydroperoxide formation at benzylic sites, sulfoxide/sulfone formation, imine formation and cleavage to form the corresponding aldehyde and amine, N-oxide formation, and elimination reactions. Some functional group transformations that CAMEO is not particularly strong at predicting are: cleavage of ether groups, amide hydrolysis under acidic conditions, decarboxylation, aryl amine hydrolysis, oxidation of the benzylic hydroxyl group to the corresponding ketone, dimerization reactions, and epimerization of benzylic hydroxyl centers. In addition, if there is more than one functionality, CAMEO will typically outline the reactivity at the theoretically most labile site. In actuality, this may not be the site of degradation or more than one degradant may be observed in actual studies. For an API with more than one amide linkage, CAMEO will only show the most labile position of amide hydrolysis, whereas more than one amide hydrolysis reaction may be observed in actual degradation studies.

Another problematic area for CAMEO is secondary degradation. As mentioned above, CAMEO typically correctly predicts benzylic oxidation to the hydroperoxide precursor; however, reactivity halts at the peroxide. In actual studies, the secondary ketone degradant is typically observed and this is not reported with CAMEO.

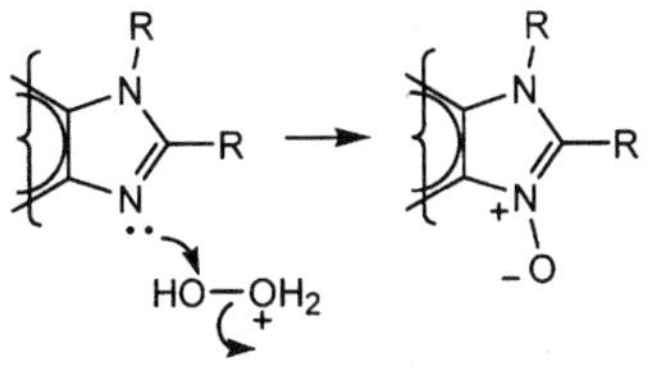

CAMEO understands that the nitrogen is nucleophilic and looks for something to react with. In this case, hydrogen peroxide is the reagent. CAMEO can adapt to new reagents and substrates.

Figure 142 CAMEO prediction example.

Due to these limitations with this prediction program, tracking historical degradation data in terms of functional groups in conjunction with CAMEO prediction data provide a more thorough approach to degradation prediction exercises. A CAMEO prediction example is provided in Figure 142.

IV. CONCLUSION

In this chapter we have highlighted some of the important drug degradation reactions that have been documented in the literature. It is important to consider the contrasts between degradation and synthetic chemistry. Synthetic chemistry is focused on stoichiometric reactions with high yields. In contrast, drug degradation chemistry is focused on reactions that are often slow, low yielding (e.g., 0.1%), and complex, where unexpected and non-obvious degradation products may form, often without literature precedent. Structure elucidation and degradation pathway delineation can be very challenging, especially when degradation products prove to be unstable. Advances in spectroscopic characterization, separation science, and analytical detection methodologies have only recently allowed for economically feasible assessments of low level impurities and degradation products. It is hoped that the examples and discussions provided in this chapter will serve as a stimulus to further explore, document, and understand the important and burgeoning field of degradation chemistry.

ACKNOWLEDGMENTS

The authors acknowledge Giovanni Boccardi, Patrick Jansen, and Dinos Santafianos for review of chapter content and mechanistic suggestions.

REFERENCES

1. March J. Advanced Organic Chemistry. Reactions, Mechanisms, and Structure. 4th ed. New York: John Wiley and Sons, 1992.

2a. Stewart PJ, Tucker IG. Prediction of drug stability—Part 1: mechanisms of drug degradation and basic rate laws. Aust J Hosp Pharm 1984; 14:165–170.

2b. Stewart PJ, Tucker IG. Prediction of drug stability—part 2: hydrolysis. Aust J Hosp Pharm 1985; 15:11–16.

2c. Stewart PJ, Tucker IG. Prediction of drug stability—part 3: Oxidation. Aust J Hosp Pharm 1985; 15:111–118.

2d. Stewart PJ, Tucker IG. Prediction of drug stability—part 4: isomerisation. Aust J Hosp Pharm 1985; 15:181–188.

3. Reynolds DW, Facchine KL, Mullaney JF, Alsante KM, Hatajik TD, Motto MG. Available guidance and best practices for conducting forced degradation studies. Pharm Tech February 2002; 2(26).

4. Zui Rappoport, Series ed. The Chemistry of Functional Groups. The Hebrew University, Jerusalem, Israel. The Patai Series was founded by Professor Saul with over 120 volumes covering all aspects of organic chemistry.
5. March J. Advanced Organic Chemistry. Reactions, Mechanisms, and Structure. 3rd ed. New York: John Wiley and Sons, 1985:334–338.
6. Florey K, ed. Analytical Profiles of Drug Substances. Vol. 8. New York: Academic Press, 1979:30.
7. Brittain HG, ed. Analytical Profiles of Drug Substances and Excipients. Vol. 21. San Diego: Academic Press, 1992:151.
8. Florey K, ed. Analytical Profiles of Drug Substances. Vol. 5. New York: Academic Press, 1976:545.
9. Brittain HG, ed. Analytical Profiles of Drug Substances and Excipients. Vol. 21. San Diego: Academic Press, 1992:280.
10. Florey K, ed. Analytical Profiles of Drug Substances. Vol. 20. New York: Academic Press, 1991:231.
11. Florey K, ed. Analytical Profiles of Drug Substances. Vol. 3. New York: Academic Press, 1974:39.
12. Florey K, ed. Analytical Profiles of Drug Substances. Vol. 4. New York: Academic Press, 1975:68.
13. Florey K, ed. Analytical Profiles of Drug Substances. Vol. 13. New York: Academic Press, 1984:229.
14. Florey K, ed. Analytical Profiles of Drug Substances. Vol. 14. New York: Academic Press, 1985:227.
15. Florey K, ed. Analytical Profiles of Drug Substances. Vol. 4. New York: Academic Press, 1989:23.
16. Florey K, ed. Analytical Profiles of Drug Substances. Vol. 20. New York: Academic Press, 1991:716.
17. Brittain HG, ed. Analytical Profiles of Drug Substances and Excipients. Vol. 28. San Diego: Academic Press, 2001:155.
18. Waterman KC, Adami RC, Alsante KM, Antipas AS, Arenson DR, Carrier R, Hong J, Landis MS, Lombardo F, Shah JC, Shalaev E, Smith SW, Wang H. Hydrolysis in pharmaceutical formulations. Pharm Dev Technol 2002; 7(2):113–146.
19. Florey K, ed. Analytical Profiles of Drug Substances. Vol. 14. New York: Academic Press, 1985:227.
20. Florey K, ed. Analytical Profiles of Drug Substances. Vol. 14. New York: Academic Press 1985:539.
21a. Baertschi SW, Dorman DE, Occolowitz JL, Spangle LA, Collins MW, Bashore FN, Lorenz LJ. Isolation and characterization of degradation products arising from aqueous degradation of cefaclor. J Pharm Sci 1997; 86(5): 526–539.
21b. Dorman DE, Lorenz LJ, Occolowitz JL, Spangle LA, Collins MW, Bashore FN, Baertschi SW. Isolation and structure elucidation of the major degradation products of cefaclor in the solid state. J Pharm Sci 1997; 86(5):540–549.
21c. Skibic M, Taylor KW, Occolowitz JL, Collins MW, Paschal J, Lorenz LJ, Spangle LA, Dorman DE, Baertschi SW. Aqueous acidic degradation of the carbacephalosporin loracarbef. J Pharm Sci 1993; 82(10):1010–1017.

21d. Bontchev PR, Papazova P. Hydrolysis of cephalosporins in strongly acidic medium. Pharmazie 1978; 33(H.6):346–348.
21e. Fuentes-Robinson VA, Jeffries TM, Branch SK. Degradation pathways of ampicillin in alkaline solutions. J Pharm Pharmacol 1997; 49:843–851.
22. Flynn EH, ed. Cephalosporins and Penicillins: Chemistry and Biology. New York: Academic Press, 1972.
23. Waxman DJ, Strominger JL. Penicillin-binding proteins and the mechanism of action of beta-lactam antibiotics. Ann Rev Biochem 1983; 52:825–869.
24. Page MI. The mechanisms of reactions of beta-lactam antibiotics. Adv Phy Organ Chem 1987; 23:65–270.
25. Smith H, Marshall AC. Polymers formed by some β-lactam antibiotics. Nature 1971; 232:45–46.
26. Larsen C, Bundgaard H. Polymerization of penicillins. J Chromatography 1978; 147:143–150.
27. Baertschi SW, Boyd DB, Cantrell AS, Jaskunas SR, Kuhfeld MT, Lorenz LJ. Inhibition of HIV-1 reverse transcriptase by degradation products of ceftazidime. Antiviral Chem Chemother 1997; 8(4):353–362.
28. Florey K, ed. Analytical Profiles of Drug Substances. Vol. 7. New York: Academic Press, 1978:35.
29. Florey K, ed. Analytical Profiles of Drug Substances. Vol. 1. New York: Academic Press, 1972:263.
30. Florey K, ed. Analytical Profiles of Drug Substances. Vol. 5. New York: Academic Press, 1976:163.
31. Florey K, ed. Analytical Profiles of Drug Substances. Vol. 7. New York: Academic Press, 1978:377.
32. March J. Advanced Organic Chemistry. Reactions, Mechanisms, and Structure. 3rd ed. New York: John Wiley and Sons, 1985:229–230.
33. March J. Advanced Organic Chemistry. Reactions, Mechanisms, and Structure. 3rd ed. New York: John Wiley and Sons, 1985:562–565.
34. Florey K, ed. Analytical Profiles of Drug Substances. Vol. 13. New York: Academic Press, 1984:319.
35. Florey K, ed. Analytical Profiles of Drug Substances. Vol. 14. New York: Academic Press, 1985:513.
36. Florey K, ed. Analytical Profiles of Drug Substances. Vol. 20. New York: Academic Press, 1991:588.
37. Florey K, ed. Analytical Profiles of Drug Substances. Vol. 20. New York: Academic Press, 1991:717.
38. Brittain HG, ed. Analytical Profiles of Drug Substances and Excipients. Vol. 24. San Diego: Academic Press, 1996:433.
39. Lowry TH, Richardson KS. Reactions of carbonyl compounds. Mechanism and Theory in Organic Chemistry. 2nd ed. New York: Harper and Row, 1981: 596–598.
40a. Wirth DD, Baertschi SW, Johnson RA, Maple SR, Miller MS, Hallenbeck DK, Gregg SM. Maillard reaction of lactose and fluoxetine hydrochloride, a secondary amine. J Pharm Sci 1998; 87(1):31–39.
40b. Maillard LCC. R Acad Sci Ser 1912; 2(154):66.
40c. Maillard LCC. R Acad Sci Ser 1912; 2(155):1554–1556.

40d. Ellis GP. The Maillard reaction. Adv Carbohydr Chem 1959; 14:63–134.

40e. Hodge JE. Dehydrated foods: chemistry of browning reactions in model systems. J Agric Food Chem 1953; 1:928–943.

41. March J. Advanced Organic Chemistry. Reactions, Mechanisms, and Structure. 3rd ed. New York: John Wiley and Sons, 1985:829–831.

42. Florey K, ed. Analytical Profiles of Drug Substances. Vol. 9, New York: Academic Press, 1980:357.

43. Albini A, Fasani E. Drugs: Photochemistry and Photostability. An Overview and Practical Problems Cambridge, UK: The Royal Society of Chemistry, 1998:2.

44. Florey K, ed. Analytical Profiles of Drug Substances. Vol. 1. New York: Academic Press, 1972:411.

45. Payne GB, Deming PH, Williams PH. Reactions of hydrogen peroxide VII. Alkali-catalyzed epoxidation and oxidation using nitrile as co-reactant. J Org Chem 1961; 26:659–663.

46. Laus G. Kinetics of acetonitrile-assisted oxidation of tertiary amines by hydrogen peroxide. J Chem Soc Perkins Trans 2001; 2:864–868.

47. Florey K, ed. Analytical Profiles of Drug Substances. Vol. 13. New York: Academic Press, 1984:164.

48. Riesz P, Kondo T, Carmichael AJ. Sonochemistry of acetone and acetonitrile in aqueous solutions. A spin-trapping study. Free Rad Res Comm 1993; 19:S45–S53.

49. Wender PA, DeLong MA. Synthetic studies on arene-olefin cycloadditions. XII. Total synthesis of (±)-subergorgic acid. Tetrahedron Lett 1990; 31(38): 5429–5432.

50. Florey K, ed. Analytical Profiles of Drug Substances. New York: Academic Press 1978:165.

51. Qin X-Z, Ip DP, Chang KH-C, Dradransky PM, Brooks MA, Sakuma T. Pharmaceutical application of LC-MS. 1—Characterization of a famotidine degradate in a package screening study by LC-APCI MS. J Pharm Biomed Anal 1994; 12(2):221–233.

52. Francolic JD, Lehr GJ, Barry TL, Petzinger G. Isolation of a 2:1 hydrochlorothiazide-formaldehyde adduct impurity in hydrochlorothiazide drug substance by preparative chromatography and characterization by electrospray ionization LC-MS. J Pharm Biomed Anal 2001; 26:651–663.

53. Schick MJ, ed. Nonionic Surfactants Physical Chemistry. Chapter 18. Stability of the Polyoxyethylene Chain. New York: Marcel Dekker, 1987:1011.

54a. Hartauer K, Arbuthnot G, Baertschi SW, Johnson R, Luke W, Pearson N, Rickard E, Tsang P, Wiens R. Influence of peroxide impurities in povidone and crospovidone on the tablet stability of raloxifene hydrochloride. Identification and control of an oxidative degradation product. Pharmaceut Dev Tech 2000; 5(3):303–319.

54b. Vermeire A, Remon JP. Stability and compatibility of morphine. Int J Pharm 1999; 187(1):17–51.

54c. Qin X, Freeh P. Liquid chromatography/mass spectrometry (LC/MS) identification of photooxidative degradates of crystalline and amorphous MK-912. J Pharm Sci 2001; 90(7):833–844.

55. March J. In: Advanced Organic Chemistry. Reactions, Mechanisms, and Structure. 3rd ed. New York: John Wiley and Sons, 1985:909.
56. Zhao ZZ, Qin X-Z, Wu A, Yuan Y. Novel rearrangements of an N-oxide degradate formed from oxidation of a morpholine acetal substance P antagonist. J Pharm Sci 2004; 93(8):1957–1961.
57. Joule JA, Mills K, Smith GF. Heterocyclic Chemistry. 3rd ed. Cheltenham, UK: Stanley Thornes (Publishers) Ltd. 1988:101.
58. Florey K, ed. Analytical Profiles of Drug Substances. Vol.12. New York: Academic Press, 1983:122.
59. Brittain HG, ed. Analytical Profiles of Drug Substances and Excipients. Vol. 28. San Diego: Academic Press, 2001:111.
60. Brittain HG, ed. Analytical Profiles of Drug Substances and Excipients. Vol. 26. San Diego: Academic Press, 1999:86.
61. Brittain HG, ed. Analytical Profiles of Drug Substances and Excipients. Vol. 26. San Diego: Academic Press, 1999:312.
62. Brittain HG, ed. Analytical Profiles of Drug Substances and Excipients. Vol. 22. San Diego: Academic Press, 1993:86.
63a. Smith MB, March J. Advanced Organic Chemistry. Reactions, Mechanisms, and Structure. 5th ed. New York: John Wiley and Sons, 2001:729.
63b. Ogata Y, Takagi K. Photochemical reactions of N-alkylanilines. J Organic Chem 1970; 35(5):1642–1645.
64. Chafetz L, Hong W-H, Tsilifonis DC, Taylor AK, Philip J. Decrease in the rate of capsule dissolution due to formaldehyde from polysorbate 80 autoxidation. J Pharm Sci 1984; 73(8):1186–1187.
65. Bindra DS, Williams TD, Stella VJ. Degradation of O^6-benzylguanine in aqueous polyethylene glycol 400 (PEG 400) solutions: concerns with formaldehyde in PEG 400. Pharm Res 1994; 11(7):1060–1064.
66a. Houminer Y, Hoz S. Formation of formaldehyde in the thermal decomposition of D-glucose labelled with ^{14}C at various positions. Israel J Chem 1979; 8:97–98.
66b. Ferrier RJ, Severn WB, Furneaux RH, Miller IJ. Isotope studies of the transfer of the carbon atoms of carbohydrate derivatives into aromatic compounds (especially xanthene) under degradation conditions. Carbohydrate Res 1992; 237:87–94.
66c. Ponder GR, Richards GN. Pyrolysis of inulin, glucose, and fructose. Carbohydrate Res 1993; 244:341–359.
67a. Walker JF. Formaldehyde. American Chemical Society Monograph Series. 2nd ed. Baltimore, Maryland: Waverly Press, 1953:311–317.
67b. Kirk-Othmer. Encyclopedia of Chemical Technology. 3rd ed. New York: Wiley Vol. 11. 1980:911.
68. Marks EM, Toutellote D, Andux A. The phenomenon of gelatin insolubility. Food Technol 1968; 22:1433.
69a. Ofner CM III, Zhang Yu-E, Jobeck VC, Bowman BJ. Cross-linking studies in gelatin capsules treated with formaldehyde and in capsules exposed to elevated temperature and humidity. J Pharmaceut Sci 2001; 90(1):79–88.
69b. Digenis GA, Gold TB, Shah VP. Cross-linking of gelatin capsules and its relevance to their in vitro-in vivo performance. J Pharm Sci 1994; 83(7):915–921.

69c. Desai DS, Rubitski BA, Varia SA, Huang MH. Effect of formaldehyde formation on dissolution stability of hydrochlorothiazide bead formulations. Int J Pharmaceut 1994; 107(2):141–147.
70. Desai DS, Rubitski BA, Bergum JS, Varia SA. Effects of different types of lactose and disintegrant on dissolution stability of hydrochlorothiazide capsule formulations. Int J Pharm 1994; 110:257–265.
71. Stephenson SA, Bryant DK, Thomson CM, Walsgrove TC, Webb ML. An analytical study of the interaction of low levels of formaldehyde with active Pharmaceuticals. Pharm Pharmacol 1998; 50(suppl):122.
72a. Belongia EA, Hedlberg CW, Gleich GJ, White KE, Mayeno AN, Loegering DA, Dunnette SL, Pirie PL, MacDonald KL, Osterhohn MT. An investigation of the cause of the eosinophilia–myalgia syndrome associated with tryptophan use. N Engl J Med 1990; 323:357–365.
72b. Smith MJ, Mazzola EP, Farrell TJ, Sphon JA, Page SW, Ashley D, Sirimanne SR, Hill RH Jr, Needham LL. 1,1′-Ethylidenebis(L-tryptophan) structure determination of contaminant 97—implicated in the eosinophilia–myalgia syndrome (EMS). Tetrahedron Lett 1991; 32(8):991–994.
72c. Toyoda M, Saito Y, Uchiyama M, Troy AL, Trucksess MW, Page SW. Formation of a 3-(phenylamino)alanine contaminant in EMS-associated L-tryptophan. Biosci Biotech Biochem 1994; 58(7):1318–1320.
73. Mayeno AN, Lin F, Foote CS, Loegering DA, Ames MM, Hedberg CW, Gleich GJ. Characterization of "Peak E", a novel amino acid associated with eosinophilia–myalgia syndrome. Science 1990; 250:1707–1708.
74. Hill RH Jr, Caudill SP, Philen RM, Bailey SL, Flanders WD, Driskell WJ, Kamb ML, Needham LL, Sampson EJ. Contaminants in L-tryptophan associatedwith eosinophilia–myalgia syndrome. Arch Environ Contam Toxicol 1993; 25:134–142.
75. Castello RA, Mattocks AM. Discoloration of tablets containing amines and lactose. Pharm Sci 1962; 51:106–108.
76a. Yaylayan VA, Huyghues-Despointes A. Chemistry of amadori rearrangement products: analysis, synthesis, kinetics, reactions, and spectroscopic properties. Cri Rev Food Sci Nutr 1994; 34(4):321–369.
76b. Colaco C, Collett M, Roser B. Pharmaceutical formulation instability and the Maillard Reaction. Chem Oggi 1996; 14:32–37.
77. Hodge JE. The Amadori rearrangement. Adv Carbohydr Chem 1955; 10: 169–205.
78. Hurley TR, Lovdahl MJ, Priebe SR, Tobias B. Synthesis and characterization of pregabalin lactose conjugate degradation products. Presented at conference session. Detecting, Identifying, and Quantitating Impurities. Princeton, New Jersey: Institute for International Research, 2002:20–21.
79. Tjan SB, van den Ouweland GAM. PMR investigation into the structure of some N-substituted 1-amino-l-deoxy-D-fructoses (Amadori rearrangement products). Tetrahedron 1974; 30:2891–2897.
80. Florey K, ed. Analytical Profiles of Drug Substances, Vol. 20. New York: Academic Press, 1991:395.
81. Florey K, ed. Analytical Profiles of Drug Substances. Vol. 20. New York: Academic Press, 1991:557.

82. Schildcrout SA, Risley DS, Kleeman RL. Drug–excipient interactions of seproxetine maleate hemi-hydrate: isothermal stress methods. Drug Dev Indust Pharm 1993; 19(10):1113–1130.
83. Baertschi SW, et al. Eli Lilly and Company, unpublished results.
84. Jansen PJ, Oren PL, Kemp CA, Maple SR, Baertschi SW. Characterization of impurities formed by interaction of duloxetine HC1 with enteric polymers hydroxypropyl methylcellulose acetate succinate (HPMCAS) and hydroxypropyl methylcellulose phthalate (HPMCP). J Pharm Sci 1998; 87(1):81–85.
85. Almarsson Ö, Kaufman MJ, Stong JD, Wu Y, Mayr SM, Petrich MA, Williams MJ. Meropenem exists in equilibrium with a carbon dioxide adduct in bicarbonate solution. J Pharm Sci 1998; 87:5.
86. Alsante KM, Salisbury JJ, Hatajik TD, Snyder KD. Investigation of ICH photostability for purposeful degradation studies: option 1 vs option 2. Pharmaceutical Photostability '01. Research Triangle Park North Carolina. 19 July 2001.
87. Florey K, ed. Analytical Profiles of Drug Substances. Vol. 4. New York: Academic Press, 1975:259.
88. Florey K, ed. Analytical Profiles of Drug Substances. Vol. 19. New York: Academic Press, 1990:615.
89. Florey K, ed. Analytical Profiles of Drug Substances. Vol. 1. New York: Academic Press, 1972:93.
90. Florey K, ed. Analytical Profiles of Drug Substances. Vol. 14. New York: Academic Press, 1985:148.
91. Florey K, ed. Analytical Profiles of Drug Substances. Vol. 3. New York: Academic Press, 1974:323.
92. Florey K, ed. Analytical Profiles of Drug Substances. Vol. 4. New York: Academic Press, 1975:109.
93. Florey K, ed. Analytical Profiles of Drug Substances. Vol. 6. New York: Academic Press, 1977:73.
94. Florey K, ed. Analytical Profiles of Drug Substances. Vol. 4. New York: Academic Press, 1975:259.
95. Florey K, ed. Analytical Profiles of Drug Substances. Vol. 5. New York: Academic Press, 1976:417.
96. Smith MB, March J. Advanced Organic Chemistry. Reactions, Mechanisms, and Structure. 5th ed. New York: John Wiley and Sons, 2001:787.
97. Smith MB, March J. Advanced Organic Chemistry. Reactions, Mechanisms, and Structure. 5th ed. New York: John Wiley and Sons, 2001:1178.
98. Florey K, ed. Analytical Profiles of Drug Substances. Vol. 19. New York: Academic Press, 1990:42.
99. Florey K, ed. Analytical Profiles of Drug Substances. Vol. 18. New York: Academic Press, 1989:245.
100. Albini A, Fasani E. Drugs: Photochemistry and Photostability. An Overview and Practical Problems. Cambridge, UK: The Royal Society of Chemistry, 1998:21.
101. Smith MB, March J. Advanced Organic Chemistry, Reactions, Mechanisms, and Structure. 5th ed. New York: John Wiley and Sons, 2001:576.

102. Horspool WM. CRC Handbook of Photochemistry and Photobiology. Chapter 61. CRC Press, 1995:758.
103. Brittain HG, ed. Analytical Profiles of Drug Substances and Excipients. Vol. 26. San Diego: Academic Press, 1999:87.
104. Florey K, ed. Analytical Profiles of Drug Substances. Vol. 6. New York: Academic Press, 1977:539.
105. Florey K, ed. Analytical Profiles of Drug Substances. Vol. 7. New York: Academic Press, 1978:414.
106. Florey K, ed. Analytical Profiles of Drug Substances. Vol. 10. New York: Academic Press, 1981:345.
107. Florey K, ed. Analytical Profiles of Drug Substances. Vol. 10. New York: Academic Press, 1981:345.
108. Hovorka SW, Schoneich C. Oxidative degradation of Pharmaceuticals: theory, mechanisms, and inhibition. J Pharm Sci 2001; 90(3):253–269.
109. Florey K, ed. Analytical Profiles of Drug Substances. Vol. 16. New York: Academic Press, 1987:676.
110. Florey K, ed. Analytical Profiles of Drug Substances. Vol. 9. New York: Academic Press, 1980:138.
111. Florey K, ed. Analytical Profiles of Drug Substances. Vol. 13. New York: Academic Press, 1984:318.
112. Florey K, ed. Analytical Profiles of Drug Substances. Vol. 2. New York: Academic Press, 1973:256.
113. Florey K, ed. Analytical Profiles of Drug Substances. Vol. 13. New York: Academic Press, 1984:165.
114. Brittain HG, ed. Analytical Profiles of Drug Substances and Excipients. Vol. 21. San Diego: Academic Press, 1992:375.
115. Florey K, ed. Analytical Profiles of Drug Substances. Vol. 19. New York: Academic Press, 1990:421.
116. Brittain HG, ed. Analytical Profiles of Drug Substances and Excipients. Vol. 21. San Diego: Academic Press, 1992:409.
117. Florey K, ed. Analytical Profiles of Drug Substances. Vol. 6. New York: Academic Press, 1977:163.
118. Florey K, ed. Analytical Profiles of Drug Substances. Vol. 9. New York: Academic Press, 1980:138.
119. Florey K, ed. Analytical Profiles of Drug Substances. Vol. 16. New York: Academic Press, 1987:383.
120. Louden GM. Organic Chemistry. 2nd ed. Menlo Park, Carolina: Benjamin/Cummings Publishing Co. Inc., 1988:319–367.
121. Brandl M, Wu X, Liu Yanzhou, Pease J, Holper M, Hooijmaaijer E, Lu Yvonne, Ping W. Chemical reactivity of R0-26-9228, l-α-fluoro-25-hydroxy-16,23E-diene-26,27-bishomo-20-epi-cholecalciferol in aqueous solution. J Pharm Sci 2003; 92(10).
122. Bontchev PR, Papazova P. Hydrolysis of cephalosporins in strongly acidic medium. Pharmazie 1978; 33(6):346–348.
123. Brittain HG, ed. Analytical Profiles of Drug Substances and Excipients. Vol. 21. San Diego: Academic Press, 1992:299.

124. Ahuja S, Aisante KM, eds. Handbook of Isolation and Characterization of Impurities in Pharmaceuticals. Vol. 5. Separation Science and Technology Alsante KM, Hatajik TD, Lohr LL, Santafianos D, Sharp TR. Solving Impurity/Degradation Problems: Case Studies. Chapter 14. San Diego, CA: Academic Press 2003:361–400.
125. Mihailović, Ĉekovic. Oxidation and reduction of phenols. In: Patai S, ed. The Chemistry of the Hydroxyl Group. Part 1. Chapter 10. New York, Interscience Publishers, 1971.
126. Florey K, ed. Analytical Profiles of Drug Substances. Vol. 7. New York: Academic Press, 1970:215.
127. Albini A, Fasani E. Drugs: Photochemistry and Photostability. An Overview and Practical Problems. Cambridge, UK: The Royal Society of Chemistry, 1998:23.
128. Florey K, ed. Analytical Profiles of Drug Substances. Vol. 11. New York: Academic Press, 1982:562.
129. March J. Advanced Organic Chemistry. Reactions, Mechanisms, and Structure. 4th ed. New York: John Wiley and Sons, 1992:860.
130. Florey K, ed. Analytical Profiles of Drug Substances. Vol. 13. New York: Academic Press, 1984:289.
131. Florey K, ed. Analytical Profiles of Drug Substances. Vol. 4. New York: Academic Press, 1975:68.
132. Moore DE, Roberts-Thompson S, Zhen D, Duke CC. Photochemical studies on the anti-inflammatory drug diclofenac. Photochem Photobiol 1990; 52: 685–690.
133. Paillous N, Verrier M. Photolysis of amiodarone, an antiarrhythmic drug. Photochem Photobiol 1988; 47:337–343.
134. Fasani E, Barberis Negra FF, Mella M, Monti S, Albini A. Photoinduced C–F bond cleavage in some fluorinated 7-amino-4-quinolone-3-carboxylic acids. J Org Chem 1999; 64:5388–5395.
135. Albini A, Fasani E. Drugs: Photochemistry and Photostability. An Overview and Practical Problems. Cambridge, United Kingdom: The Royal Society of Chemistry, 1998:7.
136. Albini A, Fasani E. Drugs: Photochemistry and Photostability. An Overview and Practical Problems. Cambridge, United Kingdom: The Royal Society of Chemistry, 1998:20.
137. Walling C. Some properties of radical reactions important in synthesis. Tetrahedron 1985; 41:3887–3890.
138. Russell GA. Deuterium-isotope effects in the autoxidation of aralkyl hydrocarbons. Mechanism of the interaction of peroxy radicals. J Am Chem Soc 1957; 79(14):3871–3877.
139. March J. Advanced Organic Chemistry. Reactions, Mechanisms, and Structure. 3rd ed. 1985:164.
140. Florey K, ed. Analytical Profiles of Drug Substances. Vol. 14. New York: Academic Press, 1985:59.
141. Waterman KC, Roy MC. Use of oxygen scavengers to stabilize solid pharmaceutical dosage forms: a case study. Pharmaceut Dev Technol 2002; 7(2): 227–234.

142. Florey K, ed. Analytical Profiles of Drug Substances. Vol. 20. New York: Academic Press, 1991:405.
143. Brittain HG, ed. Analytical Profiles of Drug Substances and Excipients. Vol. 21. San Diego: Academic Press, 1992:163.
144. Brittain HG, ed. Analytical Profiles of Drug Substances and Excipients. Vol. 27. San Diego: Academic Press, 2001:293.
145. Smith MB, March J. Advanced Organic Chemistry. Reactions, Mechanisms, and Structure. 5th ed. New York: John Wiley and Sons, 2001:1049.
146. Florey K, ed. Analytical Profiles of Drug Substances. Vol. 7. New York: Academic Press, 1978:125.
147. Florey K, ed. Analytical Profiles of Drug Substances. Vol. 17. New York: Academic Press, 1988:177.
148. Florey K, ed. Analytical Profiles of Drug Substances. Vol. 18. New York: Academic Press, 1989:553.
149. Brittain HG, ed. Analytical Profiles of Drug Substances and Excipients. Vol. 21. San Diego: Academic Press, 1992:299.
150. Lowry TH, Richardson KS. Mechanism and Theory in Organic Chemistry. 3rd ed. New York: Harper & Row, 1987:903.
151. Smith MB, March J. Advanced Organic Chemistry. Reactions, Mechanisms, and Structure. 5th ed. New York: John Wiley and Sons, 2001:903.
152. Wang Y, Taylor J-S, Gross ML. Nuclease P1 digestion combined withtandem mass spectrometry for the structure determination of DNA photoproducts. Chem Res Toxicol 1999; 12:1077–1082.
153. Saitou M, Hieda K. Dithymine photodimers and photodecomposition products of thymidylyl-thymidine induced by ultraviolet radiation from 150 to 300 nm. Radiation Res 1994; 140(2):215–220.
154. Lowry TH, Richardson KS. Mechanism and Theory in Organic Chemistry. 3rd ed. New York: Harper & Row, 1987:1009.
155. Reddy M, Reddy V, Srinivas U, Reddy M, Rao V. Regioselective E(*trans*)-Z(*cis*) photoisomerization in napthyldiene derivatives. Proc Indian Acad Sci (Chem Sci) 2002; 114(6):603–609.
156a. Morliere P, Avice O, Melo T, Dubertret M, Giraud M, Santus R. A study of the photochemical properties of some cinnamate sunscreens by steady state and laser flash photolysis. Photochem Photobiol 1982; 36:395–399.
156b. Broadbent J, Martincigh B, Raynor M, Salter L, Moulder R, Sjoberg P, Markides M. Capillary supercritical fluid chromatography combined with atmospheric pressure chemical ionization mass spectrometry for the investigation of photoproduct formation in the sunscreen absorber 2-ethylhexyl-*p*-methoxycinnamate. J Chromatography 1996; 732:101–110.
157. Porter NA, Caldwell SE, Mills KA. Mechanisms of free radical oxidation of unsaturated lipids. Lipids 1995; 30(4):277–289.
158a. Porter NA, Caldwell SE, Mills KA. Mechanisms of free radical oxidation of unsaturated lipids. Lipids 1995; 30(4):277–290.
158b. Porter NA. Mechanisms for the autoxidation of polyunsaturated lipids. Acc Chem Res 1986; 19:262–268.
158c. Rouzer CA, Marnett LJ. Mechanism of free radical oxygenation of polyunsaturated fatty acids by cyclooxgenases. Chem Rev 2003; 103(6):2239–2304.

159. Morrow JD, Awad JA, Boss HJ, Blair IA, Roberts LJ II. Non-cyclooxygenase-derived prostanoids (F2-isoprostanes) are formed in situ on phospholipids. Proc Nat Acad Sci USA 1992; 89(22):10721–10725.
160. Morrow JD, Roberts LJ. II, The isoprostanes: unique bioactive products of lipid peroxidation, Progr in Lipid Res 1997; 36(1):1–21.
161. Roberts LJ II, Montine TJ, Markesbury WR, Tapper AR, Hardy P, Chemtob S, Dettbam WD, Morrow JD. Formation of isoprostane-like compounds (neuroprostanes) in vivo from docosahexaenoic acid. J Biol Chem 1998; 273(22):13605–13612.
162. Florey K, ed. Analytical Profiles of Drug Substances. Vol. 4. NewYork: Academic Press, 1975: 399.
163. Brittain HG, ed. Analytical Profiles of Drug Substances and Excipients. Vol. 26. San Diego: Academic Press, 1999:87.
164. Florey K, ed. Analytical Profiles of Drug Substances. Vol. 12. New York: Academic Press, 1983:393.
165. Florey K, ed. Analytical Profiles of Drug Substances. Vol. 9. New York: Academic Press, 1980:411.
166. Florey K, ed. Analytical Profiles of Drug Substances. Vol. 16. New York: Academic Press, 1987:617.
167. Florey K, ed. Analytical Profiles of Drug Substances. Vol. 20. New York: Academic Press, 1991:588.
168. Brittain HG, ed. Analytical Profiles of Drug Substances and Excipients. Vol. 22. San Diego: Academic Press, 1993:254.
169. Florey K, ed. Analytical Profiles of Drug Substances. Vol. 18. New York: Academic Press, 1989:141.
170. Pop E, Huang MJ, Brewster ME, Bodor N. On the mechanism of cephalosporin isomerization. J Mol Struct (Theochem) 1994; 315:1–7.
171. Richter WF, Chong YH, Stella VJ. On the mechanism of isomerization of cephalosporin esters. J Pharm Sci 1990; 79(2):185–186.
172. Florey K, ed. Analytical Profiles of Drug Substances. Vol. 8. New York: Academic Press, 1979:383.
173. Voet D, Voet JG. Biochemistry, 2nd ed. New York: John Wiley and Sons, Inc., 1995:251–259.
174. Louden GM. Organic Chemistry. 2nd ed. Reading, MA: The Benjamin Cummings Publishing Company, Inc.,1988:1210.
175. Juaristi E. The Anomeric Effect. CRC Press, 1994.
176. Carey FA, Sunberg RJ. Advanced Organic Chemistry, Part A: Structure and Mechanism. 3rd ed. 1990; 147–149.
177. Brittain HG, ed. Analytical Profiles of Drug Substances and Excipients. Vol. 23. San Diego: Academic Press, 1994:305.
178. Miller PS. A brief guide to nucleic acid chemistry. Bioconjugate Chem. 1990; 1:187–191.
179. Pogocki D, Schoenich C. Chemical stability of nucleic acid-derived drugs. J Pharm Sci 2000; 89(4):443–456.
180. Lindahl T. Instability of the primary structure of DNA. Nature 1993; 362: 709–715.

181a. Anliker SL, McClure MS, Britton TC, Stephan EA, Maple SR, Cooke GG. Degradation chemistry of gemcitabine hydrochloride, a new antitumor agent. J Pharm Sci 1994; 83(5):716–719.

181b. Jansen PJ, Akers MJ, Amos RM, Baertschi SW, Cooke GG, Dorman DE, Kemp CAJ, Maple SR, McCune KA. The degradation of the antitummor agent gemcitabine hydrochloride in an acidic aqueous solution at pH 3.2 and identification of degradation products. J Pharm Sci 2000; 89(7):885–891.

182. Waterman KC, Adami RC, Alsante KM, Hong JH, Landis MS, Lombardo M, Roberts CJ. Stabilization of Pharmaceuticals to oxidative degradation. Pharm Dev Technol 2002; 7(1):1–32.

183. Yu J. Intentionally degrading protein pharmaceuticals to validate stability-indicating analytical methods. Bio Pharm November 2000; 13(11):46–50.

184. Niu CH, Chiu Y. FDA Perspective on peptide formulation and stability issues. J Pharm Sci 1998; 87(11).

185. Geiger T, Clark S. Deamidation, isomerization, and racemization at asparaginyland aspartyl residues in peptides. J Biol Chem 1987; 262(2):785–794.

186. Capasso S, Kirby AJ, Salvadori S, Sica F, Zagari A. Kinetics and mechanism of the reversible isomerization of aspartic acid residues in tetrapeptides. J Chem Soc Perkin Trans 1995; 3:437–442.

187. Capasso S, Mazarella L, Zagari A. Deamidation via cyclic imide of asparaginyl peptides: dependence on salts, buffers, and organic solvents. Peptide Res 1991; 4(4):234–238.

188. Patel K, Borchardt RT. Chemical pathways of peptide degradation.II. Kinetics of deamidation of an asparaginyl residue in a model hexapeptide. Pharm Res 1990; 7(7):703–711.

189. Xie M, Vander Velde D, Morton M, Borchardt RT, Schowen RL. pH-induced change in the rate-determining step for the hydrolysis of the Asp/Asn-derived-cyclic-imide intermediate in protein degradation J Am Chem Soc 1996; 118:8955–8956.

190. Aswad DW. Stoichiometric methylation of porcine adrenocorticotropin by protein carboxyl methyltransferase requires deamidation of asparagine 25. Evidence for methylation at the alpha-carboxyl group of atypical L-isoaspartyl residues. J Biol Chem 1984; 259:10714–10721.

191. Johnson BA, Shirokawa J, Hancock W, Spellman M, Basa L, Aswad D. Formation of isoaspartate at two distinct sites during in vitro aging of human growth hormone. J Biol Chem 1989; 264:14262–14271.

192. Kwong M, Harris R. Identification of succinimide sites in proteins by N-terminal sequence analysis after alkaline hydroxylamine cleavage. Protein Sci 1994; 3:147–149.

193. Moorhouse KG, Nashabeh W, Deveney J, Bjork NS, Mulkerrin MG, Ryskamp T. Validation of an HPLC method for the analysis of the charge heterogeneity of the recombinant monoclonal antibody IDEC-C2B8 after papain digestion. J Pharm Biomed Anal 1997; 16:593–603.

194. Battersby IE, Hancock WS, Canova-Davis E, Oeswein J, O'Connor B. Diketopiperazine: formation and N–terminal degradation in recombinant human growth hormone. Int J Peptide Protein Res 1994; 44(3):215–222.

195. Niedernhofer LJ, Riley M, Schnetz-Boutaud N, Sanduwaran G, Chaudhary AK, Reddy GR, Marnett LJ. Temperature-dependent formation of a conjugate between tris-(hydroxymethyl)aminomethane buffer and the malondialdehyde-DNA adduct pyrimidopurinone. Chem Res Toxicol 1997; 10:556–561.
196. Bubb WA, Berthon HA, Kuchel P. Tris buffer reactivity with low molecular-weight aldehydes, NMR characterization of the reactions of glyceraldehyde 3-phosphate. Bioorg Chem 1995; 23:119–130.
197. Richter S, Fabris D, Binaschi M, Gatto B, Capranico G, Palumbo M. Effects of common buffer systems on drug activity: the case of clerocidin. Chem Res Toxicol 2004; 17:492–501.
198. Alsante KM, Friedmann RC, Hatajik TD, Lohr LL, Sharp TR, Snyder KD, Szczesny EJ. Degradation and impurity analysis for pharmaceutical candidates. In: Ahuja S, Scypinski S, eds. Handbook of Modern Pharmaceutical Analysis. Separation Science and Technology. Vol. 3. New York: Academic Press, 2001:113.
199. Jorgensen WL, Laird ER, Gushurst AJ, Fleischer JM, Gothe SA, Helson HE, Paderes GD, Sinclair S. CAMEO: a program for the logical prediction of the products of organic reactions. Pure Appl Chem 1990; 62:1921–1932.
200. Luo D, Smith S, Anderson BD. Kinetics and mechanism of the reaction of cysteine and hydrogen peroxide in aqueous solution, J Pharm Sci 2005; 94(2):314–314.

4

Stress Testing: Analytical Considerations

Patrick J. Jansen, W. Kimmer Smith, and Steven W. Baertschi
Eli Lilly and Company, Lilly Research Laboratories, Lilly Corporate Center, Indianapolis, Indiana, U.S.A.

I. STRESS-TESTING CONDITIONS AND SAMPLE PREPARATION

A. Introduction

Although there are some guidelines for stress testing given in the ICH guideline on the stability testing of drug substances and drug products, the guidance given is very general and not particularly useful for designing a stress-testing study. The following is an excerpt from the revised guideline [Q1A(R2)] (1):

> Stress testing is likely to be carried out on a single batch of the drug substance. It should include the effect of temperatures [in 10°C increments (e.g., 50°C, 60°C, etc.) above that for accelerated testing], humidity (e.g., 75% RH or greater) where appropriate, oxidation, and photolysis on the drug substance. The testing should also evaluate the susceptibility of the drug substance to hydrolysis across a wide range of pH values when in solution or suspension. Photostability testing should be an integral part of stress testing.

Additional guidance is given only for photostability testing (2). Since there is very little guidance on stress testing, the goal of this chapter is to provide the reader with general guidance on the design, set up, and analytical aspects of carrying out stress-testing studies. The main focus of this chapter is chemical degradation, therefore, the assessment of the physical stability of solid drug substances is not discussed. Although a significant amount of detail is given in this chapter, the reader is reminded that these are only suggestions from the experience of the authors and that there are many acceptable ways to perform these studies.

B. Data Gathering

The first task before beginning stress-testing studies is to gather all the relevant information about the compound. Information such as molecular structure, solubility, p*K*(s), known chemical instability, hygroscopicity, enantiomeric purity, etc. is important. In addition, previously established analytical methods may provide a starting point for development of more discriminating methods required for the separation of the complex mixtures which may result from stress degradation.

The molecular structure of a compound is very important. For example, one can usually deduce from the structure whether or not the compound will absorb UV radiation and be detectable with a UV detector. The molecular structure also reveals if the compound has ionizable functional groups and will require a mobile phase modifier if HPLC analysis is used. Examination of the molecular structure may also tell something about the chemical reactivity of the molecule. The molecular structure indicates whether the molecule contains any chiral centers. If the molecule is chiral and non-racemic, then an assay to determine chiral stability may be required.

Knowledge of the solubility of the compound, particularly the aqueous solubility, is required in order to design the study. If the aqueous solubility is too low, then an organic co-solvent may be utilized to achieve solutions for stressing.

C. Designing Stress-Testing Studies

1. Preliminary Studies

Unless a significant amount of information about the stability of the molecule is known, it will probably be necessary to conduct some preliminary studies to gain some basic information about the stability of the compound. The samples generated in this preliminary study can also be used to aid in the development of an analytical method, if needed. Generally, the goal of stress testing is to facilitate an approximate 5–20% degradation of the sample under any given condition (if possible after reasonable limits of stressing). In the preliminary investigation, observations are made regarding sample stability including exposure of solid state samples to heat, humidity, and light and exposure of solutions to pH extremes, oxidative conditions (hydrogen peroxide and a radical initiator such as 2,2′ -azobisisobutyroni-

Table 1 Typical Stress Conditions for Preliminary Studies

Sample condition	Time/exposure
Solid/70°C	1 week
Solid/70°C/75% RH	1 week
Solid/simulated sunlight	2–3 × ICH confirmatory exposure
Aqueous solution/simulated sunlight	2–3 × ICH confirmatory exposure
0.1 N HCl solution/ up to 70°C	1–7 days
Aqueous Solution/up to 70°C	1–7 days
pH 8 Solution/up to 70°C	1–7 days
0.1 N NaOH solution/up to 70°C	1–7 days
0.3% H_2O_2 solution/ambient in the dark	1–7 days
Solution with radical initiator/40°C	1–7 days

trile (AIBN)), light and heat. Table 1 lists some typical stress conditions for preliminary studies.

2. Stress Test Screen

After conducting some preliminary studies and developing analytical methods (the development of appropriate stress testing methods is dealt within Section II of this chaper) it is time to design the stress test screen. Unfortunately, it is impossible to devise a universal set of stress conditions since there is significant variability in the stability of drugs. What can be defined, however, are suggested upper limits for the various stress conditions that can be used as starting points for stress-testing studies. If no degradation can be induced at these proposed maximum stress conditions, then it is concluded that the molecule is stable. The proposed upper limits are listed in Tables 2 and 3. Refer to Chapter 2 for a discussion of the rationale used to establish the maximum stress conditions.

Table 2 Proposed Maximum Stress Conditions for Solid State Drug Substance

Storage condition	Time
70°C	4 to 6 weeks
70°C NaCl ~75% RH	28 days
Photostress	Exposure 2–5 times ICH exposure levels defined in Q1B, Photostability Testing of New Drug Substances and Products

Table 3 Proposed Maximum Stress Conditions for Solutions or Suspensions of Drug Substances

Solution or suspension	Storage condition	Time
0.1 N HCl, water, NaOH, and any buffers between pH 1 and 14	70°C	14 days
80/20 ACN/H_2O containing a radical initiator such as AIBN	40°C	7 days
Water (consider buffering compounds which have ionizable functional groups both below and above p*K*a)	Photostress	Exposure 2–3 times ICH exposure levels defined in Q1B, Photostability Testing of New Drug Substances and Products
Dilute hydrogen peroxide (0.3–3%)	25°C	7 days
Solutions containing dilute metal salt (e.g., Fe(III), Cu(II))	40°C	1 day

3. Design of Study

Taking into account the information derived from the preliminary study, one can devise a more detailed stress test study. Tables 4 and 5 list the proposed conditions and analytical time points for stress testing of a drug substance that appeared to be reasonably stable at the proposed upper stress conditions. Additional conditions can be added if deemed necessary.

D. Sample Preparation General

1. Solid-State Samples

Solid-state samples can be prepared by accurately weighing the drug substance into a container that can be stored under the appropriate condition. Suitable containers include volumetric flasks, scintillation vials, etc. The amount of drug substance used is usually dictated by the availability of material, accuracy of balances, and the final concentration desired for analysis. Typical amounts used for solid-state samples would be between 2 and

Table 4 Proposed Conditions and Time Points for a Detailed Study (Solid-State Stress)

Storage condition	Time points
70°C	7, 14, 28 days
70°C NaCl ~75% RH	7, 14, 28 days
Photostress	Exposure 2–3 times ICH guideline

Table 5 Proposed Conditions and Time Points for a Detailed Study (Solution Stress)

Solution or suspension	Storage condition	Time points
0.1 N HCl, pH 3, pH 5, pH 7, pH 9, pH 11, 0.1 N NaOH, and water	70°C	3, 7, 14 days
80/20 ACN/H_2O containing a radical initiator such as AIBN	40°C	3, 7 days
Water (consider buffering compounds which have ionizable functional groups both below and above p*K*a)	Photostress	Exposure 1 and 3 times the ICH exposure levels defined in Q1B
Dilute hydrogen peroxide (0.3–3%)	25°C	3, 7 days
Solutions containing dilute metal salt (e.g., Fe, Cu)	40°C	1 hr, 1 day

20 mg. For example, if the final analytical concentration desired is 0.3 mg/mL, solid-state samples of approximately 3 mg in 10 mL volumetric flasks could be stressed and then simply diluted to volume at the time of assay. Alternatively, samples could be prepared in scintillation vials, stressed, and then diluted with a known amount of solvent.

Solid-state samples can be pre-weighed into the respective containers before stressing. Pre-weighing the samples simplifies the analysis of stressed samples by eliminating any concerns about changing levels of volatile constituents such as water or organic solvents during thermal stress. The ICH guideline on photostability indicates that samples for photoexposure be less than 3 mm in depth.

Occasionally, one will have to deal with hygroscopic drug substances or drug substances containing a significant level of a volatile compound (e.g., solvates). These types of drug substances can pose significant issues when preparing samples for quantitative analysis. Fortunately, most of these issues can be overcome by using a simple approach. A simple method for eliminating volatile content issues is to allow samples to come to equilibrium with the environment and then conducting all of the weighing of samples and standards over as short a time frame as possible. Performing a volatiles analysis (i.e., TGA) both before and after sample weighing will provide assurance that no significant change in volatiles content occurred over the weighing period.

2. Solution Samples

Solution samples can be prepared in a number of different ways. One way is to prepare a single stock solution at a known concentration for each stress condition and then pull aliquots at the desired time points. This method requires that the container used for the solution be tightly closed to prevent evaporation. If evaporation is a problem, it can be overcome by preparing a separate sample for each time point at a concentration higher than the analytical concentration. For example, if the final analytical concentration desired is 0.3 mg/mL, solutions could be prepared at a concentration of approximately 1 mg/mL by adding 3 mL of the appropriate solvent to samples of approximately 3 mg in 10-mL volumetric flasks. Prior to assay, the samples can then be diluted to volume to achieve the final analytical concentration.

3. Suspension or Slurry Samples

Suspensions or slurries pose a problem since by definition they are not homogeneous. The problem is how to obtain reliable quantitative results from suspensions. One method for dealing with suspensions is to prepare individually weighed samples and stress them at concentrations greater than the final analytical concentration. Prior to analysis the samples are then diluted to the final analytical concentration with a solvent that completely dissolves the sample. For example, if the final analytical concentration desired is 0.3 mg/mL, suspensions could be prepared at a concentration of approximately 1 mg/mL by adding 3 mL of the appropriate solvent to samples of approximately 3 mg in 10-mL volumetric flasks. Prior to assay, the samples can then be diluted to volume with a solvent capable of completely dissolving the sample.

4. Standards

The assay of stressed samples will usually require the use of some type of external standard. The external standard could be an established reference standard, however, the preferred method is to use the same material/lot as is being stressed. This is easily accomplished by weighing additional samples (that will not be stressed) for use as "standards" at the same time as the stress test samples are weighed. The "standards" should then be stored under conditions that will assure that no degradation will occur (e.g., freezer). At the time of analysis, the stressed samples are simply assayed vs. the freshly prepared unstressed "standards" and the results calculated as percent initial.

5. Solution and Buffer Preparation

Typically 0.1 N HCl and 0.1 N NaOH are used for the pH extremes of aqueous solution stressing (i.e., pH 1 and 13). Since neither of these solutions possesses significant buffering capacity, the pH of the solution should be verified following addition of the drug to these solutions. In order to obtain solutions at pH values between 1 and 13, a buffer must be used. It is desirable to use the same buffer for all the pH levels to avoid chemical differences between different buffers, since buffers are not always inert and can sometimes act as catalysts for drug degradation or even react with the

Table 6 Some Common Buffers and Their Buffering Ranges

Buffer	p*K*a	Buffer range
Phosphate	2.1	1.1–3.1
	7.2	6.2–8.2
	12.3	11.3–13.3
Citrate	3.1	2.1–4.1
	5.4	4.4–6.4
Formate	3.8	2.8–4.8
Succinate	4.2	3.2–5.2
	5.6	4.6–6.6
Acetate	4.8	3.8–5.8
Citrate	3.1	2.1–4.1
	4.7	3.7–5.7
	5.4	4.4–6.4
Tris	8.3	7.3–9.3
Borate	9.2	8.2–10.2

drug being studied (3). Unfortunately, no single buffer provides buffering capacity across this wide pH range. A common practice is to make the buffer of sufficient ionic strength such that it still offers some pH stability even outside of its normal buffering range (e.g., 50 mM phosphate). For example, if pH values of 3, 5, 7, 9, and 11 are desired, a phosphate buffer can be used keeping in mind that the buffering capacity will be low at pH 5 and pH 9. If more buffering capacity is required, then other buffers or a combination of buffers can be used. The buffering range for several common buffers is given in Table 6.

E. Example Stress Test Screen

The following sections describe a stress-testing study conducted on LY334370 hydrochloride. The structure of LY334370 hydrochloride is shown below in Figure 1. This stress-testing example illustrates many of the concepts discussed in the previous paragraphs. An important detail that should be pointed out is that this work did not include the use of transition metals [e.g., iron(III) or copper(II)], therefore, no results from these conditions are given.

1. Data Gathering

Examination of the structure of the example compound clearly indicates that it possesses both a phenyl and an indole moiety and should therefore be amenable to UV detection. The compound has a tertiary amine, which is an ionizable functional group with a p*K*a of approximately 9, therefore, a buffered mobile phase will likely be required if HPLC is chosen as the analytical method. Since the compound does not contain a chiral center, there is

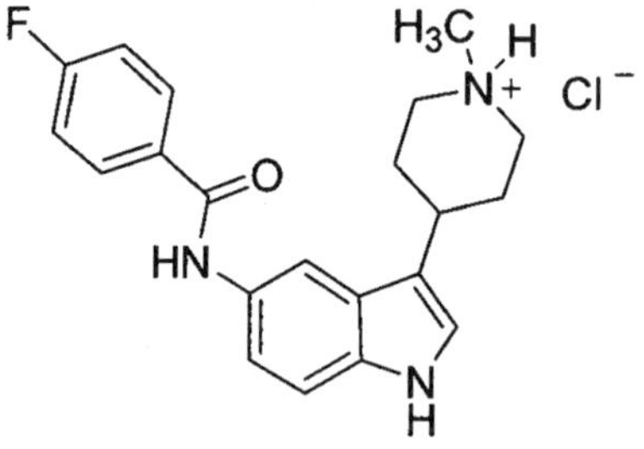

LY334370 Hydrochloride

Figure 1 The chemical structure of LY334370.

no need for chiral analysis. Since there was no available solubility information on LY334370 hydrochloride, a simple and semi-quantitative solubility study was performed. Table 7 gives the results of this study. The solubility values were obtained by adding a specified amount of solvent to a known quantity of the drug and visually observing whether all the material dissolved. Although the solubility numbers are only rough estimates of solubility, they are very useful for designing the stress-testing study. The solubility results indicate that an organic co-solvent will be necessary to achieve solutions at pH values of 8 and higher and in 0.1 N HCl.

2. Preliminary Studies

In the case of LY334370 hydrochloride, an analytical method needed to be developed and very little was known about its degradation chemistry. Solid-state and solution samples of LY334370 hydrochloride were prepared

Table 7 Semi-Quantitative Solubility Study Results

Solvent	Solubility
Water	>2.75 mg/mL
Methanol	>5 mg/mL
Acetonitrile	<0.5 mg/mL
Water/acetonitrile 50/50 (v/v)	>4.4 mg/mL
Water/acetonitrile 80/20 (v/v)	>4.4 mg/mL
0.1 N HCl	<0.5 mg/mL
pH 2 phosphate buffer	>3.2 mg/mL
pH 4 phosphate buffer	>2 mg/mL
pH 6 phosphate buffer	>1.5 mg/mL
pH 8 phosphate buffer	<0.5 mg/mL
0.1 N NaOH	<0.5 mg/mL
0.1 N NaOH	<0.5 mg/mL

Table 8 Preliminary Sample Descriptions and Results

Sample description	Stress condition	Result related substances increase (%)
Approximately 2 mg in an open 10-mL volumetric flask	70°C for 21 days	0.0
Approximately 2 mg in an open 10-mL volumetric flask which was stored in a sealed container over a saturated NaCl solution	70°C for 21 days (75% RH)	0.0
Approximately 2 mg in a 20-mL scintillation vial covered with polyethylene film	Irradiate with simulated sunlight produced by a xenon arc lamp for 20 hr. Visible exposure: ~3 million lx hr UV exposure: ~1500 W hr/m^2	0.0
Approximately 2 mg dissolved in 2 mL of 70/30 0.1 N HCl/ acetonitrile	70°C for 7 days	20.4
Approximately 2 mg dissolved in 2 mL of water	70°C for 7 days	0.2
Approximately 2 mg dissolved in 2 mL of 70/30 pH 8 phosphate/acetonitrile	70°C for 7 days	10.7
Approximately 2 mg dissolved in 2 mL of 70/30 0.1 N NaOH/ acetonitrile	70°C for 7 days	27.0
Approximately 2 mg dissolved in 2 mL of 0.3% hydrogen peroxide	Ambient temperature protected from light for 7 days	2.2
Approximately 2 mg of drug and a molar equivalent of AIBN dissolved in 2 mL 20/80 water/acetonitrile	40°C for 7 days	16.5
Approximately 2 mg dissolved in 2 mL of water	Irradiate with simulated sunlight produced by a xenon arc lamp for 20 hr Visible exposure: ~3 million lx hr UV exposure: ~1500 W hr/m^2	8.1

and stressed under the conditions described in Table 8. The samples were then analyzed by HPLC using the preliminary HPLC conditions given in Table 9. Calculation of the area percent of the impurity peaks provided an estimate of the amount of degradation that occurred in each sample. The results indicate that LY334370 appears to be stable in the solid state but

Table 9 Preliminary HPLC Screening Method for LY334370

	Related Substances Method	
Mobile phase A	0.025 M KH_2PO_4, adjust pH to 2.5 with H_3PO_4	
Mobile phase B	Acetonitrile	
Column	150 × 4.6 mm Zorbax SB-C18, 3.5 μm, 40°C	
Detection	UV-PDA (205 nm)	
Flow	1.5 mL/min	
Gradient	Time (min)	% acetonitrile
	0.0	3
	5	14
	20	21
	30	75

degrades significantly under acidic, basic, and oxidative conditions. Some of the samples generated in this preliminary study were used to further develop the analytical method used for the final study. More details on the development of the method can be found in the next section. The results of this preliminary study were also used to design the time points and conditions of the final stress testing study where the objective was to induce 5–20% degradation, if possible.

3. Stress-Testing Study

The results of the preliminary study were used to design the final stress testing study. Examination of the preliminary solid-state results indicates that the molecule appears to be stable under all of the solid-state conditions and therefore can be stressed at the maximum temperature (70°C) with a minimum number of time points. The preliminary solution results indicate that the molecule is susceptible to degradation particularly at the pH extremes at the upper temperature limit of 70°C. The temperature of 70°C appears to be appropriate for most conditions but will require time points shorter than seven days. The final screen was designed keeping these preliminary results in mind. Tables 10–12 list the final stress-testing conditions, time points, and results. The HPLC method used for the final screen is given in Table 13.

4. Experimental Details

Solid-state samples were prepared in duplicate and consisted of approximately 3 mg of material accurately weighed into a 10-mL volumetric flask. Samples were subjected to heat at 70°C under both ambient and high humidity. High humidity conditions were maintained by storing samples in open flasks over a saturated $NaCl/H_2O$ solution in a closed glass container. Solid-state samples were exposed to simulated sunlight generated using a xenon arc lamp in a separate experiment. These samples consisted of approximately 3 mg of

Table 10 LY334370 Hydrochloride Solid-State Stress Conditions and Results

Storage condition	Container	Time point (days)	Assay (% initial)	Related substance increase (%)	Physical appearance
70°C	Open 10-mL volumetric flask	14	98.0	0.1	No change
		28	98.4	0.1	No change
70°C 75% RH	Open 10-mL volumetric flask	14	99.1	0.1	No change
Simulated sunlight	Glad wrap sealed 20-mL scintillation vial	20 hr	99.3	0.3	No change
Simulated sunlight (control)	Glad wrap sealed 20-mL scintillation vial wrapped with foil	20 hr	99.7	0.3	No change

Table 11 LY334370 Hydrochloride Solution and Slurry Stress Conditions and Results

Storage condition	Container	Time point (days)	Assay (% initial)	Related substances increase (%)	Physical appearance
Slurry in 0.1 N HC1 at 70°C	Closed 10-mL volumetric flask	3	92.6	5.8	Faint pink, clear
		7	81.5	14.2	Faint pink, clear
		14	60.6	27.4	Amber, clear
Solution in 80/20 0.1 N HCl/ACN at 70°C	Closed 10-mL volumetric flask	3	96.7	2.0	Faint pink, clear
		7	90.8	5.9	Faint pink, clear
		14	71.3	14.8	Amber, clear
Solution in pH 2 phosphate buffer at 70°C	Closed 10-mL volumetric flask	3	99.4	0.5	Faint pink, clear
		7	98.4	1.0	Faint pink, clear
		14	93.8	3.1	Faint yellow, clear
Solution in pH 4 phosphate buffer at 70°C	Closed 10-mL volumetric flask	3	100.4	0.1	No change
		7	99.8	0.1	No change
		14	98.9	0.2	No change
Solution in unbuffered water at 70°C	Closed 10-mL volumetric flask	3	99.8	0.2	No change
		7	100.0	0.1	No change
		14	97.1	1.0	Faint yellow, clear
Solution in pH 6 phosphate buffer at 70°C.	Closed 10-mL volumetric flask	3	99.9	0.0	Faint yellow, clear
		7	100.1	0.2	Faint yellow, clear
		14	99.0	0.5	Faint yellow, clear

Slurry in pH 8 phosphate buffer at 70°C	Closed 10-mL volumetric flask	3	99.2	0.6	Faint yellow, clear
		7	95.2	1.7	Faint yellow, clear
		14	87.7	8.2	Yellow, clear
Solution in 80/20 pH 8 phosphate buffer/ACN at 70°C	Closed 10-mL volumetric flask	3	95.5	3.0	Faint pink
		7	89.3	6.3	Faint yellow, cloudy
		14	81.9	10.6	Yellow, clear
Slurry in 0.1 N NaOH at 70°C	Closed 10-mL volumetric flask	3	63.9	21.1	Amber, cloudy
		7	40.5	20.2	Amber, cloudy
		14	6.8	32.7	Dark amber, ppt
Solution in 80/20 0.1 N NaOH/ACN at 70°C	Closed 10-mL volumetric flask	3	91.1	5.2	Faint yellow, Clear
		7	88.8	9.0	Faint yellow, cloudy
		14	85.6	13.4	Faint yellow, cloudy

Table 12 LY334370 Hydrochloride Solutions Oxidative Conditions and Light Exposure

Storage condition	Container	Time point (days)	% initial	Related substances increase (t-t_o)	Physical appearance
Solution in 0.3% H_2O_2 stored in dark	Closed 10-mL volumetric flask stored in the dark	3	98.9	0.8	No change
		7	97.4	1.6	No change
		14	96.7	3.2	No change
Solution in 80/20 ACN/H_2O containing AIBN at 40°C	Closed 10-mL volumetric flask	3	87.9	8.8	Faint yellow, clear
		7	74.7	18.2	Faint yellow, clear
		14	58.9	25.6	Yellow, clear
Solution in unbuffered water exposed to fluorescent light at an intensity of ~16,000 lx	Closed 10-mL volumetric flask	14	80.2	19.3	No change
		28	64.6	33.6	No change
Solution in unbuffered water exposed to fluorescent light at an intensity of ~16,000 lx (control)	Foil wrapped closed 10-mL volumetric flask	14	99.9	0.0	No change
		28	99.1	0.4	No change
Solution in pH 2 buffer irradiated with simulated sunlight	Closed 10-mL volumetric flask	10 hr	96.7	0.9	Faint tan, clear
Solution in pH 2 buffer irradiated with simulated sunlight (control)	Foil wrapped closed 10-mL volumetric flask	10 hr	99.3	0.3	No change

Solution in unbuffered water irradiated with simulated sunlight	Closed 10-mL volumetric flask	10 hr	95.5	6.7	No change
Solution in unbuffered water irradiated with simulated sunlight (control)	Foil wrapped closed 10-mL volumetric flask	10 hr	100.2	0.3	No change
Solution in pH 6 buffer irradiated with simulated sunlight	Closed 10-mL volumetric flask	10 hr	97.4	2.6	No change
Solution in pH 6 buffer irradiated with simulated sunlight (control)	Foil wrapped closed 10-mL volumetric flask	10 hr	100.5	0.2	No change

Table 13 Final HPLC Conditions Developed for Stress Testing of LY334370

0.025 M KH_2PO_4	adjust pH to 2.0 with H_3PO_4	
Mobile Phase B	Acetonitrile	
Column	250 × 4.6 mm Zorbax SB-Ph 5.0 μm, 40°C	
Detection	UV-PDA at 205 nm (260 nm for assay)	
Flow	1.0 mL/min	
Gradient	Time (min)	% acetonitrile
	0	3
	5	15
	25	27
	35	75

material in a clear 20-mL scintillation vial that was sealed with Glad Wrap(TM) (i.e., polyethylene film). In all cases, the thickness of the samples was significantly less than 1 mm. Control samples were prepared in the same manner except that they were completely wrapped in aluminum foil.

The solution and slurry samples were prepared in duplicate and consisted of approximately 3 mg of material accurately weighed into a 10-mL volumetric flask. Three milliliters of the appropriate solvent was added to each sample and the flasks were tightly stoppered prior to placing the flask in the given storage condition. Immediately prior to analysis, after equilibration to room temperature, all samples were diluted to volume with 77/23 (v/v) 0.025 M KH_2PO_4 pH 2.0 buffer/ACN. The solution samples could have been prepared as stock solutions with removal of a sample aliquot at the appropriate time points; however, evaporation of the solution at the stress temperature (70°C) was a major concern. Preparation of individual samples with partial dilution prior to stressing eliminated the evaporation concern.

All the buffers (pH 2, 4, 6, 8) were prepared from 0.05 M KH_2PO_4 adjusted to the proper pH with either 5 N NaOH or 85% H_3PO_4. The 0.3% H_2O_2 solution was prepared by diluting 10 mL of fresh 3% H_2O_2 to 100 mL with water. The AIBN solutions contained approximately 1 molar equivalent of AIBN with respect to LY334370 hydrochloride.

The photostability chamber was a Suntest CPS+ manufactured by Atlas Material Testing Technology, LLC, Chicago, IL. It was set up to simulate natural sunlight and contained a xenon long-arc lamp with an infrared filter and a UV filter with a cutoff of ~295 nm. The photostability chamber was set at an intensity of 765 W/m^2 (300–800 nm). Manufacturer measurements indicate that this setting corresponds to a visible intensity of ~150,000 lx, and a UVA intensity (320–400 nm) of ~78 W/m^2. Thus, a 10 hr sample exposure corresponds to ~1.5 million lx-hr visible and ~780 W-hr/m^2 UVA. For comparison, the ICH guideline on photostability specifies a minimum exposure for confirmatory studies of 1.2 million lx-hr in the visible and not less than 200 W-hr/m^2 in the near UV.

The fluorescent light chamber consisted of 8 Sylvania fluorescent bulbs (Octron, 4100K, 32 W) in a 19″ ×21″× 50″ box. The average intensity of the light with measurements taken at the level of the samples was approximately 16,000 lx. The average temperature of the light box was approximately 26°C. Fluorescent light exposure was included in the study in addition to simulated sunlight to enable the assessment of the potential for photodegradation from visible light exposure only (e.g., in the laboratory environment, manufacturing facilities, etc.).

The stressed samples were assayed vs. unstressed LY334370 hydrochloride prepared at concentrations corresponding to approximately 50%, 80%, and 110% of the nominal concentration of the samples (0.3 mg/mL). A three point standard curve was constructed using the standards and the concentration of LY334370 in the stressed samples was determined using the curve. All samples and standards were weighed out at the same time to eliminate any concerns about volatiles content changes during stressing. The undiluted standards were stored in a refrigerator at approximately 5°C prior to use. TGA analyses run on this material prior to the weighing of samples and following the weighing of samples indicated no change in volatile content during the weighing process.

The related substances results were calculated vs. an external standard prepared at a concentration of approximately 1% (0.003 mg/mL) of the nominal sample concentration using the equation given below. Total related substances on the unstressed material were measured to be 0.34%. All of the related substances results were corrected for this initial related substances level and are reported as related substances increase.

$$\%\ \text{Rel Subs} = \frac{(\text{Area of Related Substances}) \times (\text{Concentration of Standard})}{(\text{Area of Standard}) \times (\text{Concentration of Sample})} \times 100\%$$

5. Results

Refer to Tables 10–12 for the stress testing results. LY334370 hydrochloride was stable under all of the solid-state conditions studied. No significant loss of potency or increase in related substances was detected for any of the solid-state samples. These results suggest that LY334370 hydrochloride should be stable under typical ambient conditions and should not require any special handling or storage conditions. Since no significant degradation occurred in the solid-state samples, none of the solid-state chromatograms are shown.

Selected chromatograms of suspension and solution samples are shown in Figures 2–5. Examination of Figure 2 indicates that LY334370 undergoes degradation to two major degradation products (A and B) at

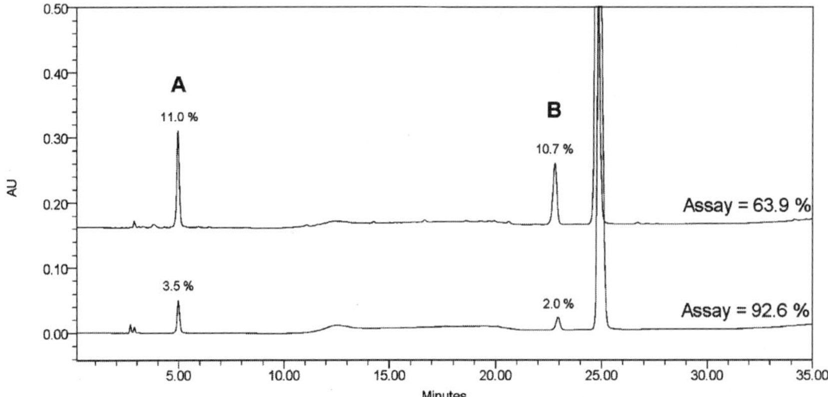

Figure 2 HPLC-related substances chromatograms (UV detection, 205 nm) obtained on slurries of LY334370 hydrochloride in 0.1N NaOH (top) and 0.1N HCl (bottom) held at 70°C for 3 days.

the pH extremes of 0.1 N HC1 and 0.1 N NaOH. It is likely that peaks A and B are the result of hydrolysis, but confirmation of this assumption would require characterization of these degradation products. The chromatograms in Figure 3 indicates that LY334370 is relatively stable at pH 2 and in unbuffered water but does degrade to a number of new peaks in pH 8 buffer containing a co-solvent. Some degradation is apparent in solutions containing hydrogen peroxide or a radical initiator (Fig. 4), suggesting that LY334370 maybe susceptible to oxidative degradation. The chromatograms shown in

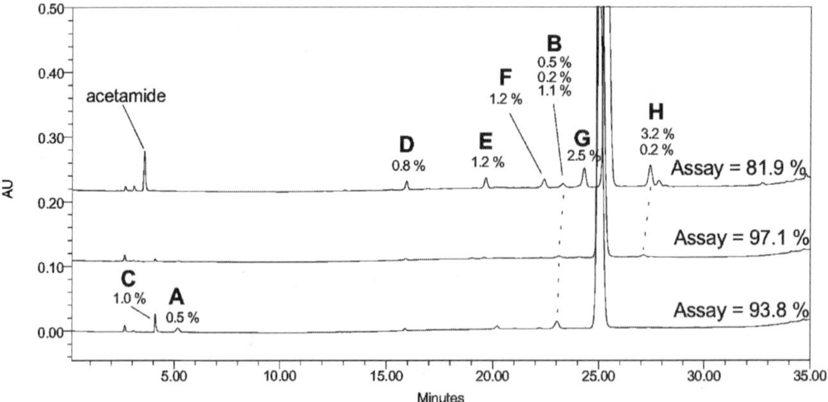

Figure 3 HPLC-related substances chromatograms (UV detection, 205 nm) obtained on solutions of LY334370 hydrochloride in pH 2 phosphate buffer (bottom), water (middle), and pH 8 phosphate buffer/acetonitrile (top) held at 70°C for 14 days.

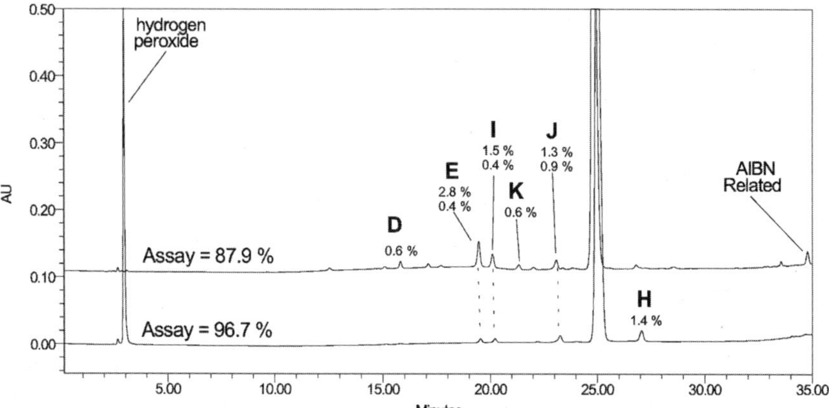

Figure 4 HPLC-related substances chromatograms (UV detection, 205 nm) obtained on solutions of LY334370 hydrochloride in 0.3% hydrogen peroxide at ambient temperature for 14 days (bottom) and a water/acetonitrile solution containing the radical initiator AIBN held at 40°C for three days (top).

Figure 5 suggests that solutions of LY334370 are susceptible to light-catalyzed degradation. The stress testing studies on LY334370 indicate that the major potential degradation products are peaks A through K. Which of these peaks are relevant degradation products (i.e., form under normal storage conditions) is determined using the results of formal stability studies.

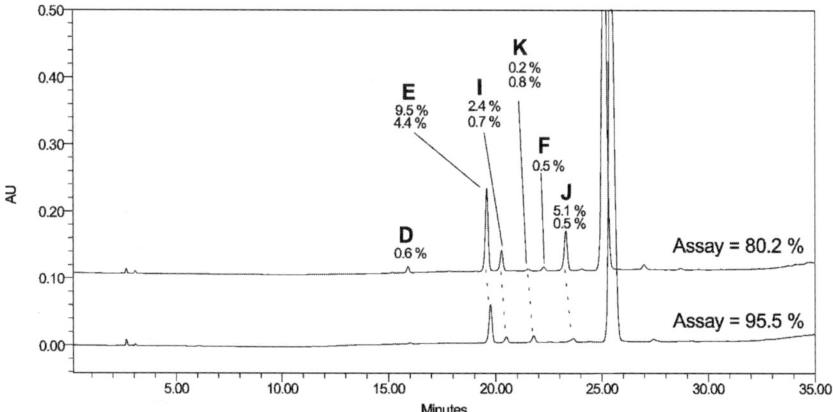

Figure 5 HPLC-related substances chromatograms (UV detection, 205 nm) obtained on solutions of LY334370 hydrochloride in water exposed to intense fluorescent light for 14 days (top) or simulated sunlight produced by a xenon arc lamp (bottom).

II. METHODS OF ANALYSIS

A. Introduction

When developing a method for stress-testing studies, it is useful to think about what would constitute an ideal method. An ideal method would enable the accurate quantification of the parent compound as well as all of its degradation products. While this sounds simple in theory, it is nearly impossible to develop an ideal method early in the development cycle of a new drug when few if any of the potential degradation products are known. After all, one of the reasons for conducting stress-testing studies is to discover the potential degradation products.

The ideal chromatographic method will resolve all degradation products from the parent as well as from each other, all degradation products will be detected, and the relative response of the degradation products with respect to the parent will be known. Since it is difficult to develop a chromatographic method that satisfies all of these requirements, the focus should be on developing a primary screening method that has the highest likelihood of resolving and detecting a diverse set of degradation products. In many cases, it may be impossible to come up with an ideal method; however, the use of two "orthogonal" analysis methods often will give adequate results in these cases.

Most of the following discussion on method development assumes that one is trying to develop an analytical method for a specific compound. Another viable approach, however, is to develop generic analytical methods that can be used for the analysis of stress-testing samples from multiple compounds. A short discussion of the development of generic methods is provided later in the section.

B. Reversed-Phase HPLC

Since a large majority of pharmaceutical products are amenable to reversed-phase HPLC, this is usually the method of choice. The development of reversed-phase HPLC methods is a broad subject with many research articles and books devoted to it and it is not practical to try to cover this topic in depth in this chapter. There are, however, some major points to consider when developing an HPLC method for analyzing stress test samples.

1. Isocratic vs. Gradient Elution

Since one does not know what degradation products will form, gradient elution should be used. This significantly increases the chances that degradation products which are much more polar than the parent compound will be pulled away from the solvent front and those which are much less polar than the parent will elute from the column. Often the use of a multi-step gradient is particularly beneficial. The first segment of the multi-step gradient

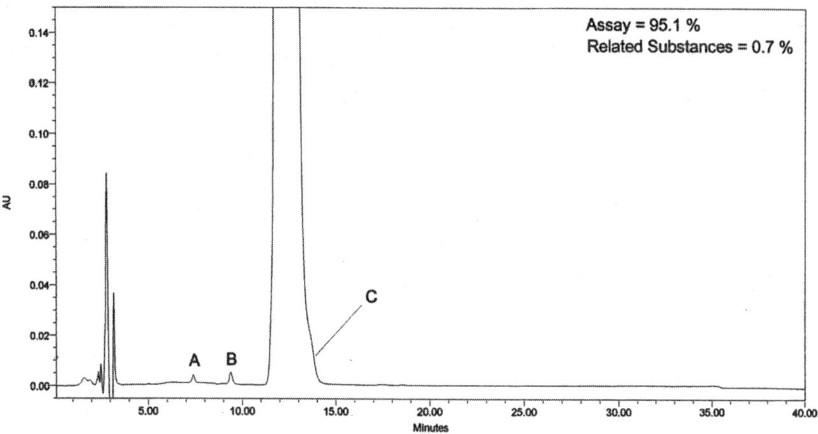

Figure 6 Isocratic HPLC chromatogram obtained on a sample of drug substance stressed in pH 7 phosphate buffer/ACN.

starts at very low organic concentration and ramps rapidly to the second segment in which the parent is eluted either under essentially isocratic conditions or with a very shallow gradient in order to maximize resolution of the degradation products from the parent compound. The third segment of the gradient begins after the parent elutes and is a rapid ramp to high organic concentration to elute any less polar degradation products.

The following example illustrates the benefits of using gradient elution for stress testing. Figure 6 illustrates a chromatogram obtained under isocratic conditions on a sample of drug substance in 50/50 acetonitrile/pH 7 phosphate buffer stressed at 70°C for 14 days. The assay result of 95.1% indicates that significant degradation has occurred. The related substances result of only 0.7%, however, suggests a potential mass balance problem. Reanalysis of the same sample using gradient elution enabled the detection of a number of degradation products not visible with the isocratic method (Fig. 7).

C. Detection

There are many types of HPLC detectors available today with the most popular ones including UV and UV-photodiode array (PDA), fluorescence, refractive index, evaporative light scattering (ELSD), charged aerosol (CAD), and the mass spectrometer. Of these, the most commonly used detector for pharmaceutical analytical methods is the UV detector since a majority of pharmaceutical compounds have some type of chromophore. Multiple detectors in series can also be utilized in order to obtain more information per chromatographic run. For example, a PDA detector can

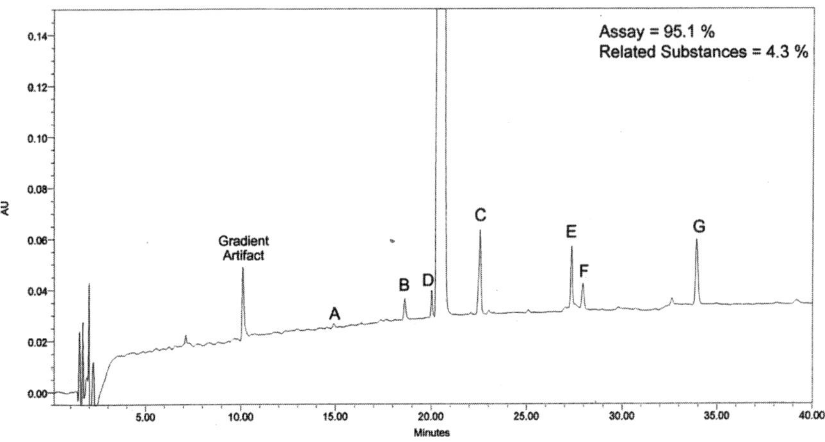

Figure 7 Gradient HPLC chromatogram obtained on a sample of drug substance stressed in pH 7 phosphate buffer/ACN.

be combined with a mass detector to give both UV and mass spectral information on impurities. For compounds that do not have any UV absorbance, the ELSD and mass spectrometric detectors are generally the most useful and can be used individually or in series. The CAD is a recently introduced detector that is described as a nearly universal detector for non-volatile and semi-volatile compounds, with a response that is reflective of the total mass passing through the detector. Fluorescence detection is not desirable because there is no guarantee that the degradation products of a fluorescent molecule will fluoresce. Most refractive index detectors are best suited for isocratic elution and are therefore not particularly useful for stress-testing methods that utilize gradient elution. Since the UV detector is the most widely used, the remainder of this discussion will focus on the aspects of UV detection.

The use of UV-transparent buffers and organic modifiers (e.g., phosphate buffers and acetonitrile or methanol) for the HPLC mobile phase is desirable since it enables chromatograms to be acquired at relatively low wavelengths near 200 nm. Typically, monitoring at these low wavelengths increases the likelihood that all of the degradation products will be detected since most compounds possessing a chromophore will absorb at these low wavelengths. The use of a PDA UV detector significantly increases the amount of information obtained from the chromatographic run. The use of the PDA detector allows the extraction of chromatograms at multiple wavelengths from a single chromatographic run as well as provides the UV spectra of individual peaks. These UV spectra can be used to correlate peaks arising from different stress conditions or from different chromatographic systems. The use of a PDA detector also enables the determination of the UV homogeneity of individual peaks thereby giving an indication of their purity.

D. Assay Methods vs. Impurity Methods

Frequently, two methods are developed for pharmaceuticals: an assay method to measure the loss of active and an impurity method to detect and measure levels of impurities. One of the major reasons for developing two methods is the common practice of using two different UV detection wavelengths for the dual methods. Assay methods typically use a wavelength that is a λ_{max} for the compound being analyzed, while impurity methods may require a different wavelength to enable detection of impurities with different absorption characteristics than the parent compound. As discussed in the previous paragraph on detection, low wavelength detection (e.g., 205–210 nm) is recommended for screening methods since this increases the likelihood that all degradation products will be detected. The use of a PDA detector enables the extraction of chromatograms at any wavelength and eliminates the need for two separate chromatographic analyses.

Another common reason for having separate assay and impurity methods is the need to use more concentrated samples with the impurity assay to increase sensitivity for minor impurities. Modern HPLC systems have been shown to adequately detect low-level impurities (i.e., ~0.05%) in chromatograms where the parent peak is still on scale (that is, within the linear range of the detector). This level of detection is usually adequate for screening methods; therefore, the assay for loss of parent compound and the measurement of the increase in impurities can typically be done using a single HPLC method.

E. Development of Method

Assuming that reversed-phase HPLC is chosen, an appropriate method must then be developed. There are numerous approaches that can be and are used to develop HPLC methods. The approach advocated here is similar to that described by Dolan (4) for development of stability indicating methods. The first requirement is a sample or samples that can be used to develop and optimize the separation. Typical samples of drug substance are often quite pure and do not contain impurity peaks that can be used for method development. In cases like this, it is necessary to either generate a partially degraded sample or samples or to prepare a sample containing impurities related to the drug substance being studied. There are advantages and disadvantages to both types of samples.

Some advantages to using partially degraded samples include: (1) actual degradation products are used, which should give additional confidence that the method developed is truly stability-indicating; (2) samples can be easily reproduced by simply preparing new samples and stressing under previously determined conditions; (3) a number of different stress conditions can be used. Some disadvantages to using partially degraded samples include: (1) there is no way to know how many degradation products are present, therefore, some may be missed under the main peak or may elute outside of the analysis window; (2) samples may degrade too much resulting in secondary and tertiary degradation products that would not be formed under normal storage conditions; (3) samples may not degrade enough or the correct conditions for degradation may not be known; and (4) peaks may be difficult to track when changing method conditions because there are too many peaks. Some advantages to using samples containing only known impurities include: (1) the number of impurities are known, therefore, one knows how many peaks should be detected; (2) the levels of the impurities can be easily adjusted making peak tracking by peak size easier. Some disadvantages of using samples containing only known impurities include: (1) the separation of the impurities from the parent compound may be significantly easier than the separation of the degradation products, resulting in methods that are not stability-indicating, and (2) there may not be suitable impurities available.

Obviously, the best way to develop a good method is to use all of the information that is available and not to rely solely on available impurities or partially degraded samples. For example, perhaps one or two impurities are available or are present in the drug substance. In this case the best strategy to develop a stability-indicating method is to use these impurities and to also generate partially degraded samples.

1. Preparation of Method Development Samples

Sometimes the task of preparing a method development sample can be accomplished by examining the functionality present on the parent compound, predicting degradation products based on known chemistry, and preparing them using common procedures. For example, if a molecule contains a tertiary amine, a common oxidative degradation product is the amine oxide. The amine oxides can often be rapidly produced by reacting the free base of the tertiary amine with an oxidizing agent such as hydrogen peroxide, peracetic acid, or *m*-chloroperoxybenzoic acid. Another functional group easily oxidized is a sulfide. These groups are often readily oxidized to the corresponding sulfoxides and sulfones. Of course if the molecule contains other easily oxidized functional groups, it may be difficult to achieve selective oxidation of specific functional groups.

For samples containing multiple chiral centers, the use of a diastereomer, if available, for method development is a good option. Diastereomers are often difficult to separate so their use in method development may lead to a more highly resolving method that, therefore, may have a higher probability of being stability-indicating.

The goal when producing partially degraded samples is to produce as many of the degradation products as possible with a minimum number of samples. Since the stability of drug substances varies widely, it is impossible to come up with a single set of conditions that are appropriate for all drugs; however, the sample conditions listed in Table 1 are a reasonable starting point.

2. Method Development Example

LY334370 hydrochloride will be used as an example to illustrate the stress-testing method development process. Ten stressed samples of LY334370 hydrochloride were prepared as described in Table 8 and used to develop the stress-testing analytical method.

We have found in our laboratory that HPLC methods utilizing a phosphate buffer at low pH and acetonitrile as an organic modifier work for a large percentage of the drug compounds we have tested. Therefore, our typical starting point for a new method uses the phosphate buffer/acetonitrile combination with a C8 or C18 reversed-phase column. In the case of LY334370, the phosphate buffer was 0.025 M potassium phosphate adjusted to pH 2.5 with phosphoric acid and the column a 4.6×150 mm Zorbax SB-C18 with an average particle size of 3.5 μm. The initial conditions settled upon are given in Table 9.

All 10 samples were analyzed using the initial HPLC method. Examination of the chromatograms indicated that none of the three solid-state samples exhibited degradation, suggesting that LY334370 hydrochloride is relatively stable as a solid. The lack of degradation of these samples also suggested that they would not be very useful for development of the method. A number of the solution samples, however, exhibited significant degradation. Chromatograms of the solution samples are shown in Figures 8 and 9. It is apparent from the chromatograms that the method needs some improvement since one of the major degradation products (A) elutes just after the void volume. Also, the chromatograms are fairly "crowded" around the main peak for a number of samples and it is desirable to improve the separation for this reason. Further optimization was conducted on samples 1 and 7 using HPLC modeling software. The final HPLC method conditions derived from the modeling are given in Table 13. These HPLC conditions moved peak A away from the solvent front and increased resolution between the parent peak and peak G.

F. Generic Screening Methods Vs. Compound-Specific Methods

Most of the previous discussion on method development assumes that one is trying to develop an analytical method for a specific compound. Another viable approach, however, is to develop generic analytical methods that can be used for the analysis of stress-testing samples from multiple

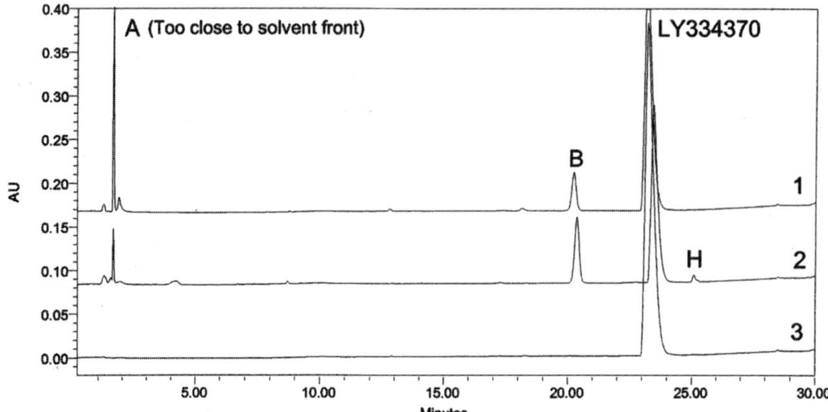

Figure 8 HPLC chromatograms (UV detection, 205 nm) obtained on solutions of LY334370 hydrochloride in (1) 0.1 N HCl/acetonitrile, (2) 0.1 N NaOH/acetonitrile, and (3) water held at 70°C for 8 days.

compounds. The major advantage to using a generic method is the reduced amount of method development time for each compound. This is something that can be particularly important for laboratories that conduct stress testing on many compounds. Some of the disadvantages include a less-specific method and the greater likelihood that major degradation products may be missed. If one is developing a generic HPLC method for stress testing, gradient elution will almost certainly be required since different

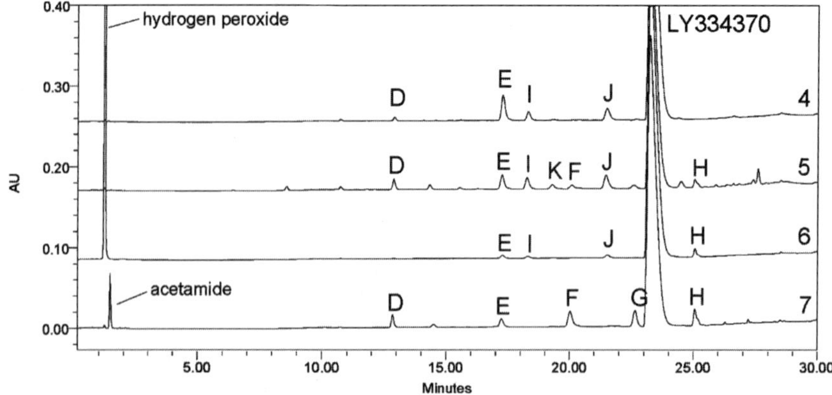

Figure 9 HPLC chromatograms (UV detection, 205 nm) obtained on solutions of LY334370 hydrochloride in (4) water exposed to simulated sunlight for 20 hr, (5) water/acetonitrile containing the radical initiator AIBN held at 40°C for 8 days, (6) 0.3% hydrogen peroxide held in the dark at 23°C for 8 days, (7) pH 8 buffer/acetonitrile held at 70°C for 8 days.

compounds likely will have different polarities. If UV detection is to be used, the use of a PDA detector in combination with UV transparent solvents will enable the extraction of UV chromatograms at the appropriate wavelengths for different compounds. One approach when using generic methods is to use two "orthogonal" generic methods. For example, generic HPLC methods could be developed using different column chemistries (e.g., C8 and phenyl) or different mobile phase pH if the compounds being analyzed contain ionizable functional groups.

G. Validation of Methods

According to the ICH guideline on validation of analytical methods (5), the objective of validation of an analytical procedure is to demonstrate that it is suitable for its intended purpose. The reader should keep in mind that stress-testing methods are screening methods to be used to help understand the degradation chemistry of a drug and therefore do not need to (nor, in general, can they) be validated to the extent of final control methods. In addition, stress-testing methods are usually only used in a limited number of laboratories without a formal method transfer. The concepts in the ICH guideline on validation of analytical methods are a good starting point for validation of stress-testing methods. The ICH guideline gives parameters to be considered when validating methods. These parameters include accuracy, precision, specificity, detection limit, quantitation limit, linearity, and range. All of these parameters should be addressed to some extent when validating stress-testing methods, however, the overall validation should be significantly abbreviated when compared to the validation of final control methods, since stress-testing methods are investigational methods. Accuracy normally should not be a problem with stress-testing methods as long as the response of the detector is linear and samples are completely dissolved prior to analysis. The specificity of methods cannot be fully validated since one normally does not know all of the possible degradation products during initial stress-testing. Specificity can be addressed by using any known impurities and the degradation products produced in the method development samples. Precision (repeatability) of the assay of the main component can be evaluated by preparing a limited number of assay samples (e.g., 5–10) and using simple statistics to estimate the standard deviation. Estimation of intermediate precision and reproducibility should normally not be necessary for stress-testing methods. Detection and quantitation limits for degradation products can be determined by using the parent compound and assuming that the responses of degradation products will be similar. Although there is no requirement to reach any specific detection limit, a reasonable goal is 0.1% since the goal of stress testing is to detect the major degradation products in samples approximately 10–20% degraded. The linearity of the method should be validated over ranges for both assay and impurity determination. A typical assay range might be from 50% to 110% of nominal sample concentration, while a typical range for impurity determination might cover a range from the quantitation limit to a few percent. If one wishes to quantitate impurities vs. the parent peak, then linearity (range) should be demonstrated from the quantitation limit to at least 100% of nominal sample concentration.

H. Alternate Methods

There are numerous analytical techniques besides reversed-phase HPLC that can be used to analyze stress test samples. Some of the more common ones include normal-phase HPLC, thin layer chromatography (TLC), capillary electrophoresis (CE), and gas chromatography (GC). The following paragraphs contain brief discussions on the use of these techniques for analysis of stress test samples.

1. Normal-Phase HPLC

Normal-phase HPLC is a good complementary technique to reversed-phase HPLC in that it often gives different selectivity. It is also more effective in separating geometric isomers than reversed-phase HPLC. The main problem with normal-phase HPLC is that aqueous samples are not normally compatible with the technique. Since many of the stress-testing samples contain water, normal-phase HPLC is rarely used as the primary analytical technique for stress test samples. Nonetheless, normal phase can be a useful complementary technique to reversed-phase HPLC. A detailed discussion on the development of normal-phase HPLC methods is beyond the scope of this chapter.

2. Thin-Layer Chromatography (TLC)

TLC is one of the oldest chromatographic methods and is widely used in the pharmaceutical industry. TLC and high-performance TLC (HPTLC) are complementary to reversed-phase HPLC. TLC and HPTLC are typically carried out under normal-phase conditions and therefore can be very useful for separating impurities that cannot be easily separated under reversed-phase conditions. One significant advantage of TLC is that detection is carried out on the entire plate following development. This ensures that all of the impurities can be detected whether or not they migrate from the origin, as long as they are separated from the parent and the correct visualization technique is used. Another significant advantage of TLC is the possibility of running multiple samples in parallel rather than running sequentially as is done in HPLC. Some of the disadvantages of TLC include generally decreased sensitivity and resolving power as compared to HPLC. For additional details on TLC and HPTLC, see one of the many literature references (6).

3. Capillary Electrophoresis (CE)

Capillary electrophoresis (CE) is another complementary technique to reversed-phase HPLC. Since there are a significant number of resources available describing CE, a detailed discussion of CE will not be presented. Although a number of detectors are available for CE, the most useful detector for analysis of stress-testing samples is the UV detector. Commercial CE instruments are also available with a PDA detector, which helps when correlating peaks between CE and HPLC. A number of articles have been published describing the use of CE for detection of pharmaceutical impurities (7). A significant amount of work has been done to develop "generic" CE methods that can be used for a wide variety of compounds. For basic solutes, Altria has suggested the use of a phosphate buffer at pH 2.5 (8) and for acidic solutes a borate buffer at a pH of 9.3 (9). Hilhorst has suggested a MEKC strategy for impurity profiling which involves the use of an SDS system and a CTAB system (7a). Analysis of samples on these two systems guarantees, in principle, that all compounds will pass the detector in at least one of the two systems. Altria has also developed a generic MEKC method utilizing lithium dodecyl sulfate and beta cyclodextrin (10).

One of the major benefits of CE is that its separation mechanism is different from that of HPLC and it will often give different selectivity. This is illustrated in the analysis of a partially degraded drug sample (Fig. 10). The drug contains two carboxylate groups and is therefore negatively charged under the CE analysis conditions. The top trace is a reversed-phase HPLC chromatogram and the bottom trace is a CE electropherogram. The analysis conditions are given on the figures. The peaks detected using the two techniques were correlated by comparing UV spectra obtained using PDA detectors. Clearly, the two techniques give significantly different selectivities.

4. Gas Chromatography (GC)

Gas chromatography is a good choice for analysis of volatile drug substance stress test samples. It is also a complementary technique to HPLC when volatile degradation products are suspected. For example, see the LY297802 example described in Chapter 6, where volatile and non-chromophoric degradation products were missed by the HPLC-UV detection scheme but readily detected by extraction and analysis using GC with a flame ionization detector (FID). The FID is usually the GC detector of choice for analysis of stress test samples since it is a nearly universal detector for carbon-containing compounds and has the required sensitivity. The mass spectrometer is another widely used GC detector and can give structural information on the peaks as they elute from the column. One major difference between HPLC and GC is the typical requirement of an internal standard for quantitative analysis using GC.

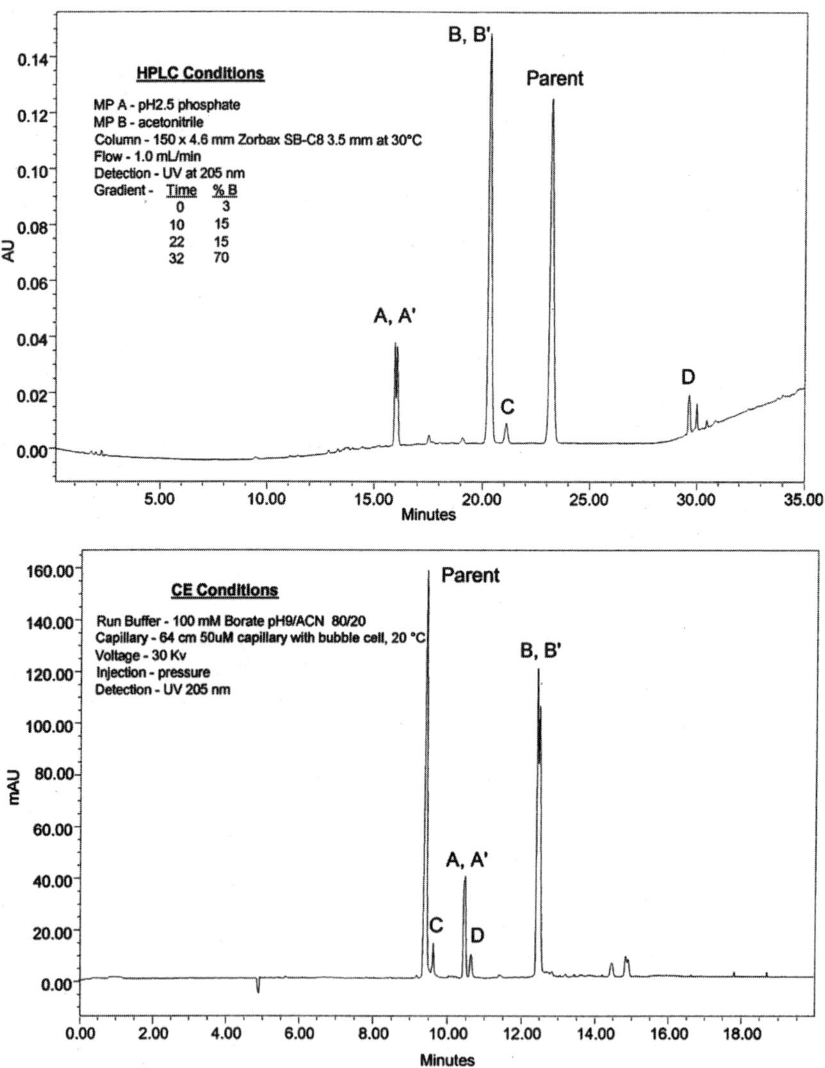

Figure 10 HPLC chromatogram (top) and CE electropherogram (bottom) obtained on a partially degraded drug sample. Peaks A,A′ and B,B′ are difficult to separate, diastereomeric pairs.

III. CONCLUSIONS

Stress testing is an important part of the drug development process as it provides knowledge about the degradation chemistry of drug compounds. This knowledge is used primarily to develop stability-indicating analytical methods but is also useful for other purposes such as formulation development, package development, and the design of official stability studies. Very little formal guidance is available for the design and execution of stress-testing studies and this chapter provides some practical guidance on these topics. Typical stress-testing studies involve exposing solid samples of drug substance to heat, heat with humidity, and photostress and solutions or suspensions of the drug substance to hydrolysis conditions at various pH values, oxidative reagents, and photostress. One of the most important aspects of stress testing is the analysis of stressed samples using a suitable analytical method which, in many cases, is reversed-phase HPLC. This necessitates the development of an HPLC method capable of measuring both the loss of the parent compound as well as the levels of degradation products or impurities formed under the stress conditions. General guidance is provided for the development of HPLC methods appropriate for analysis of stress-testing samples.

REFERENCES

1. International Conference on Harmonisation, Stability Testing of New Drug Substancesand Products, Ql A(R2), February 2003.
2. International Conference on Harmonisation, Photostability Testing of New Drug Substances and Products, Q1B, November 1996.
3. Richter S, Fabris D, Binaschi M, Gatto B, Capranico G, Palumbo M. Effects of common buffer systems on drug activity in the case of Clerocidin. Chem Res Toxicol 2004; 17(4):492–501.
4. Dolan JW. Stability indicating assays. LC/GC N Am 2002; 20(4):346–349.
5. International Conference on Harmonisation, "Text on Validation of Analytical Procedures", Q2A, October 1994.

6a. Gorman PM, Jiang H. Isolation methods I: thin-layer chromatography. In: Ahuja S, Alsante KM, eds. Handbook of Isolation and Characterization of Impurities in Pharmaceuticals. Separation Science and Technology. Vol. 5. San Diego, CA: Academic Press, 2003.

6b. Sherma J. Planar chromatography. Anal Chem 2000; 72(12):9–25.

7a. Altria KD, Chen AB, Clohs L. Capillary electorphoresis as a routine analytical tool in pharmaceutical analysis. LCGC 2001; 19(9):972–985.

7b. Hilhorst MJ, Derksen AF, Steringa M, Somen GW, DeJong GJ. Towards a general approach for the impurity profiling of drugs by micellar electrokinetic chromatography. Electrophoresis 2001; 22:1337–1344.

8. Altira KD, Frake P, Gill I, Hadgett T, Kelly MA, Rudd DR. J Pharm Biomed Anal 1995; 13:951–957.
9. Altria KD, Bryant SM, Hadgett T. Validated capillary electrophoresis method for the analysis of a range of acidic drugs and excipients. J Pharm Biomed Anal 1997; 15:1091–1101.
10. Altria KD, McLean R. Development and optimisation of a generic micellar electrokinetic capillary chromatography method to support analysis of a wide range of pharmaceuticals and excipients. J Pharm Biomed Anal 1998; 18: 807–813.

5

Stress Testing: Relation to the Development Timeline

Steven W. Baertschi
Eli Lilly and Company, Lilly Research Laboratories, Lilly Corporate Center, Indianapolis, Indiana, U.S.A.

Bernard A. Olsen
Eli Lilly and Company, Lilly Research Laboratories, Lafayette Indiana, U.S.A.

Karen M. Alsante
Pfizer Global Research & Development, Analytical Research & Development, Groton, Connecticut, U.S.A.

As has been discussed elsewhere (1,2), for a novel drug candidate that progresses from discovery through pre-clinical and clinical stages of development and eventually to the market, stress testing is not a "one-time" event. Instead, stress testing is typically performed at several stages in the "life cycle" of a novel drug candidate with different goals (and therefore often different strategies and levels of thoroughness) depending on the stage of development. For example, stress testing of a solid drug substance requires the testing of material that is representative—i.e., the material that will be used during clinical trials or the material that will be marketed. Thus, the drug substance should be the same solid form (e.g., same polymorphic form) with similar solid characteristics (e.g., particle size, surface area, etc.). Since early lots of a drug candidate are generally obtained from synthetic routes and processes that will not be the same as that used for the final marketed form, stress testing of early lots may not accurately reflect potential stability issues with new routes and processes. A significant factor in the design of stress testing studies at different stages is the reality that only a small percentage of novel drug candidates make it to the market—the vast majority fail at some point during the drug development process due to factors such as unexpected toxicity, poor absorption or bioavailability (or other biopharmaceutical or metabolism problems), or lack of efficacy (3,4). Since there is a high attrition rate (approximately 90% of compounds entering development will fail), it is not cost-effective to perform the kind of thorough research needed for a marketed product for every new drug candidate. Thus, it is worth discussing stress testing in the context of typical life cycles of a novel drug candidate: (1) drug discovery, (2) pre-clinical/early phase, (3) "commercialization" or late phase, and (4) line-extensions and products on the market.

I. DRUG DISCOVERY STAGE (STRUCTURE–ACTIVITY RELATIONSHIP AND COMPOUND SELECTION STAGE)

During drug discovery, compounds with the desired biological activity (-ies) are identified and structure-activity relationships are determined. In addition to biological activity, compounds need to have appropriate biopharmaceutical properties (3), stability being one of the critical properties. The goal of stress testing or stability studies at this stage is to determine whether or not a compound has stability sufficient for the desired routes of administration and would be able to have a reasonable shelf life as a marketed product. Such stress testing studies are typically very short in duration and are limited in scope (with an emphasis on high throughput), and analytical methodologies are typically generic (i.e., not specifically designed for the individual compound) and therefore are usually less thorough and rugged than would be expected for regulatory submissions. The goal of these studies is to provide rapid guidance to discovery efforts geared toward designing compounds with the desired biological activities and biopharmaceutical properties. Degradation prediction analyses from software programs such as CAMEO (5) are useful at this stage when the resources are not available for time-consuming experimental degradation studies. Also useful at this stage is knowledge gained from previous studies on compounds with similar structures. Database storage and retrieval of such information can be valuable in focusing efforts on the most critical degradation experiments (6). In addition, communications with discovery scientists can play a critical role. For example, predicted degradation products for a candidate may be available as samples from discovery research. Such degradation samples can be run as standards during early method development efforts to provide degradation information when time cannot be invested in LC/MS structural elucidation studies. It is critical to capture as much learning as possible on candidates since the majority will have a short life cycle. Any learning on degradation (e.g., degradation conditions where the compound demonstrates instability, mechanistic data, and/or structural data) can be applied to future candidates in the same class of compounds or with similar structure, etc.

II. PRE-CLINICAL/EARLY PHASE (PRE-CLINICAL TO PHASES I/II)

Once a compound with the desired biological activities and biopharmaceutical properties has been identified and selected for clinical evaluation, information about the stability of the compound needs to be gathered in a more rigorous process. At this stage, the primary goals of stress testing are to develop valid stability-indicating analytical methods that are specifically developed for the compound being evaluated. These methods must be able to separate the analyte from the degradants and impurities that are specific to the compound being evaluated.

The goal of these studies should be to ensure that the stability of the compound can be maintained throughout the clinical trial period. In addition, stress-testing studies should provide basic stability information to aid early formulation development. Generally, identification of degradation products observed during stress testing is not critical during this stage, although there are many times when such information can be very useful to the further development of the compound.

It is worth mentioning that there are various philosophies in the pharmaceutical industry at this time regarding the amount of stress testing (and development work in general) that is needed during the various phases of pre-clinical and clinical development. The differences in approaches to stress testing are documented by Alsante et al. in a benchmarking study of current stress-testing practices in 20 pharmaceutical companies (7).

Most companies (out of 20 surveyed, Fig. 1) first perform degradation studies in the pre-clinical phase of development. Five companies out of 20 first perform stress testing in the discovery stage. Most companies conduct additional stress studies as the clinical trials progress through phases 1 through 3. The practice of repeating or conducting additional stress-testing studies varies by stage of development. Repeating or conducting additional stress-testing studies is typically associated with factors such as analytical methodology improvements, changes in the drug substance (e.g., changes in salt or polymorph, solid-state physical changes, etc.), or changes in the drug product formulation as the compound progresses through the development process. Of those companies that repeat or conduct additional stress-testing studies, eight do so in more than one phase.

For the drug product, 18 out of 20 companies perform stress-testing studies (Fig. 2). Companies first perform these studies between discovery

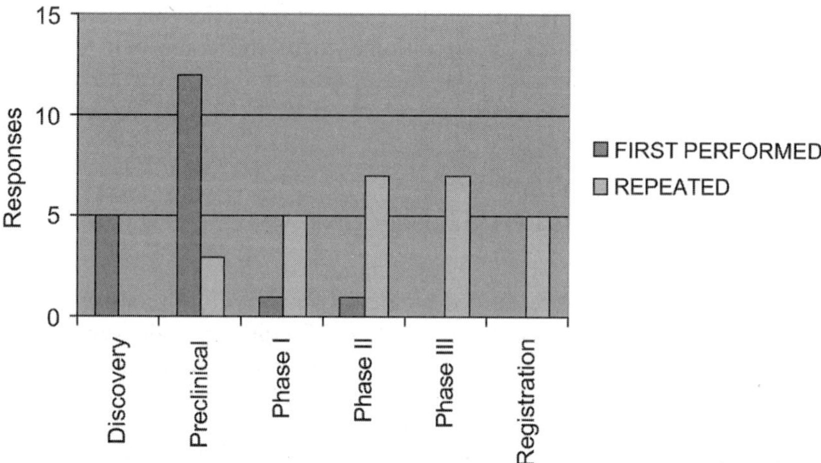

Figure 1 Drug substance stress testing studies performed by phase of development ($n = 19$ first performed, $n = 17$ repeated).

and phase II but mostly in pre-clinical. Phases in which the studies are repeated vary across companies from phase I through registration. Of those that repeat drug product stress-testing studies, eight companies do so in more than one phase.

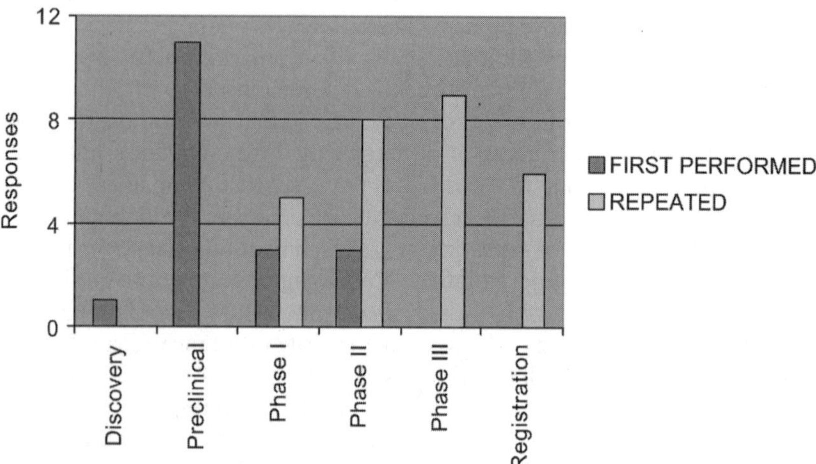

Figure 2 Drug product stress testing studies performed by phase of development ($n = 18$ first performed, $n = 16$ repeated).

III. "COMMERCIALIZATION" STAGE OR LATE-PHASE DEVELOPMENT (PHASE II/III TO REGULATORY SUBMISSION)

Once a drug candidate has shown an acceptable safety profile and has also shown appropriate efficacy (e.g., during phase II clinical trials), larger-scale clinical trials (i.e., phase III) are warranted. At this stage of development, it is apparent that the regulatory authorities expect the pharmaceutical companies to do the needed research to fully characterize and understand the drug compound. The FDA has published a guidance for industry for phase 2 and phase 3 studies conducted under INDs (8). Quoting from the guidance for phase 2 (drug substance) studies:

> Performance of stability stress studies with the drug substance early in drug development is encouraged, as these studies provide information crucial to the selection of stability indicating analytical procedures for real time studies.

It is noteworthy that stress testing is not mentioned for the drug product for phase 2 studies. With regard to phase 3, the guidance indicates the following (for the drug substance):

> If not performed earlier, stress studies should be conducted during phase 3 to demonstrate the inherent stability of the drug substance, potential degradation pathways, and the capability and suitability of the proposed analytical procedures. The stress studies should assess the stability of the drug substance in different pH solutions, in the presence of oxygen and light, and at elevated temperatures and humidity levels. These one-time stress studies on a single batch are not considered part of the formal stability program. The results should be summarized and submitted in an annual report.

With regard to the drug product studies during phase 3, the guidance indicates the following:

> For certain drug products, one-time stress testing can be warranted to assess the potential for changes in the physical (e.g., phase separation, precipitation, aggregation, changes in particular size distribution) and/or chemical (e.g., degradation and/or interaction of components) characteristics of the drug product. The studies could include testing to assess the effect of high temperature, humidity, oxidation, photolysis and/or thermal cycling. The relevant data should be provided in an annual report.

The goals of stress testing at this stage go beyond ensuring stability during the clinical trials since the intention is to bring the product to the market. The goals are therefore to understand all potential stability issues including storage, distribution, short-term temperature excursions, and formulation issues (and even potential patient "in-use" stability issues), as well as to provide a thorough foundation for validation of stability-indicating analytical methods for the marketed life of the compound. A thorough understanding of potential degradation products and pathways should be developed during this stage, keeping in mind that this information will form "an integral part of the information provided to regulatory authorities" in the marketing authorization submission.

IV. LINE-EXTENSIONS (NEW FORMULATIONS, NEW DOSAGE FORMS, NEW DOSAGE STRENGTHS, ETC.), OLDER PRODUCTS ALREADY ON THE MARKET (UPDATING METHODS, ASSESSING PROCESS CHANGES)

After registration, changes to the drug substance or drug product manufacturing process are often desired to reduce cost, increase quality or reliability, or reduce environmental impact. Manufacturing site and scale changes are also common. Stability studies need to be conducted to demonstrate that the proposed changes do not adversely impact the already established stability characteristics of the product. This assessment is usually desired in a much shorter period of time than that required for long-term studies or even the 3–6 months required for accelerated conditions. A rapid stability assessment is also needed for line-extensions involving new formulations or different strengths of an existing product. In Chapter 8, the use of "highly accelerated" conditions is described for comparative stability studies or for developing stability models useful for a broad range of conditions. In this mode, elevated temperatures and/or humidities beyond the ICH accelerated stability conditions are used to compare the stabilities of products made in different ways or to develop predictive models. Such highly accelerated or stress studies can be useful in evaluating process changes where a baseline of knowledge about the stability characteristics of the compound already exists. Information about the stability of new formulations of existing active components can also be obtained quickly using highly accelerated conditions. These studies may reveal stability issues much more rapidly than traditional methods and lead to more efficient and effective drug development.

Another important consideration during the lifecycle of a drug is the development of new dosage strengths, new dosage forms, new formulations, and alternate routes of administration. Each new development will require new or modified stress testing and stability studies, as it cannot be assumed that degradation rates and pathways will remain the same as the original product. New or modified analytical methodologies may also be required, and therefore new or revised stress testing studies will need to be performed as part of the analytical method development process. New or modified analytical methodologies can also lead to the discovery of new impurities (in line-extensions and even in existing products) that were not detected with previous methods.

REFERENCES

1. Alsante KM, Friedmann RC, Hatajik TD, Lohr LL, Sharp TR, Snyder KD, Szczesny EJ. Degradation and impurity analysis for pharmaceutical drug candidates (Chapter 4). In: Ahuja S, Scypinski S, eds. Handbook of Modern Pharmaceutical Analysis. Boston: Academic Press, 2001.
2. Reynolds DW, Facchine KL, Mullaney JF, Alsante KM, Hatajik TD, Motto MG. Available guidance and best practices for conducting forced degradation studies. Pharm Tech 2002; 26(2):48–54.
3. Lipper RA. How can we optimize selection of drug development candidates from many compounds at the discovery stage? Modern Drug Discovery 1999; 2: 55–60.
4. Prentis RA, Lis Y, Walker SR. Pharmaceutical innovation by the seven U.K. owned pharmaceutical companies. Br J Clin Pharmacol 1964–1985; 25:387–396.
5. Jorgensen WL, Laird ER, Gushurst AJ, Fleischer JM, Gothe SA, Helson HE, Paderes GD, Sinclair S. Pure Appl Chem 1990; 62:1921–1932.
6. Alsante KM, Snyder KD, Swartz M, Parks C. Application development using out-of-the-box-software: a structure searchable degradation/impurity database. Sci Comp Instrument 2002; 30–37.
7. Alsante KM, Martin L, Baertschi SW. A stress testing benchmarking study. Pharma Technol 2003; 27(2):60–72.
8. FDA, INDs for phase II and III studies of drugs, including specified therapeutic biotechnology derived products. Federal Register (Notices) 1999; 64(76): 19543–19544.

6

Role of "Mass Balance" in Pharmaceutical Stress Testing

Mark A. Nussbaum
Chemistry Department, Hillsdale College, Hillsdale, Michigan, U.S.A.

Patrick J. Jansen and Steven W. Baertschi
Eli Lilly and Company, Lilly Research Laboratories, Lilly Corporate Center, Indianapolis, Indiana, U.S.A.

I. INTRODUCTION

The assessment of degradation in pharmaceutical products involves two aspects of analytical measurement. First, a selective analytical method must be available for accurate assay of the parent drug compound, in order to correctly measure any loss. Second, methodology should be in place for quantification of the degradation products formed. Ideally, when degradation occurs, the measured amount of parent drug lost should correlate well with the measured increase in degradation products. This correlation is referred to as "mass balance"(1). More recently, the International Conference on Harmonization (ICH) has provided a definition of "mass balance; material balance" as follows:

> The process of adding together the assay value and levels of degradation products to see how closely these add up to 100% of the initial value, with due consideration of the margin of analytical precision. This concept is a useful scientific guide for evaluating data, but it is not achievable in all circumstances. The focus may instead be on assuring the specificity of the assay, the completeness

of the investigation of routes of degradation, and the use, if necessary, of identified degradants as indicators of the extent of degradation via particular mechanisms (2).

Clearly, from a theoretical standpoint, any true decrease in the mass of parent compound (and other reactants involved) upon degradation is necessarily equivalent to the total mass of all degradation products formed. In a closed system, mass balance would thus be assured if sufficient analytical methods were in place to accurately quantify all species present in the original and degraded material and their environment. However, such is almost never the case. The requirement for a "closed system" is rarely met (2). For example, degradation may produce volatile substances that escape from the sample matrix. Adsorption or other physical losses may also result in inaccurate assessment of amounts of material degraded or produced. That is, it is not typically practical to assay a sample's entire environment (e.g., container, atmosphere, etc.). Finally, one may deliberately choose not to quantify certain degradation products if the given degradation pathway can be monitored by assessing a limited number of key substances. As always, the analyst must balance time and resource demands to provide the information necessary to understand degradation without going to extreme measures to quantify components of little interest.

II. WHY IS MASS BALANCE IMPORTANT?

Mass balance in pharmaceutical analysis is important for several reasons. By demonstrating that degradative losses of parent drug correlate well with the measured increase in degradation products, an analyst confirms that there are no significant degradation products unaccounted for. Conversely, if one observes, for example, a 20% loss of parent drug but only measures a 5% increase in degradation products, it is likely that additional degradation products are formed that are not accurately determined by the given method(s). Because unknown degradation products could potentially be toxic or otherwise compromise the safety of the drug, it is important to have methods that detect all major degradation products. Thus, safety is the primary reason for evaluating mass balance.

Mass balance is also useful in method validation (1,3,4). In order to demonstrate that analytical methods are stability indicating, unstressed and stressed materials are often compared. An increase in degradation products that correlates well with loss of parent drug aids in demonstrating that the methods can be used to accurately assess degradation.

Mass balance is also important in understanding alternative degradation pathways (5). For example, consider a situation where both acid-catalyzed degradation and oxidative degradation produce substantial loss of parent compound in stress-testing studies. If good mass balance is achieved for the acid-catalyzed degradation, but not for the oxidative degradation, further work to better understand the oxidative degradation pathway(s) is warranted. It may be that the poor mass balance in the latter case results from important oxidative degradation products that are unaccounted for or from structures which need to be more fully elucidated to understand response factor differences.

III. HOW IS MASS BALANCE MEASURED AND EXPRESSED?

Mass Balance can be calculated and expressed in a variety of ways. The amount of parent compound lost and of degradation products formed can be expressed in terms proportional either to weight or to number of moles. The term "mass balance" is suggestive of a straightforward correlation of mass or weight lost and gained. If all starting materials and degradation products are accounted for, then a correlation in terms of weight is appropriate. However, if degradation involves the formation of products of substantially different molecular weight, or which are not all readily measured, it may be more appropriate to consider molar mass balance.

For the purposes of this discussion, then, the following definitions will be used (examples are given below the set of definitions). Let P be the parent drug and I be the impurity or degradation product. Assume that $M_{\mathrm{P},0}$ and $M_{\mathrm{P},x}$ are the mass of parent compound (and other starting reactants) initially and at time X, respectively; $M_{\mathrm{I},0}$ and $M_{\mathrm{I},x}$ are the total mass of impurities initially and at time X, respectively. Similarly, $N_{\mathrm{P},0}$, $N_{\mathrm{P},x}$, $N_{\mathrm{I},0}$, and $N_{\mathrm{I,x}}$ are the analogous number of moles of each.

Mass balance: The situation in which the measured mass of parent and other reactant(s) consumed is equivalent to the measured increase in mass of degradation product(s); i.e., $M_{\mathrm{P},0} - M_{\mathrm{P},x} = M_{\mathrm{I}},x - M_{\mathrm{I},0}$

Molar mass balance: The situation in which the measured increase in moles of degradation product(s) is equivalent to that predicted via a balanced chemical reaction from the number of moles of parent consumed. For a degradation reaction:

$$aP + \cdots \rightarrow bI + \cdots$$

molar mass balance at time x can be expressed as:

$$\frac{N_{\mathrm{P},0} - N_{\mathrm{P},x}}{a} = \frac{N_{\mathrm{I},x} - N_{\mathrm{I},0}}{b}$$

Furthermore, an observed deviation from mass balance can be expressed in either absolute or relative terms, as described below.

Absolute mass balance deficit (AMBD): The difference between the measured amount of parent compound consumed and of degradation product(s) formed; i.e., $\mathrm{AMBD} = (M_{\mathrm{P},0} - M_{\mathrm{P},x}) - (M_{\mathrm{I},x} - M_{\mathrm{I},0})$. Although

AMBD can be expressed in units of mass, it is commonly expressed in percentage (see example below).

Relative mass balance deficit (RMBD): The absolute mass balance deficit expressed as a percentage of the total amount of parent consumed; i.e.,

$$\text{RMBD} = 100\% \times \frac{(M_{\text{P},0} - M_{\text{P},x}) - (M_{\text{I,x}} - M_{\text{I},0})}{M_{\text{P},0} - M_{\text{P},x}}$$

The absolute and relative molar mass balance deficit can be analogously calculated using the number of moles—in place of mass—of parent and degradation product(s).

Example 1: Stress-testing studies indicate a loss of parent compound from 100 to 86 μg/mL (a loss of 14.0%) and an increase in total related substances from 2.0% to 11.5% (relative peak area). The AMBD is thus 14.0 – (11.5–2.0) = 4.5% (or 4.5 μg/mL). The corresponding RMBD is 4.5/14.0 = 32.1%.

Example 2: Stress-testing studies indicate a loss of parent compound from 100 to 86 μg/mL (a loss of 14.0%) but no corresponding increase in related substances. Now, AMBD = 14– 0 = 14.0%, and the RMBD = 14.0/14.0 = 100%.

Example 3: Stress-testing studies indicate a loss of parent compound (P) from 200 to 180 μmol/mL (a loss of 10.0%) and an increase in one key degradation product from 2.1 to 15.5 μmol/mL. The degradation product (*I*) is believed to be formed from a dimerization reaction of the type:

$$2\text{P} \rightarrow \text{I}$$

Thus, the loss of 20 μmol/mL of P would be expected to produce 10 μmol/mL of I. In this case, the measured increase of I exceeds what would be expected from molar mass balance. The AMBD in this case is [(200−180)/2] – (15.5−2.1) = 10−13.4 = −3.4 μmol/mL. The RMBD is therefore (−3.4/10) = −34%.

AMBD and RMBD are both zero in the case of perfect mass balance, positive when the measured increase in degradation products is less than the loss of parent, and negative when the measured increase in degradation products exceeds the loss of parent. The RMBD is particularly useful in assessing how significant a mass balance issue is, as it is independent of the extent of degradation (in contrast to AMBD). The RMBD, in other words, expresses the relative inaccuracy of the measured increase in degradation products.

Often, stress-testing results from HPLC assays are reported in terms of percentages lost or gained upon degradation, on the basis of peak areas. Consideration should be given to exactly what the reported percentages mean, in order to understand mass balance. Generally, for stress-testing, any counter-ion or other inorganic impurity present is ignored, and percentages are with respect to the total sum of parent compound and related impurities. In addition, for solid-state samples, changes in water or other volatile components should be accounted for. One way to address this is to analyze samples using thermogravimetric analysis (TGA) or Karl–Fischer titration (for water content) to account for loss or gain of volatiles. Another app roach is to perform the analyses such that volatiles lost or gained are compensated for in the procedure. This can be accomplished using a method that involves individually weighing samples for each time point to be analyzed (from a lot with a known volatile content) into separate containers to be placed under the stress condition. At the prescribed time point, the individual container (with a known preweighed amount of sample) is completely dissolved and diluted to a specified volume. Any changes in volatile content are irrelevant to the assay result. Thus, when reporting changes in parent content after stress testing, it is important to clearly state what a percentage change refers to and whether changes in overall mass (e.g., due to water loss or gain) are normalized.

Typically, organic degradation products ("related substances") are determined by HPLC. It is important to know whether degradation products are quantified against an external standard or, more commonly, by relative peak area. HPLC peak areas are integrated and the results are, in the simplest case, reported as a percentage of the total of all integrated peaks. Of course, this assumes uniform response factors (e.g., UV absorptivity) for degradation products and parent, and such an assumption may not be valid (6–8). Even when valid, or when response factor corrections are used, it is important to remember what the total of the HPLC peak areas excludes. Clearly, any substances that do not respond to the given HPLC detector will not be included in the total. In addition, the assumption is made (and presumably tested) that all degradation products are eluted from the column.

Finally, if multiple analytical methods are required in order to quantify all the relevant degradation products, then the meaning of relative peak areas becomes more complex. For example, consider a compound that undergoes racemization in addition to achiral degradation. Suppose compound Y, initially 95% parent and 5% related substances, is also initially purely R-isomer. After stress testing, an achiral assay yields the result of 80% parent, and a chiral assay shows that the parent is now 2:1 R:S. Thus, if we had started with 100 mg of sample, we should now have 20 mg of related substances, and of the remaining 80 mg parent, 53 mg is R-isomer- and 27 mg is S-isomer. Overall, then, there has been a 44% loss (by weight) of the R-form of compound Y (95 –53 mg). Given mass balance, the related substance assay should show an increase from 5% to 20% relative peak area, and the chiral assay gives an increase from 0% to 33% S-isomer (relative to the total of R- and S-isomers). Hence, it is important that results be clearly stated. For example, in this case, one could report a 20% loss in compound Y (total enantiomers) or a 44% loss of the R-enantiomer of Y after stress testing.

IV. STRESS TESTING AND MASS BALANCE

The relation of mass balance to stress testing is apparent from the respective definitions found in the ICH guidelines. As defined by ICH, stress testing is designed to determine the "intrinsic stability of the molecule by establishing degradation pathways in order to identify likely degradation products and to validate the stability-indicating power of the analytical procedures" (2). Thus, an assessment of mass balance is an important part in achieving the goals of understanding degradation pathways and evaluating the capability of the analytical procedures to detect all the relevant degradation products.

When carrying out stress-testing studies during development of analytical methods for a particular drug, there are practical problems to consider. If degradation is observed under some stress condition (as inferred by a loss of parent in the analytical assay), how does one determine whether all of the degradation products are being detected when most, if not all, are unknown? It is the intent of this chapter to provide a practical guide for making this assessment.

It is important to remember that the goal of stress testing is not primarily to achieve mass balance in the analytical results, but rather to achieve a full understanding of the degradation chemistry. That is, if the degradation pathways are fully understood, then it is relatively straightforward to determine whether all relevant degradation products are being accurately determined. Typically, this kind of understanding cannot be achieved unless the *structures* of the main degradation products are known. Correlation of the degradation product structures with scientifically reasonable pathways then enables one to assess whether or not any major products are unaccounted for. This mechanistically driven approach (also referred to as a chemistry-guided approach, see Chapter 2, Section XI) can provide an assessment of "the completeness of the investigation of the routes of degradation and the use, if necessary, of identified degradants as indicators of the extent of degradation via particular mechanisms" (2). A practical example of utility of this scientifically guided approach is given below, in the case of LY297802 [see Section V.A, (b)].

V. CAUSES OF AND APPROACHES TO SOLVING MASS BALANCE PROBLEMS

There are several potential causes of poor mass balance. The list of considerations below covers the most common difficulties and suggests ways to diagnose and resolve them.

A. Positive Mass Balance Deficit

In these cases, the increase in mass (or number of moles) of degradation products is less than the corresponding decrease in parent. Potential sources and resolution of the problem are described as follows.

1. Degradation Product(s) are Not Eluted from the HPLC Column

The are a number of pratical ways to diagnose this problem: (a) the HPLC method can be modified to elute any additional impurities; (b) samples can be analysed using UV spectrophotometric analysis; (c) samples can be analyzed using the HPLC system without the column present (flow injection analysis); or (d) an alternate/orthognal separation can be used.

(a) The HPLC method can be modified to elute any additional impurities

Reversed-phase methods can be modified to elute retained, non-polar compounds by increasing the strength of the mobile phase or increasing the analysis time. This can be done using either gradient or isocratic elution.

(b) Stressed, partially degraded samples can be analyzed against a standard using UV spectrophotometric analysis and the results compared to the results obtained by HPLC analysis of the same samples and standard.

This method is useful for HPLC methods utilizing UV detection. Because UV spectrophotometric analysis involves no separation, there is no chance that compounds are being missed due to retention on a column. Using this approach, a partially degraded sample is dissolved (in the case of solid samples) or diluted (in the case of solution samples) in the mobile phase solvent. The full UV (and/or VIS) spectrum for the partially degraded sample is obtained and compared to the spectrum of the undegraded sample. (If this is a gradient HPLC method, it is recommended that the samples be dissolved in the approximate mobile phase composition under which the parent elutes.) The ratio of the absorbance of the partially degraded sample to that of the undegraded sample is obtained at the wavelength used in the HPLC method. This absorbance ratio is then compared to the ratio of total peak area obtained by the HPLC method for the partially degraded sample compared to the undegraded sample. If all of the impurities are detected with the HPLC method, then the total HPLC peak area from the partially degraded sample divided by the HPLC peak area from the undegraded sample should be equivalent to the absorbance ratio. If the HPLC method utilizes a photodiode array detector, comparisons can be determined at multiple wavelengths, if desired. If the HPLC area ratio is significantly less than the spectrophotometric absorbance ratio, then the HPLC method must be omitting some of the degradation products.

(c) The sample can be analyzed using the HPLC system without the column present (flow injection analysis)

In this experiment, the column is removed from the HPLC system and the total peak area compared to the total peak area obtained when using a column. If the total peak area obtained with the column present is significantly less than that when the column is absent, then the HPLC method must be missing some of the total mass. In the absence of the column, all related substances and parent compound co-elute, giving a single unretained peak with an area proportional to the total amount of detectable material. The total area of all peaks should be the same when the column is present, assuming all species are eluted. If the total area is less when the column is present, then it is likely that one or more compounds are not eluted under the given conditions. One potential difficulty with this diagnosis tool is the impact of the sample solvent. If significantly different from the mobile phase, the solvent effects on sample response may make accurate integration difficult in the absence of the column. In addition, it is important that the quantity of sample injected does not produce peak area(s) that are off-scale or outside the linear range. Finally, if a mobile-phase gradient is used when the column is persent, the changing solvent composition can affect analyte response and, consequently, the peak area of eluting species. One can determine if the gradient has such an impact by comparing the total areas obtained, without the column, when each extreme of the gradient mobile-phase composition is used isocratically.

(d) An alternate/orthogonal separation can be used and the results compared to the HPLC results

The use of RP-TLC can aid in the investigation by revealing slowly migrating compounds or compounds at the origin. The orthogonal techniques of normal phase HPLC, normal phase TLC, and capillary electrophoresis (CE) can be powerful investigative tools in determining whether the original HPLC method fails to elute all products (1).

2. Degradation Product(s) Not Detected by the Detector Used

Ultraviolet absorbance is the most common detection technique for HPLC. Although widely applicable, UV detectors do not detect all compounds. Degradation may produce compounds without chromophores, in which case the observed increase in degradation products will be smaller than the loss in parent compound. The diagnosis (as well as the solution) for the problem may be to use a shorter wavelength or an alternative detector [e.g., evaporative light-scattering detection (ELSD), mass spectrometry (MS), or flame ionization detection (FID)]. It is important to keep in mind that most such detectors, while broadly applicable, are—like UV—not uniform in their response. For example, compounds with significant vapor pressure give poor response by ELSD, and MS response varies greatly with ionizability. However, such detectors can be very useful in confirming the presence of degradation products undetected by the original method (9–13).

As an example of this type of mass balance issue, consider drug candidate LY297802 (Fig. 1). Stress testing of aqueous solutions of LY297802 under cool-white fluorescent lighting (~17,000 lux) produced a 5.4% loss after 3 days and a 42% loss after 7 days (overlaid chromatograms, Figure 2). However, the corresponding increases in degradation products were only

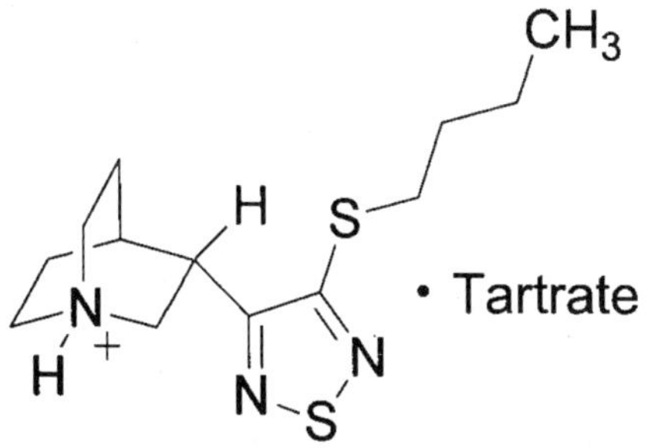

Figure 1 Structure of LY297802.

0.4% and 1.3%, respectively, by the gradient HPLC–UV-related substance method, revealing a significant analytical mass balance deficit. Careful inspection of the containers in which the samples were exposed revealed an insoluble hazy film deposited on the surfaces. Collection of this insoluble film and subsequent analysis by probe EI–MS revealed that the film was elemental sulfur (S_8). As the sulfur was likely originating from degradation of the thiadiazole ring, the potential for formation of non-chromophoric products was considered. LC–MS analyses of the solutions were unfruitful, and the potential for formation of volatile products was considered. Hexane extraction (of the aqueous light-degraded solution, basified to give the free base of LY297802) followed by GC–FID revealed two major degradation

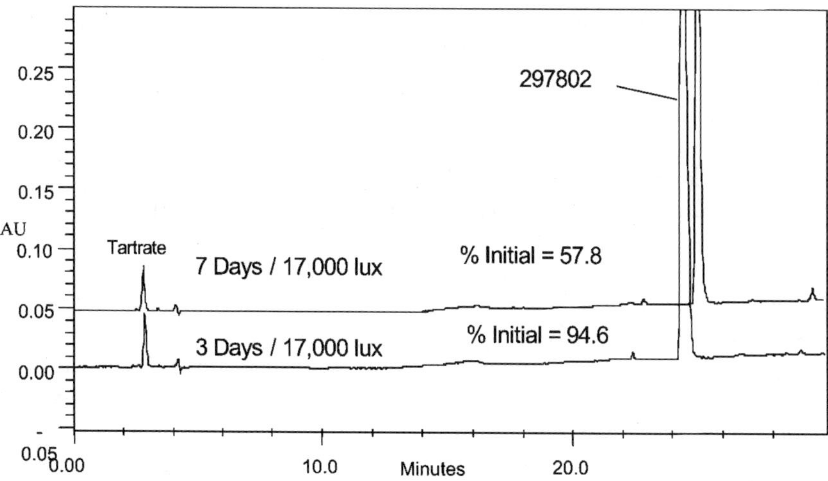

Figure 2 HPLC-related substance chromatograms (UV detection) of 297802 tartrate aqueous solution exposed to cool-white fluorescent light (~17,000 lux) for 3 and 7 days.

products in the degraded samples. Analysis using GC–MS (with accurate mass measurements) provided molecular formula information. As a result, structures were elucidated, providing an understanding of the degradation chemistry and the reason for the lack of detectability with HPLC–UV (i.e., the degradation products were volatile and non-chromophoric) (14).

3. Degradation Product(s) Lost from the Sample Matrix

In some cases, degradation products are inadvertently excluded from the sample tested because of insolubility, volatility, or adsorption losses. Instances of insolubility are usually the most obvious and straightforward to solve. In such cases, visual observation or turbidity measurements may reveal the problem. Use of a different sample solvent or isolation and specific testing of the insoluble material may then be necessary. For example, in the degradation of compound LY297802 described earlier (14), some insoluble material was observed and determined to be elemental sulfur, providing a valuable clue to the mass balance problem. Of course, insoluble degradation products are less obvious when present in drug products containing insoluble excipients. Isolation and examination of the insoluble material, compared to placebo or undegraded drug product, is appropriate in such cases.

If degradation products are lost because of their volatility, other analytical techniques can be utilized. In such instances, it may be appropriate to extract the sample using solvent–solvent extraction (as in the LY297802 example mentioned earlier) or to degrade material in a manner in which the headspace is captured. Gas chromatography (GC–FID or GC–MS) can then be used to compare the headspace from degraded and undegraded samples. In limited cases, if the degradation is thermally induced and rapid, TGA with associated vapor spectral analysis (e.g., IR, MS) may be a useful approach. Finally, if the degradation can be generated at low temperatures, it may be possible to minimize volatility simply by keeping the sample cold.

Degradation products may also adsorb to the sample container or to insoluble excipients. In the latter case, the diagnosis and resolution of the problem is the same as if the degradation product were insoluble (see above). If adsorption to the container is a potential issue, then the most straightforward approach is to compare results using different container materials (e.g., glass, polypropylene). In some cases, changing the sample solvent (e.g., pH, solvent strength) may minimize the adsorption. Occasionally, it may be necessary to use particularly strong solvents to remove the adsorbed material.

4. Parent Compound Lost from the Sample Matrix

In rare cases, the parent compound may itself be lost from the sample matrix due to volatility or adsorption. Often, even if such losses occur, they will be insignificant in proportion to the quantity of parent present. However, if significant, the decrease in assay results would not be due to degradation and so would not correspond to any increases in degradation products. Generally, information obtained prior to stress testing (e.g., melting and/or boiling point, vapor pressure, tendency to adsorb to various materials) should provide indications of this potential problem. Diagnosis and resolution are approached as described earlier (c).

5. Degradation product(s) Co-eluting with the Parent Compound in the Related Substance Method

If a degradation product co-elutes with the parent compound in both assay and related substance methods, then the resulting mass balance depends on the response factor of the impurity relative to that of the parent compound under the given conditions. If the impurity formed has a lower response factor, then there will be a "positive" mass balance deficit. If the response factor of the impurity is greater than that of the parent, then there will be a "negative" mass balance deficit. Examination of the parent compound peak by photodiode array (PDA)–UV detection (and using UV-homogeneity algorithms) or by MS detection may reveal the co-eluting impurity as peak heterogeneity. Of course, PDA detection is effective only for impurities that have distinct UV spectra and that do not perfectly co-elute with the parent. In addition, the *sensitivity* of PDA to detecting peak heterogeneity is dependent on how different from the parent the spectral properties of the impurity are. For some related substances, PDA detection may be unable to detect impurities at levels below a few percent. LC–MS may provide greater sensitivity to a wider range of potential co-eluting impurities; however, LC–MS is more expensive and more restrictive in the types of mobile phase that can be used. Alternatively, an orthogonal separation technique (e.g., CE) can be used to check for co-eluting impurities. If a co-elution problem is discovered, the related substance method should be modified to separate the co-eluting impurity.

6. Degradation Products are Not Integrated Due to Poor Chromatography

Some degradation products may not chromatograph well (e.g., due to adverse interations with residual silanols, on-column conversion or interconversion from one product to another, etc.) and, although they may elute from the HPLC column, the resulting broad peaks can easily be "missed" and remain unintegrated, especially when the broad peak area is present at low levels. Alternatively, if the parent drug degrades to a large number of products that are poorly resolved, the chromatogram observed upon analysis may not reveal discrete peaks but rather an elevated baseline. At low levels, such an elevated baseline can easily escape detection. Situations such as this are not uncommon, especially when isocratic HPLC methods are used. Running a blank (and overlaying the chromatogram) can be very helpful in determining if a baseline elevation is from the sample or simply an artifact of the chromatography. Experiments to determine if low mass balance results are from poor chromatography are the same as those that would be performed to determine if degradation products are not eluting from the column (see Sec. V.A.1).

An example of a drug that degrades to numerous poorly resolved species is shown in Figure 3. In this example, a partially degraded sample was analyzed by RP-HPLC (with a relatively "shallow" gradient of 5–70% acetonitrile over 25 min), and a number of known degradation products, with known response factors, were detected, but the RMBD was 69.1% (83.5% assay, 5.1% total impurities). The possibility of degradation products not eluting from the column was considered, and an experiment was designed to test this hypothesis. In this experiment, the stressed material was assayed without a column in place (flow injection). If all of the degradation products were detected with the RP-HPLC method, then the sum of the HPLC assay and related substance results (i.e., 83.5 + 5.1 = 88.6%) should be equivalent to the flow injection result. The flow injection result was 97.3% indicating that a significant amount of the total mass (degradation) was not being detected with the RP-HPLC method, consistent with degradation products either not eluting from the column or not being integrated. In order to investigate whether products were not eluting from the column, the gradient RP-HPLC method was modified to ramp to a very high organic content (i.e., 90% acetonitrile) and held at this high organic content for 1 hr. This did not result in the elution of any additional degradation

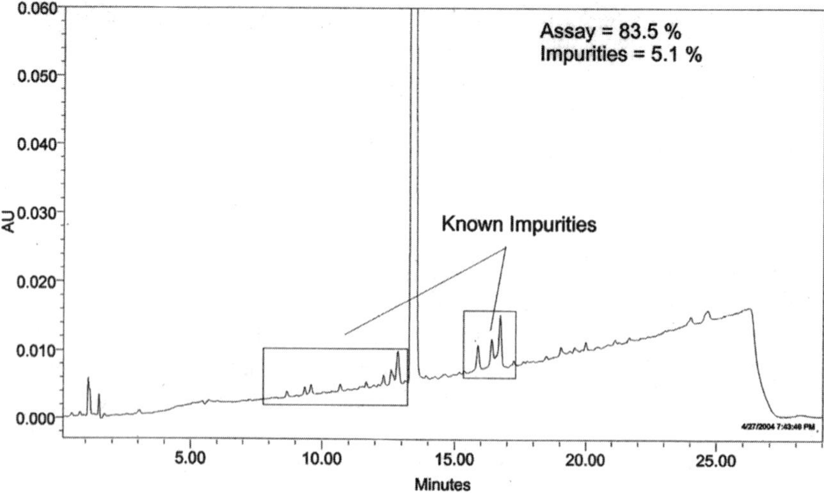

Figure 3 HPLC chromatogram obtained on a thermally stressed drug product using gradient HPLC ("shallow" gradient method).

products, suggesting that there were not any highly retained, nonpolar degradation products. To test the possibility of poorly chromatographing degradation products, another experiment was conducted. In this experiment, the sample was assayed using an isocratic HPLC method with a high organic content to elute the parent drug and the degradation products as a single peak. The result obtained was comparable to the result from the flow injection analysis, suggesting that all degradation products were being eluted from the column. This result is consistent with the hypothesis of poorly chromatographing degradation products that are not being detected/integrated with the original RP-HPLC method. This hypothesis was confirmed by modifying the original RP-HPLC gradient to a steep gradient (0–90% acetonitrile over 25 min). The resulting chromatograms, comparing unstressed samples and degraded stressed samples (with poor mass balance), are shown in Figure 4. Note the elevated baseline in the region of approximately 3–8 min for the stressed sample that is not observed with the control sample. Integration of this baseline "hump" and inclusion in the total peak area (parent and total impurities) provided results that were similar to those obtained using flow injection analysis. This baseline "hump" could also be recognized in samples that were not as extensively degraded when the chromatograms were overlaid with unstressed and blank sample chromatograms (as shown in Figure 5). Thus, the low mass balance was attributed to poorly chromatographing species that were not previously integrated because they were disregarded as mere fluctuations in baseline.

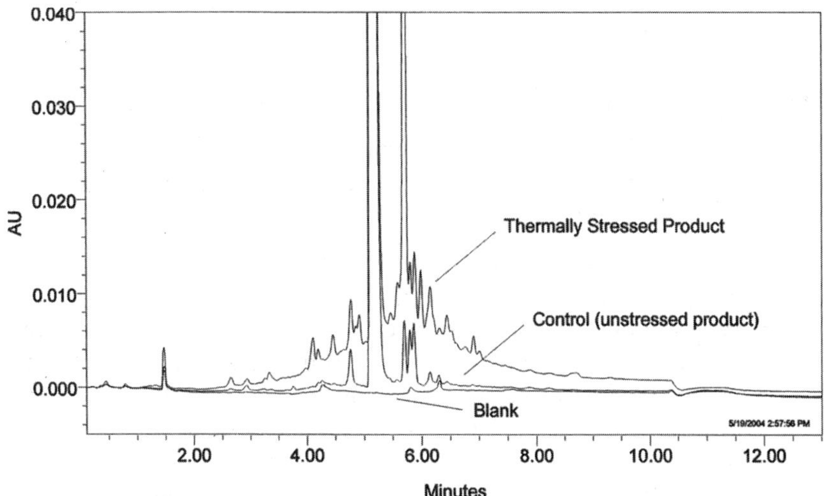

Figure 4 Overlaid HPLC chromatograms obtained on a thermally stressed drug product, a control (unstressed sample), and a blank using a steep-gradient HPLC method.

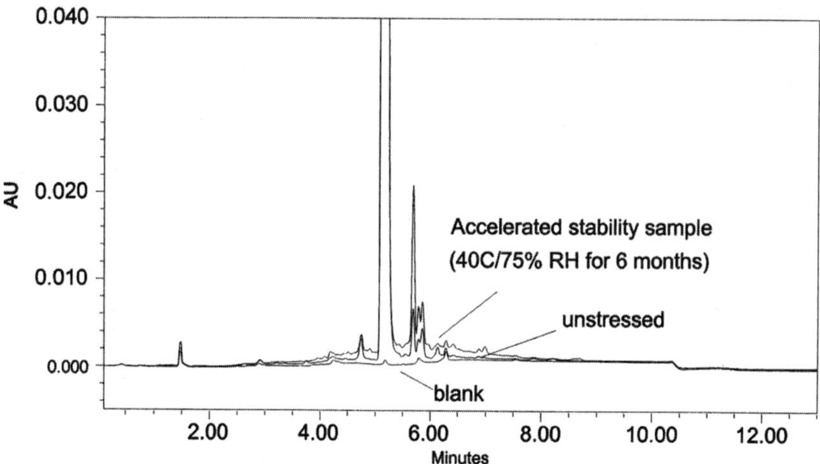

Figure 5 Overlaid HPLC chromatograms obtained on a drug product sample exposed to 6 months of accelerated stability conditions, an unstressed drug product sample, and a blank, analyzed using a steep-gradient HPLC method.

7. Inaccurate Quantification Due to Differences in Response Factors

The importance of response factors to mass balance issues is such that a separate section of this chapter (see Sec. VI.) is devoted to a more comprehensive discussion of this topic.

B. Negative Mass Balance Deficit

In these cases, the increase in mass (or number of moles) of degradation products is greater than the corresponding decrease in parent. Potential sources of the problem are described below.

- Inaccurate quantification of degradation product(s) due to differences in response factors. See Section VI.
- Unaccounted-for reactants involved in addition reaction(s) to the parent compound. Consider reactants from matrix (oxygen, excipients, container ingredients). Compare molar mass balance to weight mass balance; i.e., molar mass balance may be more appropriate in this case.
- Impurities arising from source(s) other than degradation of the parent compound. Such impurities could be present in the mobile phase, sample solvent, or column or could be from the sample matrix. Run a blank sample matrix, or one with varying concentrations of parent

under the same conditions, to determine which—if any—impurities are unrelated to amount of parent present.

- Degradation product(s) co-eluting with the parent compound in the parent compound assay. Check for peak homogeneity via PDA–UV, LC–MS, and/or use an orthogonal separation technique, as discussed earlier. Modify conditions to separate if necessary.

VI. PRACTICAL APPROACHES TO SOLVING RESPONSE FACTOR PROBLEMS

Poor mass balance is inevitable if response factors (e.g., absorptivity at the given wavelength) differ significantly between impurities and the parent compound when uncorrected peak areas are assumed to represent actual relative amounts (6). A positive mass balance deficit results if the response factors of the degradation products are less than that of the parent. A negative mass balance deficit results when the degradation products have larger response factors. Thus, relative response factors (RRFs) of impurities are an important consideration in assessing mass balance.

Occasionally, the UV response factors can be reasonably assumed to be quite similar; for example, the parent and degradation product(s) share the same chromophoric backbone, with structural differences only in regions unassociated with the chromophore. Favorable comparison of UV spectra (e.g., from a PDA array detector) can help confirm such a situation (15).

More often, structures are unknown or differ significantly in the chromophoric region of the molecule such that the assumption of similar response factors is questionable at best. Traditionally, the process for establishing response factors involves the use of isolated samples of individual impurities. For accurate determinations, the purity of each such sample must be known. For synthetic samples, the purity is generally estimated using a combination of HPLC (with UV, light-scattering, or other appropriate detection), NMR, and some method to determine volatile impurities (e.g., TGA, Karl–Fischer). This process involves a significant amount of time and effort (i.e., expense). The effort required is typically even greater for impurities that are not readily synthesized (e.g., low–level process impurities and degradation products). Such impurities need to be isolated and purified using standard techniques such as preparative TLC or HPLC. The risk of having contaminants in the isolated impurities is magnified when compared with synthetic samples because of the large amounts of solvents used, the possibility of non-chromophoric components (e.g., solvents or column bleed), the presence of counterions (e.g., trifluoroacetic acid, acetate, etc.), and the impracticality of using crystallization (with the low levels isolated) to enhance the purity. Moreover, in some cases, the degradation products are unstable and thus very difficult to purify. In order to assess sample purity, amounts of $\geq$50 mg are often needed. Isolation of these amounts of impurities can be very time consuming and costly. Once material of known purity is available, the determination of the response factor(s) is straightforward. A measured concentration is prepared and processed as per the analytical method, to determine the detector response (under the given conditions) per unit weight or molar concentration.

A potential alternative for determining UV response factors is to use two HPLC detectors: a standard UV absorbance detector and a second detector that has a response uniformly proportional to weight or concentration. For example, if a detector could provide accurate information on the relative amounts of the impurities and parent compound, then this information, combined with the UV peak areas, would supply the desired RRF information without the need for a purified impurity sample. One could reasonably question the need for a UV detector and RRF values at all if such an alternative detector was available, as it would directly provide information on relative amounts of impurities/parent. However, UV detectors are inexpensive, rugged, and readily available; therefore, RRF values, once determined, are widely applicable to situations in which no other detector is available.

Some "universal" HPLC detectors will give a response for nearly any compound, but that response is not always related to weight or concentration. For example, ELSD allows detection of most non-volatile substances, but the response depends on the quantity and nature of the particles produced upon drying. For compounds of similar structures and vapor pressures, one can expect similar responses per unit mass by ELSD ($\pm$10–20%) (16). Under such circumstances, the ELSD can be used in conjunction with a UV detector to determine RRF values by peak area ratios:

$$\mathrm{RRF}_{\lambda} = \frac{[(\text{UV peak area})/(\text{ELSD peak area})]_{\mathrm{i}}}{[(\text{UV peak area})/(\text{ELSD peak area})]_{\mathrm{p}}} \tag{1}$$

where i is the impurity and p is the parent compound.

The assumption for Eq. (1) is that the ELSD peak area is directly proportional to mass. For compounds of widely varying structures, charges, or vapor pressure, or for varying mobile phase compositions (e.g., gradient HPLC), the ELSD response can vary markedly (16–22). Thus, Eq. (1) is limited in its applicability. Similarly, mass spectral (MS) detectors are universal, but the response per unit weight depends greatly on the ionization type (e.g., electrospray, fast-atom bombardment, etc.) and on the ionization efficiency of the analyte. Refractive index is another universal detector, but it too suffers from variability in response depending on the mobile phase composition, temperature, and dissolved gases; furthermore, it is relatively insensitive (19,22). In some cases, then, the earlier-mentioned detectors may be used to estimate relative amounts but only when there is reason to believe that the responses are consistent for parent compound and impurities. Similarly, NMR may be used in some cases to quantify the components in a simple mixture, provided the concentrations are high enough and the chemical shifts are well resolved.

A more widely applicable detector for RRF determinations of nitrogen-containing compounds is the chemiluminescent nitrogen-specific HPLC detector (CLND). This detector is based on combustion of the HPLC effluent in an oxygen-rich furnace to convert all organic species to oxides of carbon, nitrogen, sulfur, etc., and water. The nitric oxide produced from nitrogen-containing compounds is then reacted with ozone to produce nitrogen dioxide in an excited state, which emits photons upon return to the ground state (Figure 6 for a schematic of the instrument). This chemiluminescent response is proportional to the number of moles of nitric oxide and correspondingly to the number of moles of nitrogen originally present in the analyte. For virtually any nitrogen-containing compound (with the exception of N_2 and compounds containing N=N bonds), the signal is independent of structure. Thus, amines, amides, nitrates, nitrogen-containing heterocycles (except those with N=N bonds), etc., all produce a signal directly related to the number of moles of nitrogen present. Provided the molecular formula of the analyte is known, one can thereby determine its

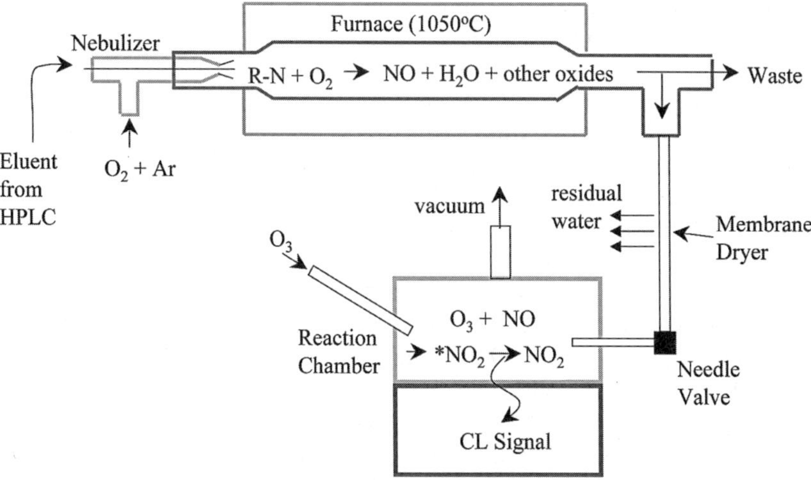

Figure 6 Schematic of CLND Instrumentation.

relative weight in the sample from the amount of nitrogen in the HPLC peak.

Quantification, then, requires only a single nitrogen-containing standard, which need not be structurally related to the analyte. Thus, the CLND opens a new avenue for concentration determinations in the absence of standards of the given analyte (23,24). Moreover, for determination of relative amounts, no standard whatsoever is necessary. All that are needed are the relative CLND peak areas and the molecular formulas of the analytes. Once the relative amounts are found, it is a simple matter to use UV peak areas (e.g., from a UV detector in series with the CLND) to determine the RRFs. Thus, UV response factors (per unit weight) for impurities relative to parent compounds can be determined by means of the following equation:

$$\mathrm{RRF}_\lambda = \frac{[(\text{UV peak area})/(\text{CLND peak area})]_\mathrm{i}}{[(\text{UV peak area})/(\text{CLND peak area})]_\mathrm{p}} \times \frac{(\mathrm{M.}W./\#Nitrogen)_\mathrm{p}}{(\mathrm{M.}W./\#Nitrogen)_\mathrm{i}} \tag{2}$$

where i is the impurity, p is the parent compound, M.W. is the molecular wt., and #Nitrogen is the number of nitrogens in the molecular formula.

Note that for unknown impurities, high resolution LC—MS may be used to determine the molecular formula (25–27). For molar (rather than weight) RRF values, one needs only the relative number of nitrogens per molecule and not the molecular weight.

Thus, RRF information can be obtained without fraction collection or purification, without standards, and without even knowing the concentration of analyte. As a result, sample preparation is greatly simplified, and the stability of the impurity is not an issue.

The CLND is limited, of course, to mobile phases that do not contain nitrogen. Acetonitrile and amine modifiers, commonly used in HPLC, are therefore precluded. In addition, the CLND is not readily amenable to non-volatile buffers in the mobile phase. However, it is still possible to determine RRF values for samples run under these non-CLND-compatible HPLC conditions. In such cases, a two-step process is used. First, a CLND-compatible mobile phase (e.g., methanol/water/trifluoroacetic acid) is used to separate the compounds of interest and determine RRF values under those conditions (RRF_1). Separately, the UV peak areas obtained using both the CLND-compatible and non-compatible HPLC conditions are compared by analyzing a common sample by both sets of HPLC conditions (apart from the CLND). The peaks of interest must, of course, be tracked to avoid misassignment (e.g., through UV spectra comparison). The relative response factor (RRF_1) obtained for the CLND-compatible method can then be used to determine the relative response factor (RRF_2)

for a different set of conditions by multiplying by the ratio of the relative UV areas obtained under each:

$$\mathrm{RRF}_2 = \mathrm{RRF}_1 \times \frac{(\text{UV peak area})_{i,2}/(\text{UV peak area})_{i,1}}{(\text{UV peak area})_{p,2}/(\text{UV peak area})_{p,1}} \tag{3}$$

where i is the impurity, p is the parent compound, and 1 and 2 represent CLND-compatible and non-compatible HPLC conditions, respectively.

Alternatively, one can analyze a sample with the CLND to determine the relative amounts of the analytes present. Then the identical sample can be analyzed with UV detection using non-CLND-compatible HPLC conditions, and the RRF calculated using Eq. (2). This approach requires that the non-CLND-compatible HPLC conditions be defined and run at the time of the CLND analysis, using the same sample. The approach described with Eq. (3) permits running a separate sample at any time at a site removed from the CLND, albeit that sample must be run with UV detection under both sets of HPLC conditions.

VII. RESPONSE FACTOR EXAMPLE: NIFEDIPINE

As a simple example of a positive mass balance deficit caused by different response factors, and corrected by use of the CLND, consider the photodegradation of nifedipine. Nifedipine [4(-2′-nitrophenyl)-2,6-dimethyl-3,5-dimethoxycarbonyl-1,4-dihydropyridine] is a well-characterized light-sensitive pharmaceutical compound. Upon exposure to sunlight or even room light, it rapidly oxidizes in solution to form 4-(2′-nitrosophenyl)-pyridine (see structures in Figure 7) (28). This degradation product has a significantly different UV absorption spectrum than nifedipine. As a result, the RRFs of the two compounds are dissimilar at most wavelengths. Thus, mass balance by HPLC–UV

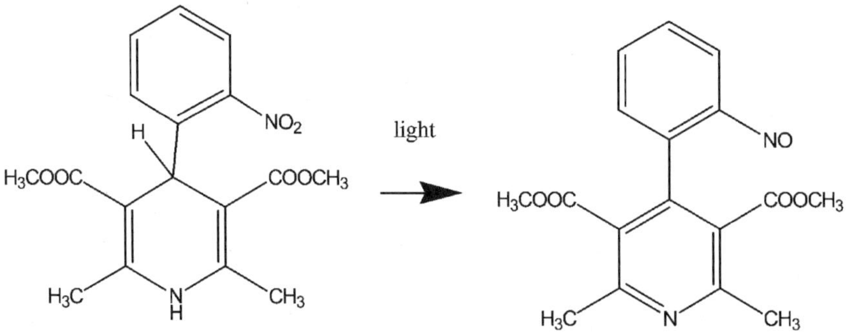

H
NO_2
H_3COOC
$COOCH_3$
H_3C
N
H
CH_3
light
NO
H_3COOC
$COOCH_3$
H_3C
N
CH_3

Figure 7 Photodegradation of Nifedipine (28).

is unlikely unless these RRF values are taken into consideration. Use of the CLND allows one to determine both the true mass balance and the RRF values, as described below (29).

A sample of nifedipine with minimal exposure to light was analyzed at its λ_{max} (237 nm) in order to get a precise measure of the CLND and UV peak areas for the parent compound. The sample solution was then degraded by exposing to a projector lamp over the course of 6 hr. Aliquots were analyzed regularly throughout this time period by HPLC–UV-CLND. After 6 hr of degradation, the lamp was turned off and the sample was analyzed at this final time-point. Sample chromatograms show the progress of conversion to the oxidation product over time (Fig. 8). Each peak was integrated with both UV and CLND detectors.

With UV detection at 237 nm, the total peak area (i.e., sum of the peak areas of nifedipine and its oxidation product) decreased throughout the photodegradation of the nifedipine sample. For example, the total UV peak area after 6 hr was only 65% of its initial value, suggesting a mass balance deficit. However, the total peak area by CLND was consistent throughout, with an overall RSD of 2.5%. Thus, the CLND indicated that the decrease in total UV peak area was due to different RRF values for the two compounds. Furthermore, the RRF value for the oxidation product was readily calculated using Eq. (2): $RRF_{237\,nm} = 0.534$ on a weight basis.

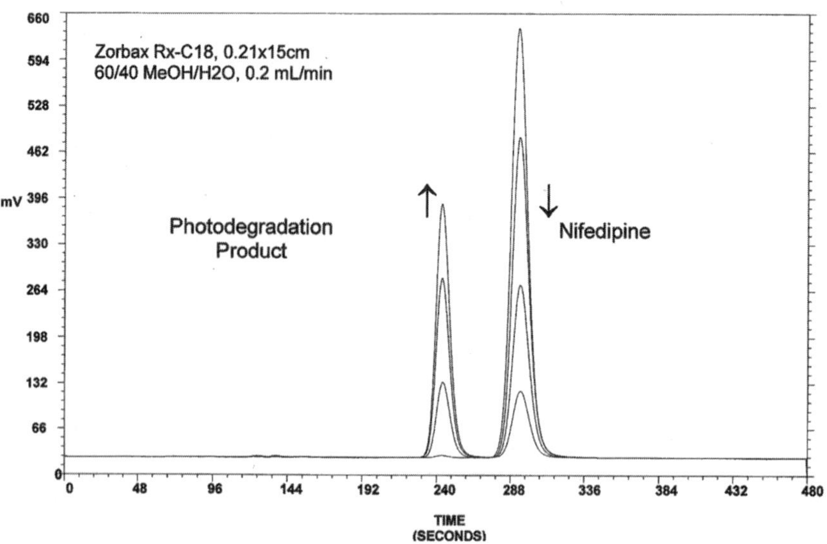

Figure 8 Photodegradation of nifedipine as monitored by HPLC/UV. HPLC conditions: Zorbax Rx-C18, 0.21 × 15 cm; mobile phase: 60/40 MeOH/H_2O, 0.2 mL/min; 5 μL inj. Detection: UV = 237 nm. Arrows indicate the progression of peak areas with time.

Table 1 Mass Balance of Photodegraded Nifedipine: Before and After RRF Correction from CLND Data

Sample	Nifedipine peak area	Oxidation product raw peak area	Total peak area	AMBD (area units)	RMBD (%)	Oxidation product corrected area	Total peak area	AMBD (area units)	RMBD (%)
Initial	13,658	105	13,763	n/a	n/a	168	13,826	n/a	n/a
Partially degraded	7,558	4,070	11,628	2,135	16%	6,491	14,049	−223	−1.6%
Fully degraded	16	8,977	8,993	4,770	35%	14,318	14,334	−508	−3.7%

Omitting the molecular weight information gives the RRF value on a molar basis: 0.563. By using this RRF value, the UV results were readily corrected. Finally, the appropriate RRF_2 for non-CLND-compatible conditions can be easily determined and broadly applied (e.g., in other laboratories). For example, the USP monograph assay for nifedipine uses a mobile phase of water:acetonitrile:methanol (50:25:25). By running a partially degraded sample via HPLC–UV under both sets of conditions, the molar RRF_2 value for the USP monograph conditions was calculated from Eq. (3) to be 0.627. Thus, peak areas obtained for the oxidation product using these conditions were corrected by dividing by 0.627. As a test case, initial, partially, and fully degraded nifedipine samples were run under the USP HPLC conditions. The corrected and uncorrected results are shown in Table 1. The AMBD and RMBD values were calculated as shown in the earlier definitions.

Note from Table 1 that, without RRF correction, the apparent mass balance is quite poor, with a consistent RMBD of 35%. Thus, in the absence of RRF information, one might conclude that mass balance was not achieved and that other, undetected degradation products were being formed or that parent compound was being lost (e.g., via adsorption, volatilization). Use of the RRF_2 value mentioned earlier, however, indicates excellent mass balance, even for a fully degraded sample (RMBD = −3.7%).

VIII. CONCLUSIONS

Mass balance is an important consideration in assessing degradation pathways of pharmaceutical products. Absolute and relative mass balance deficits are useful means of expressing deviations from true mass balance. Many of the most common sources of mass balance discrepancies and approaches to resolving them have been discussed. Often, response factor differences between degradation products and the parent compound are responsible for mass balance problems. RRFs should therefore be incorporated, when possible, in the quantification of degraded samples. Such response factor information can be obtained from purified samples of degradation products or by the use of specialized detectors such as ELSD (for compounds of similar structure and vapor pressure) or chemiluminescent nitrogen-specific detection (for most nitrogen-containing compounds). Alternatively, a lack of detection (e.g., from loss of chromophore with UV detection or from long elution times on HPLC) may be encountered. In these cases, the use of different detectors and alternate separation techniques can help to uncover the source of the problem. By incorporating the concepts and techniques outlined in this chapter, the analytical chemist can begin to assess whether mass balance issues are truly indicating a need to further elucidate degradation pathway information.

ACKNOWLEDGMENTS

The contributions of Bernd Riebesehl and Heiko Brunner (Lilly Research Laboratories, Hamburg, Germany) to the development of the concepts of absolute mass balance deficit and relative mass balance deficit are gratefully acknowledged.

REFERENCES

1. Kirschbaum JJ. Synergistic use of multiple assays and achievement of mass balance to validate analytical methods. Trends Anal Chem 1988; 7:16–20.
2. International Conference on Harmonization Tripartite Guideline: Stability Testing of New Drug Substances and Products, ICH Q1A, September, 1994.
3. Riley CM, Rosanske TW, eds. Development and validation of analytical methods. In: Prog Pharm Biomed Anal. Pergamon Press, 1996.
4. Priestner AA. Use of radiolabeled drug substance to investigate mass balance during validation of a high-performance liquid chromatography method for impurities. Anal Proc 1993; 30:374–377.
5. Conner KA, Amidon GL, Stella VJ. In: Chemical Stability of Pharmaceuticals—A Handbook for Pharmacists. 2nd ed. New York: John Wiley and Sons, 1986.
6. Newton MP, Mascho J, Maddux RJ. Chromatography of pharmaceuticals: natural, synthetic, and recombinant products. In: Ahuja S, ed. Chromatography of Pharmaceuticals. ACS Symposium Series 512. New York: ACS Publications, 1991.
7. Olsen BA, Argentine MD. Investigation of response factor ruggedness for the determination of drug impurities using high-performance liquid chromatography with ultraviolet detection. J Chromatogr A 1997; 762:227–233.
8. Guillemin CL, Gressin JC, Caude MC. The deferred standard method—a technique for quantitative analysis in laboratory and process HPLC. J High Res Chrom Chrom Com 1982; 5:128–133.
9. McCrossen SD, Bryant DK, Cook BR, Richards JJ. Comparison of LC detection methods in the investigation of non-UV detectable organic impurities in a drug substance. J Pharm Biomed Anal 1998; 17:455–471.
10. Righezza M, Guiochon G. Effects of the nature of the solvent and solutes on the response of a light-scattering detector. J Liq Chromatogr 1988; 11:1967–2004.
11. Cech NB, Krone JR, Enke CG. Predicting electrospray response from chromatographic retention time. Anal Chem 2001; 73:208–213.
12. Tang L, Kebarle P. Dependence of ion intensity in electrospray mass spectrometry on the concentration of the analytes in the electrosprayed solution. Anal Chem 1993; 65:3654–3668.
13. Cheng ZL, Siu KW, Guevremont R, Bergman SS. Dependence of ion intensity in electrospray mass spectrometry on the concentration of the analytes in the electrosprayed solution. J Am Soc Mass Spectrom 1992; 3:281–288.
14. Baertschi SW. The role of stress testing in pharmaceutical product development. (oral presentation). AAPS Midwest Regional Meeting, Chicago, IL, May 19, 1996.

15. Olsen BA, Baertschi SW, Riggin RM. Multidimensional evaluation of impurity profiles for generic cephalexin and cefaclor antibiotics. J Chromatogr 1993; 648:165–173.
16. Fang L, Wan M, Pennacchio M, Pan J. Evaluation of evaporative light-scattering detector for combinatorial library quantitation by reversed phase HPLC. J Comb Chem 2000; 2:254–257.
17. Cebolla VL, Membrado L, Vela J, Ferrando AC. Understanding evaporative light scattering detection for high-performance liquid chromatography. Sem Food Anal 1997; 2:171–189.
18. Hopia AI, Ollilainen VM. Comparison of the evaporative light scattering detector (ELSD) and refractive index detector (RID) in lipid analysis. J Liq Chromatogr 1993; 16:2469–2482.
19. McNabb TJ, Cremesti AE, Brown PR, Fischl AA. High-performance liquid chromatography/evaporative light-scattering detector techniques for neutral, polar, and acidic lipid classes: a review of methods and detector models. Sem Food Anal 1999; 4:53–70.
20. Kibbey CE. Quantitation of combinatorial libraries of small organic molecules by normal-phase HPLC with evaporative light-scattering detection. Mol Divers 1995; 1:247–258.
21. Hsu BH, Orton E, Tang S, Carlton RA. Application of evaporative light scattering detection to the characterization of combinatorial and parallel synthesis libraries for pharmaceutical drug discovery. J Chromatogr B 1999; 725: 103–112.
22. Snyder LR, Kirkland JJ, Glajch JL. Practical HPLC Method Development. 2nd ed. New York: John Wiley & Sons, 1997:80–81.
23. Fitch WL, Szardenings AK, Fujinari EM. Chemiluminescent nitrogen detection for HPLC: an important new tool in organic analytical chemistry. Tetrahedron Lett 1997; 38:1689–1692.
24. Taylor EW, Qian MG, Dollinger GD. Simultaneous online characterization of small organic molecules derived from combinatorial libraries for identity, quantity, and purity by reversed-phase HPLC with chemiluminescent nitrogen, UV, and mass spectrometric detection. Anal Chem 1998; 70:3339–3347.
25. Haskins NJ, Eckers C, Organ AJ, Dunk MF, Winger BE. The use of electrospray ionization with Fourier transform ion cyclotron resonance mass spectrometry in the analysis of trace impurities in a drug substance. Rapid Commun Mass Spectrom. 1995; 9:1027–1030.
26. Perkins G, Pullen F, Thompson C. Automated high resolution mass spectrometry for the synthetic chemist. J Am Soc Mass Spectrom 1999; 10:546–551.
27. Palmer ME, Clench MR, Tetler LW, Little DR. Exact mass determination of narrow electrophoretic peaks using an orthogonal acceleration time-of-flight mass spectrometry. Rapid Commun Mass Spectrom 1999; 13:256–263.
28. Pietta P, Rava A, Biondi P. High-performance liquid chromatography of nifedipine, its metabolites and photochemical degradation products. J Chromatogr 1981; 210:516–521.
29. Nussbaum MA, Baertschi SW, Jansen PJ. Determination of relative UV response factors for HPLC by use of a chemiluminescent nitrogen-specific detector. J Pharm Biomed Anal 2002; 27:983–993.

7

Oxidative Susceptibility Testing

Giovanni Boccardi
Discovery Analytics, Discovery Research, Sanofi-Aventis, Milano, Italy

I. MECHANISTIC BACKGROUND

A. General Considerations

Water and molecular oxygen (dioxygen) are the two ubiquitous molecules that frequently affect the stability of a drug substance. Though acids and bases are the catalysts that control the hydrolytic behavior of organic compounds, they are not the principal factors in oxidations. In many cases, oxidation by dioxygen (autoxidation) is hard to understand and may also seem hard to reproduce. The reason, as we will see, is that the reaction is often catalyzed by impurities, whose presence is normally variable. The aim of oxygen susceptibility tests is to detect the factors that control these reactions and to identify the most important degradation products.

At first, it may be useful to define the oxidant involved in autoxidations: dioxygen (1a-c). In the orbital diagram of molecular oxygen, the highest occupied molecular orbitals are two degenerate π^* orbitals in which there must be two electrons (Fig. 1). The ground state, according to the Hund rule, is when these orbitals are occupied by one electron and the spins are parallel: this is the triplet ground state ($^3\Sigma_g$) of atmospheric molecular oxygen (Fig. 1). Triplet oxygen can be excited, either chemically or by photochemical sensitizers, to singlet oxygen, $^1\Delta_g$, the first excited state, 92 kJ mole^{-1} higher than the ground state. The triplet ground state is the species involved in autoxidation (and in this chapter dioxygen is understood to be in this

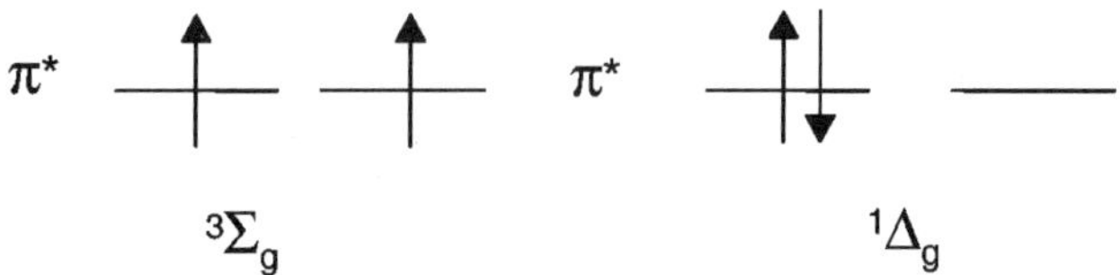

Figure 1 Electronic configurations of molecular oxygen: triplet ground state and the singlet first excited state. The figure shows the highest occupied molecular orbitals.

state if not otherwise specified) whereas singlet oxygen is involved in many photochemical reactions.

Secondly, we will look at some of the factors that govern autoxidation by examining its well-established mechanism. A molecule in its triplet state is a biradical, and an organic chemist expects a radical to be highly reactive. In fact, triplet oxygen does react very fast only with radicals, whereas the vast majority of organic molecules are in the singlet state, and the reaction

$$RH + (^3\Sigma_g)O_2 \rightarrow ROOH \tag{1}$$

is spin-forbidden. For this reason, a large number of organic molecules, in spite of the large negative value of the Gibbs free energy of oxidation, are kinetically inert toward triplet oxygen.

Under "normal" room temperature conditions, the mechanism of autoxidation of hydrogen bearing sp^3 carbon atoms is

$$RH + In^{\bullet} \rightarrow R^{\bullet} + InH \qquad \text{Initation (rate}=R_i\text{)} \tag{2}$$

$$R^{\bullet} + O_2 \rightarrow ROO^{\bullet} \tag{3}$$

$$ROO^{\bullet} + RH \rightarrow ROOH + R^{\bullet} \text{ Propagation (rate constant } = k_p\text{)} \tag{4}$$

$$2ROO^{\bullet} \rightarrow \text{Inert products} \qquad \text{Termination (rate constant } = k_t\text{)} \tag{5}$$

Let us examine the different elementary steps of the mechanism. Initiators [$In^{\bullet}$ in Eq. (2)] can be chemical species of different origins. Very often they are peroxy ($ROO^{\bullet}$) and oxy ($RO^{\bullet}$) radicals produced by thermal homolytic decomposition of organic peroxides,

$$ROOR \rightarrow 2RO^{\bullet} \tag{6}$$

or by photochemical reactions. Heavy metal ions can initiate autoxidation through different mechanisms. Initiators can also be produced by radiolysis (2) or as by products of ozonolysis (3). All these are not normal components of drug substances, but rather are impurities or environmental contaminants: this means that oxidative degradation is often catalyzed by minor components that are very often beyond our control. A small concentration of the initiator can also destroy all the starting organic substrate, because for each radical formed in reaction (2) several molecules may be oxidized according to Eqs. (3) and (4) until a termination reaction (5) occurs. In the light of these facts, a high interbatch variability in degradation rates (when oxidation is the dominant degradation pathway) is not surprising (4).

Rate constants of Eq. (3), radical scavenging of carbon radicals by oxygen, are very high (of the order of 10^9 M sec^{-1} or higher at 300K) regardless of the organic radical (5). A direct consequence is that the radical $R^•$ can only react with dioxygen, so direct attack of organic molecules by this radical can be dismissed, at least at ambient oxygen partial pressure conditions.

Nevertheless, in the case of stable $R^•$ radicals, like pentadienyl radicals, reaction (3) is reversible (6,7):

$$ROO^• \rightleftharpoons R^• + O_2 \tag{7}$$

The backward reaction of Eq. (7) is an example of β-fission of a radical. When this occurs, an equilibrium is established between all possible stereo- and regioisomers of a given peroxy radical and the most stable product is favored, despite the very low selectivity of reaction (3):

$$ROO^• \rightleftharpoons R^• + O_2 \rightleftharpoons R'OO^• \tag{8}$$

where $ROO^•$ and $R'OO^•$are two different regio- or stereoisomeric radicals obtained from the same molecule RH.

The hypothesis of the occurrence of Eqs. (7) and (8) was one of the key elements in the interpretation of the autoxidation of polyunsaturated fatty acids (6).

β-Fission described in Eq. (7) can be inhibited by strong H-radical donors, like cyclohexadiene or phenol antioxidants, that competes with Eq. (4), to give the hydroperoxide ROOH. This quenching prevents the attainment of the equilibrium between different peroxy radicals and therefore limits the selectivity of the hydroperoxidation.

The propagation step, Eq. (4), is much slower than Eq. (3); as an example, its rate constant k_p is 0.18 M^{-1} sec^{-1} for cumene at 303K. Values of k_p can vary considerably for different substrates, as shown by the oxidation rates of substituted toluenes (8). With respect to toluene, taken as 1.0, the reactivity of 4-nitrotoluene toward $ROO^•$ is 0.33 and that of *p*-xylene is 1.6. A homolytic process like the fission of the C–H bond should be essentially apolar, but data for substituted toluenes correctly suggest that the hydrogen radical abstraction is favored by electron-donor substituents and that in the transition state the carbon atom involved has a partial positive charge. The difference in k_p between different molecules or different groups of the same molecule is the reason of the selectivity of autoxidation.

It is interesting to review some very simple kinetic concepts. In the case of a stable hydroperoxide, the kinetic equation of autoxidation is (9)

$$-\frac{d[O_2]}{dt} = -\frac{d[RH]}{dt} = k_p[RH]\sqrt{\frac{R_i}{2k_t}} \tag{9}$$

where R_i is the rate of the chain initiation [Eq. (2)], k_p is the rate constant of propagation [Eq. (4)] and k_t is the rate constant of termination [Eq. (5)]. There is no oxygen partial pressure on the right side of Eq. (9). It is therefore not surprising that very often the oxidation rate does not depend on the oxygen partial pressure (10), at least at high substrate/oxygen ratio. Furthermore, it is not surprising that often carrying out the reaction "in an oxygen atmosphere" or at even higher oxygen partial pressure does not accelerate autoxidation. The main step that must be controlled in order to obtain reproducible data is initiation.

This chapter does not deal with the kinetics of oxidative degradation, treated elsewhere in detail (11), because the author believes degradation kinetics is a more advanced task in drug development than the stress test; however, the need to control the initiation rate cannot be neglected if one is to obtain interbatch and interlaboratory reproducible kinetics parameters.

Another important kinetic feature of autoxidation is autocatalysis. One of the oxidation products is the hydroperoxide, while peroxides can also be produced in termination. Peroxides and hydroperoxides are stable within a limited temperature range, but at higher temperatures they decompose homolytically giving alkoxy radicals:

$$ROOR' \rightarrow RO^{\bullet} + R'O^{\bullet} \tag{10}$$

Outside the range of temperatures at which they are stable, these radicals catalyze the reaction and the rate, initially low during an induction time in which peroxides accumulate, then rises sharply. This nonlinearity must be kept in mind in order to avoid extrapolating the rate of degradation from too short a period, especially when no initiator is added to the system.

The temperature effect is another important feature of the radical chain mechanism and is the consequence of autocatalysis. Peroxides produced by autoxidation can be stable under mild conditions and decompose outside this range, participating in the catalysis of the reaction. What happens if the temperature is raised fast or far in order to accelerate degradation? The first result is that hydroperoxy impurities, though relatively stable at room temperatures, are lost. Moreover, their thermal degradation leads to oxy radicals (especially $OH^{\bullet}$), which are much more reactive and thus less selective than peroxy radicals; there may therefore be a change in the degradation profile compared to oxidation under milder conditions. Another way temperature can affect autoxidation mechanism is mentioned at the end of Section I.C. The overall result is that a stress test at too a high temperature may be poorly predictive of the room temperature degradation and the analyst performing such tests must always bear this conclusion in mind.

We will not go in depth into the subject of antioxidants (12), which is more a part of preformulation than a stress test, but the autoxidation mechanism does suggest that oxidation can be inhibited by peroxy radical scavengers (chain-breaking antioxidants) like "phenol" antioxidants, by heavy metal chelating agents, and by peroxide inactivating substances (preventive antioxidants).

B. The Fate of the Unstable Peroxy Species: The Origin of the Stable Degradation Impurities

The degradation pattern of an organic molecule due to autoxidation is often a complex process, and is one of the reasons why molecular oxygen is seldom the preferred reagent of the synthetic organic chemist. Now that the main features of the autoxidation mechanism have been stated, it is appropriate to analyze the fate of the reactive species afforded by the reaction, in order to understand the whole degradation profile.

Hydroperoxides are the early products of autoxidation and can be found as degradation impurities, but the most stable products develop in side reactions involving hydroperoxides and peroxy radicals. Some of these processes surrounding the formation and decomposition of hydroperoxides will be summarized here.

- *Termination reactions.* A very common termination reaction, known as the Russel mechanism from its discoverer, is the recombination of two peroxy radicals to form an unstable tetroxide that decomposes through a concerted mechanism to yield a hydroxy moiety and a carbonyl moiety (13):

$$2\ \text{PhCH(CH}_3\text{)OO}^\bullet \longrightarrow [\text{tetroxide: PhCH(CH}_3\text{)–O–O–O–O–CHCH}_3\text{Ph}] \longrightarrow \text{PhC(O)CH}_3 + \text{PhCH(OH)CH}_3 + {}^1\text{O}_2 \quad (11)$$

  The oxygen molecule produced by this mechanism is in the singlet state and the reaction gives the carbonyl group in its excited state: its relaxation produces chemiluminescence that can be used for kinetic measurements (14).
- *Epoxide formation.* Acyl- (15) and alkylperoxy (16,17) radicals can react with carbon–carbon double bonds to produce epoxides:

$$\text{R–O–O}^\bullet + \text{C=C} \longrightarrow \text{R–O–O–C–C}^\bullet \longrightarrow \text{R–O}^\bullet + \text{epoxide} \quad (12)$$

This reaction introduces the concept of cooxidation. A substrate that is inert under given conditions can decompose under the same conditions in the presence of an oxygen-sensitive molecule. Pure *cis*-stilbene is inert in the presence of oxygen even at a high temperature, whereas *trans*-stilbene is oxygen-sensitive under the same conditions. In a mixture of the two stereoisomers, *cis*-stilbene reacts at the same rate as its isomer, because it is sensitized by the autoxidation of *trans*-stilbene. This is because *cis*-stilbene is inert toward oxygen, but not toward radicals produced by *trans*-stilbene autoxidation (18).

Aldehydes are easily oxidized (19) and are well-known sensitizer compounds: benzaldehyde enhances oxidation of linear alkenes producing the corresponding epoxides (15). An interesting feature of radical epoxidation is the generation of the alkoxy radical $RO^{\bullet}$, which is more reactive and less selective than the peroxy radical (16)

- *Acid decomposition.* Hydroperoxides are decomposed by acids (Fig. 2). The first step is protonation, but two paths are possible for the development of the protonated hydroperoxide. The first is elimination of a water molecule, giving the oxonium ion (I) that can rearrange, yielding an alcohol and a ketone. This path is favored by substituents on the carbon atoms that can migrate. A well-known example is cumene oxidation, which is the basis of the industrial phenol–acetone process. The second path is the elimination of hydrogen peroxide to yield the carbocation (II). The carbocation can add a nucleophile such as water or an alcohol, or other carbocation scavengers. Carbocations can also rearrange causing ring expansion, or elimination of a proton to give a carbon–carbon double bond (21).

Peroxides can also arise from the following reaction:

$$R_3C^+ + R'OOH \rightarrow R_3C{-}OOR' + H^+ \tag{13}$$

- *Decomposition during isolation.* Silica gel is a Lewis acid: this helps account for the difficulties of isolating hydroperoxides by column chromatography.
- *Base decomposition.* Peroxides and hydroperoxides are decomposed by bases to produce the same products as the tetroxide rearrangement (22).
- *Oxidation and reduction reactions.* Hydroperoxides can be reduced by reducing agents but also oxidized, for instance by heavy metal ions, to the corresponding alkoxy radicals. This is an important initiation reaction and is discussed later.

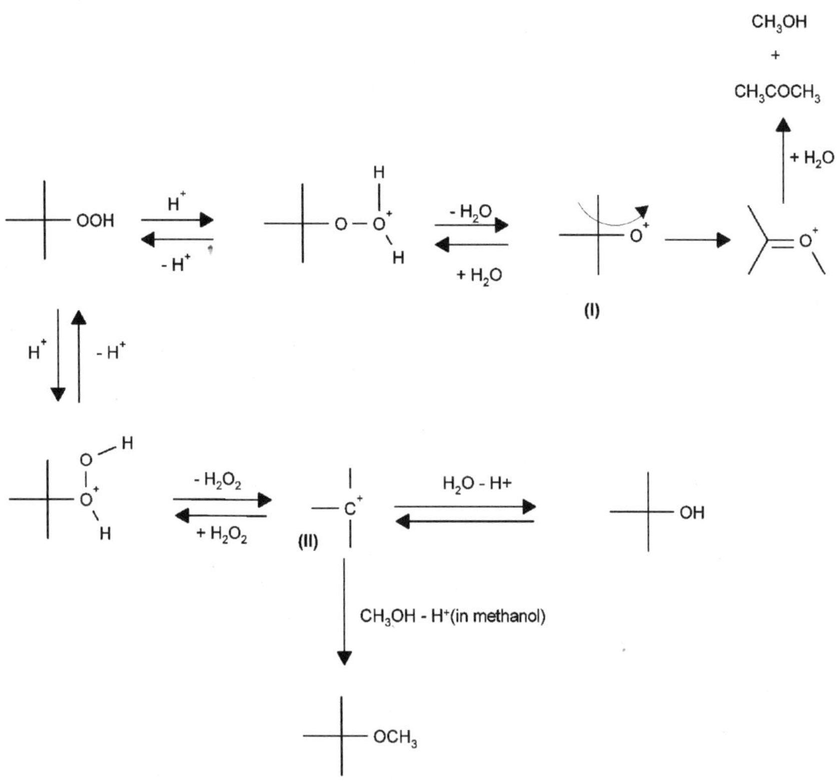

Figure 2 Acid decomposition of hydroperoxides (20): main pathways. Dehydration and rearrangement (upper), loss of H_2O_2, and nucleophilic attack of the solvent (bottom).

- *Reactions with electrophilic substrates.* Oxygen peroxide formed during the development of the early products and hydroperoxides can attack electrophilic substrates according to an ionic, nonradical reaction. In this way, carbon–carbon double bonds can be transformed into epoxides and tertiary amines into N-oxides. These are cooxidations with an ionic mechanism.
  Polyethylene glycol (PEG) is an excipient used in the formulation of liquid pharmaceutical forms of poorly soluble drugs. As an ether, PEG is easily oxidized, and its degradation often facilitates the oxidation of otherwise stable drug substances.

C. Spontaneous Oxidation

The radical-initiated mechanism outlined above can explain a large number of autoxidations, but some particular substrates can apparently be directly oxidized by molecular oxygen, despite the fact that this reaction is spin-forbidden (1c). Directly oxidized organic substances are electron-rich compounds, such as pyrroles (23), α,β-unsaturated enamines (24), carbanions (1a), sterically strained cyclic olefins (25), and strained aromatic polycyclic compounds (26). Direct oxidation involves a charge-transfer step:

$$R^- + {}^3O_2 \rightarrow R^\bullet + O_2^{\bullet -} \tag{14}$$

The carbon radical can react with molecular oxygen and then initiate a radical chain as shown in Section I.A.

The driving forces for electron transfer are a high-energy level of the highest occupied molecular orbital or a steric strain of the starting molecule. Complexation of oxygen by the electron-rich organic molecule has often been indicated as the first step of the mechanism.

In studying the reactivity of a new drug substance, it is obviously interesting to ascertain whether it can be directly oxidized by molecular oxygen without the need for any initiator, but this is not an easy task. An obvious step is to start by monitoring an oxygen-saturated solution of the test compound with no initiator. However, bearing in mind the number of initiators acting in Eq. (2) and their efficacy at very low concentrations, it is practically impossible to exclude them totally. Nevertheless, the first clue of the noncatalytic oxidation mechanism is just the detection of a spontaneous oxidative degradation in experiments performed with particular care using very pure reagents and very clean apparatus.

A lag time in the kinetic curve indicates that oxidation is not direct, but mediated by radical initiators. However, we cannot easily rule out the presence of a very short induction period. A first-order kinetic curve in oxygen partial pressure is strong evidence of the direct mechanism, since initiated reactions do not depend on oxygen pressure, as shown by Eq. (9).

But the best evidence is a product distribution that is not in agreement with the radical-chain mechanism. At high temperature and high partial pressure of oxygen, electron-rich compounds like sulfides, amines, and alkenes undergo direct oxidation, as indicated by products not accountable for a radical-initiated reaction (18). Normal radical oxidation leads to oxidation of the carbon atom α to the functional group. Under high temperature and partial oxygen pressure, a totally different product distribution was observed:

- Sulfides only gave sulfoxides and sulfones
- Amines selectively gave the corresponding N-oxides that are only minor impurities in the radical process
- Alkenes yielded only epoxides and the products corresponding formally to those of the ozone oxidation

These data, confirmed by physicochemical evidence, led the authors to conclude that direct oxidation was involved.

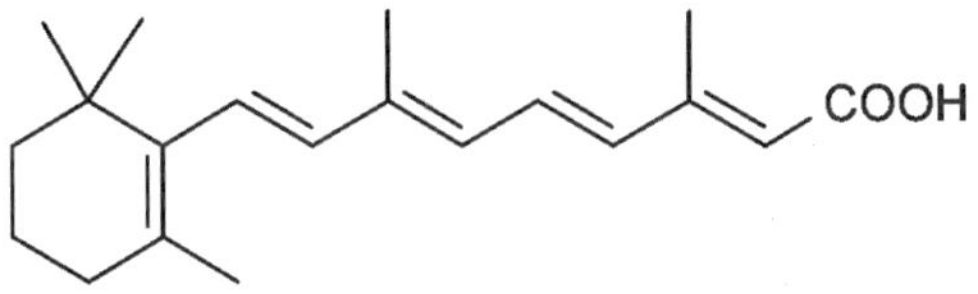

RETINOIC ACID

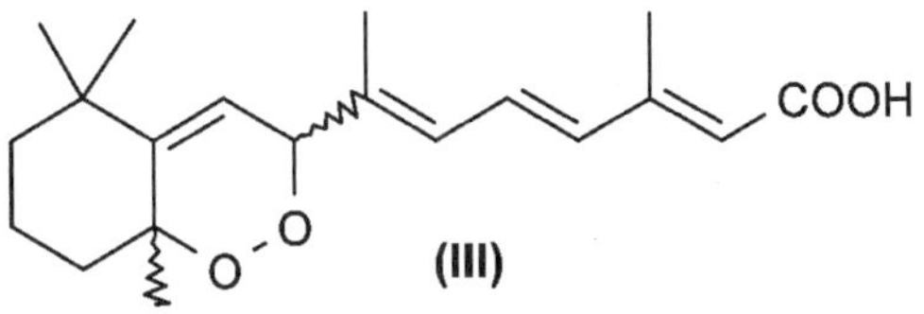

(III)

Figure 3 Retinoic acid and its cyclic peroxide supporting a spontaneous oxidation of the parent compound.

The dramatic change of selectivity at high temperature and high oxygen pressures once again imposes caution in the use of such conditions for accelerating processes that normally require milder conditions.

Retinoic acid can be oxidized by molecular oxygen without the need for radical initiators (27). The key evidence was the isolation of products like (III) that cannot be accounted for the mechanism outlined in Section I.A (Fig. 3).

II. PRACTICAL TESTS

A. Radical Chain Initiators

The aim of oxygen susceptibility studies is to accelerate "natural" oxidation so that its selectivity is maintained. Here "natural" means "occurring under the normal conditions of storage under catalysis of common impurities". Three specific goals can be identified:

1. To discover degradation mechanisms, in order to prevent degradation
2. To produce all the oxidative impurities that may be formed in accelerated and long-term degradation (qualitative prediction)
3. To predict whether the substance is particularly sensitive to oxidation or not (semiquantitative prediction)

Initiators of "spontaneous" oxidation are compounds normally occurring only at trace levels. Thus, a substance will noticeably degrade by radical oxidation only if each radical produced in reaction (2) leads to the oxidation of several molecules of the substrate through the propagation reactions (3) and (4), in other words, if the chain length is more than one. This means that

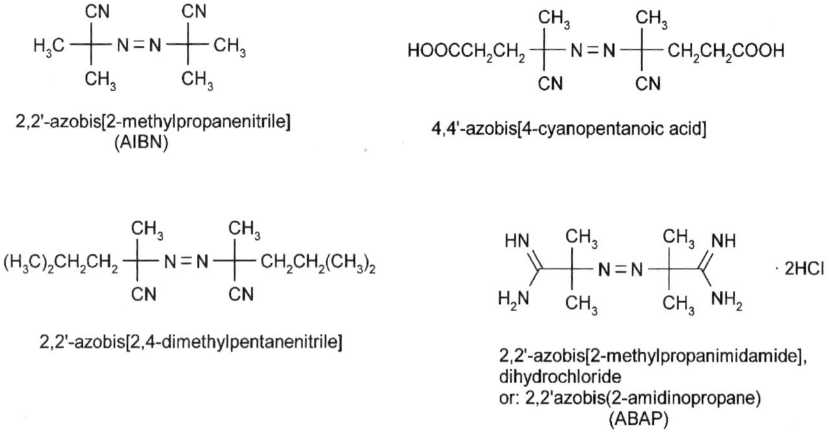

$$H_3C-C(CN)(CH_3)-N=N-C(CN)(CH_3)-CH_3$$

2,2'-azobis[2-methylpropanenitrile]
(AIBN)

$$HOOCCH_2CH_2-C(CH_3)(CN)-N=N-C(CH_3)(CN)-CH_2CH_2COOH$$

4,4'-azobis[4-cyanopentanoic acid]

$$(H_3C)_2CH_2CH_2-C(CH_3)(CN)-N=N-C(CH_3)(CN)-CH_2CH_2(CH_3)_2$$

2,2'-azobis[2,4-dimethylpentanenitrile]

$$(HN=)(H_2N)C-C(CH_3)_2-N=N-C(CH_3)_2-C(=NH)(NH_2) \cdot 2HCl$$

2,2'-azobis[2-methylpropanimidamide], dihydrochloride
or: 2,2'azobis(2-amidinopropane)
(ABAP)

Figure 4 Azocompounds used in oxidative stress testing.

most of the substrate molecules are oxidized by the peroxy radical $ROO^\bullet$ through reaction (3).

The best way to accelerate the oxidation while maintaining "natural" reactivity and selectivity is thus to catalyze the reaction by means of $ROO^\bullet$ radicals formed at a controlled rate, or by means of species with the same behavior. Azocompounds, including the very popular azobisisobutyronitrile (AIBN), are well-known organic reagents having the required properties (Fig. 4).

The thermal decomposition of AIBN yields peroxy radicals according to the following reactions:

$$R-N=N-R \rightarrow 2R^\bullet + N_2 \tag{15}$$

$$R^\bullet + O_2 \rightarrow ROO^\bullet \tag{16}$$

As preliminary examples, AIBN was reported to give a 48 hr degradation of tetrazepam very similar to that obtained in 6 months accelerated degradation of tablets (28). Similarly, the water-soluble initiator 2,2′-azobis (2-amidinopropane) dihydrochloride was shown to accelerate the natural degradation of thymidine. In contrast, systems producing the more reactive hydroxy radicals (e.g., Fenton conditions) give mainly "nonnatural" degradation products (29).

Practical example: degradation of tetrazepam. A fresh AIBN solution was prepared, containing 5.7 mg (0.035 mmol) of AIBN per mL of acetonitrile. Tetrazepam (50 mg, 0.17 mmol) was dissolved in 5 mL of the AIBN solution. The solution was placed in a 25-mL Pyrex vial with a screw cap. Two blank vials were prepared, one containing an acetonitrile solution of tetrazepam and the other initiator solution. Vials were stored at 40°C in the dark. After 48 hr, the solutions were analyzed by HPLC, using a C-18 column and a 1:1 mixture of acetonitrile: 0.1 M potassium dihydrogen phosphate as mobile phase.

The initiator blank and a tetrazepam blank were analyzed in order to detect peaks due to the reagent and its degradation products or to a spontaneous degradation of tetrazepam, respectively.

The degradation profile of tetrazepam is shown in Figure 5.

Let us discuss the experimental conditions in detail. The solution was not saturated with oxygen, as only a head-space of air is left over the solution. As Eq. (9) shows, oxygen partial pressure should not influence the oxidation rate, as it is only necessary to provide the stoichiometric quantity of oxygen.

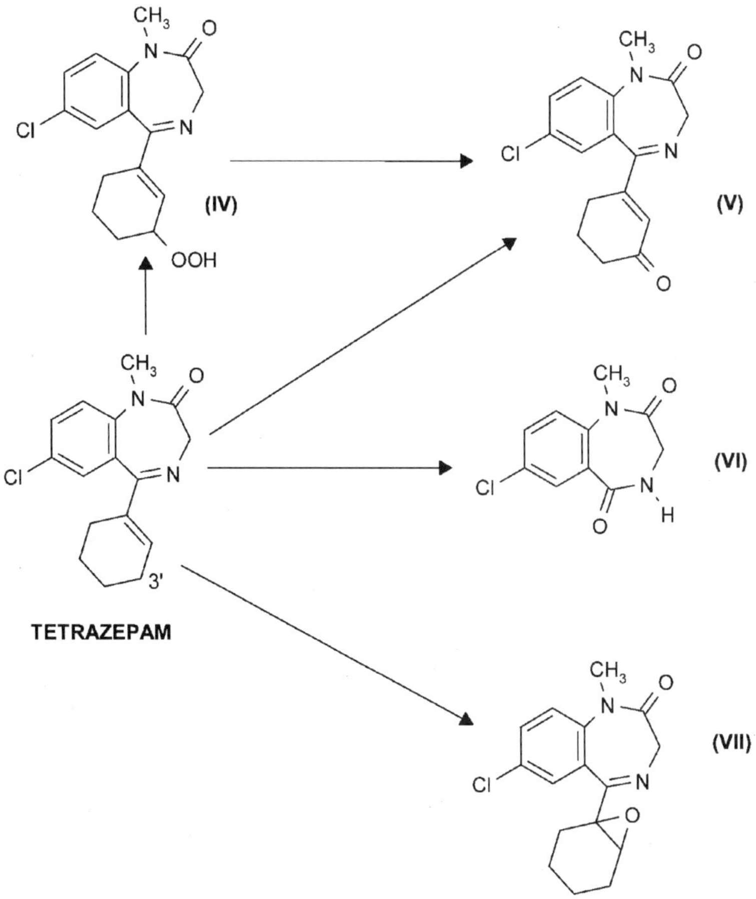

Figure 5 Degradation scheme of tetrazepam (28,30).

Though AIBN is normally used in organic synthesis at temperatures between 60°C and 80°C, tetrazepam oxidation was done at a considerably lower temperature, 40°C. There are two reasons. First, the oxidation conditions should simulate long-term, room temperature degradation and allow the isolation of labile degradation products such as hydroperoxides, which would be destroyed at higher temperatures. According to Burton and Ingold (31a,b), even antioxidants can become prooxidants at a temperature significantly higher than that at which we want to predict the behavior of our system.

The second reason is closely related to the time scale of the experiment. This merits some kinetic considerations. Arrhenius activation energy of the homolytic decomposition of AIBN in toluene is 143 kJ mol^{-1} and $\log A$ is 17.33 (32). The Arrhenius parameters are not very sensitive to the solvent (33). Not all radicals produced by AIBN decomposition yield $ROO^{\bullet}$ radicals, because of reaction (17)

$$2R^{\bullet} \rightarrow R_2 \qquad (17)$$

This side reaction also operates in the presence of oxygen, because $R^{\bullet}$ radicals can recombine before escaping the solvent cage (cage effect). The efficiency of radical production is given by the ratio between the rate of production and the theoretical value in the absence of reaction (17) and ranges between 0.43 and 0.73 in different solvents (34). Here we shall take the mean efficiency as 0.5. Using the Arrhenius data, an efficiency of 0.5 and a first-order degradation equation we can calculate the percent decomposition of the initiator and the amount of peroxy radicals generated at any time and any temperature. Assuming AIBN equimolar with the substrate, after 48 hr at 40°C the initiator will have generated 5 mol of radical per 100 mol of substrate. Thus, a very reactive test compound with a chain length more than one should be decomposed more than 5% under these conditions. The author's experience agrees with this figure: compounds showing a few percent degradation present low oxygen susceptibility, while degradations of more than 10% were normally associated with sensitive compounds. Of course, these figures are only very approximate, because there is no single "true" degradation rate of a drug molecule, as the rate is influenced by the pharmaceutical form, the manufacturing process, the packaging, and even by storage conditions. In any case, for most compounds the degradation after 48 hr should be less than 20–30%, which is the maximum amount of degradation normally desired in a stress test.

The half-life of AIBN at 40°C, calculated in the same way, is about 28 days. This means that for preparative purposes, where we have already identified the impurities to be isolated, AIBN-catalyzed oxidation at 40°C can last several days (assuming that the dissolved oxygen supply is not depleted). Shorter times at higher temperatures can also be used for preparative purposes.

The example described above used acetonitrile, which is an excellent solvent for radical oxidation because it is inert toward radicals and peroxides. Degradation of tetrazepam in acetonitrile was not affected by the presence of 20% water. As a first approximation this is not surprising, because a radical process should not be strongly influenced by the polarity of the solvent. However, this result cannot be assumed as an absolute rule, for at least two reasons. First of all, the hydrogen abstraction passes through a partially polarized transition state, as reported in Section I.A. Thus, solvents of very different polarities may give different propagation rates, although these differences should not be as important as in the case of true ionic reactions. Strong solvent effects have been described in the autoxidation of simple amines (35). The second reason is that the development of the early oxidation product yields carbocations, and these secondary processes are presumably strongly affected by the polarity of the solvent. However, in common examples the polarity of the solvent, within a reasonable range, should only quantitatively affect the degradation profile and, if we are only interested in qualitative results, we can simply adjust the solvent polarity in order to ensure a satisfactory solubility of the drug molecule we are stressing.

Alcohols have also been tested as solvents for tetrazepam degradation (30). The hydrogen atoms on the carbon atom bearing the oxy group of an alcohol can be removed by a homolysis. They can then compete with the substrate for propagation. In fact, taking the example of 2-propanol, the following reaction competes both with propagation and with termination for the common intermediate ROO$^{\bullet}$:

$$ROO^{\bullet} + (CH_3)_2CH\text{-}OH \longrightarrow ROOH + (CH_3)_2C^{\bullet}\text{-}OH \tag{18}$$

Competition of the solvent with propagation reaction sustained by the substrate slows the rate of oxidation, while competition with termination decreases the products of the Russel rearrangement and supports hydroperoxide accumulation. Depending on the covalent bond energies, competition should be in the order methanol < ethanol < 2-propanol. The oxidation rate of tetrazepam does in fact decrease in this order. But the most interesting result concerns the product distribution. In acetonitrile, the carbonyl compound (V) was the main product (11.2% of the starting tetrazepam), the hydroperoxide impurity (IV) being slightly less (9.6%). In 2-propanol only traces (0.3%) of (V) were found and the hydroperoxide (IV) amounted to 4.3% of the starting material. These results were expected. But the most surprising outcome is the rise in the impurity (VI) switching the solvent from acetonitrile to 2-propanol, where (VI) and (VI) are equally present. In mechanistic terms, this can be explained as follows (see Fig. 6). The removal of a hydrogen from carbon 3′ leads to a radical that can be attacked by oxygen at carbons 1′ or 3′. The oxygen attack is very rapid and not

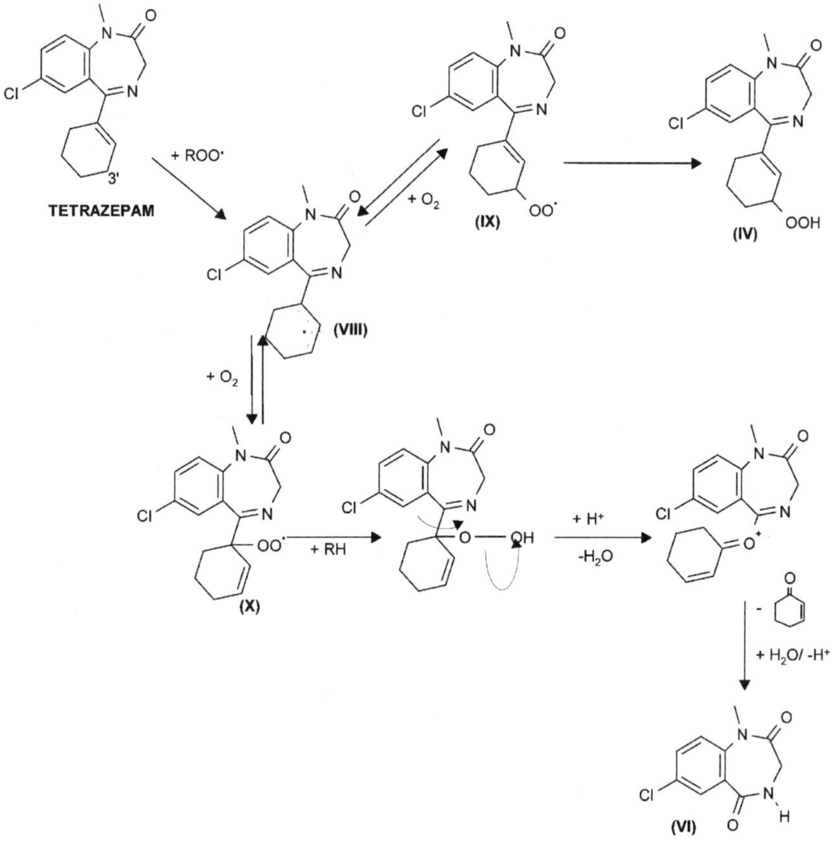

Figure 6 Proposed mechanism for the origin of the impurity (VI) of tetrazepam.

selective; nevertheless, we can assume that it is reversible because the carbon-centered radical is stabilized by conjugation with the benzodiazepine moiety. The 3′ peroxy radical is more stable than the 1′ one because of the same conjugation effect, and this isomer is favored if 1′ and 3′ peroxy radicals have the time to equilibrate, as is the case with acetonitrile solutions. By quenching ROO$^\bullet$, the hydrogen-donor 2-propanol stops the propagation of the chain and yields 1′- and 3′- hydroperoxide in a 1:1 ratio; the 1″ hydroperoxide can evolve to the impurity (VI) through a cumene hydroperoxide-like rearrangement. This rearrangement may take place in the reaction mixture or after dilution with the aqueous buffer before HPLC injection.

This example illustrates the importance of the solvent effect not only to increase the yields of some impurities for preparative purposes, but also to elucidate the mechanism of the overall degradation. It is worth noting that AIBN is toxic and can explode by heating. In general, safety informations must be read before the use of azocompounds.

Azocompounds other than AIBN can be used: 4,4′-azobis[4-cyanopentanoic acid] gives similar results and its degradation products can be separated from the reaction mixtures by simple extraction more easily than with AIBN.

According to the published Arrhenius data (32) 2,2′-azobis[2,4-dimethylpentanenitrile] at 25°C should give the same timescale as AIBN at 40°C. This could be useful for the isolation of unstable impurities, but the author has no experience with this initiator.

Autoxidation of thymidine has been elucidated by means of 2,2′-azobis[2-amidinopropane] dihydrochloride (29) (ABAP); this initiator can be employed in water solutions.

When drug degradation is monitored by HPLC with UV detection at more than 230 nm, the advantage of all these cited initiators is the UV transparency. At lower wavelengths or with nonspecific detection, the initiator and its degradation products can generate peaks in the chromatogram. It is therefore essential to run a blank containing only the initiator in parallel to the test solution. In the case of AIBN, tetramethylsuccinonitrile, the recombination product of the $R^{\bullet}$ radicals, is the most important byproduct; 3,3′,4,4′-tetramethylsuccinimidine was isolated from the oxidation with ABAP (29).

The reactive intermediates of the initiator can also give adducts with the substrate, though in my own experience this is not frequent (36).

In stress tests on a new substance, a chromatographic peak can be suspected to be due to a hydroperoxide, for instance because of a UV spectrum very similar to that of the parent compound. Isolation of hydroperoxide impurities can be difficult, because of their instability. However, it is very easy to confirm the presence of the hydroperoxide just by quenching the test solution with a reducing agent such as potassium iodide or methionine: the peak corresponding to the hydroperoxide will disappear and a peak due to the hydroxy derivative will appear or increase. Triphenylphosphine can also be employed as reducing agent, but it is very toxic. At this point, to isolate the hydroperoxide, the chemist should use the best combination of the solvent effect (e.g., 2-propanol) and mild reaction and isolation conditions. For characterization, it is worth reporting that in ^1H NMR the protons on the α-carbon atom of ROOH show a 0.3 ppm downfield shift compared with that in the corresponding alcohol (37).

Hydrogen peroxide is one of the products of autoxidation. It can be easily detected by TLC on silica gel using a mixture of acetic acid, chloroform, and methanol (10:10:1) as eluent and potassium iodide or more sophisticated reagents as the development reagent (38,39).

More suggestions and experimental details can be found in papers on the autoxidation of simvastatin (40), econazole, and miconazole nitrate (41).

In preparative work, oxidation initiated by azocompounds is convenient for isolating the main degradation products but can be difficult for the generation of significant quantities of the minor impurities. In this case, it is better to use stress test conditions that are less predictive of "natural" degradation but more selective for the synthesis of some classes of degradation products.

B. Hydrogen Peroxide and Peroxyacids

Oxidation with hydrogen peroxide is very popular in pharmaceutical development as a test for "oxidative conditions" (42). The most common reactions with organic compounds are electrophilic attack on amines and sulfides to give N-oxides and sulfoxides or sulfones, respectively, and the slower attack on carbon–carbon double bonds to give epoxides. These reaction are ionic and do not involve radicals:

$$>N: \quad H{-}O{-}O{-}H \longrightarrow >N^{+}{-}O^{-} + H_2O \qquad (19)$$

The test with hydrogen peroxide often gives degradation impurities that may arise in long-term degradation as minor impurities. This is not surprising, taking into account that hydrogen peroxide and organic hydroperoxides are among the autoxidation products. However, in some cases, the agreement between radical oxidation and H_2O_2 oxidation is a matter of chance, as in the case of the epoxidation of carbon–carbon double bonds, which has a different mechanism in the two cases. The susceptibility of electrophilic moieties to oxidation can be overestimated if the reaction with hydrogen peroxide is compared with the real stability of the drug substance. For example, amines may react quantitatively under mild conditions with hydrogen peroxide to give the N-oxide, whereas they are quite stable toward radical oxidation and their N-oxide is only a minor impurity. The reason is the different mechanism of the two processes. Nevertheless, the H_2O_2 test should always be performed in parallel to the test with radical initiator, as it gives complementary information and yields minor impurities with very clean reactions.

As an example, tetrazepam epoxide (VII) was obtained in high yields with H_2O_2 (28). The proposed experimental conditions are water, acetonitrile, or methanol as solvent, a temperature of not more that 40°C and a duration of 2–7 days. The concentration of H_2O_2 can be 0.3–3%.

Peracetic acid can produce the same degradation profile in a shorter time. The following procedure can be followed. Add 2–10 μL of peracetic acid to the solution of the drug (about 0.2 mg/mL) in dichloromethane or in the HPLC mobile phase. Wait up to 1 hr at room temperature and inject (S. Baertschi, personal communication, 1998). Caution: peracetic acid is toxic and explosive.

A totally different oxidation system is that of the Fenton reagent and analogues. In these reagents, hydrogen peroxide or organic peroxides are the oxidants, which are activated by metal ion catalysis. Fenton reagents are mixtures of iron (II) salts and either one hydrogen peroxide or an organic peroxide. The mechanism of the oxidation by these reagents is controversial (43), but the simplest proposed mechanism is as follows. Fe(II) decomposes H_2O_2 in a catalytic cycle:

$$Fe(II) + H_2O_2 \rightarrow Fe(III)OH + HO^{\bullet} \tag{20}$$

$$Fe(III)OH + H_2O_2 \rightarrow Fe(II) + HO_2^{\bullet} + H_2O \tag{21}$$

Fenton mixtures react with a radical mechanism, but the radical produced under Fenton conditions ($HO^{\bullet}$) is much more reactive than the "natural" oxidant $ROO^{\bullet}$. Even normally inert substances such as cyclohexane can be oxidized under these conditions and therefore the oxidative products formed using Fenton reagents may deviate significantly from the autoxidation profile (29). Equation (21) shows how the metal is regenerated in the catalytic cycle; this is the reason why traces of heavy metal ions combined with the presence of peroxides can have a detrimental effect on sensitive substances. But it is worth pointing out that in the case of initiation by traces of metal ions and peroxides, the extent of oxidation is detrimental for the stability of the substrate only if it is supported by a long radical chain; now, a long chain is propagated by the $ROO^{\bullet}$ radicals coming from the substrate, so the expected products are those of the usual autoxidation. With Fenton reagents, however, a high concentration of $HO^{\bullet}$ radicals are produced, and the oxidation is supported by this less selective radical. In conclusion, Fenton systems have too poor selectivity to belong to the first-line battery of tests for oxidation-susceptibility of drugs.

At least two systems can be cited as catalysts of peroxide oxidation: the first are the iron (III) porphyrins (44) and the second are the Gif reagents (45,46), based on iron salt catalysis in a pyridine/acetic acid solvent with peroxide reagents and other oxidants. The author's opinion is that more than systems for stress testing these are tools useful for the synthesis of impurities, especially epoxides. From another point of view, they are often considered as potential biomimetic systems, predicting drug metabolism. Metabolites are sometimes also degradation impurities, but this is not a general rule, because enzymes and free radicals have different reactivity; an example is the metabolic synthesis of arene oxides that never can be obtained by radical oxidation.

C. Heavy Metal Salts

We have already discussed the importance of heavy metal salts as autoxidation catalysts. Their mechanism of action may involve several pathways.

Metals can (a) directly oxidize the substrate trough a radical or ionic mechanism; (b) activate molecular oxygen by complexation; (c) decompose peroxides, as discussed in the previous section. A review of these mechanisms is beyond the scope of the present book and can be found in the literature (10). An interesting example of the effect of heavy metal salts on the stability of drugs is the oxidation of hydrocortisone, which was catalyzed by copper (II) ions at a concentration as low as 3×10^{-3} M (47).

Contamination of pharmaceutical substances and dosage forms by heavy metals is nowadays very low, and this reduces our interest in challenging the stability of candidate drugs with heavy metal ions. Nevertheless, these tests are still interesting and the author personally recommends their use in first-line screening for oxygen susceptibility for the following reason. Compounds with active methylene groups or electron-rich groups can be easily oxidized by heavy metal ions and are often directly oxidized by dioxygen. A simple test with heavy metals can prove the sensitivity to oxidation and predict the need for more demanding investigation of the mechanisms of direct oxidation.

Under mild conditions, heavy metals such as iron (III) and copper (II) are discriminating agents, because they attack organic compounds with a mechanism different from that depicted in Eqs. (2)–(5), so that substances oxidized only by that mechanism are normally inert. The word "normally" is dictated by the complexity of the processes.

Example: test with copper (II) and iron (III) salts and acetyl acetonates (48a,b). Four stock solutions were prepared in acetonitrile containing $Fe(NO_3)_3 \cdot 9H_2O$, $CuBr_2$, $Fe(acac)_3$ and $Cu(acac)_2$, respectively. Test solutions contained phenylbutazone or selegiline hydrochloride (about 10^{-2} M) in acetonitrile and the appropriate amount of the heavy metal ion or complex. For each drug substance and each metal species, three solutions were prepared, at 10, 100, 1000 ppm (mol/mol drug substance) of metal ion; 20 mL of each test solution was placed in a 150 mL flask at 40°C. A blank solution containing only the tested active substance was stored under the same conditions. Solutions were analyzed at 24, 48, and 72 hr.

Some comments about the choice of the conditions: The use of acetonitrile as solvent and the selected temperature have been already discussed. Iron (III) and copper (II) were selected for a couple of reasons. First of all, they are ubiquitous ions and typical autoxidation catalysts. Iron (III) is a hard acid and copper (II) a borderline acid according to the HSAB classification, so it is reasonable to expect they will react differently, with a different complexing power. Manganese (II) has also been proposed as a widespread catalyst of autoxidation (49).

Compared to salts, acetyl acetonates offer better solubility in organic solvents and better stability to hydrolysis. They are likely to be less reactive than salts, because complexes of either iron or copper in their highest oxidation state with acetyl acetone are more stabile than at the lower oxidation state.

Table 1 Percent Degradation of Phenylbutazone in the Presence of Heavy Metal Salts and Complexes (48a,b)

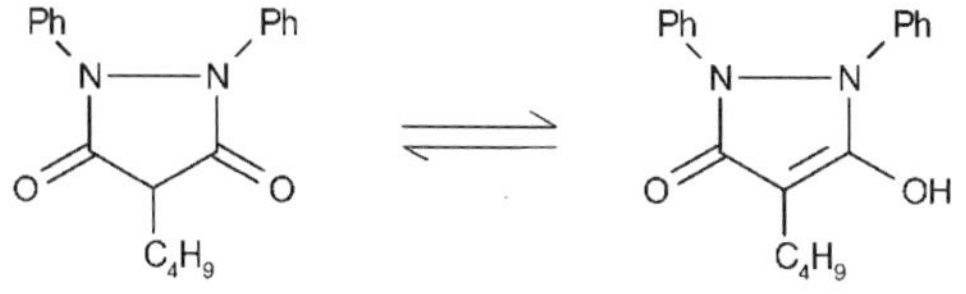

Catalyst	24 hr	48 hr	72 hr
$Fe(NO_3)_3 \cdot 9H_2O$	3.8	4.1	4.5
$Fe(acac)_3$	1.0	3.6	5.6
$CuBr_2$	82.7	90.8	95.5
$Cu(acac)_2$	72.1	82.2	92.7

Table 1 (48a,b) shows the 24 hr results of the test described above on phenylbutazone. Copper degraded phenylbutazone both as a salt and as acetyl acetonate. Iron was less aggressive, and the free salt was stronger than the complex. The degradation products were 4-hydroxy- and 4-hydroperoxy-phenylbutazone, the known oxidation impurities. The susceptibility of phenylbutazone to metal oxidation can be attributed to activation of the hydrogen on C-4 by the adjacent carbonyls. Selegiline hydrochloride, a stable compound, was not oxidized under the same conditions. This confirms the discriminating power of the experimental conditions.

D. Singlet Oxygen

Singlet oxygen is normally produced by a photochemical reaction in the presence of a sensitizer like rose bengal or methylene blue ("dye-sensitized" oxidation), although it can also arise from thermal reactions. Singlet oxygen is not the oxygen state, which is active in autoxidation, and it normally gives different degradation products from the triplet ground state. A well-known reaction of singlet oxygen is the oxidation of carbon–carbon double bonds to give hydroperoxides. The mechanism of this reaction (1b), also known as the "ene" reaction, involves a cyclic six-membered transition state:

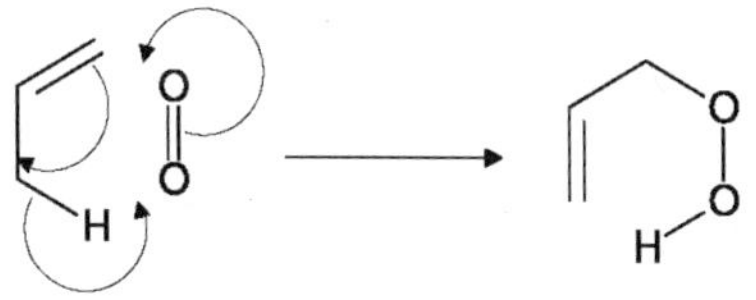

(22)

The result of the concerted process is a well-defined regiochemistry, which results from the shift of the double bond to the adjacent position.

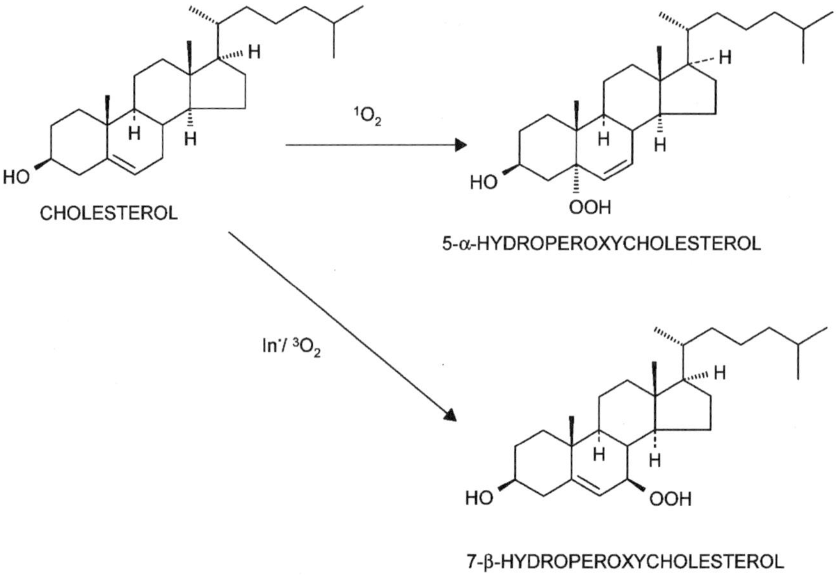

CHOLESTEROL

$^1O_2$

5-α-HYDROPEROXYCHOLESTEROL

$In^{\cdot}/\,^3O_2$

7-β-HYDROPEROXYCHOLESTEROL

Figure 7 Oxidation of cholesterol: regiochemistry of the oxidation with singlet oxygen and of autoxidation (50).

However, generally the radical oxidation by triplet oxygen leads to two regioisomers, unless specific factors stronger stabilize one of the two hydroperoxides:

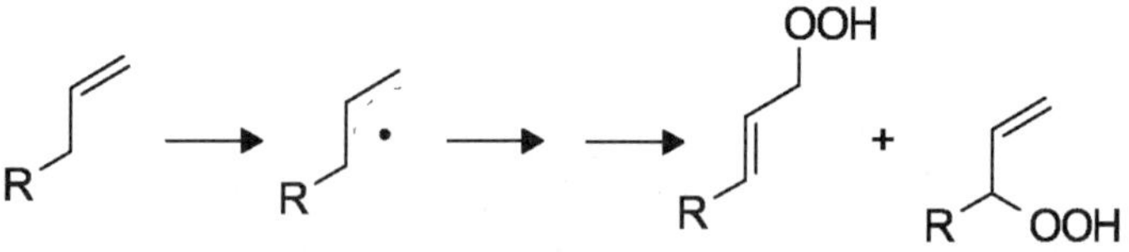

R → R → → R (OOH) + R OOH (23)

Figure 7 shows the early oxidation products of cholesterol with singlet and triplet oxygen (50). Triplet oxygen gives the 7-β hydroperoxide and small amounts of the 7-α isomer. The intermediate radical could also yield the 5-isomer, but this process is not favored because the 7-β one is more stable. Singlet oxygen gives only the 5-α hydroperoxide, because this is the only product consistent with the concerted oxidation. The hydroperoxides can then evolve to stable products.

N-Formylkynurenine is one of the 16 autoxidation products of tryptophan (51) (Fig. 8). The dye-sensitized photo-oxygenation of tryptophan in sodium carbonate - acetic acid buffer (pH 7) gave *N*-formylkynurenine as the major product (52). This is also the oxidation product of tryptophan with hydrogen peroxide (53) and with ozone (54). This is an interesting case: the same degradation impurity can be obtained in different ways, probably

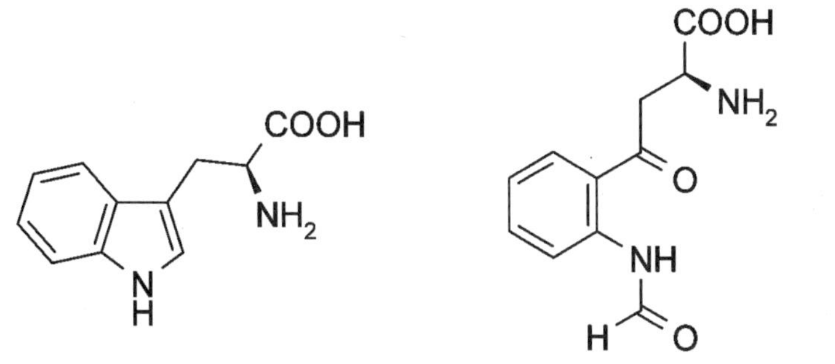

L-TRYPTOPHAN N-FORMYLKYNURENINE

Figure 8 L-Tryptophan and its oxidation product *N*-formylkynurenine.

by different mechanisms, but the "less natural" singlet oxygen condition gives an impurity with better selectivity, thereby making isolation easier. Singlet oxygen should thus be considered as an arrow in our quiver for isolation of the impurities observed in the radical-initiator test. It is important to bear in mind that degradation profiles may differ with changes in pH (52).

Procedure for dye-sensitized (singlet oxygen) oxidation (S. Baertschi, personal communication, 1999): Prepare a solution containing about 1 mg/mL of the test substance and 0.1 mg/mL of rose bengal. The solvent is preferably acetonitrile or water, or a mixture of the two. Put 10 mL of the test solution in four 20 mL scintillation vials saturated with oxygen and close with plastic caps. Place the first three vials under visible light (e.g., cool-white fluorescent or xenon long arc, intensity of 10,000–20,000 lx) for 15, 30, and 60 min, respectively. Keep the fourth vial in the dark as control. Examine a blank solution of rose bengal exposed to xenon light.

III. OXIDATION OF THE MOST COMMON ORGANIC FUNCTIONAL GROUPS

The degradation pathways of some organic molecules of pharmaceutical interest help illustrate the oxidative behavior of selected organic functional groups. This is not an exhaustive review, but only shows some significant examples.

A very important reaction is the oxidative attack on methylene $X{-}CH_2{-}$ activated by a group X (or on the corresponding methyne X–CH–). X may be any group able to stabilize the X–CH•– radical by resonance: a carbon–carbon double bond, an aromatic ring, a heteroatom possessing electron lone pairs, such as oxygen (ethers or alcohols), sulphur, nitrogen (amines), or a carbonyl group. The most common products are the hydroperoxide, the alcohol, and the ketone:

$$X - CH_2 - + O_2 \rightarrow X\text{–}CHOOH - + X\text{–}CHOH - + X\text{–}C = O- \qquad (24)$$

The degradation pattern of alkenes has been amply illustrated, particularly for tetrazepam and cholesterol. In addition to the activation of the α-sp^3 carbon atom, alkenes can give epoxidation and polymerization (40,55).

Aldehydes are very sensitive to oxidation, due to the stable carbonyl radical shown in Eq. (25):

$$R{-}CHO + In^{\bullet} \rightarrow RC^{\bullet}{=}O + InH \qquad (25)$$

$$RC^{\bullet}{=}O + O_2 \rightarrow RC(O)OO^{\bullet} \qquad (26)$$

Oxidation of aldehydes leads to peracids that are often involved in cooxidations and are finally transformed to the more stable carboxylic acids.

The amino group frequently occurs in drug substances. Figure 9 shows the main reaction pathways. Hydrogen removal in α to the nitrogen atom is promoted by radical initiators and is probably the most important initiation of oxidation. The driving force of stabilization of the N–CH$^{\bullet}$ radical is the interaction between the lone pair of the nitrogen atom and the orbital bearing the unpaired electron. For this reason, the protonated amine is normally stable to oxidation.

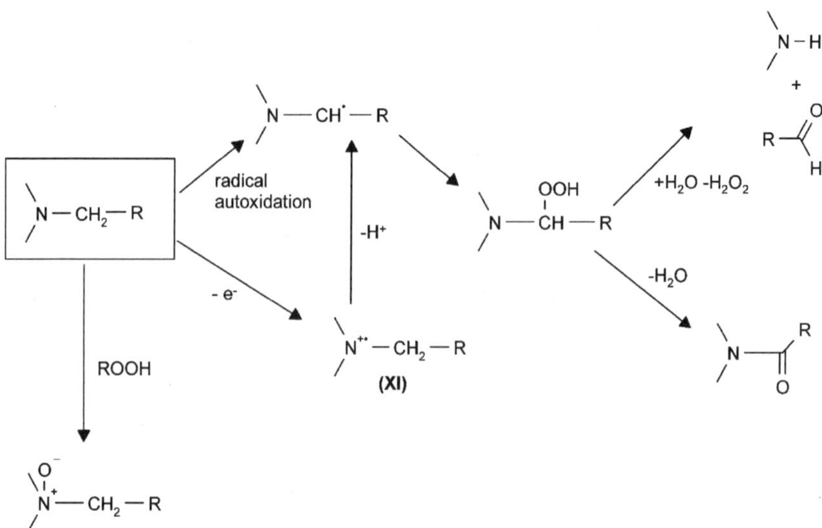

Figure 9 Oxidation pathways of amines.

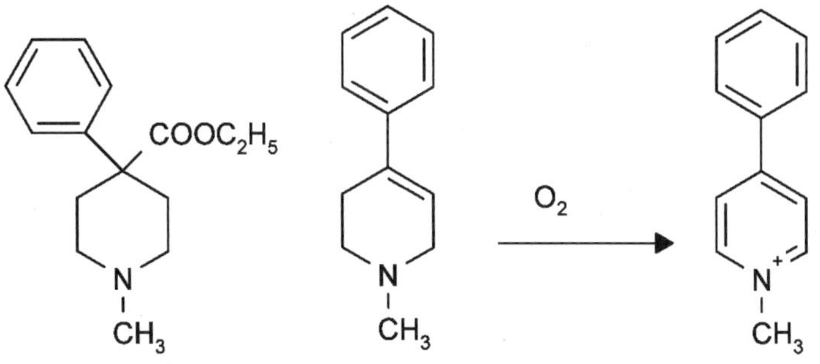

Figure 10 Meperidine, its impurity and its degradation product (57).

"Spontaneous" oxidation of amines by one-electron transfer has been reported as a key process in polar solvents (35). It is not easy to distinguish the spontaneous and initiated mechanisms, because these pathways have a common intermediate (XI, Fig. 9). Thus, potassium hexacyanoferrate (III), a one-electron oxidant, gives electron transfer oxidation of amines (56) yielding the classical radical autoxidation products.

N-oxides are always present as cooxidation impurities in tertiary amine oxidation, due to the accumulation of hydrogen peroxide during autoxidation.

Autoxidation of an impurity of meperidine (XII) leads to the aromatization product (XIII) (57) (Fig. 10). Some time ago, this was the major feature in an important criminal case, because this impurity, found in a drug manufactured illicitly, produced a severe parkinsonian syndrome in men. The tetrahydropyridine ring, not uncommon in pharmaceuticals, easily gives aromatization. In fact, the allylic methylene group adjacent to the nitrogen atom is activated and two dihydropyridine molecules formed by this oxidation may disproportionate to the finally aromatized product and to the starting material (57).

Indoles are very important in medicinal chemistry. The indole moiety is electron-rich so it is very easily oxidized. One example of severe cleavage of the indole ring is the oxidation of tryptophan to *N*-formylkynurenine. An example of milder oxidation of indoles is reserpine degradation. Reserpine, an indole alkaloid, spontaneously decomposes in chloroform solution to give oxygenated products (58) (Fig. 11). Reserpine 7-hydroperoxide (XIV) was isolated in the reaction mixture; this is the key intermediate in the oxidative pathways of many indoles (59).

Autoxidation of 9-hydroxyellypticine (60) is a good example of degradation of phenols, showing the formation of a quinone-imine (XV) and an oxidative dimer (XVI, Fig. 12). Phenols can be quite stable in the protonated

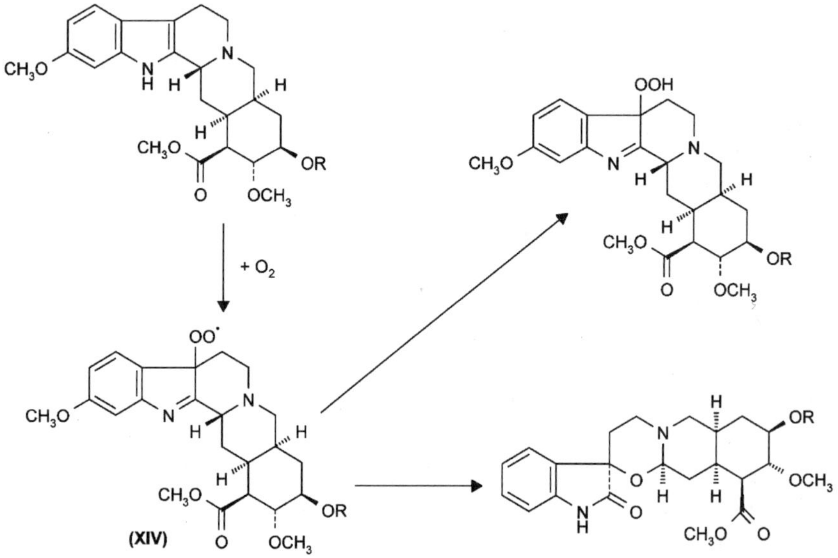

Figure 11 Reserpine autoxidation, where R = 3,4,5-trimethoxybenzoyl (59).

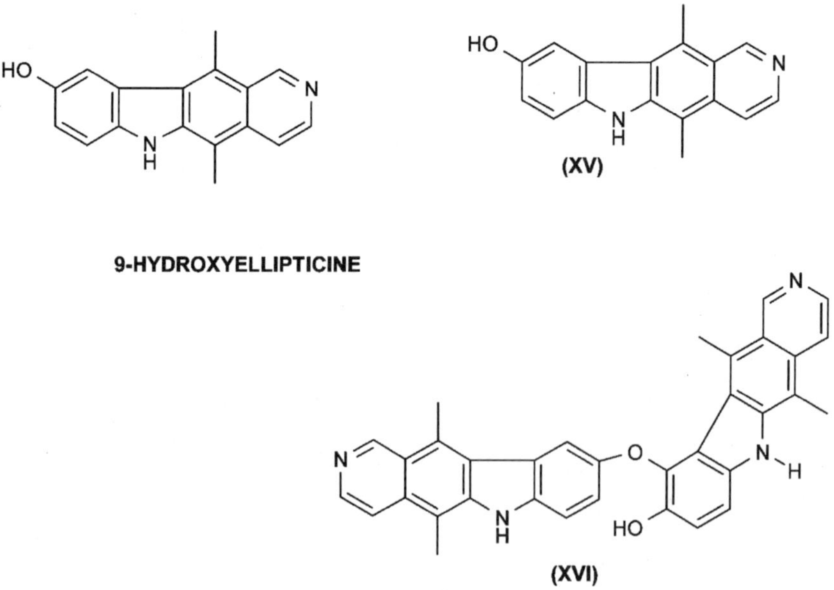

9-HYDROXYELLIPTICINE

(XV)

(XVI)

Figure 12 9-Hydroxy-ellipticine and its autoxidation products (60).

form, but are easily oxidized in the base-conjugated form. Oxidative dimers of phenols can be obtained from reaction with potassium hexacyanoferrate (III), a typical monoelectron oxidant.

Captopril degradation is a good example of oxidation of thiols, a reaction very common in protein chemistry (61).

IV. STRATEGY OF OXIDATIVE SUSCEPTIBILITY TESTING

The first step of the design of stress experiments should be to examine the molecular formula of the test compound. Does the structure resemble substances for which a degradation pattern is already known? Does it contain easy oxidizable functional groups? Do tautomers exist, that can be more sensitive to oxidants? Can pH affect the sensitivity, because prototropic equilibria can generate easily oxidizable species? Are potential degradation impurities available? Time spent in answering these questions and in collecting literature data is never lost.

The first tier of experimental tests consists in my opinion of AIBN (or other azocompounds), hydrogen peroxide, and heavy metals (at least one) tests. The blank sample must always be prepared, to confirm that the oxidant is really the cause of the observed degradation. The AIBN test very often gives the full spectrum of oxidation impurities and a semiquantitative estimation of the sensitivity of the substance to oxygen. In my opinion, a drug showing a decomposition of less than 5% after 48 hr will not probably require special considerations for solid-state formulations. A drug showing 20% or more degradation is a candidate for the use of antioxidants, inert gas filling, or other formulation techniques. The free base of amines should be tested if the selected form is a protonated salt, because basic excipients can have a detrimental effect on the stability of these compounds.

Hydrogen peroxide is a good test to produce selected degradation impurities, but also has some predictive value. Sensitivity to hydrogen peroxide can predict interaction with peroxide generating excipients. Moreover, a positive result of both AIBN and hydrogen peroxide is a strong evidence that the test substance is susceptible to oxidation.

Heavy metal testing allows us to detect substances with a low redox potential. If the test compound is sensitive to a number of different oxidants or catalysts, such as hydrogen peroxide, iron (III), and copper (II), it is advisable to consider the substance as potentially very sensitive to oxidation. In this case, it is wise to consider a preformulation involving the use of antioxidants or special protecting conditions.

A second tier of tests should be designed for compounds already detected as sensitive. The goals of the second tier are the isolation of impurities and the investigation of the degradation mechanism. It is not possible to propose general protocols, as in this case the chemistry of the substance must be fully considered. In this phase we can study, by comparison with known examples and data, solvent effect, pH effect, detection of hydroperoxides, or the use of singlet oxygen or oxidants that are more selective for the structural class of interest.

Once the degradation profile is ascertained, more in-depth studies can be recommended, in order to help preformulation studies.

The more challenging study is probably the investigation on suspected spontaneous autoxidations, but this is the matter of physical chemistry research.

A quantitative expression of the oxidative susceptibility can give an idea of the degree of protection the molecule will require in formulations. Some authors proposed kinetic methods for the quantitative evaluation of the sensitivity of a molecule to hydroxy and peroxy radicals (62).

Another challenging aspect is the dependence of the degradation pattern and rate on the solvent and on the protonation ratio. Degradation of a sulfonamide-containing 5,6-dihydro-4-hydroxy-2-pyrone was studied in aqueous/organic mixtures and effects of the solvent polarity, of the protonation and of the ion pairing were detected (63). In this study, hydrogen peroxide and *t*-butylperoxide were found to be more useful than azoderivatives for predicting degradation impurities of the investigated drug: this strongly confirms the value of running different tests in parallel.

Other approaches to the study of oxidations in stress test can obviously be proposed (64), and once again the preformulation scientist will benefit greatly by combining good science and flexible guidelines for solving specific problems related to oxidative degradation.

ACKNOWLEDGMENTS

I am deeply indebted to Giovanni Palmisano and Andrea Bertario for many discussions, to Michel Bauer, Michel Gachon and Jean-Pierre Vergnaud for encouragement and collaboration, and to Luigi Panza for useful suggestions on the manuscript. I thank Steven Baertschi for many discussions and for examples.

REFERENCES

1a. Knopf H, Mueller E, Weickmann A. Houben-Weyl Methoden der Organischen Chemie. Vol. 4. Part 1a. Stuttgart: G. Thieme, 1981:69–168.
1b. Carey F, Sundberg RJ. Advanced Organic Chemistry. Part B. New York: Plenum Press, 1990:640.
1c. Hovorka SW, Schöneich C. Oxidative degradation of pharmaceuticals: theory, mechanism and inhibition. J Pharm Sci 90 2001 253–269.
2. Simic MG. Free radical mechanisms in autoxidation processes. J Chem Ed 1981; 58:125–131.

3. Pryor WA, Prier DG, Church DF. Detection of free radicals from low-temperature ozone–olefin reaction by ESR spin trapping: evidence that the radical precursor is a trioxide. J Am Chem Soc 1983; 105:2883–2888.
4. Hansen LD, Eatough DJ, Lewis EA, Bergstrom RG, Degraft-Johnson D, Cassidy-Thompson K. Shelf-life-prediction from induction period calorimetric measurements on materials undergoing autocatalytic decomposition. Can J Chem 1990; 68:2111–2114.
5. Maillard B. Rate constants for the reactions of free radicals with oxygen in solution. KU Ingold and JC Scaiano. J Am Chem Soc 1983; 105:5095–5099.
6. Porter NA, Wujek DG. Autoxidation of polyunsaturated fatty acids, an expanded mechanistic study. J Am Chem Soc 1984; 106:2626–2629.
7. Beckwith ALJ, O'Shea DM, Roberts DH. Novel formation of bis-allylic products by autoxidation of substituted cyclohexa-1,4-dienes. J Am Chem Soc 1986; 108:6408–6409.
8. Russel GA. The rate of oxidation of aralkyl hydrocarbons. Polar effects in free radical reactions. J Am Chem Soc 1956; 78:1047–1054.
9. Walling C. J Am Chem Soc 1969; 91:7590–7594.
10. Sheldon RA, Kochi JK. Metal-Catalyzed Oxidations of Organic Compounds. New York: Academic Press, 1981.
11. Carstensen JT. Drug Stability. New York: Marcel Dekker, 1990:83–94.
12. Scott G. Antioxidants. Chichester: Albion Publishing, 1997.
13. Russel GA. Deuterium-isotope effects in the autoxidation of arylalkyl hydrocarbons. Mechanism of peroxy radicals. J Am Chem Soc 1957; 79:3871–3877.
14. Singh SK, Suurkuusk M, Eklsater C. Kinetics of decomposition of hydroperoxides formed during the oxidation of soya phosphatidylcholine by analysis of chemiluminescence generated. Int J Pharm 1996; 142:215–225.
15. Vreugdenhil AD, Reit H. Liquid-phase co-oxidation of aldehydes and olefins—radical versus non-radical epoxidation. Rec Trav Chim 1972; 91:237–245.
16. Freyaldenhoven MA, Lehman PA, Franz TJ, Lloyd RV, Samokyszyn VM. Retinoic acid-dependent stimulation of 2,2′-azobis(2-amidinopropane)-initiated autoxidation of linoleic acid in sodium dodecyl sulfate micelles: a novel pro-oxidant effect of retinoic acid. Chem Res Toxicol 1998; 11:102–110.
17. Stark MS. J Phys Chem 1997; 101:8296–8301.
18. Correa PE, Hardy G, Riley DP. Selective autoxidation of electron-rich substrates under elevated oxygen pressures. J Org Chem 1988; 53:1695–1702.
19. Clinton NA, Kenley RA, Traylor TG. Aldehyde autoxidative carbon dioxide evolution. J Am Chem Soc 1975; 97:3752–3757.
20. Turner JO. The acid-catalyzed decomposition of aliphatic hydroperoxides: reactions in the presence of alcohols. Tetrahedron Lett 1971; 14:887–890.
21. Anderson GH, Smith J. Acid-catalyzed rearrangement of hydroperoxides. II. Phenylcycloalkyl hydroperoxides. Can J Chem 1968; 46:1561–1570.
22. Kornblum N, Delamare HE. The base catalyzed decomposition of a dialkyl peroxide. J Am Chem Soc 1951; 73:880–881.
23. Beaver BD, Cooney JV, Watkins JM, Jr. Autoxidation of nitrogen heterocycles. 2. Kinetic measurements of the autoxidation of 2,5-dimethylpyrrole. Heterocycles 1985; 23:2847–2851.

24. Malhotra SK, Hostynek JJ, Lundin AF. Autoxidation of enamines and Schiff bases of α,β-unsaturated ketones. A new synthesis of unsaturated 1,4-diones. J Am Chem Soc 1968; 90:6565–6566.
25. Bartlett PD, Banavali R. Spontaneous oxygenation of cyclic olefins: effects of strain. J Org Chem 1991; 56:6043–6050.
26. Seip M, Brauer H-D. Endoperoxide formation of helianthrene with triplet molecular oxygen. A spin-forbidden reaction. J Am Chem Soc 1992; 114: 4486–4490.
27. Brady Clark K, Howard JA, Oyler A. Retinoic acid oxidation at high oxygen pressure: evidence for spin-forbidden direct addition of triplet molecular oxygen. J Am Chem Soc 1997; 119:9560–9561.
28. Boccardi G, Deleuze C, Gachon M, Palmisano G, Vergnaud JP. Autoxidation of tetrazepam: prediction of degradation impurities from the oxidative behaviour in solution. J Pharm Sci 1992; 81:183–185.
29. Martini M, Termini J. Peroxy radical oxidation of thymidine. Chem Res Toxicol 1997; 10:234–241.
30. Boccardi G. Autoxidation of drugs: prediction of degradation impurities from results of reactions with radical chain initiators. Il Farmaco 1994; 49:431–435.
31(a). Burton GW, Ingold KU. Autoxidation of biological molecules. 1. The antioxidant activity of vitamin E and related chain-breaking phenolic antioxidants in vitro. J Am Chem Soc 1981; 103:6472–6477.
31(b). Burton GW, Ingold KU. β-Carotene: an unusual type of lipid antioxidant. Science 1984; 224:569–573.
32. Engel PS. Mechanism of the thermal and photochemical decomposition of azoalkanes. Chem Rev 1980; 80:99–150.
33. Lewis FM, Matheson MS. Decomposition of aliphatic azo compounds. J Am Chem Soc 1949; 71:747–748.
34. Hammond GS, Sen JN, Bozer CE. The efficiency of radical production from azo-bis-isobutyronitrile. J Am Chem Soc 1955; 77:3244–3248.
35. Beckwith ALJ, Eichinger PH, Mooney BA, Prager RH. Amine autoxidation in aqueous solution. Aust J Chem 1983; 36:719–739.
36. Goosen A, McCleland CW, Morgan DH, O'Connell JS, Ramplin A. Heptyl 2-cyanopropan-2-yl peroxides from the AIBN-initiated autoxidation of heptane. J Chem Soc Perkin Trans I 1993; 401–402.
37. Barton D, Ollis WD. Comprehensive Organic Chemistry. Vol. 1. Oxford: Pergamon Press, 1979:917.
38. Draper WM, Crosby DG. Sensitive, enzyme-catalyzed chromogenic reagent for hydrogen peroxide and other peroxygen compounds on thin-layer chromatographic plates. J Chromatogr 1981; 216:413–416.
39. Raftery DP, Smyth MR, Leonard RG, Kneafsey BJ, Brennan MC. Identification of hydrogen peroxide as the autoxidation product of N-phenyl-2-propyl-3,5-diethyl-1,2-dihydropiridine. Anal Commun 1996; 33:375–379.
40. Smith GB, DiMichele L, Colwell LF, Dezeny GC, Douglas AW, Reamer RA, Verhoeven TR. Autooxidation of simvastatin. Tetrahedron 1993; 49:4447–4462.
41. Oyler AR, Naldi RE, Facchine KL, Burinsky DJ, Cozine MH, Dunphy R, Alves-Santana JD, Cotter ML. Characterization of autoxidation products of

the antifungal compounds econazole nitrate and miconazole nitrate. Tetrahedron 1991; 47:6549–6560.
42. Aulesa C, Castillo M, Garcia S. Scientific study of the oxidation of mestranol and ethynylestradiol. Int J Pharmaceutics 1979; 11:152–157.
43. MacFaul PA, Wayner DDM, Ingold KU. A radical account of "oxygenated Fenton chemistry". Acc Chem Res 1998; 31:159–162.
44. Traylor TG, Kim C, Richards JL, Xu F, Perrin CL. Reactions of iron(III) porphyrins with oxidants. Structure-reactivity studies. J Am Chem Soc 1995; 117:3468–3474.
45. Barton DHR. On the mechanism of Gif reactions. Chem Soc Rev 1996; 25: 237–239.
46. Minisci F, Fontana F. Free radicals in oxidation processes. La Chimica e l'Industria 1998; 80:1309–1316.
47. Hansen J, Bundgaard H. Studies on the stability of corticosteroids V. The degradation pattern of hydrocortisone in aqueous solution. Int J Pharmaol 1980; 6:307–319.
48a. Bernardi G. Thesis dissertation, Università di Torino (Italy), 1996; supervisor: Belliardo F.
48b. Rossi A. Thesis dissertation, Università di Torino (Italy), 1996; supervisor: Belliardo F.
49. Villablanca M, Cilento G. Oxidation of phenylpyruvic acid. Biochim Biophys Acta 1987; 926:224–230.
50. Smith LL, Teng JI, Kulig MJ, Hill FL. Sterol metabolism. XXIII. Cholesterol oxidation by radiation-induced processes. J Org Chem 1973; 38:1763–1765.
51. Simat TJ, Steinhart. Oxidation of free tryptophan and tryptophan residues in peptides and proteins. J Agric Food Chem 1998; 46:490–498.
52. Nakagawa M, Yokoyama Y, Kato S, Hino T. Dye-sensitized photo-oxygenation of tryptophan. Tetrahedron 1985; 41:2125–2132.
53. Timat S, Meyer K, Stoever B, Steinhart H. Oxidation of free and peptide bound tryptophan. Adv Exp Med Biol 1996; 398:655–659.
54. Masuda N, Sakiyama F. Direct formation of kynureine on oxidation of tryptophan by ozone. Jpn Pept Chem 1977; 14:41–44.
55. Van Sickle DE, Mayo F, Arluck RM. Liquid-phase oxidation of cyclic alkenes. J Am Chem Soc 1965; 87:4824–4832.
56. Lindsay Smith JR, Mead LAV. Amine oxidation. Part VII. The effect of structure on the reactivity of alkyl tertiary amines toward alkaline potassium hexacyanoferrate(III). Chem Soc Perkin II 1973; 206–210.
57. Brewster ME, Kaminski JJ, Bodor N. Reactivity of biologically important reduced pyridines. 2. The oxidation of 1-methyl-4-phenyl-1,2,3,6-tetrahydropyridine. J Am Chem Soc 1988; 110:6337–6341.
58. Awang DVC, Dawson BA, Girard M, Vincent A, Ekiel I. The product of reserpine autoxidation. J Org Chem 1990; 55:4443–4448.
59. Sundberg RJ. The Chemistry of Indoles. New York: Academic Press, 1970: 282–315.
60. Auclair C, Hyland K, Paoletti C. Autoxidation of the antitumor drug 9-hydroxyellipticine and its derivatives. J Med Chem 1983; 26:1438–1444.

61. Lee TY, Notari RE. Kinetics and mechanism of captopril oxidation in aqueous solution under controlled oxygen partial pressure. Pharm Res 1987; 4: 98–103.
62. Karki SB, Treemaneekarn V, Kaufman MJ. Oxidation of HMG-CoA reductase inhibitors by tert-butoxyl and 1,1-diphenyl-2-picrylhydrazyl radicals: model compounds reactions for predicting oxidatively sensitive compounds during preformulatiom. J Pharm Sci 2000; 89:1518–1524.
63. Hovorka SW, Hageman MJ, Schöneich C. Oxidative degradation of a sulfonamide-containing 5,6-dihydro-4-hydroxy-2-pyrone in aqueous/organic cosolvent mixtures. Pharm Res 2002; 19:538–545.
64. Alsante KM, Friedmann RC, Hatajik TD, Lohr LL, Sharp TR, Snyder KD, Szczesny EJ. Degradation and impurity analysis for pharmaceutical drug candidates. In: Satinder A, Scypinski S, ed. Handbook of Modern Pharmaceutical Analysis. San Diego: Academic Press, 2001:103.

8

Comparative Stress Stability Studies for Rapid Evaluation of Manufacturing Changes or Materials from Multiple Sources

Bernard A. Olsen
Eli Lilly and Company, Lilly Research Laboratories, Lafayette, Indiana, U.S.A.

Larry A. Larew
Eli Lilly and Company, Lilly Research Laboratories, Lilly Corporate Center, Indianapolis, Indiana, U.S.A.

I. INTRODUCTION

"Frequently, time is of the essence. It is necessary to evalulate, in a short time span, the stability of a product change, and here, the design of stress conditions which will accelerate decomposition in a meaningful way is necessary. This is a difficult task and one very particular to the stability scientist."

—J. T. Carstensen (1).

Understanding the stability characteristics of drug substances and drug products is a critical activity in drug development and the above quote by Carstensen underscores the need to learn of potential stability problems as soon as possible during development. In early phases of development, drug substances or products are exposed to stress conditions to induce degradation to gain an understanding of the drug's inherent stability and to identify degradation products and pathways. Additional studies may also be conducted to support the packaging materials used to store products. Definitive stability studies under normal storage and accelerated conditions are conducted to support use of the drug during clinical trials and ultimately for marketing applications (2). The accelerated conditions used for these purposes may or may not degrade the samples. Definitive studies on the drug substance from the commercial synthesis and the drug product in the final market formulation including packaging are necessary for product registration. Results from these studies are used to establish appropriate specifications and to justify product dating. Requirements for such studies are described in the International Conference on Harmonization (ICH) guidelines for stability (3).

As stability information becomes established it serves as a comparison for future development. If production process, formulation, or packaging changes during or after development are contemplated, the effect of the change on stability must be evaluated. This is especially important for compounds or formulations that are relatively labile. Recent guidelines or draft guidelines describe stability studies needed for postapproval changes, where the definitive stability has already been established (4). In most cases, a study under accelerated conditions for 3 months and a concurrent room temperature study are needed to support changes with the potential to impact stability behavior. Before committing the resources and time necessary to produce material and conduct such studies, it is valuable to have an indication that the studies will be successful, i.e., that the change will not have an adverse effect on stability. A rapid indication of stability impact is also helpful in guiding additional development or optimization work.

The use of stress conditions more severe than those used for normal 3–6-month studies can provide a rapid indication of relative stability behavior when comparing one sample to another. Equivalent behavior under these conditions will be an indication that the materials will behave similarly under less stringent conditions but with longer times of exposure.

Comparative studies may also be useful in evaluating the relative stability of commercial formulations of the same drug from different suppliers. In these cases, the cause(s) of differences in stability may be difficult to determine since different sources of active ingredient and different excipients may all be variables that affect stability.

In this chapter, considerations are described for conducting comparative stress stability studies. Examples are presented to illustrate considerations and approaches for using stress conditions to compare sample stability. Finally, a statistical modeling approach is described, whereby the stability of a labile compound is modeled as a function of moisture and temperature. While requiring more time than some stress condition studies, this approach allows prediction of stability behavior over a wide range of conditions and ultimately saves time by eliminating the need for additional studies.

II. CONSIDERATIONS FOR COMPARATIVE STRESS STABILITY STUDIES

Much work has gone into conducting accelerated studies as a faster means of predicting normal storage temperature degradation rates and justifying expiration dating (5–15). That is not the purpose of the approach described here. Instead, the goal here is to design rapid stress studies capable of showing stability *differences among samples* that may indicate differences under normal conditions. Likewise, if no differences are observed, more confidence is gained that the materials will display equivalent behavior under normal conditions.

Stress conditions, as defined by the ICH stability guidelines, are considered to be more severe than accelerated conditions used for marketing application stability studies. They are usually chosen to induce degradation in an amount of time that the investigator deems appropriate. There is always a compromise between obtaining results in a short time by using more extreme conditions and producing degradation that is not representative of pathways operative at less extreme conditions.

Considerations involved in planning, conducting, and interpreting comparative stress stability studies are outlined in Table 1 and discussed below.

1. *Previous knowledge*: Although it may be obvious, information such as degradation product identity, degradation pathways, stability under various conditions, and the ability of analytical methods to determine degradation products is very valuable. Without this information, more extensive preliminary experiments will be required to understand degradation behavior and aid in the choice of appropriate stress conditions.
2. *Representative degradation*: Stress conditions which produce a degradation profile similar to that observed under normal conditions

Table 1 Considerations for Stress Studies

(1) What is known about stability/degradation from previous studies?
(2) Do the stress conditions being considered produce a degradation product profile typical of that seen under normal conditions?
(3) How much degradation should be obtained?
(4) Is the analytical method suitable?
(5) Is humidity control necessary?
(6) Is packaging important?
(7) What is a significant difference?
(8) Is a kinetic model and/or Arrhenius study needed?
(9) Is confirmatory data needed?

should be used. Production of different degradation products indicates that a different degradation pathway is operative and results may not reflect comparative room temperature stability. Investigators are often cautioned against extrapolating too far between stress/accelerated and normal conditions (16). Problems with the use of extrapolations from Arrhenius studies (17) and with changes in the degradation mechanism of proteins as a function of temperature are examples that have been noted (18–20). Also, conditions that are too harsh may degrade all materials at the same rate, whether or not they would display differences under normal conditions. Conditions that are too mild, however, will require excessive time to observe differences and therefore defeat the purpose of a rapid stability comparison. When comparing drug products containing different formulation components, different impurities may arise due to drug–excipient interactions. In these cases, comparative stress testing begins to overlap with the concept of drug–excipient compatibility studies. However, such studies provide valuable information regarding the relative stability of each formulation.

3. *Extent of degradation*: Degradation levels of interest will vary depending on the compound and purpose of the study. Time/temperature combinations that produce levels of degradation products or loss of potency that would cause failure to meet specifications would be reasonable to use for comparative stress studies.

   For very stable drugs, the utility of stress comparison studies may be to show that manufacturing or formulation changes have not caused a change that could impart instability such as the presence of greater amorphous content. Showing good stability under stress conditions would add confidence that the change did not affect stability properties.

4. *Analytical method*: The method used to detect degradation must be suitable for its intended purpose. Loss of potency of the drug is often the measured response for stability studies. This may reflect a lack of specification limits and methodology for impurities in pharmacopeial monographs, especially for dosage forms and older drug substances. It is also sometimes assumed that monitoring degradation products is not necessary since it will only mirror the loss of potency.

   Analytical precision relative to the amount of degradation is the primary reason that determination of the increase in levels of degradation products rather than loss of potency is recommended. Potency results have been used when degradation well beyond the levels considered pharmaceutically acceptable were studied, usually in connection with mechanistic determinations. For more relevant amounts of degradation more typical of those observed during product shelf-life (~2–5%), the inherent variability of most potency measurements (1–2%) is on the order of the differences of interest among the samples being studied. Therefore, many assay replicates would be needed to reduce measurement variability to acceptable levels. A better approach is the measurement of degradation product levels using methods such as high-performance liquid chromatography (HPLC) which provide much better precision relative to the changes being investigated and improve the accuracy of the predictions. Of course, knowledge of the degradation products of the compound is necessary to ensure that the analytical method used can detect them adequately. Isothermal calorimetry is also a technique that may provide a rapid comparison of stability among different samples (21). Minute quantities of heat produced as a compound degrades even at normal storage temperatures can be determined and degradation rates projected. Disadvantages to this approach are the need for instrumentation that is not available in many laboratories and the inability to distinguish between degradation and other thermal events such as relaxation of a "higher energy" crystal lattice.

5. *Humidity control*: Moisture is an important factor in the stability of many pharmaceutical compounds and formulations (22,23). The decision to control moisture for comparative stress studies should depend on the characteristics of the compound and the information desired. The moisture content of typical samples, moisture sorption as a function of relative humidity, and the effect of moisture on degradation can help guide the decision to control humidity. At a minimum, samples being compared should be exposed to the same ambient humidity conditions in the storage chamber.
6. *Packaging*: Unless different packaging materials or systems are being compared, the same packaging should be used for comparative stress studies. The relative stabilities of the drug substances or products stored under similar conditions can then be ascertained.
7. *Determination of differences in results*: Sound scientific judgement, well thought out experiments and previous experience with the drug substance or product must be used to determine if an observed difference in degradation rates between samples is due to an actual difference in stability properties or whether the difference is within experimental error. Checking several containers of the same sample under the stress conditions can be used to establish the reproducibility of the observed degradation rate. This would include variability due to the individual samples and the

measurement method. Differences greater than this or some higher value set considering the desired confidence level, could then be attributed to stability differences. Data obtained at room temperature are also very useful in establishing the magnitude of difference under stress conditions that can reflect room temperature differences. If comparisons of samples not stressed at the same time are desired, a further evaluation of study-to-study variability would be required. In most cases, a direct comparison where the samples to be compared are all treated in the same study is recommended.

8. *Kinetic model/Arrhenius study*: Various kinetic models have been proposed for solid-state degradation (24). Degradation plots for several models are given in Figure 1. Most of these models display approximately linear or zero-order behavior in the pharmaceutically relevant range of up to about 10% degradation. An exception is the Avrami–Erofeev model, $n \leq 0.5$ (Fig. 1*D*) which starts to show a sigmoidal degradation pattern with an initial lag phase. For most purposes, a zero-order model provides a simple and convenient means of data comparison for stress studies. Also, it is important to remember that accurate kinetic modeling is usually

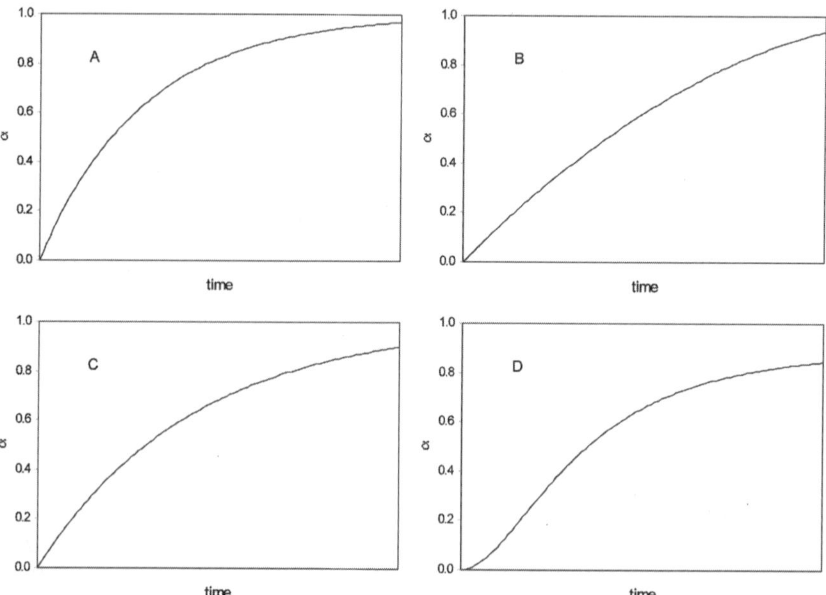

Figure 1 Solid-state degradation models. α=fraction decomposed. A = Prout–Tompkins, $kt = \ln(\frac{1}{1-\alpha})$, B = 2 dimensional phase boundary $kt = 1-(1-\alpha)^{1/2}$, C = Avrami–Erofeev, $kt = [-\ln(1-\alpha)]^n$, $n = 1$, D = Avrami–Erofeev, $n = 0.5$.

not the purpose of stress studies and accurate kinetic modeling becomes even more tenuous for solid dosage forms containing mixtures of compounds. If nonlinear degradation data are obtained, other models can be used to obtain a rate constant if desired. For most development purposes, a strictly empirical (rather than theoretical or mechanistic) approach is adequate to compare the relative stability of samples. For some studies, only initial and final time point measurements may be needed. The number of time points should be increased for more accurate determinations of rate constants. Four time points are usually sufficient for linear degradation.

For greater confidence that stress conditions are predictive of relative stability under normal conditions, an Arrhenius study of degradation rate at different temperatures can be performed and a room temperature rate calculated. At least four temperatures should be used to obtain enough points to fit to the Arrhenius equation (7). Knowledge of the observed degradation rate at room temperature from previous studies is useful for comparison. A predicted rate that is consistent with the observed rate can provide good evidence of the applicability of the stress conditions for reflecting room temperature behavior.

9. *Confirmatory studies*: In addition to consistency of Arrhenius predictions with observed room temperature data, it may be desirable to confirm that the relative stability results for samples compared under the chosen stress conditions are consistent with the relative stability for the same samples at room temperature. This provides another degree of validation that the stress conditions will provide results predictive of real differences observed at lower temperatures over a longer period of time. Since the room temperature data will take longer to obtain, this type of confirmation may be obtained at a later time after initial stress comparison studies are well over. The room temperature data may be generated for regulatory purposes and should be compared to the initial stress study predictions.

III. LITERATURE EXAMPLES

Accelerated or stress stability studies for the purpose of predicting sample shelf life at normal conditions have been investigated for many years. In addition, some examples of stress stability studies for sample comparison have been described. Goldberg and Nightingale (25) compared the stability of aspirin in a combined dosage form with propoxyphene. The hydrolysis product, salicylic acid, was monitored in samples stored at 25°C, 37°C, and 50°C at both low (< 10%) and high (90%) relative humidity. Data were reported for up to 28 days. One formulation showed instability at room temperature in this time, while the others were stable. At 50°C, different degradation rates were observed for the three samples with the fastest rate obtained for the sample that degraded at room temperature. The degradation rate differences were apparent within two weeks at 50°C. The enhanced stability of one sample was postulated as due to physical separation of propoxyphene from the aspirin in pelleted form. This separation may have prevented exposure of the aspirin to an acidic environment caused by the contact with the HCl counter ion of propoxyphene.

Furlanetto et al. (26) attempted to predict and compare the solid-state stability of cefazolin sodium and cephaloridine sterile powders using data obtained at 37°C, 45°C, and 60°C. They analyzed samples for up to 6 months and found cephaloridine to be more stable than cefazolin sodium, in contrast to the relative stability of the compounds as indicated by their respective compendial storage instructions. They attributed greater stability of the cephaloridine samples to greater crystallinity compared to the cefazolin sodium samples which appeared to be mostly amorphous. Rather than comparing different samples of the same drug, this study determined the relative stability of two different drugs and compared the results to expectations based on previous information.

An example of the use of accelerated conditions during development is given by Barthomeuf et al. (27) who compared the stability of vapreotide (an octapeptide somatostatin analog) freeze-dried preparations with lactose and glutamic acid/sodium glutamate as stabilizing agents. Studies were conducted at 50°C, 70% RH for three weeks, with HPLC monitoring of vapreotide content and levels of degradation products. The glutamate buffered formulation was more stable. The lactose formulation showed evidence of Maillard reactions leading to degradation in addition to oxidative and peptide bond-breaking mechanisms.

Concerns about degradation as a result of transporting products under uncontrolled conditions have been raised, particularly in regard to mail-order distribution and actual conditions of use by patients. For example, Black and Layloff (28) showed that mailbox temperatures could reach values as high as 58°C. Temperature cycling stability studies have been proposed to mimic temperature ranges that might be experienced during product distribution (29). Accelerated conditions have been used as a means of identifying labile products which might require greater control during distribution (30–33). In these studies, the effect of direct exposure (open-dish) to temperature/humidity combinations (30°C/75% RH or 25°C/60% RH) on properties such as appearance and dissolution was determined. The results gave an indication of products that might need special labeling or shipping requirements.

A. Detailed Example—Cefaclor Monohydrate

Most of the considerations given in Table 1 were illustrated in an investigation of the relative stability of cefaclor monohydrate drug substance and capsule formulations (34). Differences in the levels of degradation products present in several commercial cefaclor products with similar expiration dates had been noted. The goal of the investigation was to quickly determine if some cefaclor capsule formulations were less stable than others without performing long-term normal stability studies on each product.

1. *Previous knowledge*: A fairly extensive description of cefaclor degradation was available in the literature including methodology for determination of degradation products (35) and identification of degradation products and pathways under different conditions (36).
2. *Representative degradation*: Figure 2 shows the qualitative degradation product profiles obtained for cefaclor monohydrate drug substance after preparation, after storage at room temperature for 2.4 years, and after storage at 67°C for 2 weeks. The major degradation products and nearly all the minor products in the 2-year and 2-week heated samples are identical, thereby providing confidence that degradation pathways at 67°C are the same as those at room temperature.

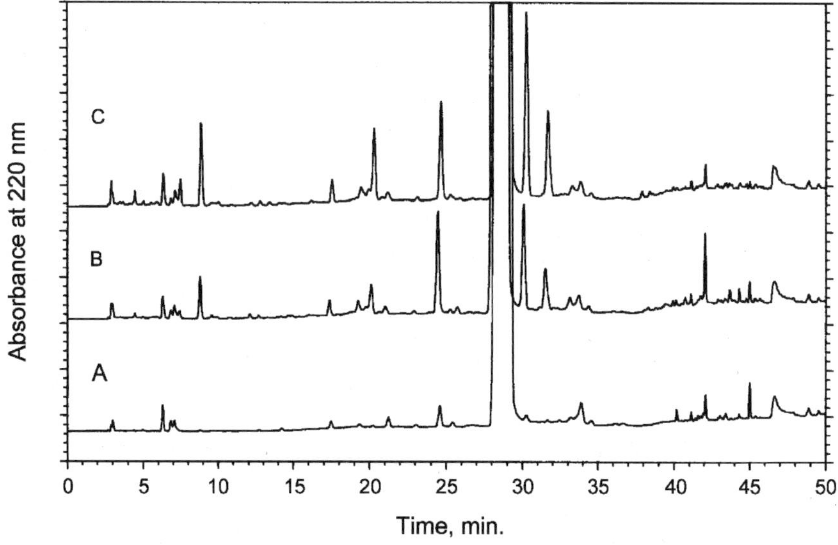

Figure 2 Degradation product profiles of cefaclor monohydrate. (A) 1 month after preparation; (B) after 2 weeks at 67°C and (C) after 2.4 years at room temperature.

3. *Degradation level*: The limit on total related substances in cefaclor monohydrate given by the United States and European Pharmacopeia is 2.0%. This establishes a level of degradation that would be considered significant. For the drug product, degradation of 10% would cause the potency to fall below the pharmacopeial minimum of 90% assuming that no overage was used initially. Taking these as benchmarks for significance, the stress conditions should target degradation levels from 2–10%.
4. *Analytical method*: Monitoring degradation product levels would provide a better indication of stability differences than a stability-indicating potency method. The relative change in degradation levels could be several fold while the potency change could be as little as 2%, which is within the variability of the potency assay and capsule content uniformity. An HPLC method for related substances was therefore used to assess the amount of degradation.
5. *Humidity control*: The question of humidity control was examined in several ways. The moisture sorption isotherm showed moisture levels from 3–6% over a relative humidity range of 20–95%. Also, samples held at 65°C for over 2 weeks remained within this range of water content, which was within pharmacopeial specification. Finally, samples which were heated did not show a change in crystal form by X-ray powder diffraction, such as partial conversion to an anhydrate. Based on these results, humidity control was not deemed necessary for comparative stress studies. Samples to be compared were all stored under identical conditions, i.e., in the same oven. Any local change in humidity around each sample was therefore a function of the sample itself.
6. *Packaging*: Most commercial samples were available in plastic bottles and similar bottles were used for comparative studies. The same type of bottle was used for all samples in order to eliminate packaging as a variable.
7. *Significant differences*: Stress degradation rate data are given in Table 2 for different batches of cefaclor monohydrate capsules from different suppliers. The average standard error in determination of the slope of the degradation plot was 0.012%/day for degradation rates covering a range of 0.04–0.22%/day. A difference of about 0.04% (three times the standard error) in the rates would indicate a significant difference in sample stability. Degradation rates for samples A-1, C-1, and B-1 were obtained in each of two separate studies. Results were very close for samples A-1 and C-1, which showed differences of 0.01% and 0.03%/day, respectively. The difference in results for different studies of sample B-1 was 0.06%/day, but the degradation rate was about twice

Table 2 Degradation Rates for 250 mg Cefaclor Monohydrate Capsules Held at 65°C for 2 weeks

Study number	Supplier-lot	Degradation rate, %/day	Std error, %/day
2	A-3	0.082	0.010
1	A-2	0.084	0.007
2	A-1	0.088	0.009
1	A-1	0.10	0.0004
2	C-1	0.10	0.010
2	C-1	0.11	0.016
1	C-1	0.13	0.013
2	C-3	0.13	0.045
2	B-1	0.16	0.016
2	B-2	0.20	0.002
1	B-1	0.22	0.006
1	C-2	0.22	0.015

that observed for the other samples (0.2% vs. 0.1%/day). Also, as discussed below, confirmatory data showed that samples with a significant room temperature stability difference showed a stress difference of 0.08%/day, which is much greater than the significance threshold identified above.

8. *Kinetic model/Arrhenius study*: Preliminary studies showed that most samples degraded in a linear fashion which would suffice for comparing degradation rates. A more detailed kinetic model was not needed but an Arrhenius study was conducted to check the agreement of the predicted room temperature degradation rate with the observed rate. Degradation rates were determined for cefaclor monohydrate stored at 45°C, 55°C, 64°C, and 70°C for a period of two weeks. This encompassed the temperature (65°C) being considered for comparative studies. The increase in degradation products vs. time for these conditions is shown in Figure 3. Zero-order degradation rates were taken from the slopes of the regression lines that included measurements at a minimum of four time points. The 45°C and 55°C conditions produced increases in degradation of less than 1%, showing that much longer times would be necessary to obtain an amount of degradation of at least 2%. As observed with other preliminary studies, storage at 65°C for about 2 weeks degraded samples by about 2%. Even though rates were faster at higher temperature, two weeks was a reasonable time to conduct studies without increasing the risk of nonrepresentative degradation at higher temperatures. The Arrhenius plot from the degradation rates obtained in

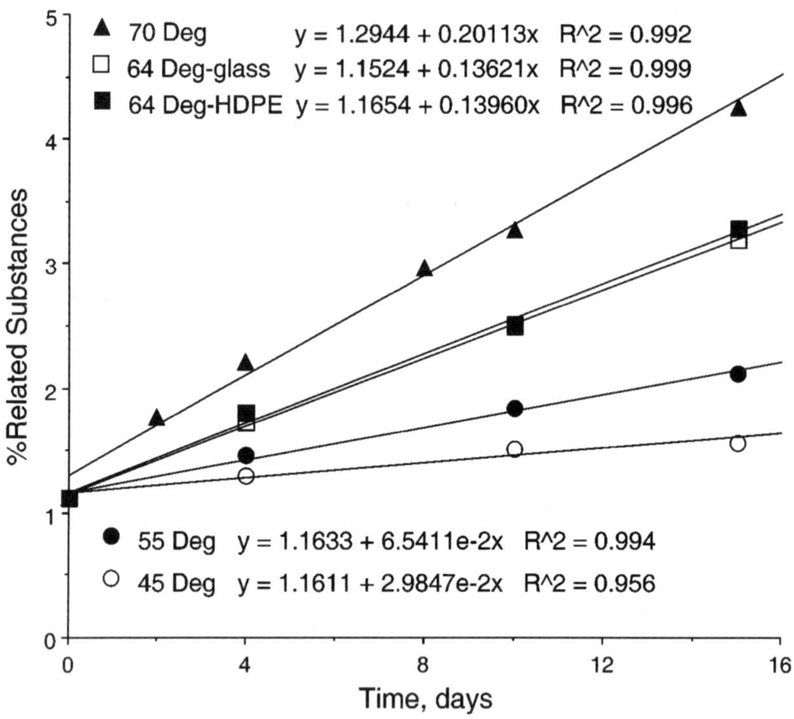

Figure 3 % Degradation vs. time at different temperatures. Data at 64°C were obtained in glass and high density polyethylene (HDPE) bottles.

Figure 3 is shown in Figure 4. From the slope of the line, the extrapolated degradation rate at 20°C was 1.1%/year with a 99% confidence range of 0.6–2.2%/year. The observed degradation rate of cefaclor monohydrate drug substance over a period of 2 years at room temperature was 0.6%/year. This is at the lower end of the range from the Arrhenius study and provides additional confidence that comparing relative stabilities at 65°C is likely to reflect their behavior at room temperature. The difference between the Arrhenius and observed rates also illustrates the danger in using Arrhenius studies alone to determine expiry dating. However, the Arrhenius results support the use of an elevated temperature such as 65°C for comparison studies to rapidly assess stability changes due to formulation or manufacturing process changes.

9. *Confirmatory data*: Two drug substance samples that had shown differences in stability at 25°C were compared under stress conditions. The degradation rates were 0.17% and 0.25%/day for the two samples. This was a significant difference, given a standard

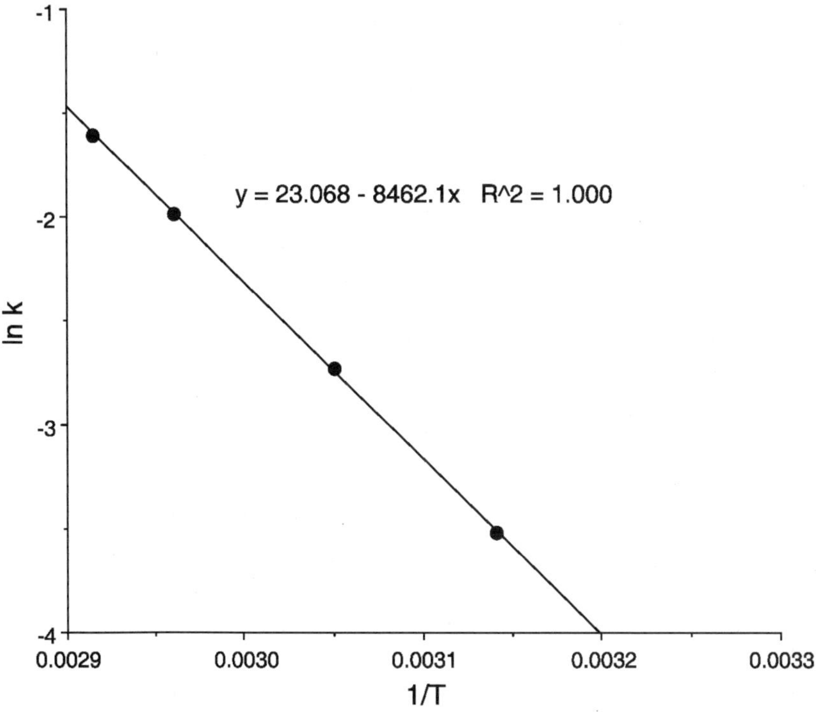

Figure 4 Arrhenius plot for cefaclor monohydrate degradation.

error of about 0.01–0.02%/day in the rates, and showed the ability of the stress results to accurately reflect the stability differences expected at room temperature. Stress degradation rates for capsule formulations were usually linear and the rates provided a basis for comparison. Sample degradation rates could be generally classified as $\leq$0.11%/day or $\geq$0.16%/day to distinguish materials with different stability behavior. This was based on the reproducibility of determining degradation rates and room temperature data showing less stability among samples in the higher rate group compared to samples with lower stress degradation rates. Greater uncertainty would accompany conclusions about the relative stability of samples falling within the same group. Some capsule formulations did not show linear degradation under stress conditions. A rapid rate was observed initially which then decreased and became more linear. The presence of rapidly degrading amorphous cefaclor was investigated and shown to be a possible explanation for this behavior. Differences in the shape of stress degradation vs. time curves could also indicate differences in the physical properties of the samples. Conclusions from these studies were that stability studies at 65°C for two weeks could be used to compare the stability characteristics of cefaclor monohydrate samples, either as bulk or in capsule formulations. Rapid observations of stability differences could be used as a tool to predict whether or not manufacturing or supplier changes might be causes for concern or investigation. Differences in relative stability of commercial formulations could explain differences in quality observed in the marketplace or in development. Decisions about the need and type of further investigations are greatly facilitated by obtaining information in only two weeks.

IV. STATISTICAL DESIGN STUDIES

In some development projects, knowledge of stability behavior over a wide range of possible storage conditions is desired. Various combinations of temperature and humidity to which a drug substance or product may be exposed are often concerns for relatively labile materials. It is very impractical to compare different samples under all conditions of interest, but statistical experimental design offers an efficient means of developing a predictive model for stability under a variety of conditions. This type of program will usually require a more significant investment of time and resources than the comparative studies described previously but can ultimately save time by directing development work toward conditions that will ensure adequate stability. Statistical design studies may also be useful for screening to identify parameters that affect stability and to help optimize the stability of a formulation. Examples are included here since accelerated or stress conditions are usually used in statistical design studies to compare many conditions in one set of experiments.

Statistical design of experiments is commonly used for optimization problems (37). Jones (38) has provided an overview of response surface methodology in the context of stability. Remunan et al. (39) used a factorial design to study the effect of tabletting force (0, 6000 N, 12,000 N), relative humidity (0% and 80%) and temperature (20°C and 40°C) on the chemical stability and dissolution behavior of sustained release nifedipine tablets. Response surfaces demonstrated the significant impact of relative humidity on dissolution behavior over time and showed the need to protect the formulations from moisture. Tabletting force also affected dissolution. Nguyen et al. (40) used a central composite design to study the effect of pH, sucrose, propylene glycol, glycerin, and EDTA, each at three levels, on the chemical stability and preservative efficacy of lamivudine liquid formulations. Samples were held at 30°C and 40°C for three months. The pH of the formulation was found to be the main factor influencing stability of the drug and preservative. Bos et al. (41) described factorial designs to assess the effect of variables such as disintegrant concentration, compression load, storage temperature, and storage humidity on the physical stability of tablets as indicated by crushing strength and disintegration time. All four variables affected the responses observed, and the ratio of a response after storage to the initial response was determined to be a useful means of comparing different batches of tablets.

The following is a detailed example of a statistically designed study to determine the effect of temperature, relative humidity, and water content on the stability of a drug substance under development in the authors' laboratory. The drug substance was obtained initially as an amorphous form, but modifications made to the method of isolating the drug substance appeared to result in greater crystallinity and improved stability properties. More detailed information concerning the stability behavior of both forms over a range of temperature and moisture content was desired.

The experimental design is given in Table 3. This is a full factorial design with duplicate center points. Of course, many other statistical designs are possible depending on the information desired, degree of precision desired, and resources available to execute the protocol. The experimental design used is usually a compromise between the completeness or precision of the results and the analytical resources required to conduct the study. Fractional factorial designs may be used to study more variables while keeping the number of experiments manageable. It is beyond the scope of this discussion, but an important consideration in fractional designs is the aliasing structure of variables and their interactions. Screening designs such as fractional factorials are useful in identifying main effect variables, but some variables and variable interaction terms may be confounded, so care should be taken in interpreting the results.

As indicated from moisture sorption data, the water content of the samples was a function of relative humidity. Storage conditions of 0%,

Table 3 Experimental Design For Stability of a Development Compound for Temperature, −1 = 5°C, 0 = 25°C, 1 = 45°C For Water Content, −1 = 3%, 0 = 6.5%, 1 = 10%

Expt. number	Temperature	Water content
1	−1	−1
2	1	−1
3	0	0
4	−1	1
5	1	1
6	0	0

45%, and 75% relative humidity were used to control water content of the samples at approximately 3, 6.5, and 10 wt/wt %, respectively. The consistency of these values was checked at each stability timepoint.

Levels of three individual degradation products and the total amount of degradation impurities were monitored at timepoints of 1, 2, 4, 8, 12, and 24 weeks. Statistical software was used to analyze the data and derive models for the rates of degradation as a function of the temperature and sample water content. The analysis showed that temperature and water content were both significant in their effect on degradation rate (Table 4). The

Table 4 Analysis of Statistical Experimental Design Data

Summary of fit					
RSquare	0.999955				
RSquare adj	0.999775				
Root mean square error	0.006435				
Mean of response	0.265283				
Observations (or sum wgts)	6				
Analysis of variance					
Source	DF	Sum of squares	Mean square	F ratio	
Model	4	0.91872124	0.229680	5547.164	
Error	1	0.00004141	0.000041	Prob > F	
C total	5	0.91876265		0.0101	
Parameter estimates					
Term	Estimate	Std. error	t ratio	Prob > |t|	
Intercept	0.08085	0.00455	17.77	0.0358	
Water	0.1954	0.003217	60.73	0.0105	
Temp	0.3575	0.003217	60.73	0.0105	
Water*temp	0.1954	0.003217	60.73	0.0105	
Curvature	0.27665	0.005573	49.64	0.0128	
Effect test					
Source	Nparm	DF	Sum of squares	F ratio	Prob > F
Water	1	1	0.15272464	3688.555	0.0105
Temp	1	1	0.51122500	12346.94	0.0057
Water*temp	1	1	0.15272464	3688.555	0.0105
Curvature	1	1	0.10204696	2464.605	0.0128

interaction term water*temperature and the curvature term temperature-*temperature were also statistically significant.

Parameter estimates for the statistical models were used to generate response surface maps for both the amorphous and crystalline forms (Figs. 5 and 6, respectively). These maps are very useful for assessing and comparing the predicted stability properties of the two forms under a range of temperature and humidity (water content) conditions. The amorphous form was stable over a much smaller temperature–humidity region than the crystalline form. The stability of the amorphous form was particularly sensitive to humidity. The crystalline form could tolerate moisture much better as long as the sample was held at an appropriate temperature. The model shows which combinations of temperature and moisture content will provide good stability.

Similar analyses for individual degradation products reveal interesting behaviors. For example, the pattern for peak B for the amorphous form (Fig. 7) is similar to the total related substances results. In contrast, the rate of peak F formation for the crystalline form is almost independent of water content (Fig. 8).

To support the accuracy of the statistical model estimates of degradation rates, Arrhenius treatments of the stability results were also performed. An additional temperature (35°C) was used for each sample form to provide

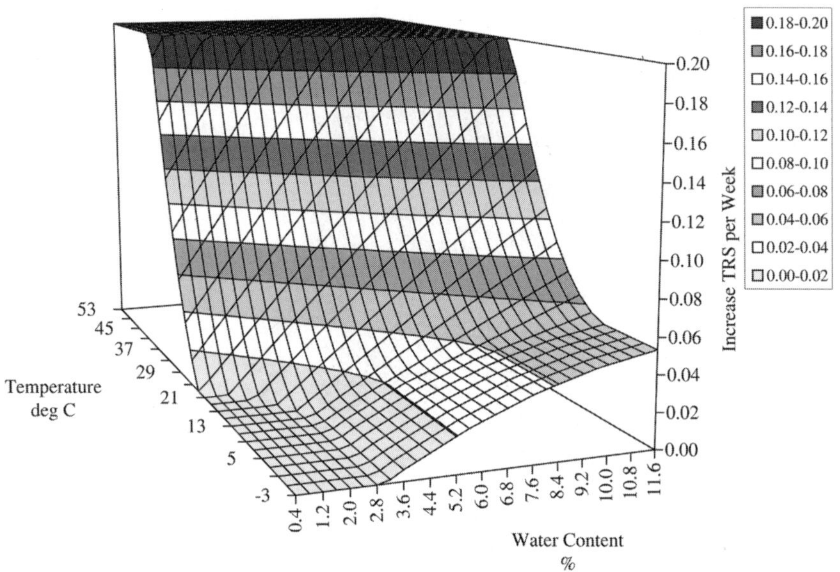

Figure 5 Response surface for amorphous form degradation. TRS = %Total degradation products formed.

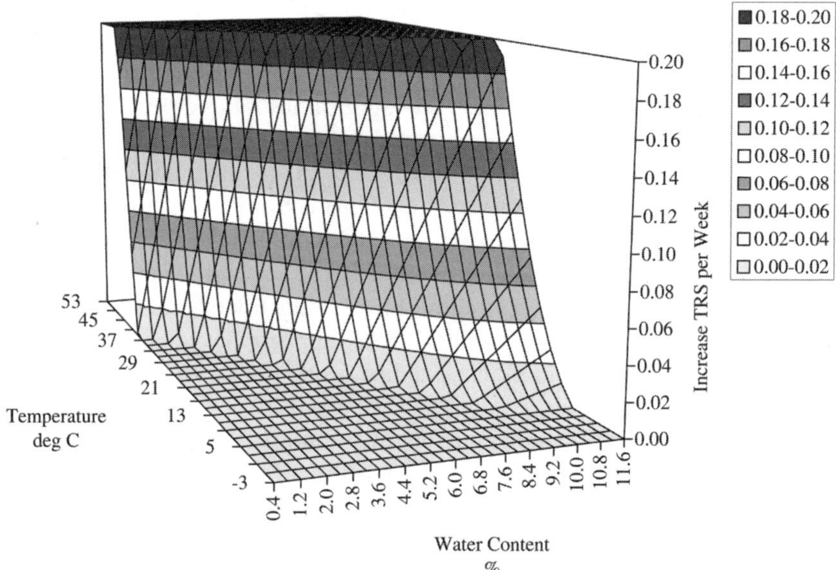

Figure 6 Response surface for crystalline form degradation. TRS = %Total degradation products formed.

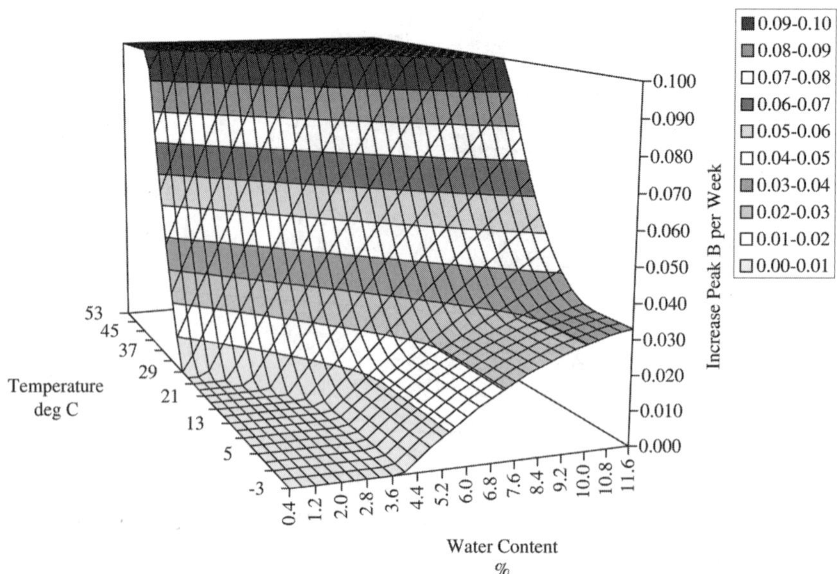

Figure 7 Response surface for peak B formation in amorphous form sample.

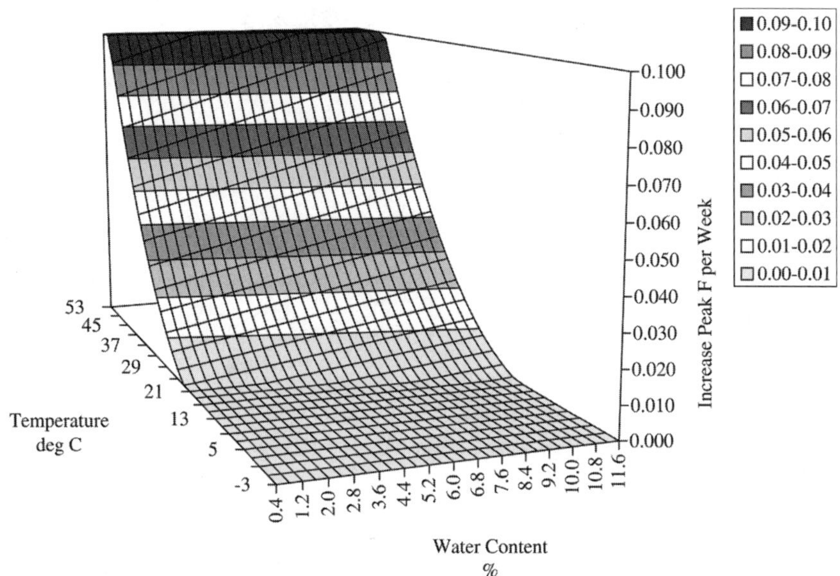

Figure 8 Response surface for peak F formation in crystalline form sample.

four points in the Arrhenius plots. Degradation rates at both high and low water content were used for the high and low temperature points. The intermediate water content was used at the intermediate temperatures. Arrhenius plots for peak B of the amorphous form and peak F of the crystalline form are shown in Figures 9 and 10, respectively. The effect of water content on degradation rate is apparent for peak B in the amorphous form by the spread of results for the two points at each of the high and low temperatures. A similar behavior was observed for total impurities.

Predicted degradation rates using the statistical models and the Arrhenius data are compared to real time stability data in Table 5. Rates were calculated assuming an intermediate water content of about 6%. The agreement of predicted and actual results is very good. Good agreement was expected for the statistical model since the center point (25°C/6% water) was used to obtain the observed degradation rate. The 5°C data from the statistical design study were not used for the observed rates, however, since higher and lower water content samples were studied.

As a final check on the accuracy of the statistical model, the observed results for total related substances and peak B obtained during stability testing of 18 different manufacturing and lab scale batches of drug substance were compared to predicted increases (Figs. 11 and 12). The stability studies represented amorphous and crystalline material with water content ranging from 3–8%. Temperatures used for stability studies were 5°C, 25°C, and 35°C. The duration of the studies was from 11 weeks to 10 months. The

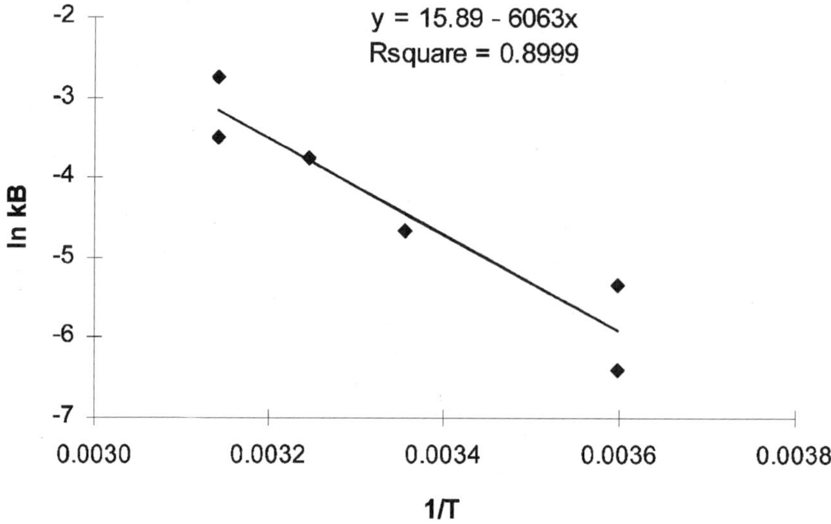

Figure 9 Arrhenius plot for peak B formation in amorphous form sample.

correlation of observed and predicted values was quite good. The intercepts were not significantly different from zero and the slopes were close to 1.0. The overall agreement and consistency of results leads to the conclusion that the estimates generated by the statistically designed models are reasonably good predictors of actual degradation rates under various conditions.

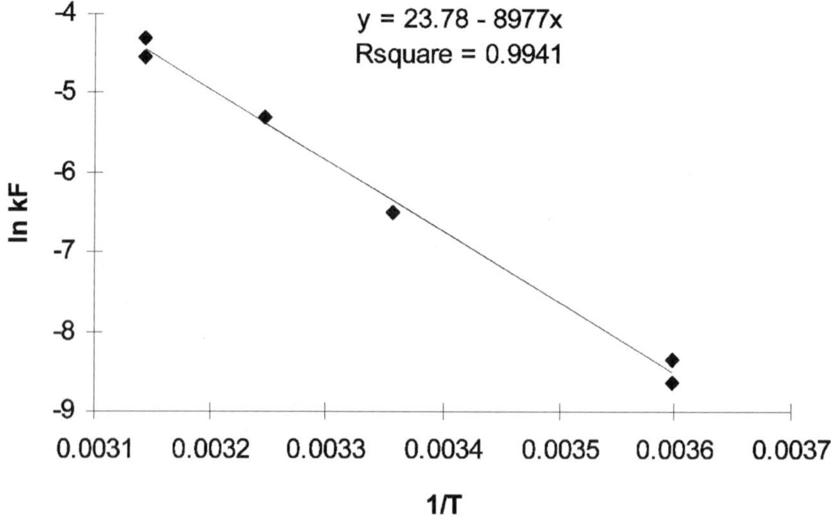

Figure 10 Arrhenius plot for peak F formation in crystalline form sample.

Table 5 Comparison of the Percent Degradation Products Formed per Year Predicted From Statistically Designed Studies, Arrhenius Studies and the Observed Rates

Product/ Temperature	Amorphous form Arrhenius	Amorphous form stat. model	Amorphous form observed	Crystalline form Arrhenius	Crystalline form stat. model	Crystalline form observed
Peak B, 25°C	4.2	3.8	3.1	0.90	1.0	1.3
Peak B, 5°C	1.0	0.8	1.0	0.04	< 0.1	0.00
Peak F, 25°C	*	*	*	0.64	0.52	0.52
Peak F, 5°C	*	*	*	0.07	< 0.1	0.09
Peak H, 25°C	*	*	*	0.12	0.10	0.09
Peak H, 5°C	*	*	*	0.02	< 0.1	0.00
TRS, 25°C	6.3	6.8	6.1	4.5	4.4	4.3
TRS, 5°C	0.9	1.3	1.1	0.58	< 0.1	0.22

*Not determined. TRS=Total degradation products formed.

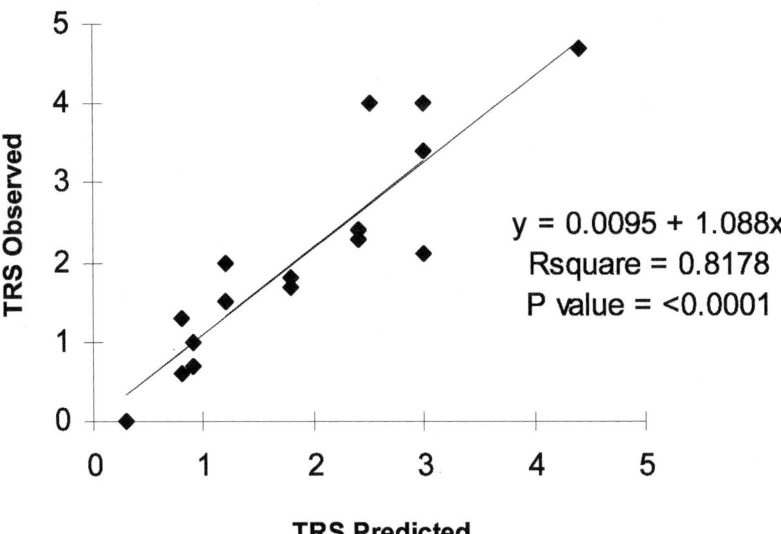

Figure 11 Comparison of results observed for total related substances (TRS) from stability testing of different lots and the predicted values using statistically derived models.

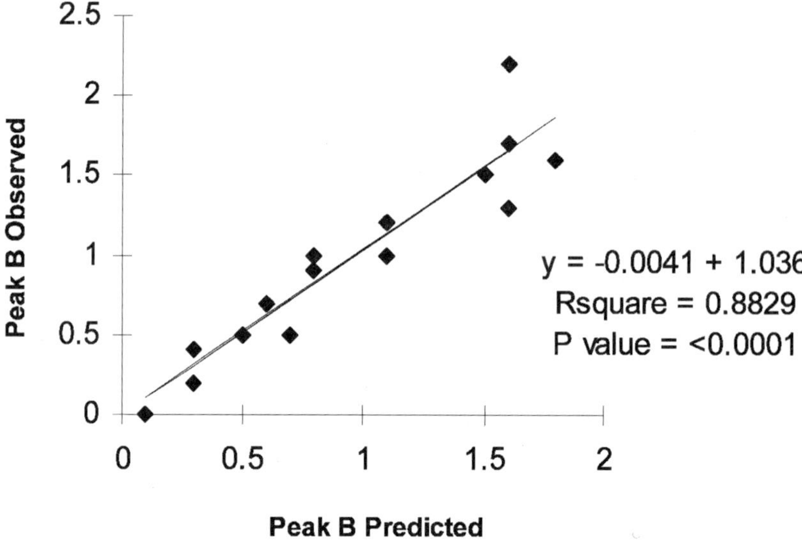

Figure 12 Comparison of results observed for peak B from stability testing of different lots and the predicted values using the statistically derived models.

V. SUMMARY AND CONCLUSIONS

Comparative stability studies done using stress conditions can be valuable in providing a rapid indication of the relative stability properties of the samples being compared. Appropriate information concerning the applicability of stress results to room temperature is necessary to draw meaningful conclusions from the stress studies. The amount of this information needed depends on the degree of confidence the investigator requires and how the results will be used. Simple studies such as direct comparisons or more complex statistical design studies can provide valuable information regarding the effects of manufacturing changes, storage conditions or sample characteristics on stability. This information can help direct further development efforts or justify processing changes appropriately.

REFERENCES

1. Carstensen JT. In: Grimm W, Schepky G, eds. Stabilitatsprufung in der Pharmazie. Aulendorf: Editio Cantor, 1980:11.
2. Grimm W. General concept for stability testing. In: Grimm W, Krummen K, eds. Stability Testing in the EC, Japan, and the USA. Stuttgart: Wissenschaftliche Verlagsgesellschaft, 1993:191–223.
3. International Conference on Harmonisation. Stability Testing of New Drug Substances and Products (Second Revision) Fed Register 1994; 59: 48754–48759.

4. FDA guidelines for Scale-up and Postapproval Changes (SUPAC) and changes to an approved NDA or ANDA.
5. Lin SL. Parenteral formulations. I. Comparison of accelerated stability data with shelf-life studies. Bull Parenter Drug Assoc 1969; 23:269–288.
6. Pope DG. Accelerated stability testing for prediction of drug product stability. Drug Cosmet Ind 1980; 127(5):54, 56, 59, 60, 62, 116.
7. Pope DG. Accelerated stability testing for prediction of drug product stability. Drug Cosmet Ind 1980; 127(6):48, 50, 55–56, 58, 60, 62, 64–66.
8. Yang W, Roy SB. Projection of tentative expiry date from one-point accelerated stability testing. Drug Dev Ind Pharm 1980; 6:591–604.
9. Kowalski K, Beno M, Bergstrom C, Gaud H. The application of multiresponse estimation to drug stability studies. Drug Dev Ind Pharm 1987; 13: 2823–2838.
10. Young WR. Accelerated temperature pharmaceutical product stability determinations. Drug Dev Ind Pharm 1990; 16:551–569.
11. Yoshioka S, Aso Y, Izutsu K, Terao T. Application of accelerated testing to shelf-life prediction of commercial protein preparations. J Pharm Sci 1994; 83:454–456.
12. Yoshioka S, Aso Y, Takeda Y. Statistical evaluation of accelerated stability data obtained at a single temperature. I. Effect of experimental errors in evaluation of stability data obtained. Chem Pharm Bull 1990; 38:1757–1759.
13. Yoshioka S, Aso Y, Takeda Y. Statistical evaluation of accelerated stability data obtained at a single temperature. II. Estimation of shelf-life from remaining drug content. Chem Pharm Bull 1990; 38:1760–1762.
14. Gneuss KD. Prediction of the stability of drug products, new techniques and strategies. In: Grimm W, Krummen K, eds. Stability Testing in the EC, Japan, and the USA. Stuttgart: Wissenschaftliche Verlagsgesellschaft, 1993: 75–94.
15. Stamper GF, Lambert WJ. Accelerated stability testing of proteins and peptides: pH-stability profile of insulinoptropin using traditional Arrhenius and non-linear fitting analysis. Drug Dev Ind Pharm 1995; 21:1503–1511.
16. Chafetz L. Practical testing of solid-state stability of pharmaceuticals. J Pharm Sci 1992; 81:107.
17. Yang W. Errors in the estimation of the activation energy and the projected shelf life in employing an incorrect kinetic order in an accelerated stability test. Drug Dev Ind Pharm 1981; 7:717–738.
18. Cleland JL, Powell MF, Shire SJ. The development of stable protein formulations: a close look at protein aggregation, deamidation, and oxidation. Crit Rev Ther Drug Carrier Syst 1993; 10:307–377.
19. Gu LC, Erdos EA, Chiang HS, Calderwood T, Isai K, Visor GC, Duffy J, Hsu WC, Foster LC. Stability of interleukin 1β in aqueous solution: analytical methods, kinetics, products, and solution formulation implications. Pharm Res 1991; 8:485–490.
20. Franks F. Accelerated stability testing of bioproducts: attractions and pitfalls. Trends Biotechnol 1994; 12:114–117.
21. Koenigbauer MJ. Pharmaceutical applications of microcalorimetry. Pharm Res 1994; 11:777–783.

22. Duddu S, Weller K. Importance of glass transition temperature in accelerated stability testing of amorphous solids: case study using a lyophilized aspirin formulation. J Pharm Sci 1996; 85:345–347.
23. Ahlneck C, Zografi G. The molecular basis of moisture effects on the physical and chemical stability of drugs in the solid state. Int J Pharm 1990; 62:87–95.
24. Byrn S. Solid State Stability of Drugs. New York: Academic Press, 1982:59–75.
25. Goldberg R, Nightingale CH. Stability of aspirin in propoxyphene compound dosage forms. Am J Hosp Pharm 1977; 34:267–269.
26. Furlanetto S, Mura P, Gratteri P, Pinzauti S. Stability prediction of cefazolin sodium and cephaloridine in solid state. Drug Dev Ind Pharm 1994; 20: 2299–2313.
27. Barthomeuf C, Pourrat H, Pourrat A, Ibrahim H, Cottier PE. Stabilization of octastatin, a somatostatin analogue: comparative accelerated stability studies of two formulations for freeze-dried products. Pharmaceutica Acta Helvetiae 1996; 71:161–166.
28. Black JC, Layloff T. Summer of 1995—Mailbox temperature excursions in St. Louis. Pharm Forum 1996; 22:3305.
29. Carstensen JT, Rhodes CT. Cyclic temperature stress testing of pharmaceuticals. Drug Dev Ind Pharm 1993; 19:401–403.
30. Bempong DK, Mirza T, Grady LT, Lindauer RF. Accelerated screening studies to identify labile preparations (1). Pharm Forum 1999; 25:8929–8938.
31. Bempong DK, Mirza T, Grady LT, Lindauer RF. Accelerated screening studies to identify labile preparations (2). Pharm Forum 1999; 25:8939–8946.
32. Bempong DK, Mirza T, Bradby S, Grady LT, Lindauer RF. Open-dish study to identify labile preparations (1). Pharm Forum 1999; 25:8947–8955.
33. Adkins RE, Mirza T, Bempong DK, Grady LT, Lindauer RF. Open-dish study to identify labile preparations (2). Pharm Forum 1999; 25:8956–8963.
34. Olsen BA, Perry FM, Snorek SV, Lewellen PL. Accelerated conditions for stability assessment of bulk and formulated cefaclor monohydrate. Pharm Dev Tech 1997; 2:303–312.
35. Lorenz LJ, Bashore FN, Olsen BA. Determination of process-related impurities and degradation products in cefaclor by high-performance liquid chromatography. J Chrom Sci 1992; 30:211–216.
36. Dorman DE, Lorenz LJ, Occolowitz JL, Spangle LA, Collins MW, Bashore FN, Baertschi SW. Isolation and structure elucidation of the major degradation products of cefaclor in the solid state. J Pharm Sci 1997; 86:540–549.
37. Box GEP, Hunter WG, Hunter JS. Statistics for Experimenters. New York: John Wiley and Sons, 1978.
38. Jones SP. Stability and response surface methodolgy. In: Hendriks MMWB, DeBoer JH, Smilde AK, eds. Robustness of Analytical Chemical Methods and Pharmaceutical Technological Products. Amsterdam: Elsevier, 1996:11–77.
39. Remunan C, Bretal MJ, Nunez A, Jato JLV. Accelerated stability study of sustained-release nifedipine tablets prepared with Gelucire. Int J Pharm 1992; 80:151–159.
40. Nguyen NAT, Wells ML, Cooper DC. Identification of factors affecting preservative efficacy and chemical stability of lamivudine oral solution through statistical experimental design. Drug Dev Ind Pharm 1995; 21:1671–1682.

41. Bos CE, Bolhuis GK, Smilde AK, DeBoer JH. The use of a factorial design to evaluate the physical stability of tablets after storage under topical conditions. In: Hendriks MMWB, DeBoer JH, Smilde AK, eds. Robustness of analytical chemical methods and pharmaceutical technological products. Amsterdam: Elsevier, 1996:309–341.

9

Physical and Chemical Stability Considerations in the Development and Stress Testing of Freeze-Dried Pharmaceuticals

Steven L. Nail

Pharmaceutical Sciences R&D, Eli Lilly and Company, Indianapolis, Indiana, U.S.A.

I. INTRODUCTION

Critical quality attributes of freeze-dried injectable pharmaceuticals include sterility, freedom from pyrogens, and freedom from extraneous particulate matter. These attributes are achieved by appropriate processing conditions. In addition, these products must completely recover their original activity when reconstituted with water, should be quickly and easily reconstituted, and should retain these attributes over the shelf life of the product. Stability assessment and shelf-life prediction is usually a major focus of a pharmaceutical scientist's attention in the development of freeze-dried dosage forms. While this is a particular concern in the development of protein pharmaceuticals, it is important in the development of small molecule drug products as well, particularly given the importance of the physical state of the drug in determining stability characteristics.

The purpose of this chapter is to present a description of the freeze drying process, an overview of the physical chemistry of freezing and freeze drying, as well as a discussion of the influence of physical state of freeze-dried solids on stability of freeze-dried pharmaceuticals, including attributes of both the drug itself and excipients. The scope of this discussion includes small molecules only, and does not include freeze drying from nonaqueous solvent systems or freeze drying of disperse systems.

II. A BRIEF DESCRIPTION OF THE FREEZE DRYING PROCESS

Freeze drying is used to remove water from heat-sensitive substances at low temperature by the process of *sublimation*, where water is removed via a phase change from a solid to a vapor without passing through a liquid state. This takes place below the triple point of water (Fig. 1), at approximately 0°C and 4.5 mm of mercury (Hg). In addition, when freeze drying is carried out properly, the freeze-dried solid has a relatively high specific surface area, which promotes rapid, complete reconstitution.

Operationally, freeze drying of a final dosage form usually consists of filling glass vials with an aqueous solution of the solutes to be freeze dried, partially inserting a special slotted rubber stopper which allows water vapor to flow through slots in the stopper when in the partially inserted position, and transferring the vials to the shelves of the freeze dryer. Temperature

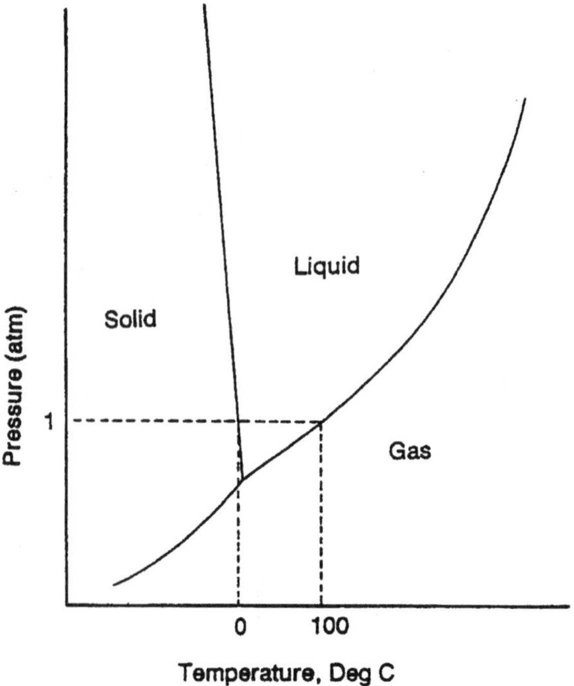

Figure 1 Phase diagram of water.

sensors are placed in a few vials to monitor product temperature during the freeze drying process. The shelves are then cooled to a temperature in the range of −40 to −50°C. The vials are held long enough to approach thermal equilibrium with the shelves, typically for a minimum of 4 hr. Pressure in the freeze dryer is then reduced to less than the vapor pressure of ice at the temperature of the product. For example, for a product temperature of −40°C, the pressure in the system would be reduced to less than 0.096 mm Hg (96 μ Hg). In order for sublimation to take place, energy must be provided in a quantity equal to the heat of sublimation of ice, ΔH_s, which is approximately 2800 joules/g. This is accomplished by heating the transfer fluid and warming the shelves to a temperature high enough to effect sublimation, but not so high as to melt the frozen material in contact with the bottom of the vial or to collapse the partially dried product. The partial pressure of water vapor in the chamber is maintained at a low level by the condenser, which typically operates at temperatures between −65°C and −80°C, and water vapor is removed from the product primarily by a process of *bulk flow* from a region of relatively high pressure (the sublimation front) to low pressure (the condenser). This phase of the process, called *primary drying*, is characterized by a visible receding boundary from the top of the frozen layer. When the ice has sublimed, the heat of sublimation is no longer needed, and the product temperature usually increases sharply toward the shelf temperature.

In general, not all of the water initially present in the product is converted to ice during freezing. The quantity of unfrozen water is a function primarily of the composition of the formulation and, to a lesser extent, the thermal history of the freezing process. This is discussed in more detail below. Removal of this "unfrozen" water, which may be 20% or more of the weight of dry solids, is called *secondary drying*. During secondary drying, the shelf temperature is usually increased, since ice is no longer present. In contrast to primary drying, where water vapor is removed by bulk flow, water vapor removal during secondary drying is largely by a process of diffusion, or flow by molecular motion from a region of high concentration to a region of lower concentration. Because secondary drying is generally slow relative to primary drying, it often represents a larger total portion of drying time than primary drying, even though the quantity of water removed is less. At the end of secondary drying, the shelf stack is compressed together, causing insertion of the lyostoppers to the fully stoppered position. This may be done under full vacuum, partial vacuum, or at atmospheric pressure. For drugs that are sensitive to oxidation in the solid state, the composition of gas in the headspace of the vial may have a critical impact on product stability.

Since the driving force for freeze drying is the vapor pressure of ice, it is important from the standpoint of process efficiency to keep the product temperature as high as practical during primary drying. However, the

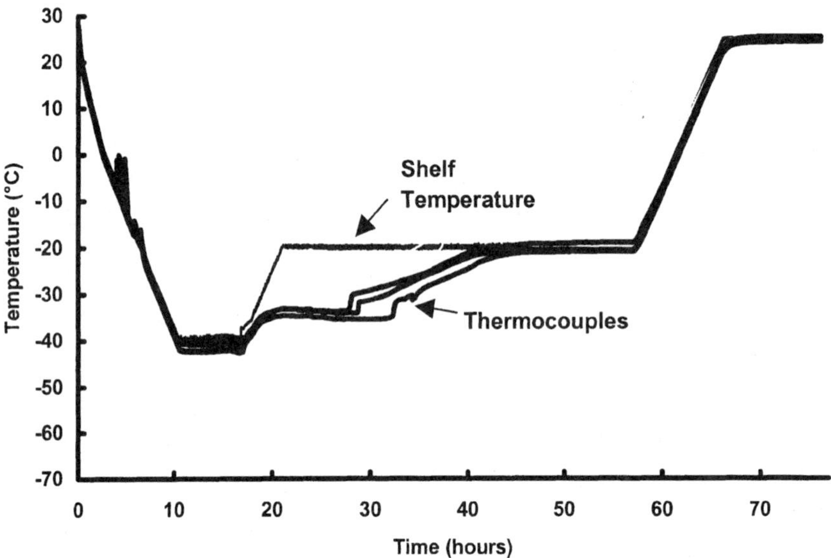

Figure 2 Representative plot of shelf temperature and product temperatures during freeze-drying.

product temperature must be maintained below the maximum allowable product temperature, which is either a eutectic melting temperature or a collapse temperature (see discussion below). Monitoring of product temperature is therefore important for establishing optimum process conditions. A typical plot of shelf temperature and product temperature during freeze drying is shown in Figure 2.

III. AN OVERVIEW OF THE PHYSICAL CHEMISTRY OF FREEZING AND FREEZE DRYING

An understanding of the physical chemistry of freezing is essential to understanding how both formulation composition and process conditions influence the quality of the freeze-dried product, including stability. A schematic diagram of the physical events occuring during freezing is shown in Figure 3. Supercooling, or retention of the liquid state below the equilibrium freezing point of the solution, always occurs to some extent—it is not uncommon for aqueous solutions to supercool by 12°C or more. This is seen in Figure 2 as a sudden "jump" in temperature during the freezing process (the smaller exothermic events seen at lower temperature are caused by crystallization of glycine). The effect of supercooling is to limit the ability to control the freezing rate by manipulation of shelf temperature, since the

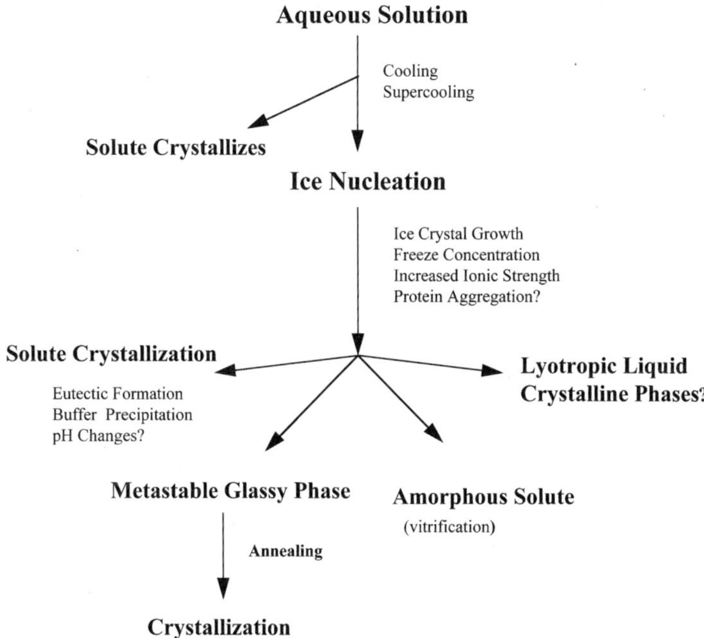

Figure 3 Schematic of physical events occurring during freezing.

greater the degree of supercooling, the faster the effective rate of freezing once ice crystals nucleate.

As indicated in Figure 3, ice may not be the first component of the solution to crystallize. As the temperature is decreased, the equilibrium solubility of one or more solutes may be exceeded, allowing nucleation and crystal growth. An example of this behavior is illustrated by the drug pentamidine isethionate where, depending on the thermal history of freezing, either drug or ice may nucleate first (1). Process validation studies should include determination of whether the thermal history of freezing (for example, placing vials on precooled shelves vs. slowly decreasing the shelf temperature during freezing) has a measureable impact on product quality, such as activity, residual moisture, appearance of solids, reconstitution time, physical state of solids, and stability characteristics.

As ice crystals grow in the freezing system, the solutes are concentrated. In addition to increased ionic strength effects, the rates of some chemical reactions—particularly second order reactions—may be accelerated by freezing through this freeze-concentration effect. Examples include reduction of potassium ferricyanide by potassium cyanide (2), oxidation of ascorbic acid (3), and polypeptide synthesis (4). Kinetics of reactions in frozen systems has been reviewed by Pincock and Kiovsky (5).

A. Solute Crystallization During Freezing—Eutectic Mixture Formation

The fate of the solute in the freeze-concentrated solution is a key concept in understanding the material science of freeze drying. As indicated in Figure 3, there are several possibilities, the simplest of which is crystallization of solute from freeze-concentrated solution to form a simple eutectic system. Direct application of the phase diagram of a binary eutectic-forming system, sodium chloride/water (Fig. 4), is not often encountered in practice, but this system is useful for a conceptual understanding of the relevance of eutectic mixtures to freeze drying. The line *ab* represents the freezing point depression curve of water in the presence of sodium chloride, and the line *bc* represents the solubility of sodium chloride in water. The intersection of these lines is the eutectic temperature, which for sodium chloride/ice is –21.5°C,

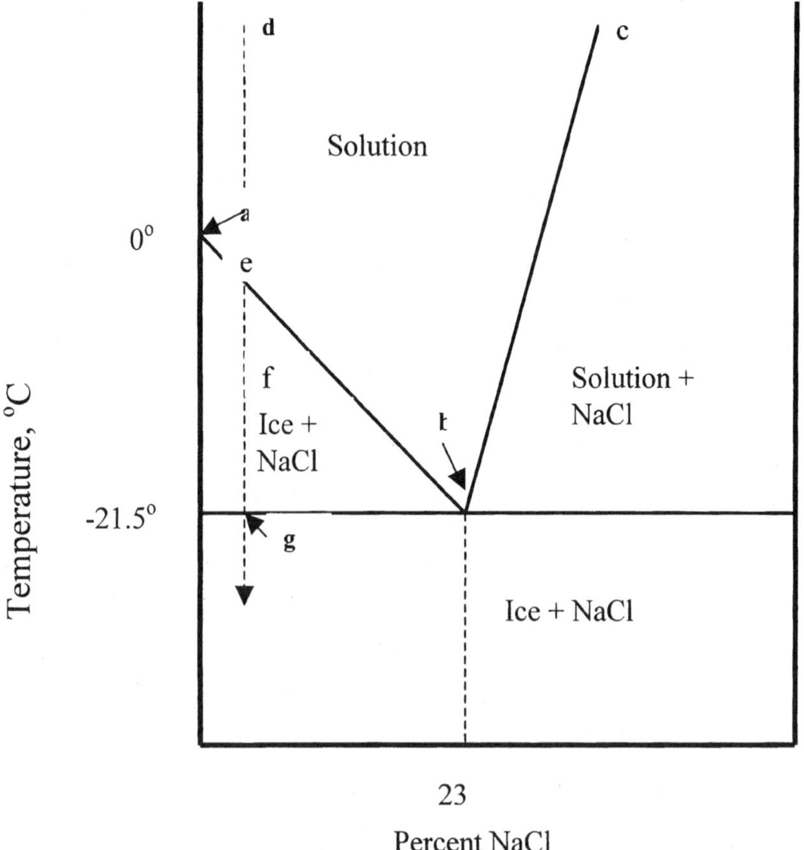

Figure 4 Phase diagram of sodium chloride/water.

and the eutectic composition is about 23.3% (w/w) sodium chloride. The freezing of a 5% solution of sodium chloride in water is represented by the line *defg* (called an *isopleth*). At room temperature (above point *d*), the system is entirely liquid. As the solution cools, ice appears at point *e* (in the absence of supercooling). As the system cools, ice continues to crystallize and the remaining solution becomes more concentrated in sodium chloride. At point *f*, two phases are present, ice and a freeze-concentrated solution of sodium chloride in water. At point *g*, the freeze-concentrate is saturated with respect to sodium chloride and (again, in the absence of supercooling) sodium chloride begins to precipitate. It is only below the eutectic temperature that the system is completely solidified. The relevance of the eutectic temperature to freeze drying is that it represents the maximum allowable product temperature during primary drying, since eutectic melting would introduce liquid water and destroy the desireable properties of a freeze-dried solid. Melting of the frozen system during primary drying is sometimes called *meltback*.

The phase diagram illustrates the degree of concentration of sodium chloride, hence the increase in ionic strength, caused by the freezing process. For example, if a solution of normal saline (0.9% w/v, or 0.15 N) is frozen, the concentration reaches 23.3% before sodium chloride crystallizes and forms a eutectic mixture, or just over 4.0 N. This increase in ionic strength associated with freezing of salt solutions is a contributing factor in osmotic dehydration of cells during freezing and has been thought to contribute to protein denaturation during freezing.

While not a thoroughly investigated aspect of freezing of pharmaceutical formulations, solutes that crystallize from freezing aqueous solutions are known to form different polymorphs during freezing at different cooling rates, or perhaps during freezing from solutions of different compositions. Examples include glycine (6,7), mannitol (8), and pentamidine isethionate (1). Mannitol has also been reported to form a hydrate during certain formulation and processing conditions (9).

B. pH Shifts During Freezing

Crystallization of phosphate buffers during freezing is a special case of eutectic mixture formation during freezing, and is worthy of mention not only because phosphate salts are the most common buffers used in freeze-dried pharmaceutical formulations, but also because the crystallization process can cause significant shifts in pH during freezing. The effect of freezing on the pH of sodium and potassium phosphate buffers has been extensively studied by van den Berg and coworkers (10,11), where the pH shift was shown to depend on the salt used. The monobasic salt of potassium phosphate, being less soluble than the dibasic salt, tends to precipitate during freezing and cause an increase in pH. For sodium phosphate, the dibasic salt is less soluble than the monobasic salt, and the opposite effect is observed. Changes in pH of as much as three units toward the acid side have been reported for the sodium phosphate system. Changes toward more alkaline pH for the potassium phosphate system are less pronounced. Gomez et al. (12) examined the influences of initial buffer solution pH and concentration on subsequent pH changes during freezing, as well as the influence of other species in solution on buffer salt crystallization. The pH changes associated with crystallization of a sodium phosphate buffer solution initially at pH 7.4 are directly related to the initial concentration of buffer in the range of 8–100 mM. Further, the lower the initial pH of the buffer, the higher the observed pH at –10°C. These investigators further reported that addition of NaCl increases the ion product of dibasic sodium phosphate, thereby leading to larger pH changes. It is important to remember that a eutectic mixture is only formed as a result of crystallization of one or more solutes, and the presence of a phosphate buffer in a formulation does not mean that the pH will shift during freezing. Gomez et al. reported that solutes such as sucrose and mannitol inhibited crystallization of buffer species, resulting in smaller pH shifts upon freezing. The presence of sucrose and mannitol at concentrations above 3 moles per mole of dibasic sodium phosphate completely prevented salt crystallization. In this case, the pH change upon freezing was only 0.5 units, which was attributed to the effect of freeze concentration.

Other pharmaceutically relevant buffer systems have not been as well characterized as phosphate with respect to pH changes accompanying freezing. Larsen (13) reported that acetate, citrate, glycine, and Tris show only small pH shifts upon freezing.

There are no published studies which examine the significance of pH shifts on quality attributes of freeze-dried formulations of small molecules. However, Costantino et al. (14) reported that lyophilized organic compounds containing protein functional groups (amino-, carboxylic-, and phenolic-) exhibit "pH memory"; that is, the ionization state of the solid, as reflected by the FTIR spectrum, is similar to that of the aqueous solution from which the compound was freeze dried.

Regardless of the lack of published data linking pH changes with freezing to loss of quality attributes of freeze-dried small molecules, the potential for significant changes exists, particularly with phosphate buffers. It is good formulation practice to minimize the concentration of buffers used, or eliminate them entirely if they are not needed.

C. Vitrification During Freezing

Many solutes do not crystallize from a freeze-concentrated aqueous solution. Modification of the temperature/composition phase diagram to illustrate this behavior was first suggested by MacKenzie (15) and termed a *supplemented* phase diagram, whereas other investigators have used the term *state* diagram (16). A supplemented phase diagram for sucrose/water is illustrated in Figure 5. The freezing curve and the solubility curve are the same as presented in Figure 4 for sodium chloride/water, and the composition of the freeze concentrate is given by the freezing curve; however, sucrose is kinetically inhibited from crystallizing at T_{eut} Instead, the composition of the freeze concentrate continues to be represented by the dotted line, which represents a supercooled liquid. Ice crystallization continues, and the freeze-concentrated system becomes more viscous, until ice crystal growth (on a practical time scale) ceases and the degree of freeze concentration of the solute reaches a maximum. The glass transition of the maximally freeze-concentrated solution is designated as T_g'. Note that T_g' is a point on the *glass transition curve*, which represents a reversible change of state between a viscous liquid and a rigid, glassy system. The viscosity of this freeze concentrate changes by three or four orders of magnitude over a temperature range of a few degrees in the region of the glass transition. The point T_{gs} represents the glass transition of amorphous sucrose (about 65°C), and

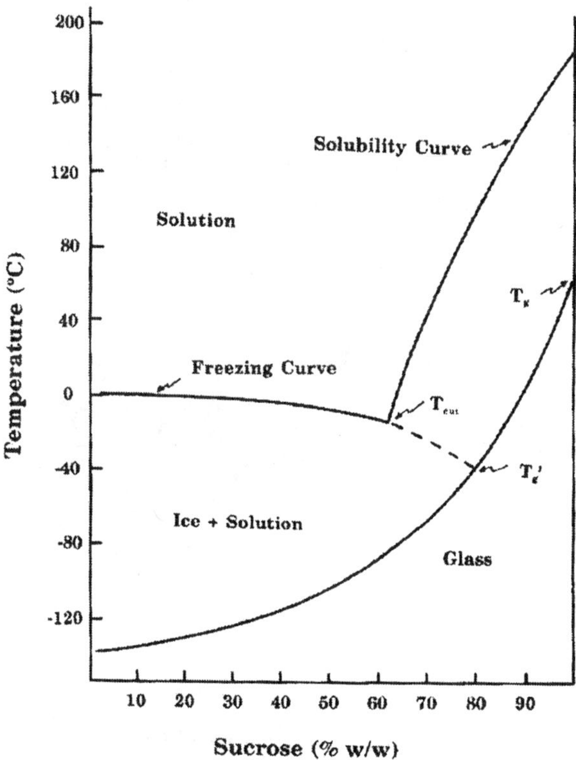

Figure 5 State diagram for sucrose.

the point T_{gw} represents the glass transition temperature of amorphous solid water, at about −135°C.

The glass transition curve in Figure 5 illustrates that only a small amount of water in amorphous sucrose causes a sharp drop in the glass transition temperature of the solid. Thus, water is acting as a *plasticizer*. The point designated as T_g', the glass transition temperature of the maximally freeze-concentrated solute, corresponds to about 20% water/80% sucrose. This glass transition is generally accepted as the physical basis for *collapse* in freeze drying. Collapse is caused by viscous flow of the freeze-concentrated solute on the time scale of freeze drying, with resultant loss of the microstructure which was established by freezing, decreased surface area of the freeze-dried solid, and loss of pharmaceutical elegance. Thus, the onset of collapse represents the maximum allowable product temperature during freeze drying of systems in which the solute(s) remain amorphous during freezing.

D. Differences in Freeze-Drying Behavior Between Amorphous and Crystalline Solutes

If the solute crystallizes completely during freezing, the microstructure of the system is illustrated by the sketch in Figure 6, where the interstitial material between the ice crystals consists of an intimate mixture of small crystals of ice and solute. For an amorphous solute, the interstitial material consists of a solid solution of solute and unfrozen water. For a eutectic-forming system, the upper product temperature limit during primary drying is the eutectic melting temperature, whereas for an amorphous system the upper temperature limit is the collapse temperature. While eutectic melting

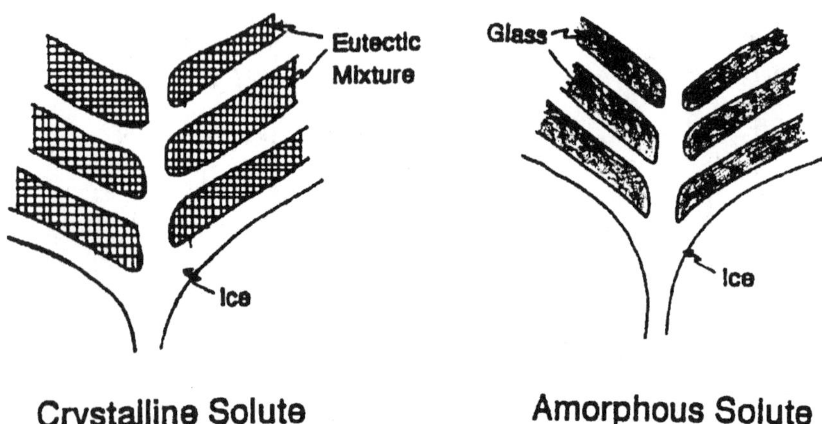

Figure 6 Cartoon of amorphous vs. crystalline solutes.

temperatures of ice/inorganic salt mixtures can be quite low (the eutectic melting temperature of calcium chloride/water is about –52°C), eutectic melting temperatures of ice and most organic compounds are in the range of just below 0°C to perhaps –12°C. These relatively high melting temperatures allow maintenance of high product temperatures during primary drying, resulting in a more efficient drying process. Collapse temperatures are generally much lower than eutectic melting temperatures. Collapse temperatures below –40°C are not uncommon, particularly for protein formulations containing sugars as protective solutes in combination with added salts. Small molecules that do not crystallize from a freezing aqueous system can also have low collapse temperatures. Given that most production-scale freeze-dryers are unable to consistently maintain product temperatures below about –40°C, freeze drying is not feasible for all formulations. Even if the product temperature can be controlled at temperatures below –40°C, the vapor pressure of ice at such low temperatures—and therefore the driving force for freeze drying, is relatively low. Since the vapor pressure of ice at –40°C is only 0.096 Torr, the system pressure must be kept well below this pressure, which can be a significant demand on the vacuum system. As a general formulation guideline, formulations with collapse temperatures of –40°C or lower should be avoided.

As illustrated in Figure 6, nearly all water is present as ice (either pre-eutectic or eutectic) when the solute crystallizes. As the sublimation front moves through the frozen system, all of the ice can be removed by a process of *bulk flow*, or transport of water vapor from a region of high pressure to lower pressure, through the porous bed of dried solid. There is essentially no secondary drying. For the sucrose/water system, representing an amorphous solute, there is 20% water associated with sucrose, which must be removed during secondary drying. This water must be removed by a process of *diffusion*, or flow by molecular motion from a region of high concentration to a region of lower concentration. This combination of a significant amount of water to be removed by secondary drying and the slower transport mechanism often means that secondary drying is a significant part of the total drying time needed.

Of course, it is common (and often desireable) to have both amorphous and crystalline phases present in a freeze-dried formulation. This is particularly relevant to freeze-dried proteins, where the lyoprotectant is present in the amorphous state, and another component, such as glycine or mannitol, is present as a crystalline solid in order to impart mechanical integrity and pharmaceutical elegance to the lyophilized solid.

E. Other Types of Freezing Behavior

In addition to eutectic crystallization and glass formation (vitrification), there are other types of freezing behavior which may be observed

(Fig. 3). A metastable glass may form which, with subsequent heating, undergoes crystallization. The most common example of metastable glass formation is mannitol, which crystallizes when heated above its T_g' (see discussion of thermal analysis below). This type of behavior is the basis for *annealing* during freeze drying (see below), which refers to warming the product after an initial freezing step, generally to a temperature above T_g' but below the onset of melting, holding for a period of perhaps 1–4 hr, then cooling the material again before starting drying.

Mannitol is one of the most commonly used excipients in freeze-dried formulations; however, the formulation scientist should be aware of problems associated with the use of mannitol. It is well known that mannitol is associated with vial breakage during freeze drying. This appears to be related to crystallization of mannitol from the metastable amorphous state. Vial breakage associated with mannitol can be minimized by keeping the depth of fill in a vial to no more than about 30% of the overflow capacity of the vial. The thermal expansion coefficient of the glass, the thermal history of freezing, and defects in the glass are also significant factors affecting vial breakage.

States of matter which have degrees of order intermediate between amorphous and crystalline are called liquid crystals. Liquid crystals are broadly categorized as *thermotropic*, which are formed by heating, and *lyotropic*, which are formed by addition of solvent to a solid. Compounds which form liquid crystals are generally surface active, and the liquid crystal represents a more ordered structure than a micelle. These higher ordered structures are a result of freeze concentration, and may be either lamellar or rod-shaped. There have been few reports of lyotropic liquid crystal formation in aqueous solutions of drugs, and even fewer which are relevant to freeze drying. Powell et al. (17) reported peptide liquid crystal formation by the luteinizing hormone releasing hormone deterelix and the effect of added salts on thermodynamic stability of the liquid crystal phase. Vadas et al. (18) reported that a leukotriene D_4 receptor antagonist forms lyotropic liquid crystalline phases when lyophilized from aqueous solution. Bogardus (19) studied the phase equilibria of nafcillin sodium-water and reported a lamellar mesophase in aqueous solutions containing more than 55% nafcillin sodium. Milton and Nail (20) extended this work by characterizing the low-temperature DSC thermogram of frozen aqueous solutions of nafcillin as well as the freeze-dried solid. Freeze drying of frozen systems containing lyotropic mesophases appears to result in a unique x-ray diffractogram consisting of a single sharp peak at low angle (less than about 5°) 2θ in addition to the "halo" which is characteristic of amorphous solids. Herman et al. (21) reported a similar x-ray powder diffraction pattern in methylprednisolone sodium succinate. The influence of liquid crystal formation during freezing on critical quality attributes of freeze-dried products is a subject which remains largely unexplored.

1. Materials Characterization

Minimizing empiricism in formulation and process development for freeze-dried products requires characterization of the formulation intended to be freeze dried. The result of such characterization should be information on the upper product temperature limit during the primary drying stage of freeze drying, knowledge of the physical state of the solute(s), and an assessment of the degree to which the characteristics of the frozen system are affected by changes in composition of the formulation.

In addition to characterizing frozen systems intended to be freeze dried, it is important to characterize the freeze-dried product. This includes determination of the physical state of the dried product; that is, crystalline, partially crystalline, or amorphous. It may also include identification of the polymorph of a crystallizing component which exhibits polymorphism and determination of whether the crystal form observed is affected by changes in formulation and processing conditions. For amorphous systems, the glass transition temperature of the amorphous solid, as well as the extent to which T_g changes with residual moisture, may be a critical attribute of the product with regard to both physical and chemical stability.

2. Thermal Analysis

Thermal transitions which are commonly observed in frozen systems are illustrated in Figure 7 where, for the sake of this discussion, a deflection upward indicates an endothermic transition. The glass transition is a shift in the baseline toward higher heat capacity. Crystallization during the DSC experiment is observed as an exothermic event, and eutectic melting is an endothermic transition which preceeds the melting of ice.

Since aqueous systems are prone to supercooling, the most common practice is to record the thermogram during the heating cycle following freezing of the sample. However, the cooling rate of an aqueous solution can have a significant influence on the thermogram recorded during subsequent heating of the sample, particularly for solutes which tend to crystallize during the time course of freezing. The term "critical cooling rate" usually refers to a cooling rate above which crystallization of solute during freezing is prevented. For example, at cooling rates less than about 2°C/min, crystallization of mannitol from a freezing solution takes place during the cooling cycle whereas, at faster cooling rates, crystallization is inhibited. In this case, complex thermal behavior is observed in the subsequent heating thermogram, which consists of a glass transition, followed by a melting endotherm and an exotherm indicating crystallization of the solute (22).

Heating rates used for thermal analysis are typically 5–10°C/min, but it is often useful to carry out experiments at lower rates in order to maximize resolution of thermal events taking place at nearly the same temperature. The choice of a heating rate for conventional DSC involves a trade-off

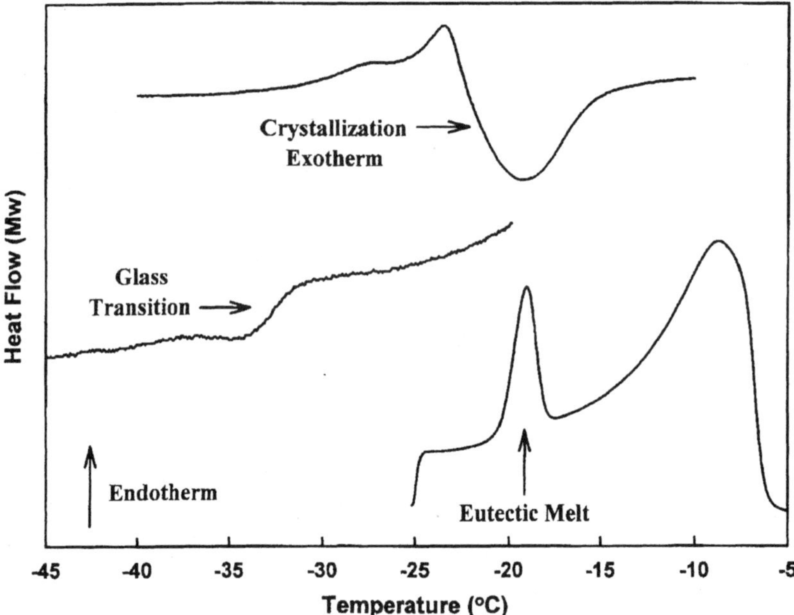

Figure 7 Thermal transitions in frozen systems.

between sensitivity and resolution, where sensitivity refers to the ability to detect a given transition, and resolution is the ability to separate two thermal events taking place at nearly the same temperature. In thermal analysis of frozen systems, particularly those in which the solute crystallizes, resolution is often a more important issue because the eutectic melting temperature may very close to the melting temperature of ice. An example of the use of slow heating rates to maximize resolution is shown in Figure 8 for the glycine–water system. In this case, three thermal events—readily apparent at a very slow heating rate—could be interpreted as simply the melting of ice if only rapid heating rates are used. In the glycine/water system, the complex thermal behavior in the region of the melting endotherm of ice arises from polymorphism of glycine.

For detection of glass transitions in both frozen systems and in freeze-dried solids, sensitivity may be more important than resolution, since glass transitions are often difficult to detect. In this case, relatively rapid heating rates are recommended. However, it should be remembered that heating rate influences the observed glass transition temperature, where faster heating rates cause observation of the transition at higher temperatures. For example, for a frozen solution of 10% dextran, the observed midpoint of the glass transition increases from about –13.5°C to about –9.5°C as the heating rate is increased from 2°C to 20°C/min.

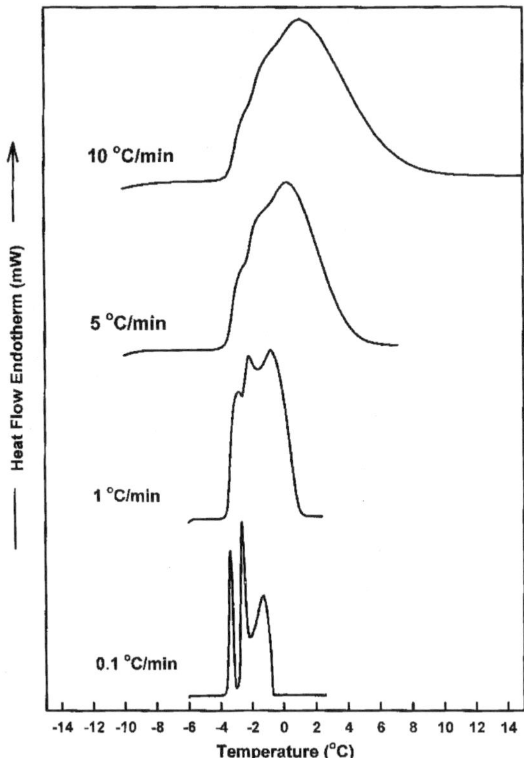

Figure 8 Effect of warming rate on the DSC thermograms of glycine/water in the melting region of ice.

While the transitions illustrated in Figure 7 are easily interpreted, uncertainties often arise. For many organic compounds which crystallize from freezing aqueous solution, the eutectic melt occurs very close to the melting temperature of ice. In this case, the eutectic melting endotherm may be partially, or completely, obscured by the ice melting endotherm even at very slow heating rates. Examples are the ice/mannitol and ice/dibasic sodium phosphate eutectic melts at about –1°C and –0.5°C, respectively. While resolution of such closely spaced endotherms is enhanced by slow heating rates, it is by no means assured.

Glass transitions, both in frozen systems and in freeze-dried solids, can be difficult to detect. This may be caused by the small heat capacity change associated with the glass transition, a broad glass transition region, or both. Interpretation is made more uncertain by baseline drift or other noise. In addition, other thermal events at temperatures close to the glass transition, such as enthalpy recovery or crystallization, may disguise the heat capacity change associated with the glass transition. Sensitivity to such transitions is enhanced by rapid heating rates. For thermal analysis of frozen solutions, it may be useful to increase the solute concentration above the intended formulation concentration in order to maximize sensitivity, particularly for glass transitions. As the state diagram predicts, the glass transition temperature is essentially independent of solute concentration. Her and Nail (22) have demonstrated this effect for solutions of lactose and related compounds.

For thermal analysis of frozen systems, it is important to remember that the time scales of the thermal analysis experiment and the freeze drying process are different by orders of magnitude. This is particularly important with respect to solute crystallization, since solutes that do not crystallize appreciably during thermal analysis may crystallize during freezing and freeze drying. Isothermal calorimetry using the DSC; that is, holding a constant temperature and monitoring heat flow, can be a useful method for monitoring solute crystallization over a longer time than conventional scanning calorimetry.

Thermal analysis of frozen solutions is a relatively small subset of the thermal analysis literature, most of which is directed toward thermal analysis of polymer systems. As a result, some phenomena which are commonly observed are poorly understood, including lyotropic liquid crystal formation during freezing and apparent multiple glass transitions in frozen systems. The glass transition region in "frozen" solutions of solutes that do not crystallize during freezing commonly appears as a multiple glass transition, particularly in concentrated solutions. Solutions of disaccharides are a common example of this behavior. The glass transition which is commonly reported at pharmaceutically relevant concentrations, perhaps 5–10%, is in the range of –32 to –35°C. Examination of higher concentrations, however, reveals another transition at a lower temperature. This apparent multiple glass transition has given rise to uncertainty regarding both the physical significance of both of these transitions and assignment of the T_g' temperature for the purpose of characterizing frozen solutions of amorphous solutes. The bulk of the evidence supports the conclusion that the lower-temperature transition is the glass transition of the maximally freeze-concentrated solution. Ablett et al. (23) reported that, in sucrose and glycerol solutions which are sufficiently concentrated that ice formation is inhibited, a single glass transition is observed at the lower temperature. However, more data are needed for a wide variety of solutes in order to better understand the physical significance of apparent multiple glass transitions, particularly in frozen system.

3. Optical Microscopy

Optical microscopy using a special low-temperature stage which can be evacuated to operate at pressures representative of freeze drying allows direct observation of materials during freezing and freeze drying, generally under a low magnification of 50–100X. Experimentally, freeze drying microscopy is usually carried out by placing a small quantity, perhaps 10 μL, of sample on a cover slip, freezing the sample, evacuating the system, then systematically varying the sample temperature and observing the resulting morphology in the dried material. This technique is particularly useful for measuring the *collapse* temperature in freeze drying, which may be different from glass transition temperatures measured by thermal analysis. Glass transitions are measured on closed systems, whereas collapse is a dynamic phenomenon taking place during freeze drying. An example of collapse phenomena is shown in the photomicrograph in Figure 9a. In addition to collapse phenomena in amorphous systems, microscopic observation is useful for studying the influence of formulation composition on ice morphology; that is, dendritic vs. spherulitic ice. Dendritic ice is normally observed; however, at high solute concentrations, spherulitic ice can form. The significance of ice morphology is that, when dendritic ice forms, open channels are created by prior sublimation of ice, providing a relatively low resistance to transfer of water vapor through the partially dried solids. Spherulitic ice, on the other hand, is associated with a high resistance to mass transfer, and inefficient freeze drying.

Another application of freeze drying microscopy is for observation of secondary, or solute, crystallization during freezing. The crystallization of nafcillin sodium during annealing at –5°C is shown in Figure 9b. The significance of crystallization of both drugs and excipients is discussed in more detail below.

F. The Influence of Physical State of Drugs on Stability

The most important factor affecting the chemical and physical stability of a drug as a freeze-dried solid is the physical state of the drug; that is, whether the drug is crystalline, amorphous, or a mixture of crystalline and amorphous forms. Amorphous solids are characterized by a glass transition temperature, T_g, which represents a reversible change in state from a solid below T_g to a fluid which exhibits viscous flow over the time frame of interest above T_g. For stability assessment, the time frame of interest is the duration of the stability study, whether at stress conditions or at the anticipated storage temperature. Viscous flow during storage can, for example, result in cake shrinkage or even collapse, with subsequent loss of pharmaceutical elegance, increased reconstitution time, and perhaps increased rates of degradation. Storage at temperatures well below T_g is generally adequate to assure physical stability of the product, but does not assure adequate chemical stability, since significant relevant molecular mobility may exist below T_g. As a result of its higher internal energy, the amorphous state has enhanced thermodynamic properties relative to the crystalline state; for example, solubility, vapor pressure, dissolution rate, and chemical reactivity. For this reason, the amorphous state tends to spontaneously crystallize at temperatures above T_g.

(a)

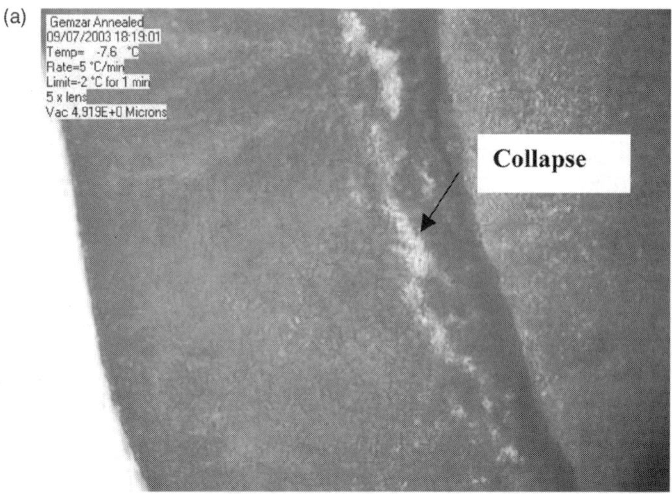

(b)

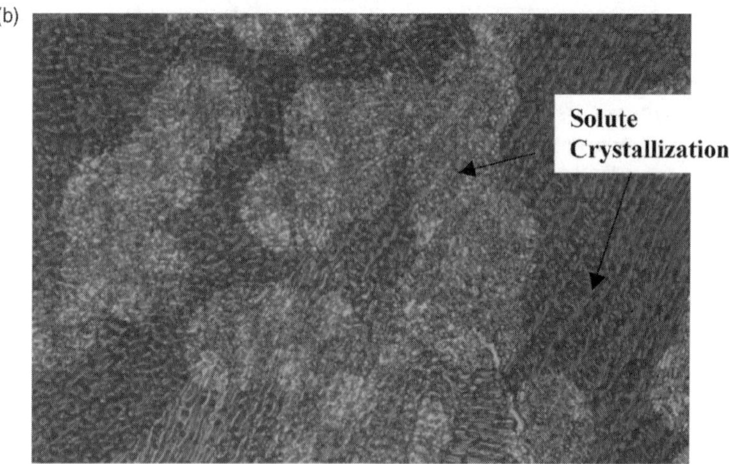

Figure 9 (a) Freeze drying photomicrograph illustrating collapse in a predominantly amorphous system and (b) Freeze drying photomicrograph illustrating crystallization of nafcillin during annealing.

Before proceeding further, it is appropriate to discuss some aspects of molecular mobility of amorphous solids as it affects stability. The temperature dependence of molecular motion in amorphous systems is described by the empirical Vogel–Tammann-Fulcher (VTF) equation:

$$\tau = \tau_0 \exp(B/T - T_0)$$

where τ is the molecular relaxation time, T is the absolute temperature, τ_0 and B are constants, and T_0 is the temperature at which the configurational entropy of the system reaches zero. T_0 is also known as the Kauzman temperature, and is believed to be roughly 50°C below the experimentally measured glass transition temperature, depending on the type of glass formed (see discussion below). Note that, when T_0 is zero, the VTF equation reduces to the Arrhenius equation, where B is analogous to the activation energy.

Glasses have been classified as "strong" or "fragile" depending on the temperature dependence of the activation energy for molecular motion in the region of T_g (24). Strong glasses exhibit an Arrhenius temperature dependence of molecular mobility, have small changes in heat capacity at T_g, and broad glass transition regions (when they can be detected at all). Proteins are good examples of strong glass formers. Fragile glasses, on the other hand, undergo much larger changes in heat capacity at T_g and have narrower T_g ranges. The molecular mobility around T_g of a fragile glass is much more temperature dependent than that described by the Arrhenius equation—the molecular mobility may change by an order of magnitude with a 10°K change in temperature, as opposed to roughly a factor of two over the same temperature range for mobility which is described by the Arrhenius relationship. The values of B and T_0 in the VTF equation are related to glass fragility. Fragile glasses are characterized by low values of B (<10), and ($T_g - T_0$) are generally less than 50. Strong glasses, on the other hand, have high values of B (>100), and ($T_g - T_0$) values are usually greater than 50. Another method for estimating the fragility of a glassy system is simply the ratio of the melting temperature to the glass transition temperature (T_m/T_g, in K), where strong glasses have ratios greater than 1.5 (25). The relevance of "strong" and "fragile" glass formation to stress testing of freeze-dried pharmaceutical solids is an area for which much more research is needed.

Dramatic differences in stability between crystalline drugs and the same drug in its amorphous form was demonstrated by Pikal et al. (26) for potassium penicillin G, cephamandole nafate, and cephamandole sodium, where the rate of degradation of the amorphous form was approximately one order of magnitude greater than that of the corresponding crystalline form, even when the amorphous form contained less than 0.1% residual moisture. This study also demonstrated large differences in stability between amorphous forms with different moisture levels. Arrhenius plots for amorphous solids were nonlinear, with activation energy decreasing with increasing temperature. Based on the discussion above, a nonlinear Arrhenius plot for solid-state stability of an amorphous system is not surprising. The curvature of the Arrhenius plot would be expected to increase as the fragility of the glass increases. This has important implications for stress testing, since incorrect predictions of shelf life at the anticipated storage temperature would be made based on stress testing data. It was further noted in this study that the energy of spray-dried amorphous drugs was less than that of the freeze-dried solid by about 2 kcal/mole. It was postulated that the spray-dried drug represents an annealed form of the amorphous drug. In this study, discoloration of the amorphous drug could be detected visually well before loss of potency could be detected by a chemical assay. The glass transition of the amorphous solid was not measured in this study, but was estimated using the general relationship that $T_g/T_m = 0.6$ (25).

Duddu and Weller (27) measured the stability of a freeze-dried aspirin formulation in the region of T_g and pointed out the significant error introduced by measuring the degradation rate above T_g and extrapolating to temperatures below T_g. For a system with a T_g of about 36°C, extrapolation of 40°, 45°, and 50°C data yielded a predicted rate constant of 0.009 day^{-1} at 22°C, whereas the observed value was 0.003 day^{-1}.

Of course, the influence of glass transition-associated mobility on rates of reaction below T_g depends on the type of reaction involved. The nonenzymatic browning reaction between xylose and lysine in a carboxymethylcellulose/lactose matrix has been reported to essentially cease below T_g, perhaps because translational motion of the reactants is needed in order for this reaction to occur to an appreciable extent (28).

Guo and coworkers (29) examined the chemical stability of lyophilized quinapril HCl as a function of initial solution pH. Lyophilization of different quinapril solutions produces mixtures of amorphous quinapril and its neutralized form, with glass transition values between the T_g values of quinapril and neutralized quinapril. As the fraction of quinapril increases the rate of chemical degradation increases relative to that of quinapril HCl alone. This is most likely caused by the plasticizing effects of neutralized quinapril.

Carstensen and Morris (30) studied chemical stability of amorphous indomethacin, largely to determine whether solid-state stability can be accurately predicted based on measurements of stability in the "molten" state; that is, above the glass transition temperature. The difference in decomposition rate between crystalline (MP 162°C) and amorphous drug at 145°C was approximately one order of magnitude. Arrhenius plots of the decomposition rate of molten solid and the amorphous solid were linear, indicating that chemical stability of the amorphous solid can be predicted by measurement of decomposition rate in the molten state. This finding is only consistent with "strong glass" behavior of amorphous indomethacin. Decomposition of crystalline indomethacin did not follow first-order kinetics, but rather a Bawn decomposition model (an S-shaped plot of fraction of drug remaining vs. time), which follows the equation $\ln(1 - ax) = -(Ak_s)\,t$, where x is the fraction decomposed and a is an iterant parameter that imposes linearity and zero intercept on the data. This underscores the importance of understanding that the kinetics of decomposition of amorphous and crystalline solids can be quite different, and a detailed study of both mechanism and kinetics of decomposition is needed in order to make meaningful stability predictions from stress testing data.

Ball (31) studied the solid-state hydrolysis of single crystals of aspirin, and also observed S-shaped plots of fraction decomposed vs. time, but found that the kinetic data fit an Avrami–Erofeyev model involving nucleation at dislocations in the crystal lattice.

The thermally induced solid-state methyl transfer of tetraglycine methyl ester was studied by Shalaev et al. (32) when the drug is subjected to lyophilization or milling relative to a highly crystalline control. Freeze drying or milling resulted in significantly reduced crystallinity, as expected, and significantly enhanced reactivity. Kinetic curves for lyophilized material were monotonic and could be treated by a first order model, whereas kinetic curves for milled material were biphasic, with a fast initial phase followed by a slower phase. Reactivity of the crystalline phase was different between milled and freeze-dried material, with a reaction rate almost two orders of magnitude greater in the freeze-dried material than in milled samples.

G. Influence of Formulation and Processing Factors on Physical State of the Drug

The physical state of a drug in a freeze-dried solid is influenced not only by the tendency to crystallize from a freezing solution, but also by processing conditions and by other components of the formulation. From a processing standpoint, the most important parameter is probably the thermal history of freezing. From a formulation perspective, the concentration of drug relative to excipients influences the ability of the drug to crystallize on the time frame of freezing and freeze drying, as well as the nature of other formulation components.

H. Thermal History of Freezing

It is important to distinguish between shelf temperature ramp rate, or cooling rate, and freezing rate. Shelf temperature ramp rate refers, of course, to the rate of change of temperature of the surface of the freeze-dryer shelf. Freezing rate, on the other hand, refers to the time between the nucleation of ice and the completion of the freezing process; that is, the time at which no further changes in the microstructure of the system or the amount of unfrozen water remaining would be observed, at least on a practical time frame. Alan MacKenzie, in a verbal communication to the author, has stated that shelf freezing of vials of pharmaceutical product is paradoxical—"slow is fast, and fast is slow." The first part of the MacKenzie paradox—slow is fast—means that a slow shelf temperature ramp rate can promote fast freezing by favoring both a high degree of supercooling and a uniform temperature throughout the volume of the supercooled liquid. This combination of maximum supercooling and uniform temperature means that, once ice nucleates, freezing proceeds rapidly. The "fast is slow" part of the paradox means that, for example, placing vials on shelves that have been precooled to a low temperature, perhaps –40°C or so, could mean that ice crystals form in product solution at the bottom of the fill volume well before thermal equilibrium is established throughout the fill volume. In essence, the solution at the bottom of the vial is "seeded" with ice, which means that only minimum supercooling takes place, and the rate of freezing at such a low level of supercooling is slow relative to a highly supercooled system. Of course, the magnitude of this effect would depend on the depth of liquid filled into a vial. That is, the greater the fill depth, the longer it would take to establish thermal equilibrium, and the greater the expected "fast is slow" effect. While this paradox is useful in underscoring the distinction between cooling rate and freezing rate, it lacks support by published experimental data.

A sometimes important difference between the freeze drying of proteins and the freeze drying of small molecules is that quality attributes of freeze-dried protein formulations are more often affected in measurable ways by differences in thermal history of freezing relative to small-molecule formulations. However, differences in quality attributes of small molecule products caused by differences in thermal history of freezing has been shown to occur. Chongprasert and coworkers (1) investigated the photostability of freeze-dried pentamidine isethionate produced at different concentrations of drug in the initial solution as well as different thermal histories of freezing. Polymorph screening revealed three anhydrates, designated A, B, and C, as well as a trihydrate (Fig. 10). Form C is a high-temperature form, and cannot be produced under lyophilization conditions. At concentrations of drug of 4% (w/v) or less, Form A is produced regardless of the freezing method used. At concentrations of 10%, the crystal forms observed are a function of the freezing method. The freezing methods examined were (1) cooling on the shelf at 2°C and holding for three hours prior to decreasing the shelf temperature to –45°C, (2) directly cooling on the shelf from room temperature to –45°C, and (3) quench-cooling in liquid nitrogen. Results showed that form A, form B, or a mixture of both forms are present in the freeze-dried solid depending on whether the trihydrate crystallizes during freezing or not. Form B can only be produced by dehydration of the trihydrate at low temperature. Photostability studies over a period of 2 weeks at 1000 ft-candles demonstrated that form B remained a white powder whereas form A turned distinctly pink after about 1 week. The results of the study underscore the point that validation studies to identify critical process variables should include thermal history of freezing, even for small molecule formulations.

Yarwood et al. (33) investigated the influence of cooling rate, initial concentration of solute, and fill volume on physical form and chemical stability of sodium ethacrynate. The freezing protocol consisted of ramping from room temperature to –25 C over four hours vs. placing vials on shelves

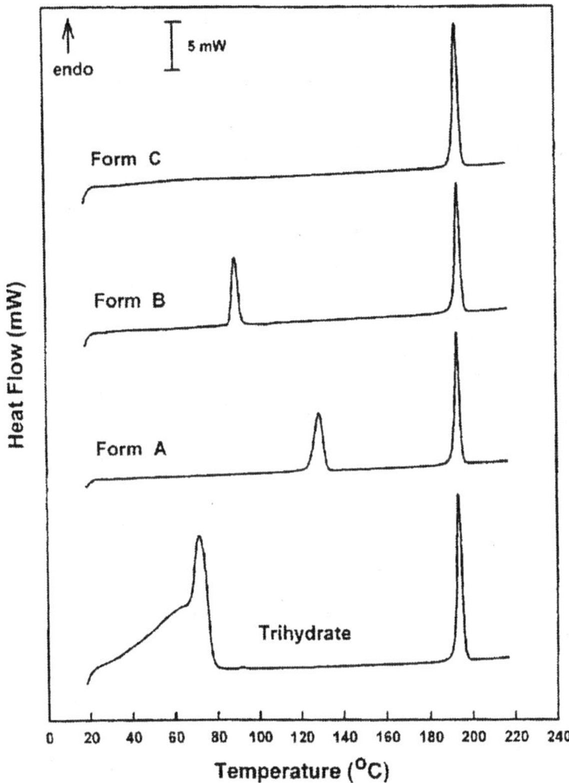

Figure 10 DSC thermograms of different crystal forms of pentamidine isethionate.

precooled to about –50 C. Drug concentration varied from 0.5% to 4% (w/v), and fill volume varied from 0.5 to 3 milliliters. Stress testing of freeze-dried solids was carried out at 60 C. Rapidly cooled samples were amorphous to x-rays, whereas slowly cooled samples were crystalline. Striking differences were observed in stability of the drug, depending on physical state. For crystalline sodium ethacrynate, 95% of the drug remained after 90 days. Amorphous drug prepared from a 1% solution at a fill volume of 0.5 mL degraded by more than half after 60 days. While no mention was made in this study of either T_g' or T_g (the glass transition temperature of the freeze-dried solid), it was noted that some samples "liquefied to produce a clear oil" at the stress testing condition, which indicates that the test was carried out above T_g of the amorphous solid. Apparently, slowly decreasing the shelf temperature results in slow freezing, which is not consistent with the above paradox. However, thermal analysis data indicate little tendency of this system to supercool, and the above paradox assumes significant supercooling. Stress testing data do show that higher fill volumes result in a slower effective rate of freezing as reflected by the relative quantity of amorphous material. For a starting solution concentration of 1% and a fill volume of 0.5 mL, only 42% of drug remained after 60 days at 60°C. For a fill volume of 3 mL and the same starting drug concentration, 79% of intact drug remained after the same time interval. This is consistent with slower freezing of higher fill volumes resulting in a higher percentage of crystalline material. Higher concentrations of drug, as expected, favor crystallization. Increasing from 1% drug to 4% favors crystallization, as reflected by 79% of drug remaining after 60 days at 60 C vs. 42% remaining for freeze-dried solid resulting from a 1% solution.

I. Residual Moisture Effects

In studying the relationship between T_g and stability, it is important to recognize that water can serve not only as a plasticizer of the amorphous phase, but also as a reactant. Bell and Hageman (34) used a freeze-dried preparation of aspartame in different molecular weights of poly(vinylpyrrolidone) in order to address the question of which is more important—the glass transition temperature or residual water activity. The solid-state degradation of aspartame via rearrangement to a diketopiperazine was measured at 25°C after equilibrating the model formulations containing different molecular weights of PVP at different relative humidities. It was found that reaction rates at constant water activity, but different T_g values, were not significantly different. However, rates at similar $(T - T_g)$ values, but different water activities, were significantly different. Therefore, in this system, water activity is more important than $(T - T_g)$. Of course, these data cannot be generalized beyond this system. The relative importance of water activity and glass transition-associated mobility would depend on the mechanism of degradation.

A subtle aspect of stability analysis of freeze-dried products in vials with rubber stoppers is the tendency for water vapor to be transferred from the stopper to the solid during storage. Representative data for residual moisture as a function of time at different temperatures are shown in Figure 11. As expected, the residual moisture level increases more rapidly at higher temperature, but the plateau level is independent of temperature as equilibrium is established between the freeze-dried solid and the stopper. The extent to which this is observed depends on several factors. First, the nature of the rubber stopper formulation affects the diffusivity of water in the rubber. Second, the processing of the stopper can affect the level of residual moisture present. It is not uncommon for extended drying of the stopper to be necessary to minimize residual moisture. Finally, the mass of the freeze-dried solid determines the extent to which the percent residual moisture is affected by water vapor transfer from the stopper, where large cakes may be relatively unaffected by the small amount of water vapor that is

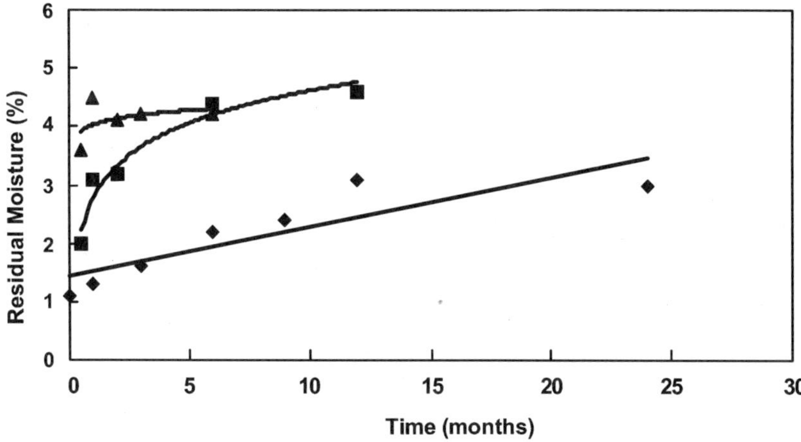

Figure 11 Changes in residual moisture during storage of freeze-dried solids due to water vapor transfer from the stopper at different storage temperatures: 5°C (diamonds), 25°C (squares), and 40°C (triangles).

transferred from the stopper. Thus, it is important to monitor residual moisture level in the product during a stability study to determine the magnitude of this effect.

J. Excipient Effects on Drug Stability in Freeze-Dried Dosage Forms

Crystallization of excipients from freeze-dried solids can affect stability of drugs as freeze-dried solids. Herman et al. (21) studied the solid-state stability of methylprednisolone sodium succinate in the presence of the bulking agents mannitol and lactose. Comparative stability data at 40°C are shown in Figure 12, where the rate of appearance of the hydrolysis product, methylprednisolone, is considerably faster for mannitol than for lactose, despite similar residual moisture levels. X-ray diffraction analysis at intervals during the stability study shows that the freeze-dried solid containing mannitol is initially amorphous, but that mannitol crystallizes during storage in the solid state (Fig. 13). The formulation containing lactose as a bulking agent remains amorphous throughout the stability study. The most likely explanation for this observation is that mannitol crystallization affects the distribution of residual moisture in the solid; that is, as mannitol crystallizes, it excludes water from the crystal lattice, thereby increasing the level of residual moisture in the remaining amorphous phase and increasing the rate of hydrolysis. This effect is enhanced by a small, but significant, increase in residual moisture during storage due to the transfer of water vapor from the rubber stopper, where this additional water is localized in the amorphous phase, thereby further increasing the water activity in the microenvironment of the drug.

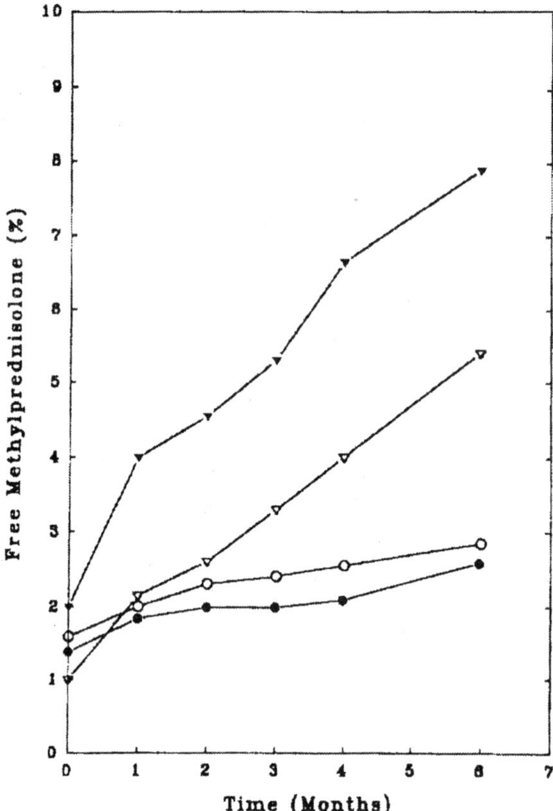

Figure 12 Rate of appearance of methylprednisolone, the hydrolysis product of methylprednisolone sodium succinate during stress testing at 40°C: control using 250 mg drug per vial with no excipient (closed circles), 40 mg of drug in 210 mg lactose (open circles), 125 mg drug in 125 mg mannitol (open triangles), and 40 mg drug in 210 mg mannitol (closed triangles).

Kirsch et al. (35) studied the effects of the excipients mannitol and lactose as well as residual moisture on the stability of lyophilized (R,R) formoterol l-tartrate under thermally stressed conditions. Although the mannitol formulations contained less than 1% residual moisture, degradation rates in mannitol were 1.3–20 times higher than rates observed for lactose formulations. At high levels of residual moisture, acetate significantly increased the degradation rate. A mechanistic interpretation of these findings was not given.

The solid-state oxidation of a freeze-dried cyclic hexapeptide was examined by Dubost et al. (36). The degradation product was identified as a benzaldehyde derivative resulting from oxidative deamidation of an

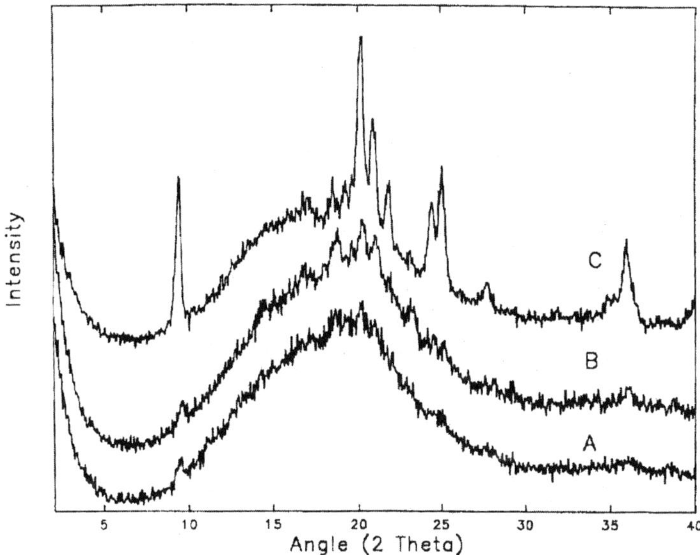

Figure 13 X-ray powder diffractograms of methylprednisolone sodium succinate in mannitol during stress testing at 40°C, showing crystallization of mannitol during storage: (A) initial freeze-dried powder; (B) two months and (C) six months.

aminomethyl phenylalanine moiety. The extent of formation of the oxidation product was influenced by the amount of mannitol used as an excipient in the formulation. This effect was attributed to reducing sugar impurities in the mannitol.

Shalaev et al. (37) examined the influence of citric acid on the acid-catalyzed inversion of sucrose in the freeze-dried solid state. Even with less than 0.1% residual moisture, the colyophilization of sucrose with acidic substances can produce reducing sugars capable of further reaction with other formulation components that are susceptible to such reactions.

The influence of surface active agents on the crystallinity of lyophilized diltiazem hydrochloride was examined by Seitakari et al. (38). As the concentration of either polysorbate 80 or poloxamer 188 was increased, the crystallinity of freeze-dried diltizem hydrochloride was found to increase.

Oguchi and coworkers examined the decarboxylation behavior of *p*-aminosalicylic acid (PAS) as a freeze-dried solid under thermal stress conditions (80°C) in the presence of the excipients pullulan (a linear polysaccharide which can not form inclusion complexes with PAS) and α-cyclodextrin (39). The solid-state stability was shown to correlate with the fraction of amorphous PAS. Increasing relative amounts of pullulan resulted in higher fractions of amorphous PAS. Rapid freezing (liquid nitrogen) was shown to result in a greater relative amount of amorphous drug, as expected.

Solid-state stability of PAS as a function of molar ratio of α-cyclodexrin (CD) to PAS was complex. At low ratios of CD to PAS, stability decreased because of inhibition of crystallization of PAS during freezing. Higher molar ratios stabilized the PAS because of formation of a crystalline inclusion complex. Again, rapid freezing resulted in higher rates of decarboxylation in the solid state.

Aso et al. (40) examined the molecular mobility of sucrose and polyvinylpyrrolidone in 1:1 lyophilized mixtures by measuring the spin-lattice relaxation times (T_1) of individual carbon atoms by NMR for systems containing residual moisture at varying levels. T_1 of the pyrrolidone ring carbon increased with residual moisture for lyophilized PVP alone. However, the mobility of these carbons did not increase with residual moisture when PVP was colyophilized with sucrose. Similarly, the mobility of sucrose did not increase with water activity as much in sucrose/PVP mixtures as much as in sucrose alone. Inhibition of sucrose crystallization by PVP in the presence of water appears to be linked to the effect of PVP on the molecular mobility of sucrose.

IV. CONCLUSION

Freeze-dried parenteral dosage forms generally offer a pharmaceutically elegant alternative to solution formulations when the drug is unstable in solution. However, it is important to understand that freeze-dried solids are not always physically and chemically stable enough to support a practical shelf life, and that the physical state of a freeze-dried solid is affected by the nature of the solute, by the thermal history of freezing, and by interaction with other components of the formulation. Characterization of the freeze-dried solids in order to determine the physical state; that is, crystalline or amorphous, is an essential element of both formulation and process development. Knowledge of the glass transition temperature of an amorphous solid, as well as how the glass transition is affected by the level of residual moisture, is essential in order to define meaningful stress testing conditions. For crystalline solids, it is important to know whether different polymorphs exist and, if so, the relative stability of these polymorphs. Monitoring for changes in physical state of the solids should be included in stress testing.

REFERENCES

1. Chongprasert S, Bottorff AT, Byrn SR, Williams NA, Nail SLThe effect of process conditions on crystallization of pentamidine isethionate during freeze drying. J Pharm Sci 1997; 87:1155–1160.

2. Hatley RHM, Franks F, Day H, Byth B. Subzero temperature preservation of reactive fluids in the undercooled state. I. The reduction of potassium ferricyanide by potassium cyanide. Biophys Chem 1986a; 24:41–46.
3. Hatley RHM, Franks F, Day H, Byth B. Subzero temperature preservation of reactive fluids in the undercooled state. II. The effect on the oxidation of ascorbic acid of freeze concentration and undercooling. Biophys Chem 1986b; 24:187–192.
4. Schuster M, Aaviksaar A, Haga M, Ullmann U, Jakubke HD. Protease-catalyzed peptide synthesis in frozen aqueous systems: the "freeze concentration" model. Biomed Biochim Acta 1991; 50:S84–S89.
5. Pincock RE, Kiovsky TE. Kinetics of reactions in frozen solutions. J Chem Ed 1966; 43:358–360.
6. Akers MJ, Milton N, Byrn SR, Nail SL. Glycine crystallization during freezing: effects of salt form, pH, and ionic strength. Pharm Res 1995; 12:1457–1461.
7. Chongprasert S, Knopp SA, Nail SL. Characterization of frozen solutions of glycine. J Pharm Sci 2001; 90:1720–1728.
8. Kim AI, Knopp S, Akers MJ, Nail SL. The physical state of mannitol after freeze-drying: effects of mannitol concentration, freezing rate, and a non-crystallizing cosolute. J Pharm Sci 1998; 87:931–935.
9. Yu L, Milton N, Groleau EG, Mishra DS, Vasickle RE. Existence of a mannitol hydrate during freeze-drying and practical implications. J Pharm Sci 1999; 88:196–198.
10. van den Berg L. The effect of addition of sodium and potassium chloride to the reciprocal system: KH_2PO_4–Na_2HPO_4–H_2O on pH and composition during freezing. Arch Biochem Biophys 1959; 84:305–315.
11. van den Berg L, Rose D. Effect of freezing on the pH and composition of sodium and potassium phosphate solutions: the reciprocal system KH_2PO_4–Na_2HPO_4–H_2O. Arch Biochem Biophys 1959; 81:319–329.
12. Gomez G, Pikal MJ, Rodriguez-Hornedo N. Effect of initial buffer composition on pH changes during far-from-equilibrium freezing of sodium phosphate buffer solutions. Pharm Res 2001; 18:90–97.
13. Larsen SS. Studies on stability of drugs in frozen systems. VI. The effect of freezing upon pH for buffered aqueous solutions. Arch Pharm Chem Sci Ed 1973; 1:433–445.
14. Costantino HR, Griebenow K, Langer R, Klibanov AM. On the pH memory of lyophilized compounds containing protein functional groups. Biotech Bioeng 1997; 53:345–348.
15. MacKenzie APThe physico-chemical basis for the freeze drying process. Dev Biol Std 1977; 36:51–67.
16. Blond G, Simatos D, Catte M. Modeling of the water–sucrose state diagram below 0°C. Carbohydr Res 1997; 298:139–145.
17. Powell MF, Fleitman J, Sanders LM, Si VC. Peptide liquid crystals: inverse correlation of kinetic formation and thermodynamic stability in aqueous solution. Pharm Res 1994; 11:1352–1354.
18. Vadas EB, Toma P, Zografi G. Solid-state phase transitions initiated by water vapor sorption of crystalline L-660,711, a leukotriene D_4 receptor antagonist. Pharm Res 1991; 8:148–155.

19. Bogardus JB. Phase equilibria of nafcillin sodium–water. J Pharm Sci 1982; 71:105–109.
20. Milton N, Nail SL. The physical state of nafcillin sodium in frozen aqueous solutions and freeze-dried powders. Pharm Dev Tech 1996; 1:269–277.
21. Herman BD, Sinclair BD, Milton N, Nail SL. The effect of bulking agent on the solid-state stability of freeze-dried methylprednisolone sodium succinate. Pharm Res 1994; 11:1467–1473.
22. Her LM, Nail SL. Measurement of glass transition temperatures of freeze-concentrated solutes by differential scanning calorimetry. Pharm Res 1994; 11: 54–59.
23. Ablett S, Izzard MJ, Lillford PJ. Differential scanning calorimetric study of frozen sucrose and glycerol solutions. J Chem Soc Faraday Trans 1992; 88:789–794.
24. Angell CA. Formation of glasses from liquids and biopolymers. Science 1995; 267:1924–1935.
25. Hancock BC, Zografi G. Characteristics and significance of the amorphons state in pharmaceutical systems. J Pharm Sci 1997; 86:1–21.
26. Pikal MJ, Lukes AL, Lang JE. Thermal decomposition of amorphous β-lactam antibacterials. J Pharm Sci 1977; 66:1312–1316.
27. Duddu SP, Weller K. Importance of glass transition temperature in accelerated stability testing of amorphous solids: case study using a lyophilized aspirin formulation. J Pharm Sci 1996; 85:345–347.
28. Hemminga MA, Roozen H, Walstra P. Molecular motions and the glassy state. In: Blanshard JMV, Lillford PJ, eds. The Glassy State in Foods. Loghborough, Leicestershire: Nottingham University Press, 1993:157–171.
29. Guo Y, Byrn SR, Zografi G. Effects of lyophilization on the physical characteristics and chemical stability of amorphous quinapril hydrochloride. Pharm Res 2000; 17:930–935.
30. Carstensen JT, Morris T. Chemical stability of indomethacin in the solid amorphous and molten states. J Pharm Sci 1993; 82:657–659.
31. Ball MC. Solid-state hydrolysis of aspirin. J Chem Soc Faraday Trans 1994; 90:997–1001.
32. Shalaev EY, Shalaeva M, Byrn SR, Zografi G. Effects of processing on the solid state methyl transfer of tetraglycine methyl ester. Int J Pharm 1997; 152:75–88.
33. Yarwood RJ, Phillips AJ, Collett JH. Processing factors influencing the stability of freeze-dried sodium ethacrynate. Drug Dev Indust Pharm 1986; 12: 2157–2170.
34. Bell LN, Hageman MJ. Differentiating between the effects of water activity and glass transition dependent mobility on a solid state chemical reaction: aspartame degradation. J Agric Food Chem 1994; 42:2398–2401.
35. Kirsch L, Zhang S, Muangsiri W, Redmon M, Wurster D. Development of a lyophilized formulation for (R,R)-formoterol (L)-tartrate. Drug Dev Ind Pharm 2001; 27:89–96.
36. Dubost DC, Kaufman MJ, Zimmerman JA, Bugusky MJ, Pitzenberger SM. Characterization of a solid state reaction product from a lyophilized form of a cyclic hexapeptide: novel example of an excipient-induced oxidation. Pharm Res 1996; 13:1811–1814.

37. Shalaev EY, Lu Q, Shalaeva M, Zografi G. Acid catalyzed inversion of sucrose in the amorphous state at very low levels of residual water. Pharm Res 2000; 17:366–370.
38. Seitakari RL, Tanninen VP, Yliruusi J. Effect of different surface active agents on the crystallinity of lyophilized diltiazem hydrochloride. S.T.P. Pharm Sci 1999; 9:365–369.
39. Oguchi T, Yonemochi E, Yamamoto K, Nakai Y. Freeze-drying of drug-additive binary systems II. Relationship between decarboxylation behavior and molecular states of *p*-aminosalicylic acid.
40. Aso Y, Yoshioka S, Zhang J, Zografi G. Effect of water on the molecular mobility of sucrose and poly(vinylpyrrolidone) in a colyophilized formulation as measured by ^{13}C NMR relaxation time. Chem Pharm Bull 2002; 50:820–826.

10

Photostability Stress Testing

Elisa Fasani and Angelo Albini
Dipartimento di Chimica Organica, Università di Pavia, Pavia, Italy

I. INTRODUCTION

Until recently the problem of photostability of drugs has received little attention in the pharmaceutical industry. Furthermore, the few degradation studies carried out involved a variety of protocols, every single issue being confronted in an independent manner. This contrasts with the general consensus in the determination of drug stability in other respects (e.g., thermal, moisture). In the case of photostability, there are many characteristic variables that can be chosen among a large number of possibilities, such as the light source, the time of exposure, and the sample presentation. Sample presentation is a determining factor since light must be adsorbed to cause an effect, and this depends on the physical state. As an example, the light sources used for photodegradation studies in the pharmaceutical industry have varied from lamps rich in UV, a choice clearly unrelated to "in use" conditions, to windowsill exposure to window-glass filtered daylight. As a consequence, data from different laboratories could not be readily compared.

The publication of the ICH guidelines as to how to carry out photostability tests on new pharmaceutical drug substances and drug products (1), introduced a reference point. This guideline is an annex to the ICH guideline for Stability Testing of New Drug Substances and Drug Products (2). Thus, there are now official guidelines to which the pharmaceutical industry should refer, and in addition a proposed publication of a general information chapter on photostability testing was recently published in the United States Pharmacopeia (3). The ICH guideline mainly concerns the determination of the photostability of drug substances and manufactured finished drug products, though not specifically addressing the problem of parametrizing "in use" conditions.

However, as it has been discussed in several instances (4–6), the guideline leaves much to be desired in terms of scientific exactness (e.g., the suggested actinometer has several disadvantages) as well as of unequivocal practical interpretation (e.g., two possibilities are presented for the light source, "Option 1" and "Option 2", but it is not clear whether these are equally appropriate).

The guideline refers to "confirmatory" testing, where a minimum dose light impinges on the sample. Such studies are analogous to "accelerated stability" studies, as defined in the parent guideline. It also hints at the possibility of carrying out "stress" testing. The latter is a scientific investigation of the "intrinsic stability characteristics" of the molecule, and is used as a predictor of "potential" photostability concerns. Thus, stress testing is analogous to forced degradation studies and, in contrast to confirmatory studies, is not part of the "formal definitive stability program." Therefore, this is not a highly regulated program, and is meant to provide suitable information to develop and validate test methods for the confirmatory studies. It should establish photodegradation pathways and allow identification of degradation products in order to validate the fitness of the analytical procedures used for confirmatory studies. Therefore, as it is general for stress testing (2), photochemical stress testing is usually carried out under more severe conditions than those chosen for the accelerated test procedures.

II. PHOTOCHEMISTRY OF DRUGS—BACKGROUND INFORMATION

A. Photochemical Reactions

Photochemical reactions involve electronically excited states that are formed through absorption of ultraviolet or visible light by molecules. As the monodimensional (Jablonski) diagram in Sch. 1 shows, the promotion of an electron from the highest occupied molecular orbital (e.g., HOMO) to an upper, more energetic, unoccupied molecular orbital, promoted by the absorption of photons of appropriate frequencies, leads to the formation of a variety of excited states. The absorption events represented in Sch. 1 are called "vertical" transitions, because they occur in a time domain shorter than that required for atomic vibrations to take place. Contrary to the ground state, excited states are open-shell species (two singly occupied orbitals), and therefore, every electronic configuration gives rise to two states of different energy, a singlet (no net total spin) and a triplet (total spin = 1) state. For

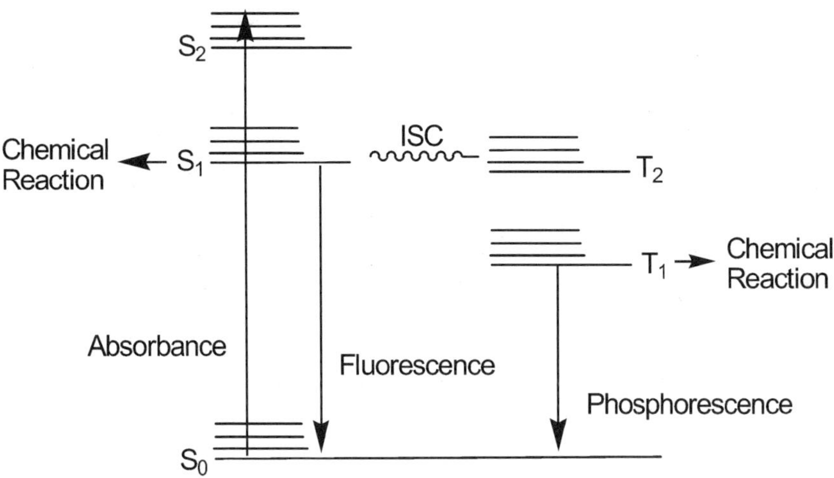

Scheme 1

every configuration, the triplet is lower in energy than the singlet. Spin inversion during absorption is forbidden, and therefore, light absorption by the ground state (S_0) leads only to singlet-excited states. $S_0 \rightarrow S_n$ transitions appear as bands of different intensity in the absorption spectrum (due to the different probability of each electronic transition, as measured by the molar absorptivity coefficient, ε, in the Lambert–Beer equation $A = \log(1/T) = \varepsilon bc$) in the absorption spectrum. Because $S_0 \rightarrow T_n$ transitions have negligible probability of occurring, the respective bands are not observed in electronic spectroscopy (a very long optical path would be required). However, triplet states may be reached through an indirect path, via a first-formed electronically excited singlet state, either the S_1 state or an upper S_n state. The latter process is known as inter-system crossing (a "horizontal"—no energy change involved—process wherein the spin is inverted). In some cases inter-system crossing occurs with a nearly unitary probability.

Excess vibrational energy within an electronically excited state is rapidly lost (vibrational relaxation), and furthermore conversion from upper (S_n or T_n) to the lowest-lying (S_1 or T_1) electronically excited states of the same multiplicity (internal conversion) is very fast (typically $>10^{12}\,\text{sec}^{-1}$). In fact, in almost every case such relaxation processes are faster than any other chemical process (i.e.,a reaction) or physical process (i.e., light emission) process. The low-lying states, though still quite short lived (typical lifetimes are $\leq 10^{-8}$ sec for S_1 and $\leq 10^{-6}$ sec for T_1) do have the time to undergo a reaction or emit light. Summing up, for all practical purposes only two excited states need to be considered: that is, the first singlet (S_1) and the first triplet (T_1) states.

The practical consequences of the above generalizations are: (1) that light needs to be adsorbed in order to cause a chemical effect and (2) that the photoreaction (or light emission) in most cases does not depend on the wavelength of the light used, provided that is adsorbed. The "action spectrum" for a photochemical effect is the relative effectiveness of different wavelengths of light in causing any kind of photochemical reaction. The "action spectrum," corresponds to the absorption spectrum of the "active" molecule and under proper conditions (typically at a low enough concentration) may be superimposable to it. This holds for a single light-absorbing species, since when different species are present (the simplest instance being that of an acid or basic compound in different ionization states) the fraction of light absorbed by each species changes with the wavelength and so does the chemistry observed.

Another concept that is used, and that has more an applied than a scientific significance, is that of "activation spectrum." This refers to the relative amount of degradation caused by a specific wavelength incident on a given material. The "activation spectrum" is affected by the presence of impurities, by any inhomogeneity of absorbance through the layer of the material, by the type of degradation measured, and as a result of the previous factors, by the type of light source used.

It is important to know whether the products from the initial photochemical reaction absorb light in the wavelength interval used. If these photoproducts are transparent, light is absorbed only by the reactant, and the photoreaction proceeds undisturbed, up to complete reagent consumption. If, as quite commonly observed, this is not the case, competitive absorption from the products increases during the photochemical reaction ("inner filter" effect) and the photoreaction slows down progressively, changes its course, or when the primary products are photoreactive themselves, leads to an increasingly complicated mixture including secondary photoproducts.

Furthermore, it is important to remember that electronic excitation can be transferred from an excited state D^* to a ground state molecule A. This is known as sensitization of A by energy donor D and is a very fast process provided that A has some excited state lower than D^*. Thus, a molecule (e.g., molecule A) may not absorb light in the wavelength range used since the $S_0 \rightarrow S_n$ transitions are too high in energy. However, if it has a low-lying triplet, such excited states may be reached through energy transfer from another light-absorbing molecule, molecule D, provided that the latter has a high enough triplet.

$$D + h\nu \rightarrow D^{1*} \rightarrow D^{3*}$$

$$D^{3*} + A \rightarrow D + A^{3*}$$

As a result, a non-absorbing molecule can react provided that a suitable sensitizer is present. When different molecules are present in solution and absorb competitively, the population of the excited states depends not only on the relative absorption at each wavelength, but also on such energy transfer processes. Therefore, while in a simple system with a single-absorbing molecule all photochemical and photophysical effects do not depend on the wavelength used, the overall result in a complex system often depends on the exciting λ.

Although this may seem unnecessarily complicated at first sight, it is important to distinguish the primary photochemical event (the one proceeding directly from the excited state) from the overall chemical process. Excited states are quite high in energy, and often lead to products that are unstable at room temperature. Highly strained (though ground state) molecules as well as unstable "intermediates," such as radicals, ions, carbenes, nitrenes, etc., may be formed from photochemical reactions. As an example, 1-phenylcyclohexene undergoes *Z–E* isomerization in the excited state, but the highly strained *E* isomer reverts to the *Z* form in microseconds (Sch. 2, path a), so that, although its formation may be demonstrated, no net change results (at least at room temperature), despite the occurrence of an efficient excited state reaction (7). However, in the presence of a protic solvent an addition to the strained *E*-cycloalkene occurs, and this highly energetic, unstable molecule reacts irreversibly, rather than reverting to the starting *Z*-isomer (Sch. 2, path b) (8). In another example, excited benzophenone abstracts a hydrogen atom from *iso*-propanol, yielding α-hydroxy radicals. The reaction of such species depends on conditions and may be driven to give either benzopinacol or benzhydrol by adding a base. The addition of a base affects the chemistry of the radicals, not that of the excited state (Sch. 3, path b) (9).

In the example above, the photodegradation product profile results from subsequent thermal reactions of the primary photoproduct, rather than from a direct effect on the formation and reactivity of molecules in

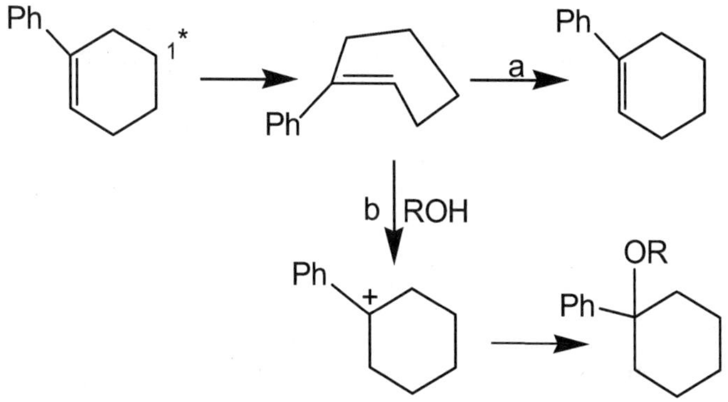

Ph 1* a Ph Ph b ROH Ph + OR Ph

Scheme 2

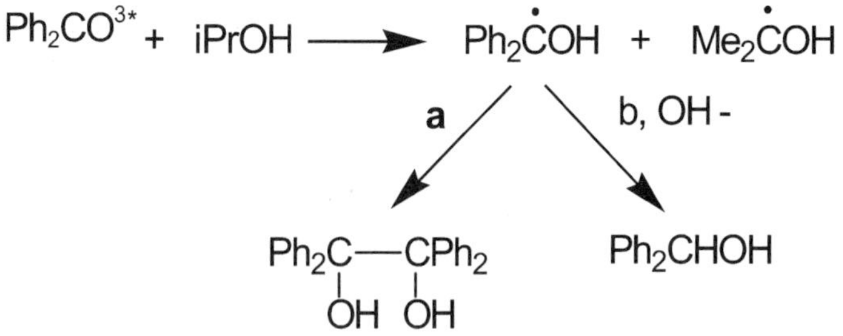

$Ph_2CO^{3*} + iPrOH \longrightarrow Ph_2\dot{C}OH + Me_2\dot{C}OH$

a: $Ph_2C(OH)—C(OH)Ph_2$

b, OH^-: Ph_2CHOH

Scheme 3

the excited state, and this is often the case. On the other hand, when a change in the medium changes the nature of a molecular orbital (e.g., by protonation of a non-bonding orbital) or deeply affects its energy (e.g., by establishing a strong hydrogen bond), the electronic structure of the excited state also changes, and so do the photochemical reactions. As a typical example, the lowest triplet state of many ketones is a $n\pi^*$ state and this triplet state abstracts hydrogen efficiently. A protic medium may sufficiently stabilize the n_O orbital to bring the $n\pi^*$ state above the $\pi\pi^*$ state. The $\pi\pi^*$ thus becomes the lowest excited state, and is, therefore, the reactive one. As a result, some ketones are much slower at hydrogen abstraction in protic than in aprotic media, and therefore the photodegradation profiles can be significantly different depending upon the solvent of the system.

Some further important peculiarities of photochemical reactions should be stressed. As an example, photochemical reactions are expected to depend little on the temperature. This is because excited states have a short lifetime, and thus, only very fast reactions with a low activation energy in the order of a few kcal M^{-1}may compete with decay to the ground state.

In contrast to a thermal reaction, the order of a photochemical reaction cannot be defined, since the observed rate of reaction depends on the rate of formation of the excited state, i.e., on the rate of *light absorption* by the reacting molecule. This is not directly related to either the substrate concentration [S] or the light flux. If light is absorbed efficiently and absorbance A remains > 1 throughout the experiment, which is quite a common occurrence taking into account that ε_{max} is 10^2 to $> 10^4$ for most organic molecules, then the fraction of light absorbed does not change appreciably up to about 90% conversion of [S], and in this case the observed rate of reaction remains constant (apparent zero order) :

$$-d[S]/dt = k$$

On the other hand, if the rate of absorption changes, because the fraction of light absorbed by the active molecule changes during the conversion, the overall rate of conversion changes and the observed order may change during the conversion. As observed earlier, changes in absorption may be the result of competitive absorption by products or due to a sensitization process. Another limiting case should be mentioned, although perhaps less frequently encountered in photostability studies, is that of poorly absorbing solutions, viz., either very dilute ones or those for which the absorptivity of the substrate is low at the λ used. In this case, the decomposition often appears to occur according to a first order rate. This is because absorbance A, and thus the rate of excitation, varies linearly with the substrate concentration for small values (e.g., $A < 0.01$) :

$$-d[S]/dt = k[S]$$

B. Carrying out a Photochemical Reaction

The first objective when attempting to induce a photochemical reaction is ensuring that light reaches the target molecule. Trivial as it may seem, this point is sometimes forgotten. Thus, the emission of the lamp and the absorption band of the substrate should contain some overlap, and no components of the system including the lamp envelope, a cooling system, the vessel containing the substrate, or the solvent should absorb competitively. It should also be ensured that a sufficient fraction of the lamp emission reaches the sample rather than being dispersed in other directions. This is easy when the lamp output is focused onto the sample by mirrors or lenses or when the lamp is immersed in the solution to be irradiated, but may not be so easy when external lamps are used.

The effect of the medium and of impurities on the course of a photochemical reaction is quite different from what is usually observed with thermal reactions. Photochemical reactions may be considered minimally affected by many experimental parameters, because reactions of excited states are so fast. Indeed, they are often less affected by impurities than are thermal reactions.

On the other hand, some impurities may specifically interact with the excited state at a very high (diffusion controlled) rate ($> 1 \times 10^{10} M^{-1} sec^{-1}$). A typical such case is that of products having low-lying triplets, which can function as acceptors in an energy transfer process and thus "quench" the photoreaction. In that case, a small amount of an impurity may effectively suppress a photoreaction. Typical examples are dienes or polyenes often present in organic solvents, and, above all, oxygen, the lowest-energy transition of which is lower than that of the excited states of practically every organic molecule. Therefore, it is recommended that one of the conditions under which photochemical tests are carried out involve "deoxygenation" by flushing for some minutes with an inert gas such as nitrogen or argon (in the case of a solution) or the use of an inert atmosphere (in the case of solids). This is sufficient for making oxygen quenching of excited state insignificant. Such experiments can be compared with non-deoxygenated tests. This is important because it is possible for oxygen to intervene at different stages of the reaction, in addition to quenching the excited state. As an example, oxygen may easily trap radicals formed in the course of the reaction.

C. Classification and Examples

1. The Chromophore

Spectroscopists are accustomed to classifying molecules according to the chromophore they contain, viz., the moiety to which the absorption(s) observed can be attributed. In terms of pharmaceutical photostability testing, absorption in the near UV or in the visible is of the greatest concern, since this is the range of wavelengths present in indoor or outdoor light. Absorption in these regions always corresponds to $n \to \pi^*$ or $\pi \to \pi^*$ transitions and thus correspond to conjugated multiple bonds and/or to aromatic systems. Recognizing the relevant chromophore(s) is also immediately relevant for the photochemistry, since this identifies the type and localization of the excited state involved. In fact, photochemical reactions are usually classified according to the chromophore present in the molecule and are rationalized on the basis of the modification of the electronic structure occurring upon excitation (10–12). The chromophores to which photochemical reactivity is usually connected have been previously reviewed with specific examples concerning the photochemistry of drugs (5,13).

2. Ketones

The lowest-lying excited state of ketones often correspond to a $n \to \pi^*$ transition, where λ_{max} for aliphatic derivatives is around 280 nm or further to the red for conjugated or aryl derivatives. The chemistry of such species is determined by the presence of an unpaired electron in the n_O orbital. This imparts a radical and electrophilic character to such species, which closely parallels that of alkoxy radicals. A typical reaction is intermolecular hydrogen abstraction resulting in reduction of the ketone function. Intramolecular abstraction is fast and usually involves the easily accessible γ position. The latter reaction is efficient whenever the geometry of the molecule allows it and yields a 1,4-biradical. This evolves through C_α–C_β bond cleavage ("Norrish Type II" reaction) or through cyclization to give a hydroxycyclobutane, "Yang reaction" (Sch. 4). Relatively weak bonds in the α-position may undergo homolytic cleavage, another reaction reminiscent of the behavior of alkoxy radicals, as exemplified in the case of metyrapone ("Norrish Type I reaction", Sch. 5) (14).

Conjugated ketones are mostly poor hydrogen abstractors. These may undergo rearrangement, which is quite common among glucocorticosteroids (Sch. 6) (15), addition reactions, and 2+2 cycloaddition reactions. The last

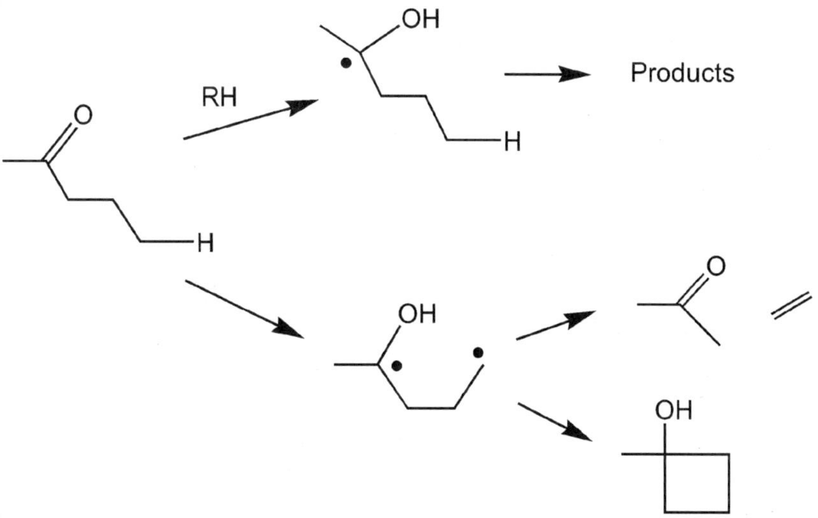

OH
RH
Products
O
H
H
OH
O
OH

Scheme 4

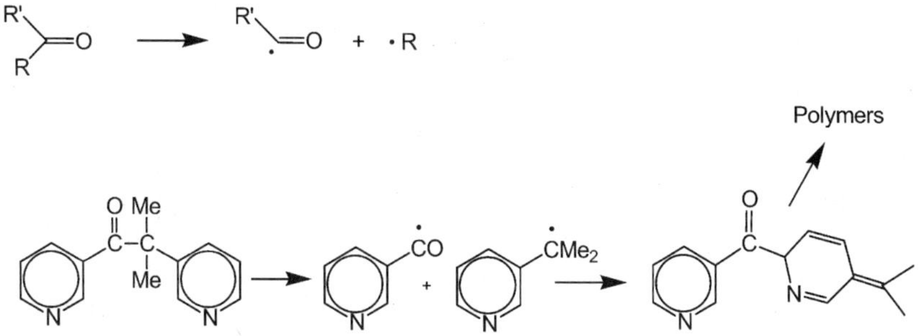

R'
O
R
R'
O
+ ·R
Polymers
O Me
C–C
Me
N
N
CO
+
CMe$_2$
N
N
O
C
N
N

Scheme 5

COCH$_2$OR
OH
X
R"
R'
O
COCH$_2$OR
OH
X
R"
O
R'

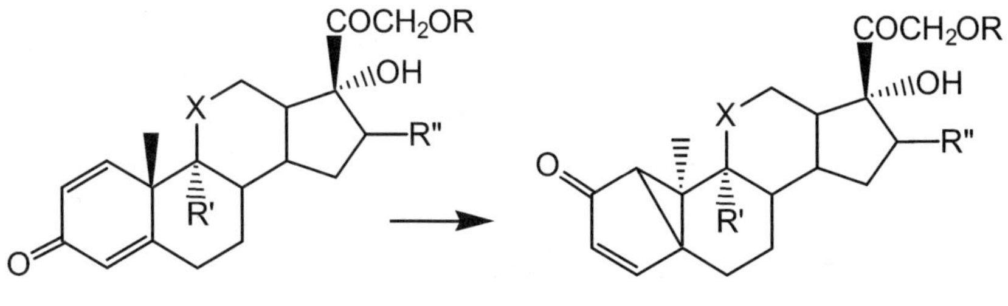

Scheme 6

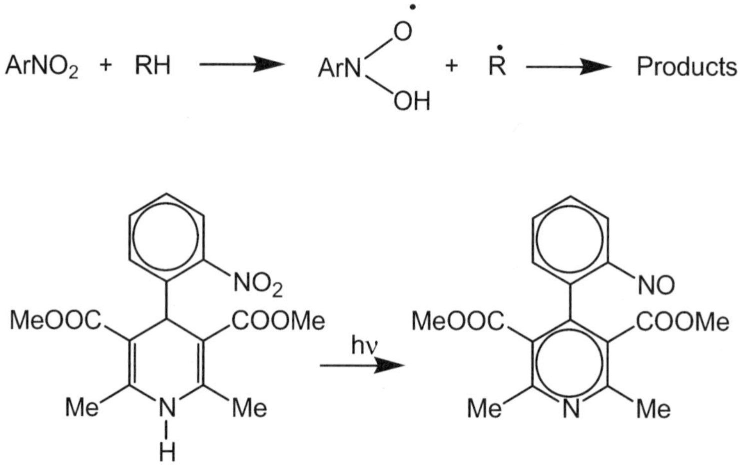

$ArNO_2$ + RH ⟶ ArN(O•)(OH) + R• ⟶ Products

MeOOC, COOMe, NO_2, Me, N, H, Me ⟶(hν) MeOOC, COOMe, NO, Me, N, Me

Scheme 7

class of reactions has often been observed both with conjugated ketones (16) and with quinones (17) following irradiation in the solid state.

3. Nitro Compounds

Nitro compounds, in particular aromatic and heterocyclic derivatives, absorb strongly in the near UV. They have properties similar to ketones in their excited state. These compounds are characterized by an unpaired electron in the n_O orbital and thus by a radical character. A typical example of this radical character is the easy intramolecular hydrogen abstraction in nifedipine and related vasodilators (Sch. 7) (18). Another manifestation of the radical character of the nitro group is the rearrangement often observed with nitrated five-membered heterocycles, as in the case of metronidazole (Sch. 8) (19).

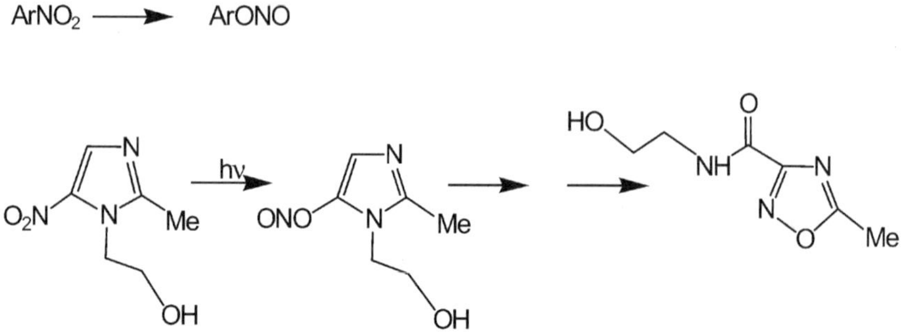

$ArNO_2$ ⟶ ArONO

O_2N, N, N, Me, OH ⟶(hν) ONO, N, N, Me, OH ⟶ ⟶ HO, NH, O, N, N, O, Me

Scheme 8

4. Alkenes

Non-conjugated alkenes do not absorb in the near UV, but polyenes or arylalkenes absorb strongly, and the absorption may extend into the visible region. Furthermore, these derivatives have low-lying triplet states that can be populated by sensitizers (including those adventitiously present). Alkenes are invariably characterized by efficient *E–Z* isomerism in the excited state, except when torsion is hindered by molecular constraint. Typical examples are synthetic estrogens (Sch. 9) (20) or vitamin A (21). Conjugated polyenes may also undergo electrocyclic reactions of the hexatriene–cyclohexadiene or of the butadiene–cyclobutene type, as observed with estrogen (20) or with vitamin D derivatives (22,23). Photochemical *E–Z* isomerism is not unique to the C = C bond; indeed, it is general with practically every A = B bond, e.g., azo compounds, oximes (24,25), hydrazones (26), etc.

5. Aromatic and Heterocyclic Derivatives

These compounds are well known for strong absorption in the UV region; higher members of the series absorb in the visible region as well. The large stabilization factor associated with aromaticity extends also to excited states, and as a result, both aromatic and heteroaromatic compounds often decay through a physical path such as re-emission of a photon, fluorescence, or phosphorescence, rather than through a chemical path. However, significant and even efficient photoreactions are known for several derivatives.

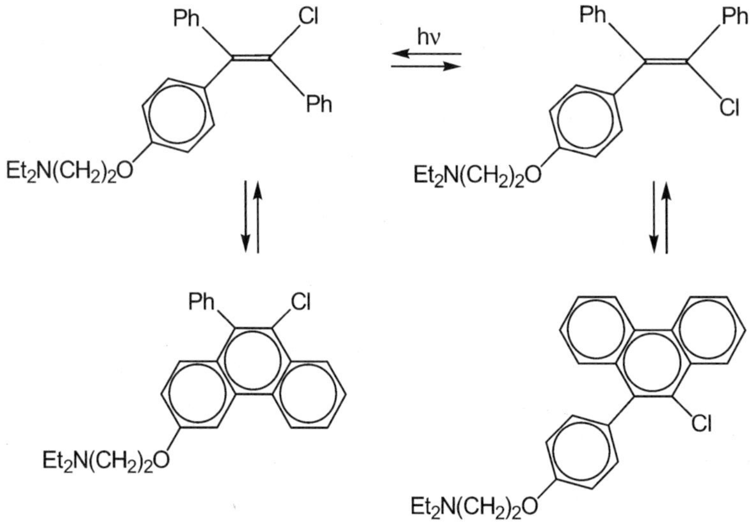

Scheme 9

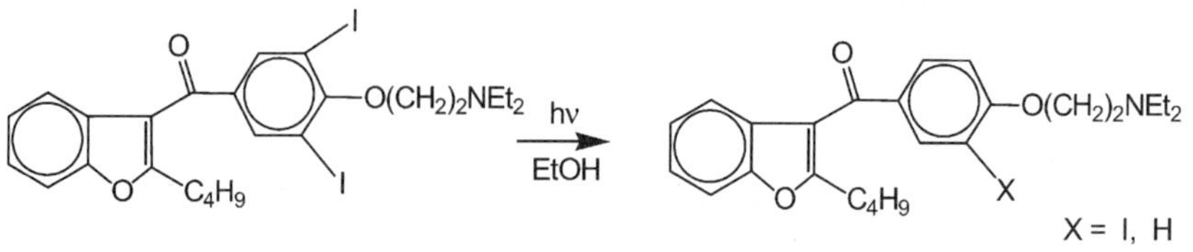

Scheme 10

Such is the case for halogen derivatives. Cleavage of the C–X bond may occur as a homolytic process, usually with low quantum yield for aryl chlorides (27) and more efficiently for bromides and iodides (Sch. 10) (28), or as a heterolytic process with a high quantum yield for some (hetero) arylfluorides, notably fluoroquinolones (Sch. 11) (29). Likewise, sulfa drugs are usually susceptible to homolytic fragmentation of the C–SO_2 bond (Sch. 12) (30).

Cleavage at the benzylic position has likewise been observed in a variety of (hetero) aromatic derivatives such as chloramphenicol (Sch. 13) (31) or methotrexate (32). An important case is that of the decarboxylation of arylacetic or arylpropionic acids used as non-steroidal anti-inflammatory agents (Sch. 14) (33–35).

Fries-type rearrangements (Sch. 15) (36) also occur photochemically; this is generally a homolytic process, in contrast to the ionic mechanism of the thermal process. Azapropazone undergoes photoinduced 1,3-acyl shift in the solid state and fragmentation in solution (Sch. 16) (37).

Among heterocycles, photoreactivity is more common than with the carbocyclic analogs. Strained rings often fragment, as it has been shown to be the case with the four-membered ring in a penem (Sch. 17). As in the case of azapropazone, notice the difference between the reaction in solution and in the solid state (38). For both five- and seven-membered rings photoinduced rearrangement or fragmentation is often observed, as exemplified by the photocleavage of pyrazolones (e.g., (dimethylamino) antipyrine) (Sch. 18) (39–41) and imidazolones (e.g., phenyltoin), (Sch. 19) (42) or the ring rearrangement typical of benzodiazepines (e.g., midazolam) (Sch. 20)

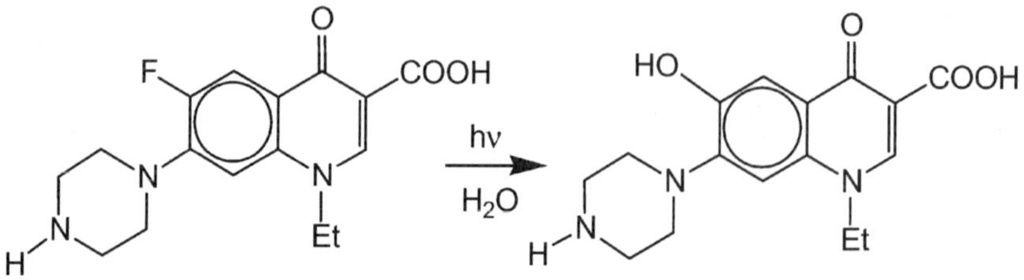

Scheme 11

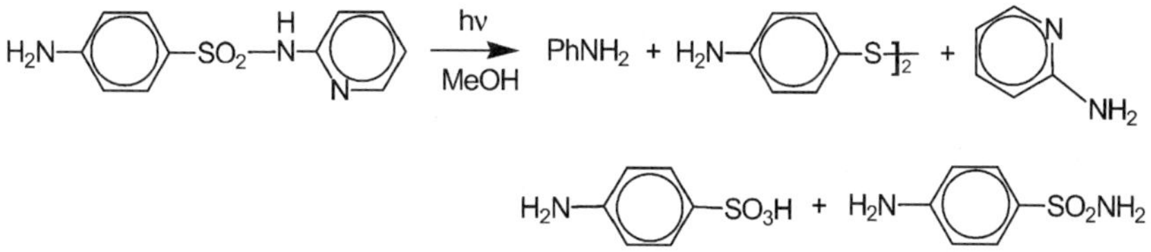

Scheme 12

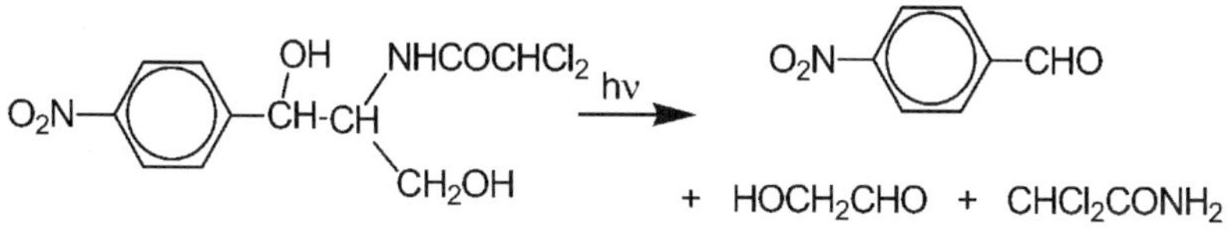

Scheme 13

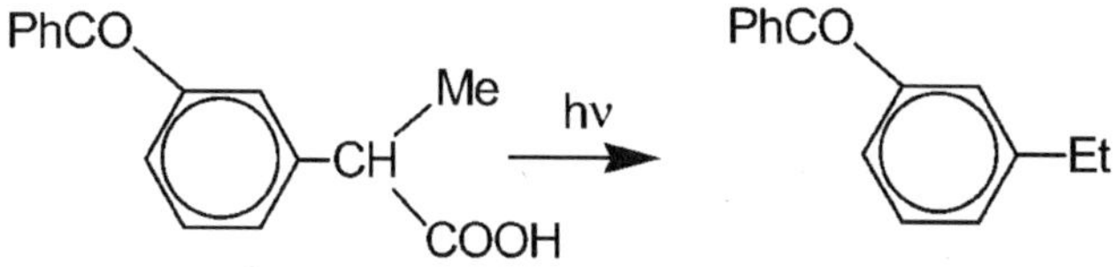

Scheme 14

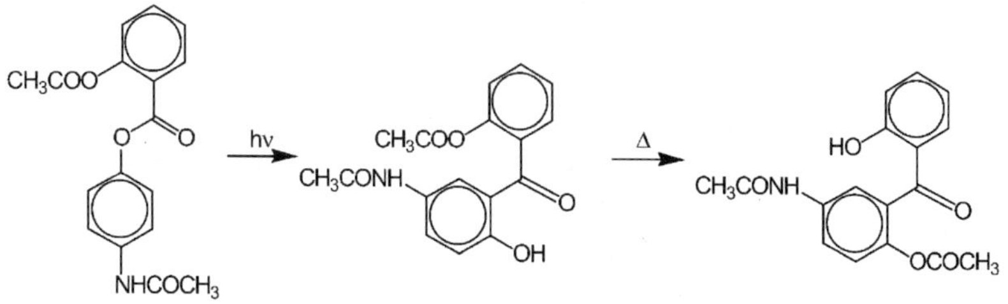

Scheme 15

(43–46). Six-membered heterocycles are generally more stable, though there are exceptions as shown by the fragmentation observed with many barbituric acid derivatives (barbital) (Sch. 21) (47–49). A class that is invariably characterized by photochemical reactivity is that of *N*-oxides such as minoxidil (50) or clordiazepoxide (44).

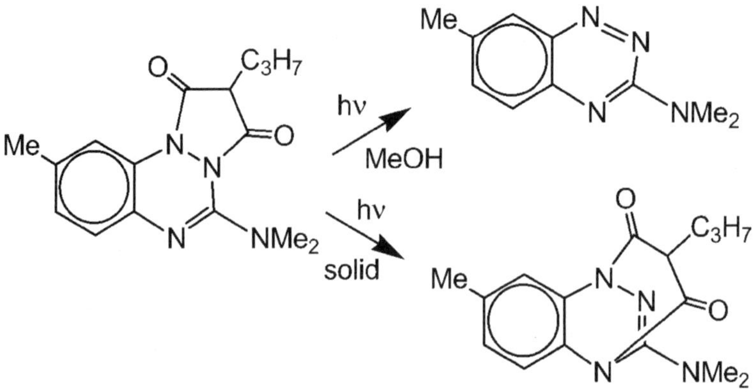

Me, C_3H_7, O, O, N, N, NMe$_2$; hν MeOH; hν solid

Scheme 16

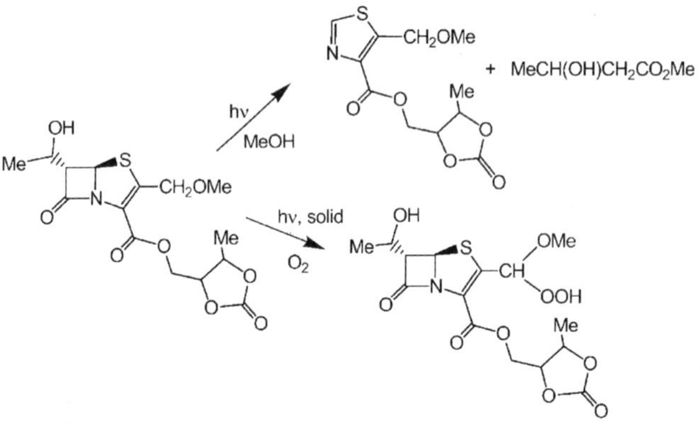

CH_2OMe; + $MeCH(OH)CH_2CO_2Me$; hν MeOH; hν, solid O_2

Scheme 17

Ph, O, N, N—Me, Me_2N, Me; hν, H_2O →

Me_2NH

MeNHCOCMe(OH)CONHPh

MeNHCHMeCONHPhCOOH

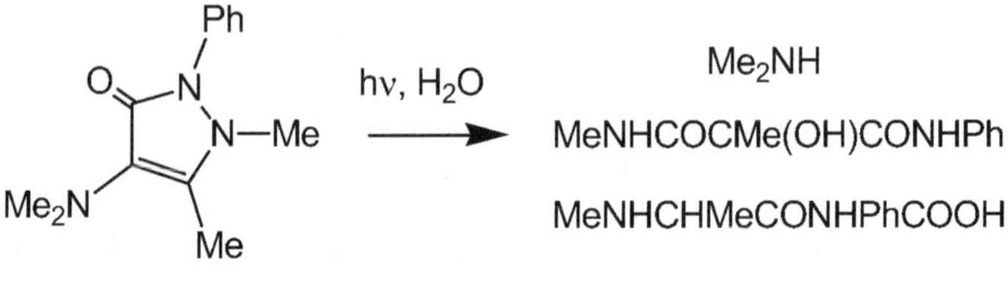

Scheme 18

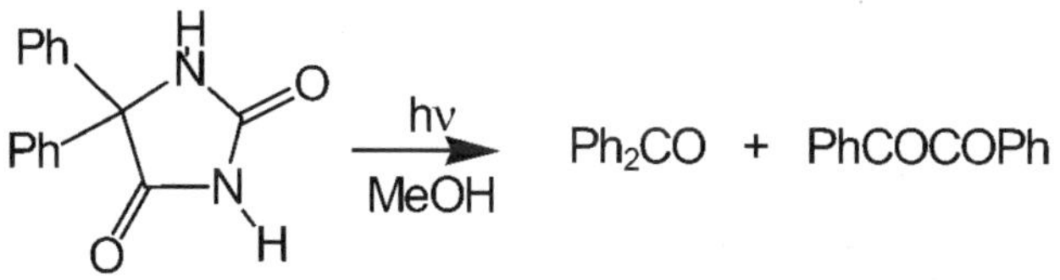

[structure] $\xrightarrow[\text{MeOH}]{h\nu}$ Ph_2CO + PhCOCOPh

Scheme 19

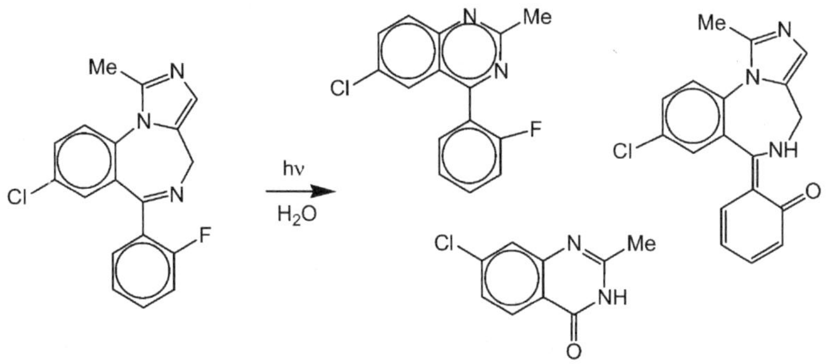

[structure] $\xrightarrow[H_2O]{h\nu}$

Scheme 20

[structure] $\xrightarrow[H_2O]{h\nu}$ $Et_2CHCONHCONH_2$

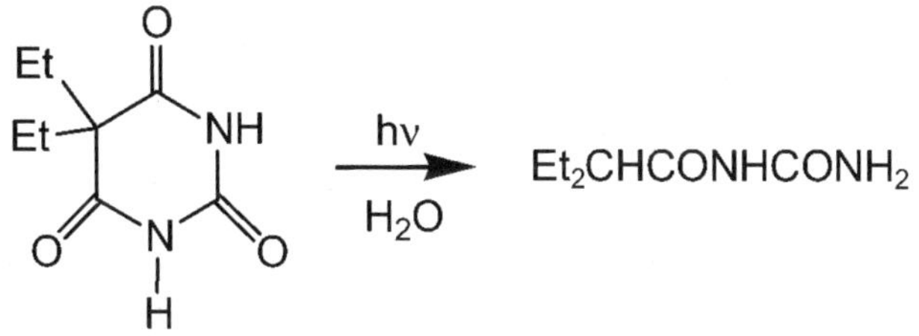

Scheme 21

6. Oxidations

Oxidation processes are common occurrences upon irradiation, in particular in the presence of oxygen. Oxygen dissolved in solution is "activated" through different sensitization processes. Consider that the role of sensitizer may be exerted by the substrate itself, by a coformulant or by an impurity. Many dyes are efficient oxygen sensitizers and due to the strong absorptivity are effective even at low concentrations. Mechanistically, oxygenations are classed into three groups. In type I oxygenations, the sensitizer interacts first with the organic substrate, e.g., leading to an alkyl radical. This radical is then trapped by ground state oxygen to give a peroxy radical that then further evolves to the end products. In type II oxygenations, the sensitizer first interacts with oxygen, which has a triplet ground state and a low-lying singlet-excited state, to produce singlet oxygen ($^1O_2$). In type II reactions, energy transfer from practically every type of organic molecule is possible (see above). Singlet oxygen is a powerful electrophile, reacting easily with alkenes. A further mechanism for oxygenation via sensitization involves electron rather than energy transfer; this electron transfer yields the radical cation of the substrate and superoxide anion, one or both of which can be involved in the subsequent reactions (Type Ia). In this case, just as in mechanism I, radicals are generated.

$$\text{Sens} + h\nu \rightarrow \text{Sens}^*$$

$$\text{Sens}^* + \text{SubstrateH} \rightarrow \text{Substrate}^{\bullet} + O_2 \rightarrow \text{SubstrateO}^{\bullet} \rightarrow \text{Products(Type I)}$$

$$\text{Sens}^* + O_2 \rightarrow {}^1O_2 \qquad {}^1O_2 + \text{Substrate} \rightarrow \text{products} \qquad \text{(Type II)}$$

$$\text{Sens}^* + \text{Substrate} + O_2 \rightarrow \text{Substrate}^{+\bullet} + O_2^{-\bullet} \rightarrow \text{Products} \qquad \text{(Type Ia)}$$

As a result, moderate or good donors often undergo oxygenation, dehydrogenation, or oxidative fragmentation by irradiation in the presence of oxygen. This is the case for good donors like amines, such as hydroxychloroquine (Sch. 22) (51), phenols, (e.g., adrenaline) (52), and some gonadotropic steroids (53), as well as for moderate donors such as aromatic hydrocarbons that react preferentially at the benzylic position if a side-chain is present. Examples include trimethoprim (Sch. 23) (54), and 9,11-dehydroestrone (Sch. 24) (55). Sulfides are easily oxidized to sulfones and/or sulfoxides, as observed with dothiepin (Sch. 25) (56) and with phenothiazines (57).

7. Inorganic Compounds

Metal complexes are often colored and usually prone to photoinduced ligand exchange, as exemplified by the well-known cases of nitroprussiate (58) and cisplatin (Sch. 26) (59).

CH_2CH_2OH

$NHCHMe(CH_2)_3N$ Et → hν $NHCHMe(CH_2)_3X$

X = NHEt, $NHCH_2CH_2OH$, H

Scheme 22

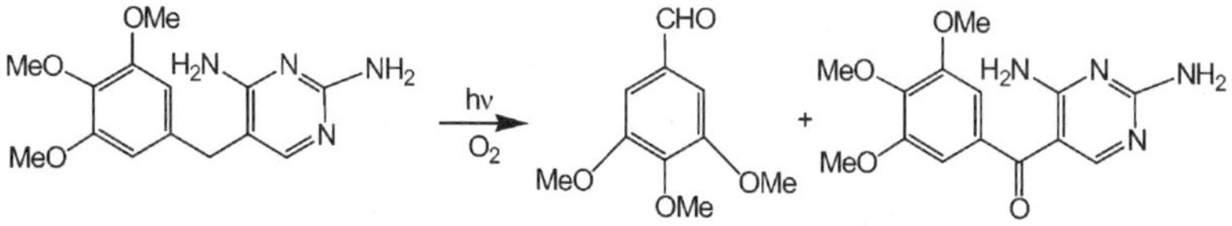

Scheme 23

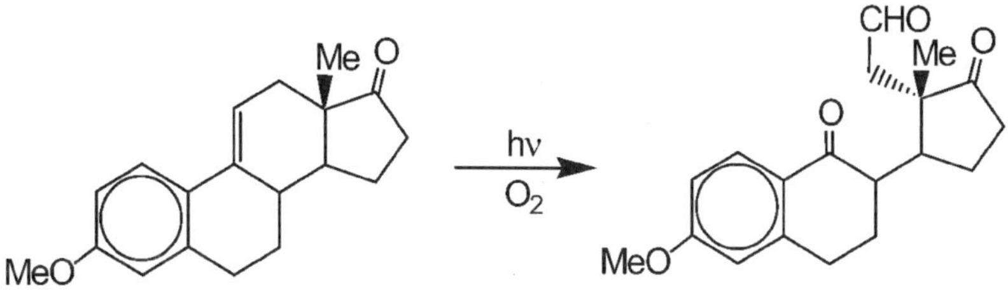

Scheme 24

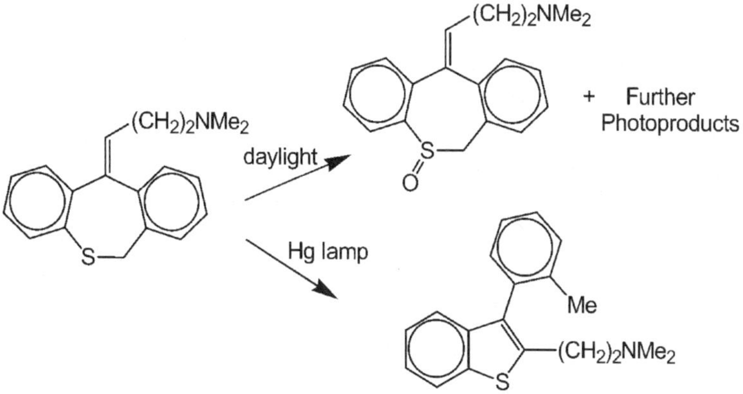

\+ Further Photoproducts

Scheme 25

$cis\text{-}Pt(NH_3)_2(Cl)_2 \xrightarrow{h\nu,\ H_2O} cis\text{-}Pt(NH_3)_2(Cl)(H_2O)^+$

$Fe(NO)(CN)_5^{2-} \xrightarrow{h\nu,\ H_2O} Fe(H_2O)(CN)_5^{3-}$

Scheme 26

III. PHOTOSTABILITY STUDIES

A. Light Sources

As seen above, the photochemistry of a considerable number of drug substances has been reported in the literature. In those works, a variety of light sources have been used, with respect both to wavelength and to intensity—from germicidal lamps (practically monochromatic, 254 nm) to solar light (emission extending from the near UV to the IR) and with intensities ranging from a few to several thousands Watts. From a scientific viewpoint, any choice of light source is correct provided that the light emitted is actually absorbed. However, from a practical viewpoint in the pharmaceutical industry, only wavelengths present in natural or artificial light and of reasonable intensity are relevant to photostability testing.

As mentioned in the Introduction, ICH describes two kinds of tests for drug photostability determination: (1) "forced degradation studies" and (2) "confirmatory studies". ICH describes two options for light sources for use in confirmatory studies (1).

Option 1 makes reference to any light source that is designed to produce an output similar to the D65/ID65 emission standard such as:

- an artificial daylight fluorescent lamp combining visible and UV outputs;
- a xenon lamp;
- a metal halide lamp.

D65 is the internationally recognized standard for outdoor daylight as defined in ISO 10977 (1993) (60). ID65 is the equivalent indoor, indirect daylight standard. For a light source emitting significant radiation below 320 nm, (an) appropriate filter(s) may be fitted to eliminate such radiation.

In option 2, the same sample should be exposed to *both* the cool white fluorescent and the near ultraviolet lamp.

- a cool white fluorescent lamp designed to produce an output similar to that specified in ISO 10097 (1993)
- a near-UV fluorescent lamp having a spectral distribution from 320–400 nm with a maximum energy emission between 350–370 nm; a significant proportion of UV should be in both bands of 320–360 nm and 360–400 nm.

In this case the question is, whether the two lamps should be used at the same time or one after the other, which may or may not give the same results. It has been suggested that carrying out two illuminations in sequence is more informative, since the effect of UV light can thus be separately established (61).

For confirmatory studies, samples should be exposed to light providing an overall illumination of not less than 1.2 million lux hours and an integrated near-ultraviolet energy of not less than 200 W hr/square meter.

As it has been remarked by many contributors (62–66), these guidelines leave a wide margin of uncertainty. The D65 and ID65 standards mentioned above are obviously different, with the indoor standard (ID65) having no contribution below 320 nm and a smaller contribution in the range 330–370 nm. The lamps listed above as a possible choice differ largely in the spectral distribution. The emission from the xenon lamps rises sharply and continuously in the 330–380 nm range and then remains essentially flat over the visible range. Metal halide lamps have bands superimposed over a continuum, and in fluorescent lamps the lines (254, 313, 365 nm, etc.) emitted by mercury vapor are transformed into a broad band by the phosphor coating deposited on the envelope of the lamp (though some bands corresponding to the Hg emissions may remain superimposed on the phosphor emission). Figures 1 and 2 show the spectral irradiance of a cool white fluorescent lamp and of a near-UV fluorescent lamp which are typically used in these studies. Lamps from different manufacturers may vary considerably in their characteristics, and indeed even lamps from the same manufacturer may yield somewhat different spectral distributions. Piechocki has shown that the coating of a phosphor deposited on the inside of the lamp walls, from which the emission originates, is not uniform and therefore the emission is not uniform over the lamp body (67,68). Since many drugs,

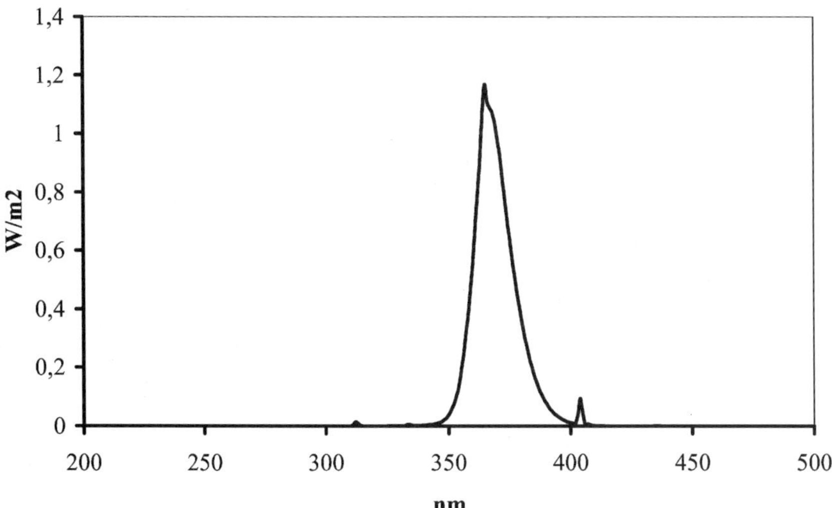

Figure 1 Spectral irradiance of a pair of near UV fluorescent lamp (Helios Italquartz, Milan, Italy, model BLB20, 60-cm long, 20 W) measured at 9-cm distance.

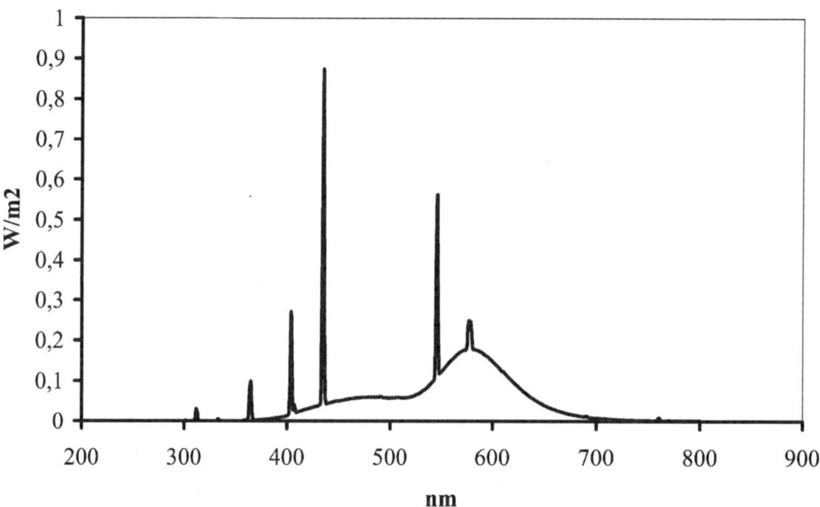

Figure 2 Spectral irradiance of a pair of cool white fluorescent lamps (OSRAM, model L18W/20, 60-cm long, 20 W) measured at 9-cm distance.

and in general many organic substances, absorb in the near UV, a different emission spectrum of the lamp in this key wavelength range can lead to dramatic differences in the rate of decomposition when different sources are used, even if the overall "UV" output is the same. Thoma has shown that the photodegradation of certain drugs may vary by over an order of magnitude when exposed to different lamps. The difference can be at least partially corrected by introducing factors accounting for the different lamp emission in the wavelength range of interest and thus obtaining values closer to the actually absorbed doses (69,70). Also, particularly for complex reactions, where different additives or the primary photoproducts absorb competitively with the starting substrate, the photodegradation rate may vary as a result of using light sources with different spectral power distributions, even if the overall light dose is the same.

ICH suggests that stress tests under forcing degradation conditions aimed at the deliberate degradation of the sample should also be carried out. Such studies, which should normally be undertaken in the development phase, are used to evaluate the overall photosensitivity of the material, for development of stability-indicating methods, and for the elucidation of the photodegradation product structure and the photodegradation pathways. Forced degradation studies are designed to induce formation of all photodegradation products that would have a reasonable chance of being formed during the confirmatory test. Forced degradation studies are not designed to establish quantitative rates of photodegradation with relation to storage, distribution, or use of the drug products. Therefore, the light dose used is not so important, except that one may consider it advisable to use a dose ten times as large as that recommended for confirmatory studies. (In fact, early drafts of the ICH photostability guideline recommended 5–10 times the confirmatory exposure for forced degradation studies.) From an academic point of view, the light source better suited for photochemical studies of a specific drug is the one better matching the absorption spectrum of the drug. From a practical point of view in the pharmaceutical industry, a sensible choice would be to use the same lamp in both confirmatory and in stress tests—one that should represent a "worst case" exposure—and to increase the intensity. A xenon lamp, an intense source rich in the short-wavelength component, is well suited for this purpose, unless it leads to extensive secondary decomposition of the primary photoproducts (see above). Sources emitting below 320 nm (UVB and C) may be excluded, unless the stability to UV sterilization must be checked. Developing the appropriate analytical method is most important in this case, since the degradation products formed in these forced degradation experiments should be looked for when carrying out confirmatory studies, where they may be formed in trace amounts. As far as it is practicable, the study should aim to establish the chemical structure of the major photoproducts, not only because this helps in choosing and developing the appropriate analytical technique, but also because knowing the structures of the photoproducts, along with information about the nature of the excited state, helps in establishing the *mechanism* of the photoreaction. In turn, an understanding of the mechanism may suggest possible ways of controlling the photostability. Therefore, analytical methods such as GC or HPLC should be complemented by techniques more informative on the structure, such as GC/MS or HPLC/MS, and, as far as possible, product isolation and identification by NMR and other appropriate spectroscopic techniques. It is also advisable that the tests are carried out under conditions aiming to maximize the photoreactivity. In the case of solids, since the photodegradation rates and pathways can change depending on the physical form of the drug, the marketed form of the drug substance should always be tested. Additionally, one may irradiate a thin film resulting from evaporation of a solution, which is often more reactive. In the case of solutions, the examination could be extended to one or two pH units above or below the p*K*a(s) of the molecule in order to assess the reactivity of the different ionic forms. Furthermore, the effect on photostability of potential excipients should be tested as a part of excipient compatibility studies.

It should be borne in mind, however, that some of the products formed in stress tests may not be formed under the less demanding conditions of confirmatory tests. In the case of highly photoreactive materials, exposure may be progressively reduced and the study terminated when extensive degradation (e.g., 5–30% degradation) still results. On the other hand, studies on photostable compounds may be terminated after the appropriate exposure has been reached.

The measurement of the light dose is particularly important in forced degradation studies, since a variety of light sources may be used. Light flux may be measured by means of a chemical actinometer, i.e., by using a substance of known quantum yield of photoreaction, or by means of a physical instrument (a phototube or a photomultiplier). For confirmatory studies, ICH suggests the photodegradation of 2% quinine monohydrochloride dihydrate in water (weight/volume) as an actinometer (1). This photoreaction has some advantage with respect to better established chemical actinometers. In particular, this has a rather low sensitivity, which is useful since long irradiation times are usually required in these measurements. Furthermore, it is simple to measure, since the measurement of the absorbance change at 400 nm is all that is required. There are, however, significant limitations. The absorption of this heterocycle declines quite abruptly at 380 nm; although it may be argued that this gives a significant evaluation of what is often the most effective wavelength range for many organic molecules, there is obviously a large number of drugs for which an actinometer of sensitivity extending into the visible would be desirable. At any rate, quinine is not appropriate for "cool white" lamps or for xenon lamps. The guideline allows the use of other validated chemical actinometers (1). A choice of well-established chemical actinometers with different wavelength range and sensitivities is available from the literature, and more of them are being evolved, some of which having specifically in mind the use for drug-photostability assessment. A few representative examples are given in Table 1 (71–76).

Alternatively, a physical detector, such as a silicon photodiode, a vacuum photodiode, or a thermopile can be chosen for the measurement of light intensity. Such instruments may either monitor the incident light

Table 1 Selected Actinometers (Refs. 71–76)

Actinometer	Wavelength range (nm)	Analytical method	Φ
Potassium ferrioxalate	250–450	UV absorbance	0.93–1.25
Azobenzene (Actinochrome 2R)	230–460	UV absorbance, HPLC	$\Phi_{trans-cis}$ 0.14 $\Phi_{cis-trans}$ 0.48
Aberchrome 540	310–375	UV absorbance	0.209
Quinine hydrochloride	300–380	UV absorbance	Low
Pyridoxine hydrochloride	250–350	UV absorbance	—
2-Nitrocinnamaldehyde	300–400	UV absorbance	0.15
2-Nitrobenzaldehyde	290–400	Titration	0.5

or integrate the incident light over a given time. Radiometers measure the total irradiance incident on the sensor. There are thermal radiometer detectors, consisting of a black surface absorbing the light and transforming it into heat; these are not very sensitive. Photonic radiometers detectors feature a photocell with a UV-sensitive cathode that converts the incident photon flow into a current. These instruments are much more sensitive, but the response depends on the wavelength and this makes it impossible to establish the irradiance of broadband emitting lamps, unless the spectral distribution of the source and the spectral sensitivity of the detector are known, and the instrument has been specifically calibrated for the light source. Higher-cost instruments with spectral resolution (i.e., spectroradiometers) are available, and UV sensors absorbing only in the UV region and insensitive to the visible light are likewise marketed.

Some confusion may arise from the use of different units for light intensity, or more precisely for flux density, which is what instruments measure. (Flux is the basic unit of optical power expressed in watts or lumens.) Irradiance (or illuminance for visible light, which is weighted to match the eye response of the "standard observer") is Flux per unit area or Flux density. Irradiance (E) is expressed in units of $W\,m^{-2}$ and illuminance is expressed in lux (lux = lumen m^{-2}). The correspondent spectral units can be defined with reference to a specific wavelength, e.g., the spectral irradiance is expressed in $W\,m^{-2}\,nm^{-1}$. Photochemists prefer units of Einsteins, the number of moles of photons. This is obviously better correlated with the mechanism, as the quantum yield of the reaction is the ratio of the number of absorbed photons to the number of reacted molecules. Since the energy of the photon changes with the wavelength, the above spectral irradiance ($W\,m^{-2}\,nm^{-1}$) can be converted to photon irradiance (E_p, Einstein $m^{-2}\,sec^{-1}$) by dividing it by the weighted average photon energy (76,77):

$$E_p = E/(hc/\lambda)N$$

As an example, an incident irradiance of $1\,mW\,cm^{-2}$ at 253.7 nm (germicidal lamp) corresponds to a photon irradiance of 2.1×10^{-9} Einstein $cm^{-2}\,sec^{-1}$, about twice as much at 500 nm, thrice as much at 750 nm and so on.

B. Sample Presentation

Presentation of the sample during photochemical studies is an all important factor, because the conditions of real use must be in some way reproduced, and this question must be confronted as soon as possible during formulation studies (78). Since the aim of stress testing is that of ascertaining the existence and the course of a photochemical reaction for the drug investigated, the presentation of the sample may be chosen freely, while keeping in mind the potential formulations for the final marketed drug product. Most mechanistic photochemical studies are carried out in dilute solutions (usually in an organic solvent), since in that case it is much easier to control the conditions (e.g., checking which species absorb the light, controlling the temperature, excluding oxygen, etc.) and to determine the role of the intermediates. Such studies can be carried out either in an immersion well apparatus fitted with a water-cooled lamp that is filtered when appropriate. The lamp commonly used for such studies is a medium pressure mercury arc, rich in the UV component. A second technique is to use external illumination in a multilamp apparatus fitted with phosphor-coated lamps (which are designed for emission in various regions of the UV and the visible). Obviously, nothing prevents mechanistic studies of this kind, although these conditions are quite far from those relevant for practical application to most pharmaceutical concerns, where solids (either pure or with an appropriate coformulant), concentrated aqueous solution, or creams or ointments are used. The course of the photoreaction may change completely under such different conditions (see below). Also, an analytical laboratory concerned with drug stability assessment may find it more expedient to use light sources that are the same as those to be used for confirmatory studies. In fact, use of the same light source for both the forced degradation studies and the confirmatory studies is recommended by many researchers, since use of the same light source will likely provide more predictive accuracy.

Particular attention must be given to obtaining a uniform absorption of the light throughout the sample. If the sample has a high absorbance (i.e., a high optical density) at the wavelength(s) employed, absorption is limited to a thin layer at the outer surface. As an example, for a solution containing a 0.1 M solution of a drug with a molar absorptivity $\varepsilon = 10^3\ M^{-1}\ cm^{-1}$, 90% of the light is absorbed in the first 0.1 mm of solution. Under such a condition, and particularly if the solution is not adequately stirred, multiple photoreactions leading to secondary products or to further degradation occur. Furthermore, a radical-initiated polymerization leading to the formation of a poorly transmitting film on the surface of the vessel often intervenes and under this condition the bulk of the solution may be scarcely affected even after prolonged irradiation, thus causing a dramatic understatement of the photolability. In this case, the only safe way is to dilute the solution and test the photoreaction in a solution more uniformly absorbing.

In the case of solid there is no simple way to ensure uniform absorption of light throughout the sample, since light absorbance is a surface phenomenon. For strongly absorbed wavelengths, light is absorbed only by the outer layer of the crystals, while weakly absorbed wavelengths penetrate further. When the photoreaction leads to a product transparent to (part of) the wavelength range used (for example, in the case of a cycloaddition process, where the chromophore in the products is less extensively conjugated than in the reagent and thus the absorption is blue-shifted), light penetrates further in the crystal as long as the reaction proceeds, extending the transformation also to the inner parts. Alternatively, it may happen that the crystals crack while the reaction proceeds and this may again allow further reaction. When the photoproducts absorb, the photochemical reaction stops, often before analytically detectable amounts of photoproducts are formed. In several cases it has been found that a conspicuous change in the appearance, e.g., yellowing, is not related to an appreciable formation of degradation products (78–80). In fact, it may be that only a small amount of colored products is formed under this condition with all of it concentrated in a thin superficial layer, due to the lack of penetration of the light. Such low a level may be undetectable by HPLC analysis of the whole sample, while resulting in a perceptible yellowing of the sample surface, both because of the localization of the reaction on the surface and of the sensitivity of human eyes to colored species.

Grinding the crystals or using a micronized material is likely to affect the sensitivity to light (78), since the exposed surface area increases. However, this does not necessarily lead to an increase in the rate of photodegradation, since the loss of light due to scattering is large for the small crystals, and this may overcome the advantage of the increased area. Stirring of a powder to expose a new surface to the light source, while not required for confirmatory studies, can help increase the photodegradation rate for forced degradation studies. A reasonably fast photochemical reaction may be conveniently monitored by irradiation of samples ground with KBr and sintered in IR pellets, but this is a poor choice for slow reactions. Further possibilities that have been examined are either mixing the crystals with an inert substrate, such as silica gel, and irradiating the mixture from outside in a rotating tube (81), or forming a film of the substrate on a glass plate by allowing a solution to evaporate. It has been also advocated that depositing solutions on a silica gel plate, irradiating it, and developing the chromatogram allows evaluation of the photolability of a substrate, although it is not clear which physical state the substrate is in under these conditions (82,83).

At present most photostability studies, at least from what can be deduced from published reports, are limited to the qualitative appreciation of the change in the aspect of an irradiated powder (78–80). It should at least be recommended that the powder is finely ground, and the thickness of the exposed material kept small (e.g., 1 mm or less). Furthermore, the sample submitted for analysis after the photoexposure should be representative (e.g., the whole sample is dissolved and examined). At any rate, with solids it remains difficult to ascertain the fraction of light absorbed vs. that lost by scattering, and this makes it more difficult to assess whether "stress" conditions are actually met when the light dose is increased. Also, it should be appreciated that different crystalline polymorphs or amorphous forms may differ a great deal both in the fraction of light scattered and in the photochemistry occurring. This has been demonstrated in a number of cases to depend on the arrangement of the molecules in the lattice (84–88). At any rate, solid dosage forms (powders, granules, pellets, tablets) are, as a general rule, less light sensitive than creams and ointments, and these in turn are more stable than solutions (infusions, injections, eye droplets), simply as a result of the different light penetration.

C. Tests on Drug Preparations

The photolability and the course of the photochemical reaction of a drug substance may be deeply affected by the presence of other substances. These may absorb light competitively, acting as internal filters, or at any rate diminish the absorbed light, e.g., by scattering. It is also possible that other substances present in the drug substance or formulated product either quench or sensitize the photochemical reaction caused by direct irradiation or interfere with some reactive intermediate formed in the course of the photoreaction, e.g., a radical intermediate. Common excipients do not absorb significantly in the near UV. When in doubt, it is advisable to check that the UV absorbance has been measured. Knowledge of the particular additives can help predict the effect that the additive might have on the photochemistry of the preparation. A good hydrogen donor or reducing agent is likely to quench either the excited states or the radicals formed from them, and likewise a molecule with a low-lying triplet, such as a polyene, is likely to quench the photoreaction, while aromatic hydrocarbon or ketones are likely to act as photosensitizers. Once again, oxygen is expected to affect the results. Experiments in the absence of oxygen may be carried out for mechanistic purposes.

D. Photoprotection

The knowledge of the photodegradation paths can be critical to the devising of a suitable protection of the drug dosage form. In principle, this can be obtained either by blocking the access of light to the drug with external protection or by the use of an additive that competitively absorbs or reflects the light reaching the sample. Finally, a more difficult method of protection that depends on a detailed knowledge of the photodegradation path can be attempted; such a method might be based on quenching the photochemical reaction in some way.

In the case of tablets or capsules, external protection from packaging is generally suitable, and can be obtained by using an opaque blister or an opaque gelatin for capsules, or covering tablets with an opaque film (89–92). The opaqueness can be obtained by adding a (pharmaceutically acceptable) dye the absorption spectrum of which is the same as that of the drug principle or by adding a reflecting pigment such as titanium dioxide.

Alternatively, absorbing excipients or opacizers can be added to the drug preparation, thus protecting the drug outside the package; this is the only choice with creams, ointments, and liquid preparations. The effectiveness of light-absorbing dyes (93–97) and of light-reflecting pigments (98) has been tested in a number of cases. Several other additives have been proved effective, even if it is not always clear whether they act as competitive absorbers, as complexing agents in the presence of which the drug is less photosensitive, or as quenchers inhibiting the photochemical reaction after absorption (99–106). Other techniques, such as minimization of solubilization of the drug in the vehicle, microencapsulation (95,107), or inclusion into cyclodextrins have been considered. In general, inclusion into cyclodextrins is not applicable since cyclodextrins are good hydrogen donors, and in some cases may increase the decomposition of the drug (108,109).

REFERENCES

1a. ICH. Harmonized Tripartite Guideline: Photostability Testing of New Drug Substances and Products, ICH-QIB, Nov. 1996.
1b. Albini A, Fasani E. Drugs: Photochemistry and Photostability. Cambridge: The Royal Society of Chemistry, 1998: 66–73.
1c. Federal Register 1997; 62:27115–27122.
2. ICH Harmonized Tripartite Guideline: Stability Testing of New Drug Substances and Products, ICH-QIA, Sep. 1994.
3. Pharmacopeial previews. Drugs and excipients — USP general information chapters. Pharmacop Forum 2000; 26:384–388.
4a. Thatcher SR, Mansfield RK, Miller RB, Davis CW, Baertschi SW. Parmaceutical photostability: a technical guide and practical interpretation of the ICH Guideline and its application to pharmaceutical stability. Pharmaceut Technol Part I 2001; 25(3):98–110.
4b. Thatcher SR, Mansfield RK, Miller RB, Davis CW, Baertschi SW. Pharmaceutical photostability: a technical guide and practical interpretation of the ICH Guideline and its application to pharmaceutical stability. Pharmaceut Technol Part II 2001; 25(4):50–62.
5. Albini A, Fasani E. Drugs: Photochemistry and Photostability. Cambridge: The Royal Society of Chemistry, 1998.
6a. Sager N, Baum R, Wolters R, Layloff T. Photostability testing of pharmaceutical products. Pharmacop Forum 1998; 24:6331–6333.
6b. Tonnesen H, Karlsen J. A comment on photostability testing according to ICH Guideline: calibration of photolysis sources. J Pharmeuropa 1997; 9: 735–736.
6c. Helboe P. The elaboration and application of the ICH Guideline on photostability: a European prospective. In: Albini A, Fasani E. Drugs: Photochemistry and Photostability. Cambridge: The Royal Society of Chemistry, 1998: 243–246.
6d. Riehl J, Maupin C, Layloff T. On the choice of a photolysis source for the photostability testing of pharmaceuticals. Pharmacopeial Forum 1995; 21: 1654–1663

6e. Anderson NH. Photostability testing design and interpretation of tests on drug substances and dosage forms. In: Tønnesen HH. Photostability of Drugs and Drug Formulation. London: Taylor and Francis, 1996:305–322.
6f. Sequeira F, Vozone C. Photostability studies of drug substances and products. Practical implications of the ICH guideline. Pharm Tech 2000; 24(7):30–35.
7. Bonneau R, Joussot-Dubien J. A trans cyclohexene. J Am Chem Soc 1976; 98: 4329–4330.
8. Kropp PJ. Photochemistry of cycloalkenes. III. Ionic behaviour in protic media and isomerization in aromatic hydrocarbon media. J Am Chem Soc 1967; 89:5199–5208.
9. Cohen SG, Sherman W. Inhibition and quenching of the light induced reduction of benzophenone to benzopinacol and to benzhydrol. J Am Chem Soc 1963; 85:1642–1647.
10. Horspool WH, Lenci F, eds. CRC Handbook of Organic Photochemistry and Photobiology. Boca Raton: CRC Press, 2004.
11. Horpool WH, Armesto D. Organic Photochemistry: A Comprehensive Treatment. New York: Ellis Horwood, 1992.
12. Turro NJ. Modern Molecular Photochemistry. Menlo Park: Benjamin Cummings, 1978.
13. Tønnesen HH, ed. Photostability of Drugs and Drug Formulation. Boca Raton: CRC Press, 2004.
14. Fasani E, Mella M, Monti S, Sortino S, Albini A. The photochemistry of metyrapone. J Chem Soc Perkin Trans 1996; 2:1889–1893.
15. Williams JR, Moore RH, Li R, Weeks CM. Photochemistry of 11α- and 11β-hydroxysteroidal 1,4-dien-3-ones and 11α- and 11β-hydroxysteroidal bicyclo[3.1.0]hex-3-en-2-ones in neutral and acidic media. J Org Chem 1980; 45:2324–2331.
16. Takàcs M, Ekiz Gücer N, Reisch J, Gergely-Zobin A. Light-sensitivity of corticosteroids in the crystalline state. Pharm Acta Helv 1991; 66:137–140.
17. Lisewski R, Wierzchowski KL. Photochemistry of 2,4-diketopyrimidines. Dimerization and stacking association of 1,3-dimethylthimine in aqueous solution. Mol Photochem 1971; 3:327–354.
18. Sadana GS, Ghogare AB. Mechanistic studies on photolytic degradation of nifedipine by use of proton-NMR and carbon 13-NMR spectroscopy. Int J Pharm 1991; 70:195–199.
19. Moore DE, Wilkins BJ. Common products from gamma radiolysis and ultraviolet photolysis of metronidazole. Radiat Phys Chem 1990; 36:547–550.
20. Frith RG, Phillipou J. Application of clomiphene photolysis to assay based on analysis of the derived phenanthrenes. J Chromatogr 1986; 367:260–266.
21. Allwood MC, Plane JH. The wavelength-dependent degradation of vitamin A exposed to ultraviolet radiation. Int J Pharm 1986; 31:1–7.
22. Mermet-Bouvier R. Photochemistry of Vitamin D_2. Bull Soc Chim Fr 1973; 11(2):3023–3026.
23. Snoeren AEC, Daha MR, Lugtenburg J, Havinga E. Studies of Vitamin D and related compounds. Part 21. Photosensitized reactions. Rev Trav Chim Pays Bas 1970; 89:261.

24. Fabre H, Ibork H, Lerner DA. Photodegradation kinetics under UV light of aztreonam solutions. J Pharm Biomed Anal 1992; 10:645–650.
25. Lerner DA, Bannefond G, Fabre H, Mandrou B, Simeon de Buochberg M. Photodegradation paths of cefatoxim. J Pharm Sci 1988; 77:699–703.
26. Quillian MA, McCurry BE, Hoo KH, McCalla DR, Weitekunas S. Identification of the photolysis products of nitrofurazone irradiated under laboratory illumination. Can J Chem 1987; 65:1128–1132.
27. Moore DE, Roberts-Thompson S, Zhen D, Duke CC. Photochemical studies on the anti-inflammatory drug diclofenac. Photochem Photobiol 1990; 52: 685–690.
28. Paillous N, Verrier M. Photolysis of amiodarone, an antiarrhythmic drug. Photochem Photobiol 1988; 47:337–343.
29. Fasani E, Barberis Negra FF, Mella M, Monti S, Albini A. Photoinduced C–F bond cleavage in some fluorinated 7-amino-4-quinolone-3-carboxylic acids. J Org Chem 1999; 64:5388–5395.
30. Golpashin F, Weiss B, Dürr H. Photochemical model studies on photosensitizing drugs: sulfonamides and sulfonylureas. Arch Pharm (Weinheim) 1984; 317:906–913.
31. Shih IK. Photodegradation products of chloramphenicol in aqueous solution. J Pharm Sci 1971; 60:1889–1890.
32. Chahidi C, Giraud M, Aubailly M, Valla A, Santus R. 2,4-Diamino-6-pteridinecarboxyaldehyde and an azobenzene derivative are produced by UV photodegradation of methotrexate. Photochem Photobiol 1986; 44: 231–233.
33. Vargas F, Rivas C, Miranda MA, Boscà F. Photochemistry of the non-steroidal anti-inflammatory drugs, propionic acid derived. Pharmazie 1991; 46: 767–771.
34. Boscà F, Miranda MA, Carganico G, Mauleon D. Photochemical and photobiological properties of ketoprofen associated with the benzophenone chromophore. Photochem Photobiol 1994; 60:96–101.
35. Moore DE, Chappuis PP. A comparative study of the photochemistry of the non-steroidal anti-inflammatory drugs, naproxen, benoxaprofen and indomethacin. Photochem Photobiol 1988; 47:173–180.
36. Castell JV, Gomez Lechon MJ, Mirabet V, Miranda MA, Morea IM. Photolytic degradation of benorylate: effects of the photoproducts on cultured hepatocytes. J Pharm Sci 1987; 76:374–378.
37. Reisch J, Ekiz-Gücer N, Takacs M, Gunaherath GM, Kamal B. The photoisomerization of azapropazone. Arch Pharm (Weinheim) 1989; 322:295–296.
38. Albini A, Alpegiani M, Borghi D, Del Nero S, Fasani E, Perrone E. Solid state photoreactivity of a dioxolenonemethyl ester. Tetrahedron Lett 1995; 36: 4633–4636.
39. Fabre H, Hussam-Eddine N, Lerner D, Mandrou B. Autoxidation and hydrolysis kinetics of the sodium salt of phenylbutazone in aqueous solution. J Pharm Sci 1984; 73:1709–1713.
40. Marciniec B. Photochemical decomposition of phenazone derivatives. Part 3: kinetics of photolysis in aqueous solutions. Pharmazie 1984; 39:103–106.

41. Reisch J, Fitzek A. Photo and radiochemical studies. V. Decomposition of aqueous amidopyrine solutions under the influence of light and γ-rays. Deut Apoth-Ztg 1967; 107:1358–1359.
42. Chiang HC, Li SY. Photochemistry of 5,5-diphenyltoin. J Taiwan Pharm Assoc 1977; 29:70–76.
43. Andersin R, Ovaskainen J, Kaltia S. Photochemical decomposition of midazolam. III. Isolation and identification of products in aqueous solutions. J Pharm Biomed Anal 1994; 12:165–172.
44. Cornelissen PJG, Beijersbergen van Henegouwen GMJ, Gerritsma KW. Photochemical decomposition of 1,4-benzodiazepines. Chlordiazepoxide. Int J Pharm 1979; 3:205–220.
45. Roth HJ, Adomeit M. Photochemistry of nitrazepan. Arch Pharm (Weinheim) 1973; 306:889–897.
46. Reisch J, Ekiz-Gücer N, Tewes J. Photostability of some 1,4-benzodiazepines in the crystalline state. Liebigs Ann Chem 1992; 69–70.
47. Barton H, Bojarski J, Mokrosz J. Photochemical ring opening of barbital. Tetrahedron Lett 1982; 23:2133–2134.
48. Barton HJ, Bojarski J, Zurowska A. Stereospecificity of the photoinduced conversion of methylphenobarbital to mephenytoin. Arch Pharm (Weinheim) 1986; 319:457–461.
49. Barton H, Mokrosz J, Boiarski J, Klimczak M. Products of photolysis and hydrolysis of pentobarbital. Pharmazie 1980; 35:155–158.
50. Ekiz-Gücer N, Reisch J. Photostability of minoxidil in the liquid and in the solid state. Acta Pharm Turc 1990; 32:103–106.
51. Tønnesen HH, Grislingaas AL, Woo SO, Karlsen J. Photochemical stability of antimalarials. I: Hydroxychloroquine. Int J Pharm 1988; 43:215–219.
52. De Mol NJ, Beijersbergen van Henegouwen GMJ, Gerritsma KW. Photochemical decomposition of cathecolamines. II. The extent of aminochrome formation from adrenaline, isoprenaline and noradrenaline under ultraviolet light. Photochem Photobiol 1979; 29:479–482.
53. Sedee AGJ, Beijersbergen van Henegouwen GMJ. Photochemical decomposition of contraceptive steroids: a possible explanation for the observed (photo)allergy of the oral contraceptive pill. Arch Pharm (Weinheim) 1985; 318:111–119.
54. Dedola G, Fasani E, Albini A. The photoreactions of trimethoprim in solution. J Photochem Photobiol A 1999; 123:47–51.
55. Lupon P, Grau F, Bonet JJ. The photooxygenation of $\Delta^{9(11)}$-dehydroestrone and its 3-methyl ether. Helv Chim Acta 1984; 67:332–333.
56. Tammilehto S, Torniainen K. Photostability of dothiepin in aqueous solution. Int J Pharm 1989; 52:123–128.
57. Glass BD, Brown ME, Drummond PM. Photoreactivity *versus* activity of a selected class of phenothiazines: a comparative study. In: Albini A, Fasani E. Drugs: Photochemistry and Photostability. Cambridge: The Royal Society of Chemistry, 1998:134–149.
58. Davidson SW, Lyall D. Sodium nitroprusside stability in light-protected administration sets. Pharm J 1987; 239:599–600.

59. Macka M, Borak J, Semenkova L, Kiss F. Decomposition of cisplatin in aqueous solutions containing chlorides by ultrasonic energy and light. J Pharm Sci 1994; 83:815–818.
60. ISO 10977:1993(E). Photography—Processed Photographic Color Films and Transmittance, Solar Direct, Total Solar Energy Transmittance and Ultraviolet Transmittance, and Related Glazing Factors. Geneva: ISO, 1993.
61. Brumfield JC. The Pharmacia and Upjohn experience in selecting a photostability guideline option. 3rd Int. Conf. Photostab. Drug Subst. Prod., Washington DC, July 10–14, 1999.
62. Matsuo M, Machida Y, Furuichi H, Nakamura K, Takeda Y. Suitability of photon sources for photostability testing of pharmaceutical products. Drug Stability 1996; 1:179–187.
63. Drew HD, Thornton LK, Juhl WE, Brower JF. An FDA/PhRMA interlaboratory study of the International Conference on Harmonization's proposed photostability testing procedures and guidelines. Pharm Forum 1998; 24:6317–6325.
64. Drew HD. Photostability of drug substances and drug products: a validated reference method for implementing the ICH photostability study guidelines. In: Albini A, Fasani E. Drugs: Photochemistry and Photostability. Cambridge: The Royal Society of Chemistry, 1998:227–242.
65. Nema S, Washkuhn RJ, Beussink DR. Photostability testing: an overview. Pharm Techn 1995; 19(3):170–185.
66. Tønnesen HH, Karlsen J. Standardization of photochemical stability testing of drugs. Pharmeuropa 1993; 5(2):27–33.
67. Piechocki JT. Selecting the right source for pharmaceutical photostability testing. In: Albini A, Fasani E. Drugs: Photochemistry and Photostability. Cambridge: The Royal Society of Chemistry, 1998:247–271.
68. Piechocki JT, Wolters RJ. Light stability studies: a misnomer. Pharm Technol 1994; 18(1):60–65.
69. Thoma K, Kerker R. Report of the behavior of substances absorbing only in the UV range during daylight simulation. Pharm Ind 1992; 54:169–177.
70. Thoma K, Kerker R. The behavior of substances absorbing visible light in daylight simulation. Pharm Ind 1992; 54:287–293.
71. Favaro G. Actinometry: concepts and experiments. In: Albini A, Fasani E. Drugs: Photochemistry and Photostability. Cambridge: The Royal Society of Chemistry, 1998:295–304.
72. Kuhn HJ, Braslawski SE, Schmidt R. Chemical actinometry. Pure Appl Chem. 1989; 61:187–210.
73. Piechocki JT, Wolters RJ. Use of actinometry in light-stability studies. Pharm Technol 1993; 17(6):46–52.
74. Sekine H, Ohta Y, Nakagawa T. Usefulness of pyridoxine hydrochloride for actinometry. Drug Stab 1996; 135–140.
75. Bovina E, De Filippis P, Cavrini V, Ballardini R. Trans-2-nitrocinnamaldehyde as chemical actinometer for the UV-A range in photostability testing of pharmaceuticals. In: Albini A, Fasani E. Drugs: Photochemistry and Photostability. Cambridge: The Royal Society of Chemistry, 1998:305–316.

76. Allen JM, Allen SK, Baertschi SW. 2-Nitrobenzaldehyde: a convenient UV-A and UV-B chemical actinometer for drug photostability testing. J Pharm Biomed Anal 2000; 24:167–178.
77. Bolton JR. Ultraviolet Applications Handbook. London, Ontario: Bolton Photosciences, 1999.
78. Merrifield DR, Carter PL, Clapham D, Sanderson FD. Addressing the problem of light instability during formulation development. In: Tønnesen HH. Photostability of Drugs and Drug Formulation. London: Taylor and Francis, 1996:141–154.
79. Nyqvist H. Light stability testing of tablets in the Xenotest and the Fadeometer. Acta Pharm Suec 1984; 21:245–252.
80. Matsuda Y, Masahara R. Comparative evaluation of coloration of photosensitive solid drugs under various light sources. Yakagaku Zasshi 1980; 100: 953–957.
81. Takacs M, Reisch J, Gergely-Zobin A, Gücer-Ekiz N. Light sensitivity investigations of some solid pharmaceutical substances. Sci Pharm 1990; 58: 289–297.
82. Reisch J. Topochemical photoreactions of drugs and drug preparations. Dtsch Apot Ztg 1979; 119:1–4.
83. Reisch J, Topaloglu Y. Is TLC chromatography suitable for the on-plate control for the light stability of drugs. Pharm Acta Helv 1986; 61:142–147.
84. Nyqvist H, Wadsten T. Preformulation of solid dosage forms: light stability testing of polymorphs as a part of a preformulation process. Acta Pharm Technol 1986; 32:130–132.
85. Matsuda Y, Akazawa R, Teraoka R, Otsuka M. Pharmaceutical analysis of carbamazepine modifications: comparative study of the photostability of cabamazepine polymorphs by Fourier-transformed reflection–absorption infrared spectroscopy and colorimetric measurements. J Pharm Pharmacol 1994; 46: 162–167.
86. Hakimoto K, Inoue K, Sugimoto I. Photostability of several crystalline forms of cianidadol. Chem Pharm Bull 1985; 33:4050–4053.
87. Hakimoto K, Nakagawa H, Sugimoto I. Photostability of several crystalline forms of cianidadol. Drug Devel Ind Pharm 1985; 11:865–889.
88. de Villiers MM, van der Watt JG, Loetter AP. Kinetic studies of the solid state photolytic degradation of two polymorphic forms of furosemide. Int J Pharm 1992; 88:275–283.
89. Matsuda Y, Inouye H, Nakanishi R. Stabilization of sulfisomidine tablets by use of film coating containing UV absorber: protection of coloration and phototolytic degradation from exaggerated light. J Pharm Sci 1978; 67: 196–201.
90. Teraoka R, Matsuda Y, Sugimoto I. Quantitative design for photostabilisation of nifedipine by using titanium dioxide and/or tartrazine as colorants in model film coating systems. J Pharm Pharmacol 1989; 41:293–297.
91. Bechard SR, Quaraishi O, Kwong E. Film coating: effect of titanium dioxide concentration and film thickness on the photostability of nifedipine. Int J Pharm 1992; 87:133–139.

92. Thoma K, Kerker R. Photodegradation and photostabilization of nifedipine in dosage forms. Pharm Ind 1992; 54:359–365.
93. Thoma K, Klimek R. Photoinstability and stabilization of drugs. Possibilities of a generally applicable stabilization principle. Pharm Ind 1991; 53:504–507.
94. Thoma K, Klimek R. Photostabilization of drugs in dosage forms without protection from packaging material. Int J Pharm 1991; 67:169–175.
95. Takeuchi H, Sasaki H, Miwa T, Hino T, Kawashima Y, Uesugi K, Ozawa H. Improvement of photostability of ubidecarenone in the formulation of a novel powdered dosage form termed redispersible dry emulsion. Int J Pharm. 1992; 86:25–33.
96. Shahjahan M. Ultraviolet light absorbers and their uses in pharmacy. East Pharm 1989; 32:37–41.
97. Thoma K, Kerker R. The photostabilization of glucocorticoids. Pharm Ind 1992; 54:551–554.
98. Desai DS, Abdelnasser MA, Rubitski BA, Varia SA. Photostabilization of uncoated tablets of sorivudine and nifedipine by incorporation of synthetic iron oxides. Int J Pharm 1994; 103:69–76.
99. Matsuda Y, Teraoka R. Improvement of the photostability of ubicarenone microcapsules by incorporating fat-soluble vitamins. Int J Pharm 1985; 26: 289–301.
100. Habib MJ, Asker AF. Influence of certain additives on the photostability of cochicine solutions. Drug Dev Ind Pharm 1989; 15:1905–1909.
101. Habib MJ, Asker AF. Photostabilization of doxorubicin hydrochloride with radioprotective and photoprotective agents: potential mechanism for enhancing chemotherapy during radiotherapy. J Parenter Sci Technol 1989; 43: 259–261.
102. Asker AF, Habib MJ. Photostabilization of menadione sodium bisulfite by glutathione. J Parenter Sci Technol 1989; 43:204–207.
103. Asker AF, Habib MJ. Effect of certain additives on photodegradation of tetracycline hydrochloride solutions. J Parenter Sci Technol 1991; 45:113–115.
104. Asker AF, Larose M. Influence of uric acid on photostability of sulfathiazole sodium solutions. Drug Dev Ind Pharm 1987; 13:2239–2248.
105. Habib MJ, Hasker AF. Complex formation between metronidazole and sodium urate: effect on photodegradation of metronidazole. Pharm Res 1989; 6:58–61.
106. Islam MS, Asker AF. Photostabilization of dacarbazine with reduced glutathione. Pharm Sci Technol 1994; 48:38–40.
107. Nasa SL, Yadav S. Microencapsulation of metoprolol tartrate using phase separation coacervation techniques. East Pharm 1989; 32:133–134.
108. Teshima D, Otsubo K, Higuchi S, Hirayama F, Uekama K, Aoyama T. Effects of cyclodextrins on degradation of emetine and cephaeline in aqueous solutions. Chem Pharm Bull 1989; 37:1591–1594.
109. Utsuki T, Imamura K, Hirayama F, Uekama K. Stoichiomety-dependent changes of solubility and photoreactivity of an antiulcer agent, 2′-carboxymethoxy-4,4′-bis(3-methyl-2-butenyloxy)chalcone, in cyclodextrin inclusion complexes. Eur J Pharm Sci 1993; 1:81–87.

11

The Use of Microcalorimetry in Stress Testing

Graham Buckton and Simon Gaisford
The School of Pharmacy, University of London, London, U.K.

I. INTRODUCTION

Isothermal calorimetry is the measurement of heat absorbed or released by a chemical or physical process, at a constant temperature, with time. Isothermal microcalorimetry is the measurement of such heats on a microwatt scale and is a technique which has been commercially available for around 15 years (1). Microcalorimetry (henceforth taken to mean isothermal in this chapter) offers a range of advantages over many other analytical techniques. For example, the instrument does not degrade nor intrude upon the sample. Neither is it dependent on the physical nature of the subject under study. The sample can be a solid, liquid or gas or, indeed, any heterogeneous mixture. This means it is possible to study most pharmaceutical preparations directly, the only consideration being to ensure the subject will fit in the microcalorimetric ampoule. Microcalorimeters measure the heat changes for *all* the reactions occurring *simultaneously* within the sample. This property has both benefits and drawbacks; it allows the study of many complex reactions that are outside the scope of other analytical tools but can lead to complexities in the analysis of the data. It also means that poor sample preparation can lead to erroneous heat-flow signals.

As a standard analytical tool microcalorimetry is not as widely employed as HPLC, for example, in stress testing, although it has found certain niche applications. Outside the pharmaceutical field, the technique is more widely accepted, for instance stress testing of propellants and explosives is routinely carried out using microcalorimetry. In the pharmaceutical sciences, however, microcalorimetry is not as widely used as one might expect it to be, and it is the purpose of this entry to illustrate the potential uses and limitations of the technique for stress testing of pharmaceuticals. While it is possible to impose most types of stress on a sample held in a microcalorimetric ampoule, it is relatively difficult to change the temperature so the role of differential scanning calorimetry (DSC) in accelerated rate stress testing will also be considered briefly. While DSC is not strictly a microcalorimetric technique, modern instruments have increased the sensitivity of some instruments such that they are just 10-fold less sensitive than an isothermal microcalorimeter.

II. MICROCALORIMETRY

A modern heat-conduction, isothermal microcalorimeter is capable of maintaining a baseline of $\pm 0.1\,\mu W$ with a temperature stability of $\pm 0.0001°C$. It conducts heat to a heat-sink surrounding the sample via semiconducting Peltier elements. The design of such an instrument has been described in detail previously (1). Examples of microcalorimeters on the market today include the Calorimetry Sciences Corp. CSC 4400, the CSC 4500, and the 2277 Thermal Activity Monitor (TAM) by Thermometric AB (formerly LKB). It is also possible to use some differential scanning calorimeters in an isothermal mode, which then offer similar performance to dedicated isothermal instruments. Examples of this type of DSC include the Microcal VP-ITC. All these instruments are capable of detecting heat-flow signals as low as $0.1\,\mu W$. Brief performance details of selected instruments are given in Table 1. A schematic representation of the TAM is given in Figure 1 (courtesy of Thermometric AB, Järfälla, Sweden). The instrument consists of a large thermostatted water bath into which are placed four or fewer calorimetric channels. Each channel comprises two chambers; a reference chamber and a sample chamber (Fig. 2; courtesy of Thermometric AB, Järfälla, Sweden). Each chamber can accept glass vials (3 mL capacity), stainless steel ampoules (5 mL capacity) or, indeed, any ampoule designed to permit the study of specific reaction systems. Usually, the reference chamber is loaded with an inert material, of similar heat capacity and in a similar quantity to the sample, and the heat flow for the sample side is compared with the heat flow (0 normally) from the reference side (differential mode). If the material used as the inert reference undergoes a very slow or unenergetic reaction, i.e. is beyond the measurement capacity of the instrument, then it can be assumed to be producing no detectable calorimetric signal. The instrument is calibrated by loading both chambers with identical ampoules and, after thermal equilibration has been achieved, the differential heat flow recorded is adjusted to read 0. The instrument is capable of

Table 1 Instrument specifications of selected currently available isothermal microcalorimeters

Instrument	2277 Thermal Activity Monitor	CSC 4400	CSC 4500	Microcal VP-ITC
Temperature control				
Temperature range	5–90°C	0–100, −40 to 80 or 20–200°C	Not stated	2–80°C
Temperature stability	±0.0001°C	±0.0005°C at 25°C	±0.0005°C at 25°C	Not stated
Sensitivity				
Baseline stability	±0.1 μW	±1 μW	±40 nW	±20 nW
Sample				
Sample size	3 mL or 5 mL	15–150 mL	1 mL	1.3 mL
Sample type	Solid, liquid	Solid, liquid	Solid, liquid	Liquid
Information				
Manufacturer	Thermometric AB, Spjutvägen 5A, S-175 61 Järfälla, Sweden	Calorimetry Sciences Corp., PO Box 799, Provo, UT 84606–0799, U.S.A.	Calorimetry Sciences Corp., PO Box 799, Provo, UT 84606–0799, U.S.A.	Microcal Inc., 22 Industrial Drive East, Northampton, MA, U.S.A.
Website	www.thermometric.-com	www.calscorp.com	www.calscorp.com	www.microcalorimetry.com

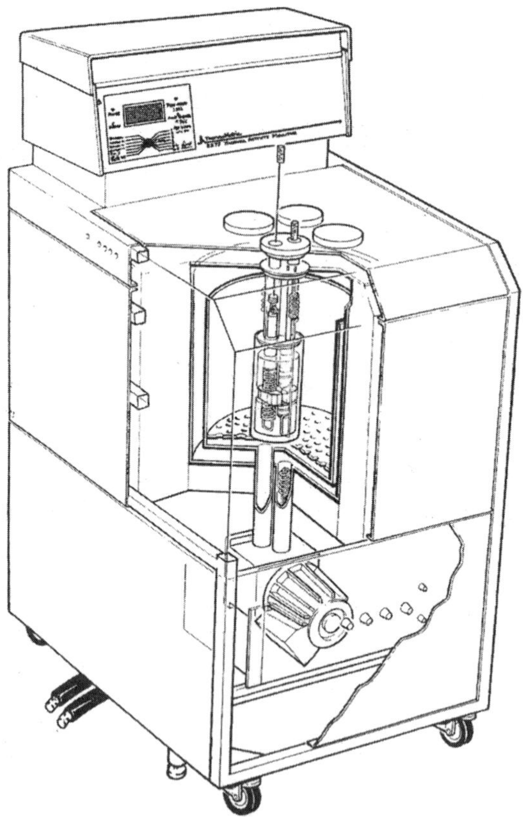

Figure 1 A schematic representation of a TAM (courtesy of Thermometric Ltd.).

recording data over a range of sensitivity scales, and must be calibrated separately for any particular setting. This is achieved using an electrical calibration. A known amount of heat passes into the sample ampoule over a period of time and, when equilibration is achieved, the heat flow recorded is adjusted until it matches the expected (calculated) value. To run a microcalorimetric experiment one simply needs to place a sample in an ampoule, seal it and place it in the instrument alongside a suitable reference.

Recently there has been considerable interest on the subject of chemical test reactions for isothermal microcalorimeters. Chemical test reactions allow a user to check if an instrument is functioning correctly because they reflect more accurately the processes under study in a real experiment. Indeed, the ideal case would be to have a universally accepted chemical test reaction for each type of experiment (perfusion, titration, etc.) one may wish to investigate. Examples of systems that have been proposed as chemical test reactions include 18-crown-6/barium sulfate (2) for titration calorimetry

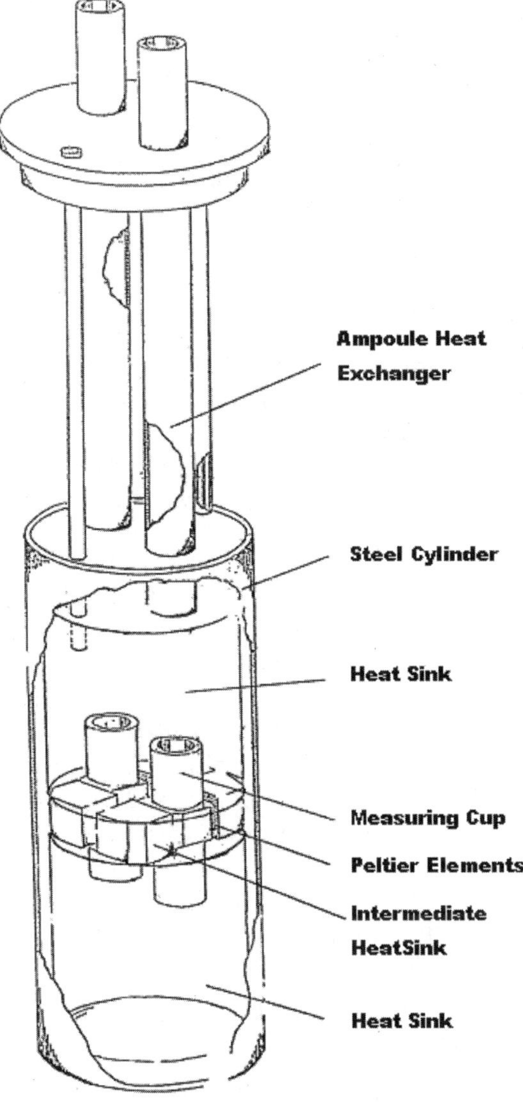

Figure 2 A schematic representation of a TAM channel (courtesy of Thermometric Ltd.).

and the acid catalyzed hydrolysis of triacetin for ampoule calorimetry (3). The latter reaction has recently been the subject of investigation (3). The reaction proceeds at a relatively slow rate with a large enthalpy and gives very reproducible power–time data. After fitting the data to a suitable model (described in detail in Section IIIA) one obtains values for the reaction rate

Table 2 Comparison of differential calorimetry and isothermal microcalorimetry (4)

	DSC	TAM
Sensitivity (mW)	10	0.1
Sample mass (mg)	10	1000
Specific sensitivity (W/g)	1	0.0001

constant order, and enthalpy. By comparing these values with accepted standards, instruments can be assessed to ensure they are functioning properly.

Isothermal microcalorimeters are usually operated at, or around, ambient temperatures and employ their inherent sensitivity to detect the heat-flow signals from any processes that are occurring in the sample ampoule. A comparison of the performance of a standard DSC (a Perkin-Elmer DSC 7, for instance) with that of a TAM gives an idea of the sensitivity of an isothermal microcalorimeter. Table 2 shows the typical performance parameters for these two instruments and shows that the TAM is of the order of 10,000-fold more sensitive than a standard DSC (4). DSC has been employed for accelerated stress testing because the rates of the processes under observation are accelerated at higher temperatures. The data that relate to any specified storage conditions are determined by extrapolation via application of the Arrhenius equation. This enforces the assumption that any processes that occur at the storage temperature are the same as that which occur over the experimental temperature range. Of course, this is not necessarily the case. Examples of processes which may lead to such problems include phase changes, moisture transfer (e.g., excipient-drug), etc.

The data in Table 3 show the temperature rise that would be required to accelerate first-order reactions with activation enthalpies of 50, 75, and

Table 3 The temperature increase, over 20°C, that would be required to accelerate a reaction by the specified factors (5)

Factor of rate increase	Activation enthalpies (kJ mol^{-1})		
	50	75	100
1	0	0	0
10	37	24	17
100	85	52	37
1000	149	85	59
10,000	239	125	85
100,000	375	175	114

100 kJ mol^{-1} by factors of between 1 and 100,000 (5). The data show, for example, that if a reaction of rate 1 (arbitrary units) and activation enthalpy of 50 kJ mol^{-1} is observable in a TAM at 20°C then for this reaction to be observed in a DSC the temperature will have to be raised by 239°C. Such an extrapolation should not be undertaken without caution.

An additional benefit of the TAM system is that it is possible to purchase a range of apparatus that fit within the calorimetric chambers. Examples of such equipment include RH vessels, titration vessels, and a solution calorimeter. It is also not outside the bounds of possibility to construct a piece of apparatus to do a specific job oneself, if no such item is commercially available.

III. ANALYSIS OF MICROCALORIMETRIC DATA

The difficulty in analysing microcalorimetric data recorded for moderately complex systems goes someway to explaining why the technique is not more commonly used. There are two principal reasons why data analysis may present some difficulty. Firstly, the microcalorimeter records the heat flows of all the processes occurring in the reaction cell simultaneously. Thus a complex signal can be obtained with what appears to be a relatively simple sample, or a simple signal can be obtained for what is expected to be a complex sample. In fact, in the theoretically possible case where two samples in equal quantity are reacting with equal rate constants, reaction order and equal (but of opposite sign) enthalpies the microcalorimeter will record no heat flow! The second problem is that the calorimeter gives no direct molecular information and it is often necessary to study the same reaction using a complimentary analytical technique such as HPLC or NMR.

However, there are numerous theoretical models available in the literature that attempt to derive meaningful values from thermal data. Solution phase reactions are generally easier to model than solid-state or heterogeneous reactions and the discussion that follows will consider the two classes separately. In all cases, it is necessary to know the time at which the reaction was initiated, t_0, in order to analyse the data correctly. Note that this does not mean the reaction must be initiated directly in the instrument—this is difficult for ampoules prepared on a bench-top—it means that the time axis on the resulting power–time curve must be corrected for the delay caused by loading. No fitting model requires the reaction to run to completion in order to return the correct reaction parameters—if this were the case it would take up to 10,000 years to model some reactions based on the sensitivity of the instrument!

A. Solution Phase Reactions

The simplest approach to modeling microcalorimetric data is to fit the data to a generic equation, i.e. an equation that conveniently fits the data but does not attempt to *model* the reaction processes occurring. A simple example would be to use an exponential decay model such as that shown in Eq. (1).

$$y = y_o + Ae^{-x/t} \tag{1}$$

For example, some microcalorimetric data are represented in Figure 3. The exact process that gave rise to these data is not important, but it shall be assumed that they represent the heat output of a partially completed reaction. These data have been fitted to the exponential model shown above to determine the equation parameters that describe them. Once these values have been determined, it is possible to extend the data to such a time as the observed heat flow (power) equals 0 (shown by the dotted line). The area under the dotted line represents the total heat, Q, which would be generated by the reaction if it went to completion. From this information, it is a simple matter to determine the extent of reaction at any time, t. Hence, some useful information can be derived by using nonspecific models.

The second approach to fitting microcalorimetric data is to base the fitting equations on kinetic models that describe the reaction(s) under study. This approach was first developed by Bakri et al. (6) and subsequently extended and developed by Willson et al. (7,8). The first stage in this case is to select a suitable kinetic model from those in the literature. The model is then converted to a calorimetric form by recognition of the fact that the

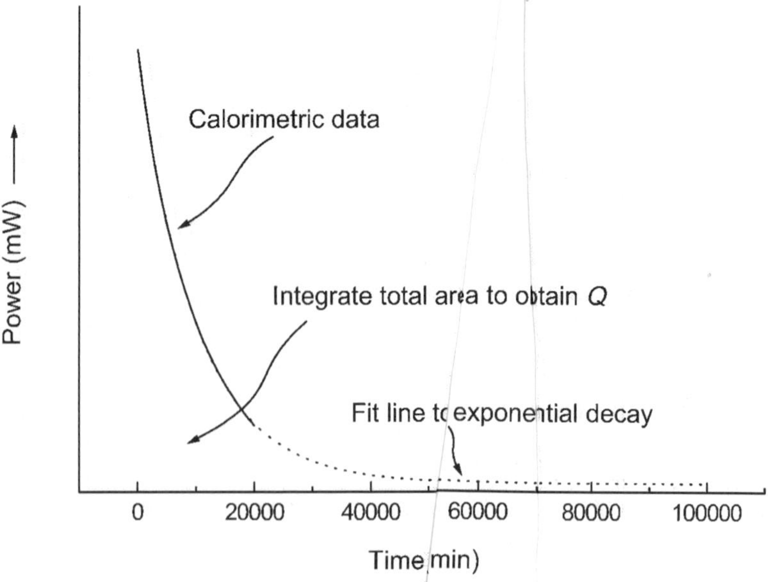

Figure 3 The modeling of microcalorimetric data using a nonspecific exponential model and the extrapolation of the data to power = 0.

total heat evolved during the course of a reaction (Q) must equal the total number of moles of material reacted (A_o) multiplied by the change in molar enthalpy for that reaction (ΔH), Eq. (2).

$$Q = A_o \Delta H \tag{2}$$

Similarly, the heat evolved at time t (q) is equal to the number of moles of material reacted (x) at time t multiplied by the change in molar enthalpy for that reaction, Eq. (3).

$$q = x\Delta H \tag{3}$$

Eq. (3) may be substituted into a general rate expression of the form dx/dt to give an expression of the form dq/dt (or power). For example, the general rate expression for a simple, solution phase, first-order, $A \rightarrow x$ process is given by Eq. (4).

$$\frac{dx}{dt} = kV(A_o - x) \tag{4}$$

where dx/dt is the rate of appearance of product x, k is the first-order rate constant, V is the volume of solution and A_o is the number of moles of reactant A available for reaction. Substitution of Eq. (3) into Eq. (4) yields,

$$\frac{dq}{dt} = k\Delta HV\left(A_o - \frac{q}{\Delta H}\right) \tag{5}$$

This modified rate expression may be used to fit power–time data recorded using the microcalorimeter by a process of iteration using a proprietary mathematical software package (for example, Origin™, Microcal Software Inc.).

The use of Eq. (5) to fit data recorded using a microcalorimeter was first demonstrated by Bakri (6), who studied the acid hydrolysis of methyl acetate in hydrochloric acid. In that experiment, 1 mmol of methyl acetate was added to 2 mL of 1 N hydrochloric acid solution in a glass ampoule. The experimental data were fitted to Eq. (5) using a least squares analysis which gave $k = 0.116 \times 10^{-3}$ sec^{-1} and $\Delta H = 1.98$ kJ mol^{-1}. In this paper, Bakri also shows how the method may be applied to both second-order, solution phase $A + B \rightarrow x$ reactions and to flow calorimetry.

More recently, Willson et al. (7,8) showed how it is possible to write calorimetric kinetic equations that describe a range of commonly encountered mechanisms. The original and transformed versions of some of these equations are given in Table 4. Many of these fitting equations have been incorporated into the thermometric operating and data capture software Digitam 4.1™.

It has also been shown that it is possible to apply this method of analysis to more complex reaction schemes (5,9,10). For example, consider the following consecutive, first-order, solution phase reaction mechanism:

Table 4 Transformed calorimetric equations for a range of reaction types (7,8)

Reaction scheme	Kinetic expression	Transformed expression
A→B	$\frac{dx}{dt} = k(A - x)^m$	$\frac{dq}{dt} = \Delta H k(A - \frac{q}{\Delta H})^m$
A+B→C	$\frac{dx}{dt} = k(A - x)^m(B - x)^n$	$\frac{dq}{dt} = \Delta H k(A - \frac{q}{\Delta H})^m(B - \frac{q}{\Delta H})^n$
A⇔B	$\frac{dx}{dt} = k\left(\frac{A}{x_e}\right)(x_e - x)$	$\frac{dq}{dt} = kA(\Delta H - \frac{q}{x_e})$
A+B⇔C	$\frac{dx}{dt} = k_1(A - x)(B - x)$	$\frac{dq}{dt} = k_1(A\Delta H - q)(B\Delta H - q) - (k_{-1}q)$
Ng* equation	$\frac{dx}{dt} = Ak(\frac{x}{A})^m(1 - \frac{x}{A})^n$	$\frac{dq}{dt} = Ak\Delta H(\frac{q}{A\Delta H})^m(1 - \frac{q}{A\Delta H})$
Autocatalytic	$\frac{dx}{dt} = k(A - x)(x_{\bar{c}} + x)$	$\frac{dq}{dt} = k(A\Delta H - q)(x_{\bar{c}}\Delta H + q)$
Coagulation	$\frac{dx}{dt} = k(n - x)^2$	$\frac{dq}{dt} = k\Delta H(n - \frac{q}{\Delta H})^2$
Michaelis–Menten	$\frac{d[ES]}{dt} = k(K_{\bar{c}}[E][S])$	$\frac{dq}{dt} = k\Delta H(k_{\bar{c}}[E][S] - \frac{q}{\Delta H})$

$$A \xrightarrow{k_1} B \xrightarrow{k_2} P$$

(first-order, ΔH_1 and ΔH_2 respectively)

It can be shown (10) that the calorimetric equation that describes this reaction is given by

$$\frac{dq_{obs}}{dt} = k_1 \Delta H_1 A_o V e^{-k_1 t} + k_1 k_2 \Delta H_2 A_o V \frac{e^{-k_1 t} - e^{-k_2 t}}{k_2 - k_1} \tag{6}$$

Similarly if the related, but slightly more complex, three-step mechanism is considered;

$$A \xrightarrow{k_1} B \xrightarrow{k_2} C \xrightarrow{k_3} P$$

(first-order, ΔH_1, ΔH_2 and ΔH_3 respectively)

It can be shown (10) that the corresponding calorimetric equation is given by

$$\begin{aligned}\frac{dq_{obs}}{dt} &= k_1 \Delta H_1 A_o V e^{-k_1 t} + k_1 k_2 \Delta H_2 A_o V \frac{e^{-k_1 t} - e^{-k_2 t}}{k_2 - k_1} \\ &+ \Delta H_3 \Bigg(A_o V k_1 e^{-k_1 t} - \frac{A_o V k_1}{(k_2 - k_1)}(-k_1 e^{-k_1 t} + k_2 e^{-k_2 t}) \\ &+ \frac{k_2^2 k_1 A_o V e^{-k_2 t}}{-k_1 k_2 - k_3 k_2 + k_2^2 + k_3 k_1} + \frac{k_2 k_1^2 A_o V e^{k_1 t}}{-k_1 k_2 + k_3 k_2 - k_3 k_1 + k_1^2} \\ &- \frac{k_2 k_1 A_o V k_3 e^{-k_3 t}}{-k_1 k_2 - k_3 k_2 + k_2^2 + k_3 k_1} - \frac{k_2 k_1 A_o V k_3 e^{-k_3 t}}{-k_1 k_2 + k_3 k_2 - k_3 k_1 + k_1^2} \Bigg)\end{aligned} \tag{7}$$

The use of these equations to analyse calorimetric data has been demonstrated using a model reaction, the acid catalyzed hydrolysis of potassium hydroxylamine trisulfonate (9,10), which reacts according to the following model (Scheme 1).

The reaction has been studied previously using a titration method that showed the hydrolysis of the trisulfonate ion is the fastest of the three steps, producing the relatively stable hydroxylamine-NO-disulfonate ion (11,12). Potassium hydroxylamine-NO-disulfonate is stable enough to be recrystallized from dilute acid solution. The disulfonate hydrolyses slowly in dilute acid solution forming the hydroxylamine-*O*-sulfonate ion and, eventually, hydroxylamine and hydrogen sulfate. Hydrogen sulfate is formed in each reaction step, and chemical assays for this ion were used to perform the early kinetic studies. The authors of the original work were unable to study the slower reaction steps at room temperature, and had to use temperatures of up to 70°C. Using the microcalorimeter, it was possible to study the reaction directly at 25, 30, and 35°C.

The power–time data obtained for the hydrolysis reactions were fitted to Eq. (7) to determine the values of the reaction parameters. A typical fit line is represented in Figure 4. The data were also fitted to the simpler Eq. (6) Figure 5). This showed whether the models possessed sufficient sensitivity to determine mechanistic information. It is apparent that the simpler model did not fit the experimental data as well as the more complex model, indicating that the data do indeed reflect a three-step process. The two-step model gives a reasonable fit over the initial section of data, where the first two hydrolysis reactions predominate, but cannot fit the section of data where all three hydrolyses are occurring.

Analysis of the data allowed estimates to be made for all the reaction parameters. The rate constant values, determined at an added acid concen-

$$(SO_3)_2N.O.SO_3^{3-} + H_2O \xrightarrow{k_1,\ \Delta H_1} SO_3.NH.O.SO_3^{2-} + HSO_4^-$$

$$SO_3.NH.O.SO_3^{2-} + H_2O \xrightarrow{k_2,\ \Delta H_2} NH_2.O.SO_3^- + HSO_4^-$$

$$NH_2.O.SO_3^- + H_2O \xrightarrow{k_3,\ \Delta H_3} NH_2.OH + HSO_4^-$$

Scheme 1

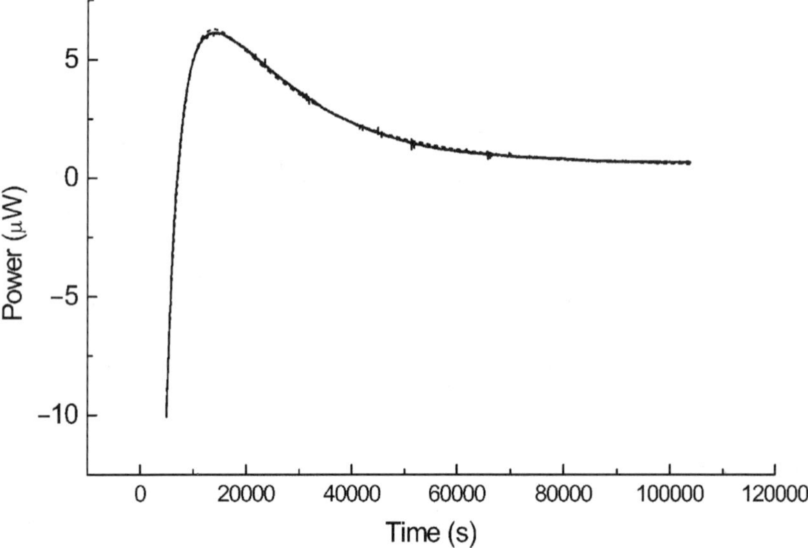

Figure 4 Power–time data for the acid-catalyzed hydrolysis of potassium hydroxylamine trisulfonate at 35°C and the fit line (dotted) obtained by application of Eq. (7) (9).

tration of 0.005 M are shown in Table 5 (9). It is apparent that, in most cases, the rate constants determined for the second and third hydrolyses are smaller than those for the first hydrolysis, an observation in accordance with expectation.

B. Solid-State and Heterogeneous Reactions

While the kinetics of solution phase reactions are well understood, the kinetics of solid-state and heterogeneous reactions are much less understood and present considerable problems (13). Solid-state reactions show complex rate behaviours that are not easily understood and cannot always be fitted to a simple kinetic model. The kinetics of solid-state degradation reactions have been studied widely, usually on pharmaceutical compounds, since these data are used to predict shelf-lives and expiry dates (14,15). An excellent review of solid-state drug stability has been published by Carstensen (16). In such cases, it is usually sufficient to obtain an equation that merely gives a satisfactory fit to the data since it is generally unnecessary to elucidate mechanistic information. This is the same as the first approach highlighted previously for solution phase reactions. There are, however, a number of kinetic treatments specifically designed for solid-state reactions. Such treatments are based on the reaction of only one substance, and all involve plotting the fraction of reactant decomposed, α, vs. time. Note that this

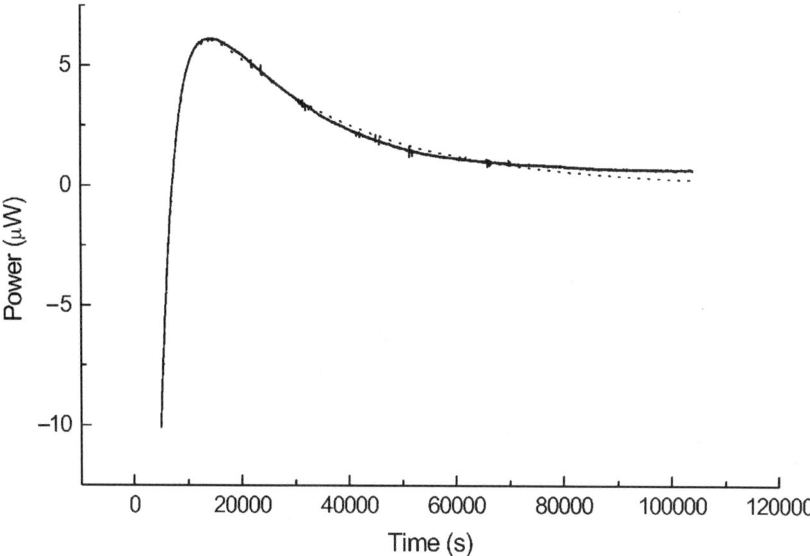

Figure 5 Power–time data for the acid-catalyzed hydrolysis of potassium hydroxylamine trisulfonate at 35°C and the fit line (dotted) obtained by application of Eq. (6) (9).

approach differs slightly from the kinetic modeling discussed previously for solution phase reactions because the equations are not considered in molar terms and, hence, not on the direct reaction mechanism, but simply on the fraction of material reacted at any specified time. This arises because concentration terms have little meaning in the solid state. Examples of such treatments include the Avrami–Erofeev equation (17) and the Prout–Tompkins equation (18).

For the purposes of fitting microcalorimetric data, one equation is perhaps of more interest than most. That is the Ng equation (19), given in Table 4, which is stated to describe all two-state solid phase reactions. If the calorimetric form of the Ng equation is used to fit suitable calorimetric data then it is possible, from knowledge of the values of the constants m and n, to infer

Table 5 Rate constant values for the acid catalyzed hydrolysis of potassium hydroxylamine trisulfonate (at an acid concentration of 0.005 M) determined from microcalorimetric data (9)

Temperature (°C)	k_1 (sec^{-1})	k_2 (sec^{-1})	k_3 (sec^{-1})
35	5.126×10^{-4}	4.751×10^{-5}	2.320×10^{-4}
30	4.381×10^{-4}	2.763×10^{-5}	6.225×10^{-5}
25	4.246×10^{-4}	4.561×10^{-6}	6.712×10^{-6}

Table 6 Reaction mechanisms described by the Ng equation with the particular variables shown (7,8)

m	n	Equation	Character
0	0	$d\alpha/dt = k$	Linear
1	0	$d\alpha/dt = k.\alpha$	Exponential
0.5	0	$d\alpha/dt = k.\alpha^{1/2}$	Square
0	1	$d\alpha/dt = k.(1-\alpha)$	Unimolecular decay
0	0.5	$d\alpha/dt = k.(1-\alpha)^{1-1/2}$	Contracting surface
0	0.66	$d\alpha/dt = k.(1-\alpha)^{2/3}$	Contracting sphere
1	1	$d\alpha/dt = k.\alpha.(1-\alpha)$	Prout–Tompkins
0.66	0.66	$d\alpha/dt = k.\alpha^{2/3}.(1-\alpha)^{2/3}$	Roginskii–Shultz

some information on the likely process by which the studied reaction occurs. Values of m and n and the related respective reaction processes are given in Table 6.

Calorimetric forms of the Ng equation were used by Willson et al. (7) to analyse the solid-state degradation of L-ascorbic acid. Known amounts (0.5 g) of dry L-ascorbic acid were placed in ampoules along with known quantities of water and the heat changes in the samples were recorded using an isothermal microcalorimeter. The power–time data obtained were analyzed using the calorimetric form of the Ng equation and the parameters obtained are shown in Table 7. It was shown that, at low added quantities of added water, the reaction could satisfactorily be described by solid-state kinetics, but at higher added quantities of water (more than 500 μL) the reaction was best described by solution phase kinetics.

Willson (8) also studied the degradation of di-benzoyl peroxide using isothermal microcalorimetry. Literature values for the degradation of di-benzoyl peroxide at 100°C are $3.8 \times 10^{-4}\ s^{-1}$ with an activation energy of

Table 7 Reaction parameters determined for the reaction between ascorbic acid and various quantities of water. If more than 500 μL of water was added, the reaction followed solution phase kinetics (7,8)

Added water (μL)	Rate constant (sec^{-1})	ΔH ($kJ\ mol^{-1}$)	A_o (mol)	m	n
Dry	3.15×10^{-6}	199	4.39×10^{-7}	−0.01	0.9
20	4.10×10^{-6}	199	2.25×10^{-6}	−0.02	0.6
30	4.35×10^{-6}	199	2.39×10^{-6}	−0.01	0.8
50	5.21×10^{-6}	197	3.93×10^{-6}	−0.01	0.8
100	5.62×10^{-6}	180	4.27×10^{-6}	−0.12	0.6
200	4.22×10^{-6}	188	8.05×10^{-6}	−0.09	0.6
Average	4.10×10^{-6}	193		−0.02	0.71

Table 8 Reaction parameters determined for the degradation of di-benzoyl peroxide at 25°C by fitting microcalorimetric data to the Ng equation (8)

	k (sec^{-1})	ΔH (kJ mol^{-1})	Quantity of material reacted (mol)	Order
	5.190×10^{-8}	−19.2	1.0×10^{-4}	1
	5.219×10^{-8}	−18.6	1.03×10^{-4}	1
	5.208×10^{-8}	−19.9	8.7×10^{-5}	1
Average	5.205×10^{-8}	−19.2±0.65	9.6×10^{-5}	1
	$\pm 1.46 \times 10^{-10}$		$\pm 8.5 \times 10^{-6}$	

125.52 kJ mol^{-1} (20). Using microcalorimetry, it was possible to study the reaction directly at 25°C. The compound was placed into an ampoule and the heat changes associated with degradation were recorded over a period of 100 hr. Since it was assumed that the degradation was mediated by water, and no attempt was made to keep the sample dry, the data were analyzed using solution phase kinetics, the results being given in Table 8. Using the Arrhenius equation, the literature data at 100°C were extrapolated to 25°C to give a rate constant of 1.37×10^{-8} sec^{-1}, a value that compares favorably with the calorimetrically determined value of 5.205×10^{-8} sec^{-1}. The enthalpy change for the reaction was determined to equal −19.2 kJ mol^{-1}. No literature value for this parameter was available, but it compares well with the value determined from gas phase bond enthalpies of −20.5 kJ mol^{-1}. These data show that it is possible to analyze relatively complex, solid phase reactions to obtain good estimates of kinetic and thermodynamic parameters. The data presented in Table 8 show that the reproducibility of the technique is excellent.

The interconversion of nitritopentamminecobalt (III) chloride to nitropentamminecobalt (III) chloride was also studied by Willson (8). Using isothermal microcalorimetry, estimates for the rate constant of interconversion and the thermodynamic reaction parameters were obtained directly, at 25°C, by fitting the data to the transformed Ng equation. The published

Table 9 Reaction parameters determined for the interconversion of nitritopentamminecobalt (III) chloride to nitropentamminecobalt (III) chloride (8)

	Rate constant	ΔH (kJ mol^{-1})	Quantity of material reacted	m	n
Analysis 1	3.99×10^{-6} sec^{-1}	−1.73	0.0035 mol	1.14	0.45
Analysis 2	3.55×10^{-6} sec^{-1}	−2.65	0.0039 mol	1.099	0.45
Analysis 3	1.4×10^{-6} sec^{-1}	−4.60	0.0045 mol	1.1	0.3
Average	2.98×10^{-6}	−2.99	0.0039	1.1	0.4
	$\pm 1.58 \times 10^{-6}$ sec^{-1}	±1.2	±0.0004 mol		

data are shown in Table 9. The interconversion of one complex to the other is regarded as a physical process whereas the reaction of ascorbic acid, discussed above, is a chemical process. Using the Willson method it is possible to study both types of reaction directly.

IV. DRUG STABILITY

Isothermal microcalorimetry is often a useful tool to investigate drug stability because of its sensitivity to processes that are occurring slowly, negating the need for a temperature increase and the associated problems with data extrapolation discussed earlier. Because the technique is noninvasive and nondestructive it is also possible to retrieve the sample after recording thermal data, which has obvious benefits for samples of new drugs that may only be available in limited quantities. A theoretical consideration of the performance capabilities of an instrument such as a TAM shows that it is possible to distinguish between first-order rate constants of 1×10^{-11} and 2×10^{-11} s^{-1} from 50 hr of power–time data, at 25° C, assuming the reaction under study possesses a reasonable ($\sim$40 kJ mol^{-1}) enthalpy change (8). Expressing this sensitivity in a more readily understandable form means that the microcalorimeter can detect the presence of a reaction that occurs with a half-life of 2200 years (0.03% $year^{-1}$). Given that the maximum rate of degradation of a pharmaceutical is usually stated to be of the order of 5% in 2 years (21), the microcalorimeter has potential for stability studies.

As highlighted in the previous section, the biggest obstacle in the widespread use of microcalorimetry to investigate drug stability is the difficulty in analysing the data quantitatively. This problem is particularly acute for drug stability, which often involves solid phases. Nevertheless, many drugs have been subjected to microcalorimetric investigation including, for instance, aspirin (22), cephalosporins (23), lovastatin (24), meclofenoxate hydrochloride (25), nifedipine (26), and ascorbic acid (7,27).

The applicability of microcalorimetry to the stability testing of drugs has, for example, been investigated using the drugs meclofenoxate hydrochloride (MF) and DL-α-tocopherol (TP) (25). MF is known to hydrolyze in aqueous solution while TP oxides in the air and hence the two drugs provide good examples of two of the main processes by which pharmaceuticals are degraded. The hydrolysis of MF was studied in aqueous solutions buffered to pH 6.4 and 2.9. Plots of ln(power) vs. time gave linear relationships, indicating the degradation followed first-order kinetics. The rate constants at the two pHs were determined to equal 1.14×10^{-4} and 9.7×10^{-7} sec^{-1}, respectively. These values concurred with results generated from HPLC data of 1.29×10^{-4} and 9×10^{-7} sec^{-1} respectively, showing that microcalorimetry can be a good match for HPLC in degradation measurements. The HPLC determination of the slower of the two rate constants required three days of work whereas the microcalorimetric data were recorded in less than a day.

Samples of TP (a slightly viscous liquid) were placed in glass ampoules that were left open to the atmosphere in ovens at 50, 40, 30, and 23°C for varying lengths of time. Each sample was then capped before being placed in the microcalorimeter. Equivalent samples were analyzed using HPLC. First-order rate constants for the samples were determined at each temperature. An Arrhenius plot of the data revealed a linear correlation and an excellent agreement between the HPLC and microcalorimetric data.

The oxidation of L-ascorbic acid in aqueous solution provides another example of the investigation of the stability of a drug by microcalorimetry (7,27). Ascorbic acid oxidizes reversibly in aqueous solution forming dehydroascorbic acid, which is subsequently hydrolyzed irreversibly to give diketogulonic acid. The rate of the reaction is affected by a number of factors including pH, oxygen concentration, ascorbic acid concentration, the presence of metal ions, and the presence of antioxidants. Using the microcalorimeter, it has been shown possible to study this oxidation reaction under varying conditions and determine the effects of altering each of the factors. This is because the power–time signal from the calorimeter is defined by the rate of the reaction under investigation, so if the rate alters, the shape of the power–time curve alters.

Angberg et al. (27) noted that the heat flow measured for solutions of ascorbic acid in pH 4.9 and 3.9 buffers was greater for those samples that were prepared with an air-space in the ampoule compared with those that were not. Furthermore, if the solution was purged with nitrogen prior to loading, the heat flow dropped nearly to 0. Similar observations were observed by Willson et al. (7) who noted, by observing a linear ln(power) vs. time plot, that the oxidation was first-order with respect to oxygen concentration. Both studies suggest that the oxygen in the ampoule is exhausted after 3–4 hr and the measured heat flow after this time falls to 0.

Similarly, the effects of varying the ascorbic acid concentration were studied in the microcalorimeter. Angberg et al. (27) noted that the measured heat flow increased with increasing ascorbic acid concentration up to a certain concentration, whereupon further increases did not increase the power response. Presumably, the reaction became limited by the oxygen concentration at higher acid concentrations. Willson et al. (7) calculated the rate constants for the oxidation at varying ascorbic acid concentrations and found that they were identical, concluding that the oxidation rate is independent of acid concentration. The presence of metal ions (copper or iron, for example) is known to affect the oxidation rate of compounds in solution and is difficult to control, because only trace amounts are required to catalyze the reaction. Both authors conducted experiments in the presence of EDTA, a metal chelating ligand and observed that the measured heat flows fell substantially compared with samples run in the absence of the metal binder.

V. DRUG–EXCIPIENT STABILITY

While hydrolysis and oxidation reactions are common degradation pathways, other factors must be considered when designing pharmaceutical preparations. Prime among these is excipient compatibility. All drugs are formulated with a range of excipients; binders, disintegrants, fillers, lubricants, etc. It is important that the drug does not interact with any of these other compounds, especially if the interaction leads to drug degradation. Microcalorimetry offers a technique with which to test for possible incompatibility. The greatest advantage of microcalorimetry is that the technique does not require the build up of a relatively large proportion of degradation products to have occurred in the way that HPLC or spectroscopy do for example. An additional benefit of the TAM in particular is that up to four experiments can be run simultaneously, further reducing screening times. A simple methodology for testing binary mixtures has recently been reported (28). The thermal behaviour of the drug alone and the excipient alone are recorded. The two heat flows are combined to produce a theoretical compatible power–time trace (the power–time data that would reasonably be expected if the two components did not interact). The theoretical compatible data are compared with those recorded for the observed binary drug–excipient mixture. Any difference between the theoretical compatible data and the observed data suggests an interaction is occurring. Typical power–time data obtained from such an experiment are shown in Figure 6, recorded at 50°C, 75% RH (courtesy of Thermometric Ltd.). It can be seen that the drug is clearly incompatible with the excipient as there is a large heat flow associated with the observed binary mixture that is not seen in the theoretical compatible case. The method can be used with a wide range of drugs and excipients and there is therefore no associated method development required for each test subject as there is with, for instance, HPLC analysis (29). Another advantage is that the experiment requires just 15 hr to complete.

Other examples of the use of microcalorimetry to study drug–excipient compatibility in the solid state are provided by Selzer et al. (30), who studied the interaction between a solid drug and a range of excipients [including potato starch, α-lactose-monohydrate, microcrystalline cellulose (MCC), and talc] and Schmitt (31) who used water slurries instead of humidified samples.

VI. WATER–DRUG, WATER–EXCIPIENT STABILITY

The study of interactions between, and reactions induced by, the introduction of water to a sample is of importance in pharmaceutical stability. This is

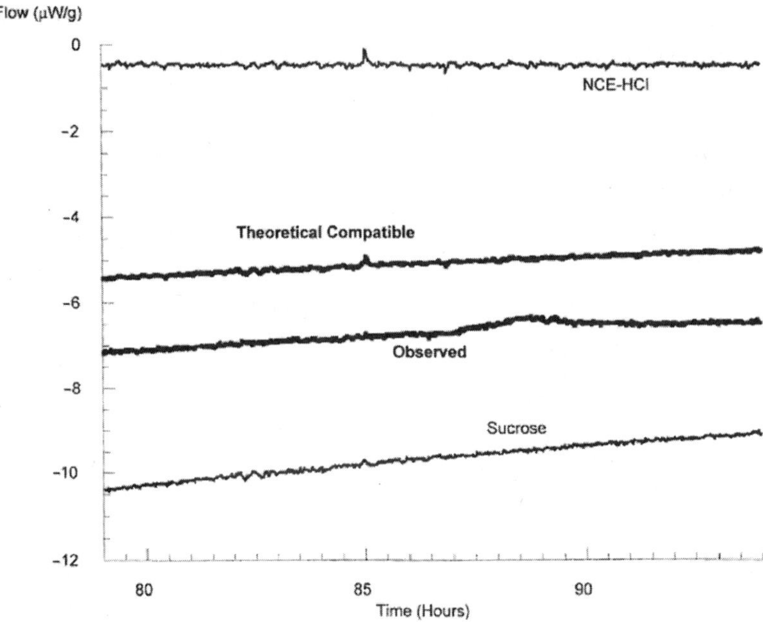

Figure 6 Heat flow vs. time data for a drug (NCE-HCl), an excipient (sucrose) and a binary mixture of the two (observed). The observed trace is different from the theoretical compatible trace, indicating a possible incompatibility (courtesy of Thermometric Ltd.).

because the presence of water can degrade a sample in several ways. For instance, water may induce a hydrolysis reaction or act as an intermediary between two solid components. The technique also allows the quantification of amorphous content. Many techniques, such as milling, grinding, or drying, used in drug manufacture induce the formation of amorphous regions in solid drugs. Above the glass transition temperature, (T_g), amorphous materials will recrystallize. Recrystallization is accompanied by a change in heat content and can therefore be followed using microcalorimetry. Water acts as a plasticizer, lowering the T_g of the material, allowing recrystallization to be investigated at room temperature. The heat output of recrystallization is directly proportional to the amorphous content of the material, and hence, microcalorimetry is an extremely sensitive technique for quantifying amorphous content. It is possible to determine amorphous content to $\pm 0.5\%$ using microcalorimetry compared with a detection limit of 10% with conventional techniques such as X-ray diffraction (32). The relative ease with which such interactions can be studied has been made easier by the commercial availability of apparatus that allow the introduction of water directly into the sample ampoule. This can be achieved in one of two ways; water vapor can be introduced to the sample (perfusion), or liquid water can be introduced to the sample (titration). A schematic representation of the commercial perfusion apparatus available from Thermometric AB is given in Figure 7 (courtesy of Thermometric AB, Järfälla, Sweden).

Of course, it is not always necessary to purchase an expensive piece of equipment in order to introduce water to a sample. If one wishes to study a

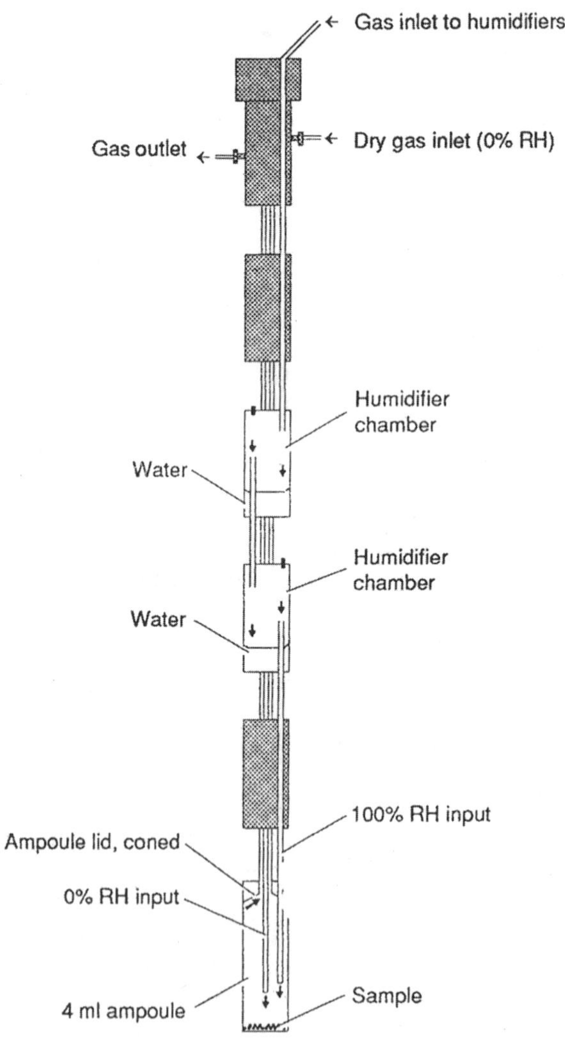

Figure 7 A schematic representation of a gas perfusion unit (courtesy of Thermometric Ltd.).

Table 10 The relative humidities (RH) obtained at various temperatures using saturated salt solutions (33)

Salt	Temperature (°C)		
	25	35	45
LiCl	11.3	11.2	11.2
$MgCl_2$	32.8	32.0	31.1
NaBr	57.5	54.0	52.0
NaCl	75.3	74.8	74.7
KCl	84.3	82.9	81.7

sample under conditions of controlled RH, then it is possible to place a small glass tube (a Durham tube or hydrostat), containing a small quantity of a saturated salt solution, directly within the ampoule. Saturated salt solutions maintain a constant RH at a specific temperature. Table 10 lists the RH obtained from various salt solutions at various temperatures (33).

An example of a reaction that can be induced by the presence of water vapor is the crystallization of amorphous lactose, a subject that has been reviewed by Buckton and Darcy (34). After a period of exposure to any particular RH amorphous lactose exhibits a crystallization exotherm (Fig. 8) (35). It can be shown that the rate of onset of crystallization varies with

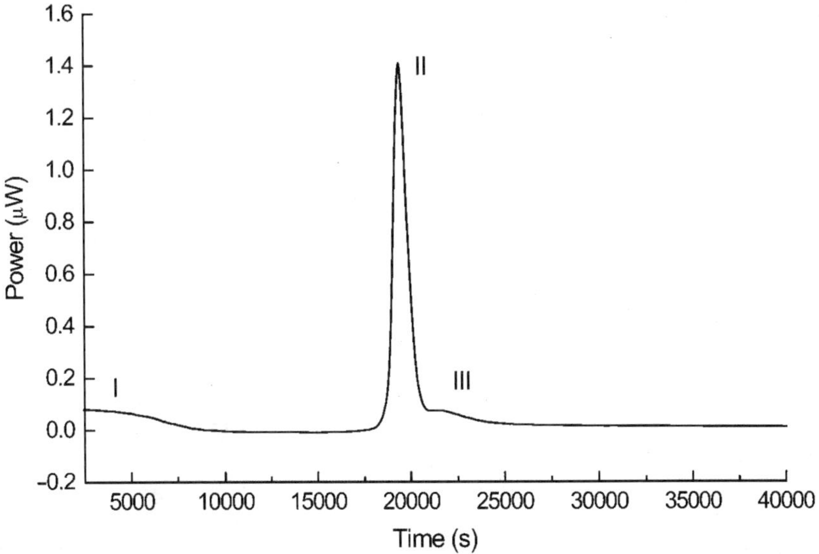

Figure 8 Power–time trace of 100% amorphous lactose exposed to 75% RH (35).

the RH in the sample ampoule. The percent crystallinity of a lactose sample of unknown composition can be deduced by measuring the area under its crystallization exotherm and comparing the result with the area obtained for a 100% amorphous sample.

Titration calorimetry can be used to introduce a liquid to a solid or a liquid to a liquid. In this case, the sample is placed in a stainless steel ampoule and the liquid to be titrated is placed in an external reservoir. To avoid problems with temperature gradients the external reservoir should be maintained at the same temperature as the sample. The titrant enters the sample ampoule via a stainless steel cannula. The injections are computer controlled, and the amounts required are entered into the software before an experiment is initiated.

An example of the use of titration calorimetry is provided by the critical micelle concentration (cmc) determination of a series of pharmaceutical excipients (poloxamers). Poloxamers are ABA block copolymers of general formula PEO_A–PPO_B–PEO_A, where PEO represents poly(ethylene oxide), PPO represents poly(propylene oxide) and A and B are the respective numbers of each monomer in each block. They are also known by the trade names Synperonic PE (Uniqema, UK) and Pluoronic (BASF, Germany). Upon an increase in solution concentration, the poloxamers are known to micellise, before clouding out and subsequently forming gels. The micellisation may be followed using titration calorimetry by injecting a concentrated poloxmer solution (one that is above its cmc) into a dilute poloxamer solution (one that is below its cmc) or into water. Following an injection the concentrated polymer solution is diluted and the poloxamers demicellise. The heat associated with these processes is recorded and plotted vs. injection number, polymer concentration or time. An example of such a trace is shown in Figure 9 (36). The experiment is referenced against a blank experiment whereby water is injected into water such that any heats associated with the injection process itself are removed. When the solution concentration in the ampoule reaches the cmc of the polymer, further injections of concentrated poloxamer will not result in a demicellisation exotherm. A first-derivative plot of the heat recorded for each injection vs. polymer concentration reveals a break point which corresponds with the cmc.

VII. ACCELERATED RATE STUDIES

Of course, there are some reactions that occur at room temperature for which microcalorimeters are not able to detect any measurable heat flow. This may be because the reaction proceeds at too slow a rate, because the reaction enthalpy is very small or simply because there may not be a sufficient number of moles of material reacting. In some of these cases, it may be possible to accelerate any reactions occurring by increasing the temperature of the sample such that a measurable signal is obtained. The data are

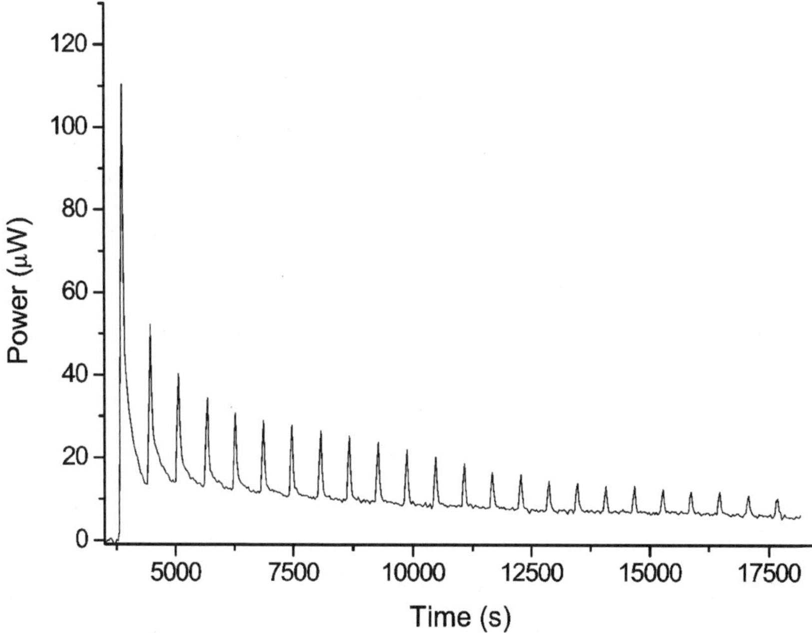

Figure 9 Power–time curve for the injection of Pluronic F127 (P407) into water using the commercial titration apparatus (36).

then extrapolated to room temperature using the Arrhenius equation, although this is not without problems (see Section 2). An easy way to study samples at high temperatures is to run a DSC in isothermal mode [a paradox of nomenclature that has not gone unnoticed (37)]. DSC instruments allow rapid changes in temperature but are usually less sensitive than microcalorimeters. This is because they utilize much smaller sample sizes (5–10 mg) than microcalorimeters. Recent developments have led to DSCs with much greater sensitivity, that are capable of holding much larger sample sizes (typically up to 1 mL) and are generally capable of detecting signals of $\pm 0.5\,\mu W$ (38–40). Such instruments are notionally referred to as high-sensitivity differential scanning calorimeters (HSDSC) although the terms used by specific manufacturers vary (for instance, some of the commercially available instruments include nano-DSCs, ultrasensitive DSCs, high-sensitivity DSCs and differential scanning microcalorimeters).

The nature of HSDSC instruments allows experiments to be run incorporating both isothermal and scanning steps. This enables rapid screens for excipient compatibility. An example is provided by the study of aspirin with two excipients using HSDSC (41). Figure 10 shows the HSDSC trace obtained for a binary mixture of acetylsalicylic acid (aspirin) with lactose and Figure 11

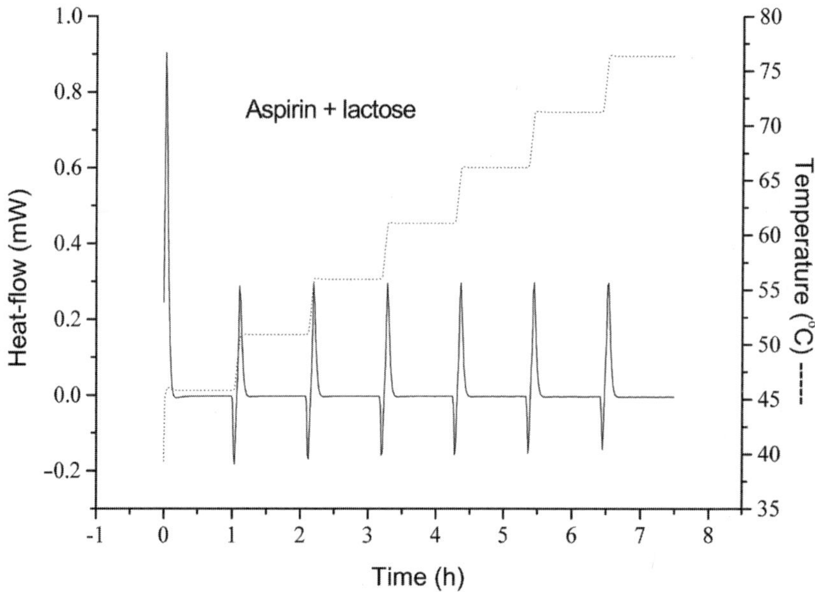

Figure 10 HSDSC trace obtained for a 1:1 mixture of aspirin:lactose over a programmed temperature ramp (42).

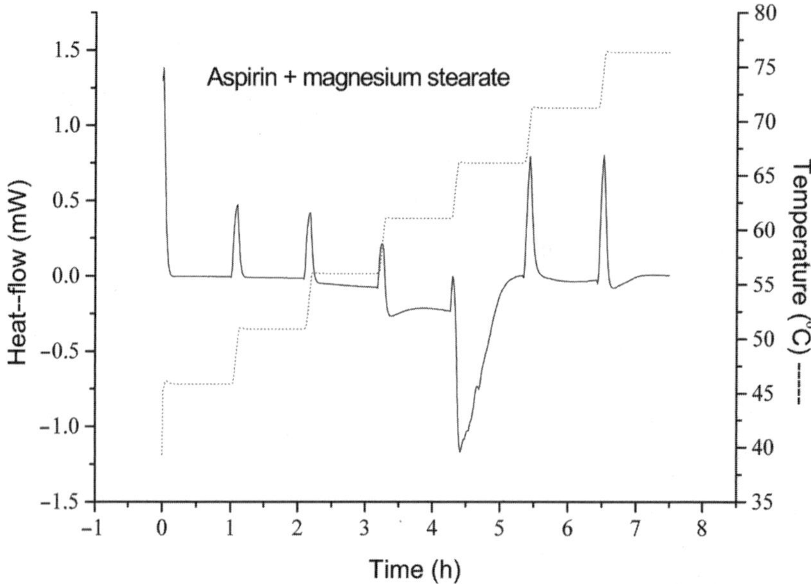

Figure 11 HSDSC trace obtained for a 1:1 mixture of aspirin:magnesium stearate over a programmed temperature ramp (42).

shows the HSDSC trace obtained for a binary mixture of acetylsalicylic acid with magnesium stearate (42). In both cases, the samples have been subjected to the same temperature program (shown on the right-hand *y*-axis). It can be seen that at lower temperatures, there is no detectable heat flow in either of the mixtures. However, at 55°C the acetylsalicylic acid/magnesium stearate mixture gives an endothermic signal. The aspirin/lactose mixture gives rise to no thermal signal over the course of the whole experiment. Such an observation suggests that acetylsalicylic acid is incompatible with magnesium stearate but not with lactose. Each experiment was completed in less than 8 hr.

VIII. FURTHER INFORMATION

There are a number of useful sources of information for pharmaceutical applications of microcalorimetry, listed below, which will hopefully be of some use to the reader.

A. Books

There are a number of excellent books that provide information on pharmaceutical thermal analysis but many do not include sections on isothermal microcalorimetry. Probably the most useful textbook in print is *The Handbook of Thermal Analysis. Vol 1: Principles and practice*, edited by ME Brown, Elsevier Science (Amsterdam), 1998, which comprehensively covers all aspects of thermal analysis. A more specialised, but now out of print, text is *Biological Microcalorimetry*, edited by AE Beezer, Academic Press (London), 1982 and an excellent chapter can be found in *Principles of Thermal Analysis and Calorimetry*, edited by PJ Haines, RSC (Cambridge), 2002. The subject of pharmaceutical uses of DSC is more widely covered with excellent texts including *Biocalorimetry*, edited by JE Ladbury and BZ Chowdhry, Wiley (Chichester), 1998 and *Pharmaceutical Thermal Analysis*, edited by JL Ford and P Timmins, Ellis Harwood, 1989 (although a new edition of this text is due, edited by JL Ford, P Timmins and G Buckton).

B. Journals

Most research papers concerned with pharmaceutical microcalorimetry can usually be found in the pharmaceutical journals *International Journal of Pharmaceutics* (Elsevier Science Publishers BV, Amsterdam) and *Pharmaceutical Research* (Plenum Publishing Corporation, New York) while more fundamental work will be found in *Thermochimica Acta* (Elsevier Science Publishers BV, Amsterdam). Excellent reviews of the field of thermal analysis have been published every two years in the fundamental reviews issue of *Analytical Chemistry* by the late D Dollimore, most recently in 1998 (43).

Reviews of the pharmaceutical applications of microcalorimetry have been published by Buckton (4,21), Koenigbauer (44), and Gaisford (45).

C. Manufacturers

Information about specific instruments and application notes can be obtained by writing directly to thermal equipment manufacturers or by visiting their websites. The addresses of selected manufacturers include:

Calorimetry Sciences Corp.; 515 East 1860 South, PO Box 799, Provo, UT, 84603–0799, U.S.A. (www.calscorp.com).

Microcal Inc.; 22 Industrial Drive East, Northampton, MA, U.S.A. (www.microcalorimetry.com).

Setaram; 7 rue de l'Oratoire, F-69300 Caluire, France (www.setaram.com).

Thermometric AB, Spjutvägen 5A, S-175 61 Järfälla, Sweden. (www.thermometric.com).

REFERENCES

1. Suurkuusk J, Wadso I. A multichannel microcalorimetry system. Chimica Scripta 1982; 20:155–163.
2. Briggner LE, Wadso I. Test and calibration processes for microcalorimeters, with special reference to heat conduction instruments used with aqueous systems. J Biochem Biophys Methods 1991; 22(2):101–118.
3. Willson RJ, Beezer AE, Hills AK, Mitchell JC. The imidazole catalysed hydrolysis of triacetin: a medium term chemical calibrant for isothermal microcalorimeters. Thermochimica Acta 1999; 325:125–132.
4. Buckton G, Beezer AE. The applications of microcalorimetry in the field of physical pharmacy. Int J Pharm 1991; 72:181–191.
5. Beezer AE, Gaisford S, Hills AK, Willson RJ, Mitchell JC. Pharmaceutical microcalorimetry: applications to long term stability studies. Int J Pharm 1999; 179(2):39–45.
6. Bakri A, Janssen LHM, Wilting J. Determination of reaction rate parameters using heat conduction microcalorimetry. J Therm Anal 1988; 33:185–190.
7. Willson RJ, Beezer AE, Mitchell JC. A kinetic study of the oxidation of L-ascorbic acid (vitamin C) in solution using an isothermal microcalorimeter. Thermochimica Acta 1995; 264:27–40.
8. Willson RJ. Ph.D. dissertation, University of Kent, Canterbury, Kent, 1995.
9. Gaisford S. Ph.D. dissertation, University of Kent, Canterbury, Kent, 1997.
10. Gaisford S, Hills AK, Beezer AE, Mitchell JC. Thermodynamic and kinetic analysis of isothermal microcalorimetric data: applications to consecutive reaction schemes. Thermochimica Acta 1999; 328(1–2):39–45.
11. Candlin JP, Wilkins RG. Sulphur-nitrogen compounds. Part I. The hydrolysis of sulphamate ion in perchloric acid. J Chem Soc 1960:4236–4241.
12. Candlin JP, Wilkins RG. Sulphur-nitrogen compounds. Part II. The hydrolysis of hydroxylamine trisulphamate and hydroxylamine-NO-disulphonate ions in perchloric acid. J Chem Soc 1961:3625–3633.

13. Byrn SR. Solid-State Chemistry of Drugs. Academic Press, 1982.
14. Carstensen JT. Stability of solids and solid dosage forms. J Pharm Sci 1974; 63:1–14.
15. Lachman L. Physical and chemical stability testing of tablet dosage forms. J Pharm Sci 1965; 54:1519–1526.
16. Carstensen JT. Drug Stability: Principles and Practices. 2nd ed. New York: Marcel Dekker, 1995.
17. Avrami M. Kinetics of phase change I. J Chem Phys 1939; 7:1103–1112.
18. Prout EG, Tompkins FC. The thermal decomposition of potassium permanganate. Trans Faraday Soc 1944; 40:488–498.
19. Ng WL. Thermal decomposition in the solid-state. Aust J Chem 1975; 28: 1169–1178.
20. Pryor WA. Free Radicals. McGraw-Hill Book Company Inc., 1966.
21. Buckton G, Russell SJ, Beezer AE. Pharmaceutical calorimetry: a selective review. Thermochimica Acta 1991; 193:195–214.
22. Angberg M, Nyström C, Cartensson S. Evaluation of heat-conduction microcalorimetry in pharmaceutical stability studies I. Precision and accuracy for static experiments in glass vials. Acta Pharm Suec 1988; 25:307–320.
23. Pikal MJ, Dellerman KN. Stability testing of pharmaceuticals by high sensitivity isothermal calorimetry at 25°C: cephalosporins in the solid and aqueous solution states. Int J Pharm 1989; 50:233–252.
24. Hansen LD, Lewis EA, Eatough DJ, Bergstrom RG, DeGraft-Johnson D. Kinetics of drug decomposition by heat conduction calorimetry. Pharm Res 1989; 6:20–27.
25. Otsuka T, Yoshioka S, Aso Y, Terao T. Application of microcalorimetry to stability testing of meclofenoxate hydrochloride and DL-α-tocopherol. Chem Pharm Bull 1994; 42(1):130–132.
26. Aso Y, Yoshioka S, Otsuka T, Kojima S. The physical stability of amorphous nifedipine determined by isothermal microcalorimetry. Chem Pharm Bull 1995; 43(2):300–303.
27. Angberg M, Nyström C, Cartensson S. Evaluation of heat-conduction microcalorimetry in pharmaceutical stability studies VII. Oxidation of ascorbic acid in aqueous solution. Int J Pharm 1993; 90:19–33.
28. Phipps MA, Winnike RA, Long ST, Viscomi F. Excipient compatibility assessment by isothermal microcalorimetry. J Pharm Pharmacol 1998; 50(suppl):9.
29. Phipps MA, Mackin LA. Application of isothermal microcalorimetry in solid state drug development. PSTT 2000; 3(1):9–17.
30. Selzer T, Radau M, Kreuter J. Use of isothermal heat conduction microcalorimetry to evaluate stability and excipient compatibility of a solid drug. Int J Pharm 1998; 171:227–241.
31. Schmitt E. Excipient compatibility screening by isothermal calorimetry. Fifty-third Calorimetry Conference, Midland, Michigan, U.S.A., 1998.
32. Giron D, Remy P, Thomas S, Vilette E. Quantitation of amorphicity by microcalorimetry. J Thermal Anal 1997; 48:465–472.
33. Nyqvist H. Saturated salt solutions for maintaining specified relative humidities. Int J Pharm Tech Prod Mfr 1983; 4(2):47–48.
34. Buckton G, Darcy P. Assessment of disorder in crystalline powders—a review of analytical techniques and their application. Int J Pharm 1999; 179(2):141–158.

35. Hogan S. Unpublished data, School of Pharmacy, University of London, 2000.
36. Ali S. Ph.D. dissertation, University of London, 2001.
37. Hansen LD. Standard nomenclature for calorimetry. Sixteenth IUPAC Conference on Chemical Thermodynamics, August 6–11, Dalhousie University, Halifax, Nova Scotia, Canada, 2000.
38. Sturtevant JM. Biochemical applications of differential scanning calorimetry. Ann Rev Phys Chem 1987; 38:463–488.
39. Chowdhry BZ, Cole SC. Differential scanning calorimetry—applications in biotechnology. TIBTECH 1989; 7:11–18.
40. Noble D. DSC balances out. Anal Chem 1995; 67(9):323A–327A.
41. Wissing S, Craig DQM, Barker SA, Moore WD. An investigation into the use of stepwise isothermal high sensitivity DSC as a means of detecting drug–excipient compatibility. Int J Pharm 2000; 199:141–150.
42. Wissing S. Unpublished data, School of Pharmacy, University of London, 2000.
43. Dollimore D, Lerdkanchanaporn S. Thermal analysis. Anal. Chem 1998; 70: 27R–35R.
44. Koenigbauer MJ. Pharmaceutical applications of microcalorimetry. Pharm. Res 1994; 11(6):777–783.
45. Gaisford S, Buckton G. Potential applications of microcalorimetry for the study of physical processes in pharmaceuticals. Thermochimica Acta 2001; 380:185–198.

12

The Power of Computational Chemistry to Leverage Stress Testing of Pharmaceuticals

Donald B. Boyd

Department of Chemistry, Indiana University–Purdue University at Indianapolis (IUPUI), Indianapolis, Indiana, U.S.A.

I. INTRODUCTION

This chapter describes an area of research that is finding new uses every day. The tools of computational chemistry—computers and software—have become so ubiquitous that there are few chemists left today who have not heard of them or used them. However, the reader may reasonably ask: Why is there a chapter on computational chemistry in a book on stress testing of pharmaceutically interesting compounds? The reason does not lie in a vast number of papers crying for review. Indeed, relatively little work has been published in this area thus far. So what is the reason? The objective of this chapter is to increase awareness of how computational chemistry can be used by pharmaceutical chemists to help confront some of the research problems they face in stress testing research. Hence, the nature of this chapter is intended to be primarily tutorial... and perhaps with a little proselytizing for increased use of the powerful techniques of computational chemistry now available.

Computational chemistry can be an aid to the experimentalist in a number of ways. These include (a) visualizing and quantifying information about molecular structure, (b) answering questions pertaining to electronic structure and hence reaction mechanisms, and (c) honing questions that can be investigated experimentally. In effect, the computer is used for learning about atomic and molecular phenomenon, just like with other laboratory instruments. A key point that pharmaceutical chemists should bear in mind is that computational chemistry's goal is not to replace experiment. Any theoretician who asserts otherwise is being naïve or worse.

Computational chemists have made their software tools increasingly easy to use so that an enlarging population of scientists may use them conveniently. These software advances generally entail implementing a user-friendly graphical user interface (GUI), which enables individuals to use a simple paradigm of point-and-click, pull-down menus, and pop-up dialog boxes to build molecular models, set up calculations, and display the results on a computer screen. Experimentalists can take advantage of these technological developments. At the same time, because the underlying theoretical models can be quite sophisticated and complex, opportunities for inappropriate use or misunderstandings or misinterpretation abound. In his book, Young (1) quotes Karl Irikura, a scientist at the National Institute of Standards and Technology, as reminding us that "Anyone can do calculations nowadays. Anyone can also operate a scalpel. That doesn't mean all our medical problems are solved."

In this chapter, we will suggest some ways to avoid common difficulties. This presentation is not intended to be a glossy sales pitch. Rather, we try to present a gentle, objective, and practical tutorial. We want to show not only where the power of the technology can be applied, but also the way around potential traps that could ensnare new users. By the end of this chapter, the readers will, hopefully, feel empowered to investigate the methodologies in applications to some of their immediate research problems. The tools to be described can give the chemist a competitive advantage in solving problems as well as in enhancing publishable work.

A. What Does Computational Chemistry Encompass?

Computational chemistry began emerging as a distinct discipline about a quarter century ago. Essentially all research-based pharmaceutical and chemical companies have come to recognize its value and have long-established groups of computational chemists (also called molecular modelers or chem-informatics experts). There are many ways to illustrate the growth of the field. About 10 years ago, it was found that about 13% of all papers in the chemical literature contained some computational chemistry work (2), and the percentage was steadily increasing. Another analysis (3) showed that in certain journals, such as *Journal of the American Chemical Society* and *Journal of Medicinal Chemistry*, about a quarter of their papers contained results of computational chemistry calculations. A further illustration of growth is shown in Figure 1 where we plot on a logarithmic scale the increase in the number of publications dealing with computational chemistry as cataloged by the Chemical Abstracts Service (CAS) (4). Use of the techniques of computational chemistry is spreading as scientists find new applications and as the methods and computers improve.

Because different people have slightly different opinions of what constitutes computational chemistry, it is useful to define its scope. Most published definitions embrace an overlapping set of ideas. Computational chemistry has been described as consisting of those aspects of chemical research that are expedited or rendered practical by computers (5). However, that scope is so broad that it would include most molecular science laboratories where modern instruments are built with programmed or programmable computers to collect and mathematically manipulate data. Such a definition is beyond the scope of this chapter.

The following definition of computational chemistry was published in 1985 (6): "quantitative modeling of chemical behavior on a computer by the formalisms of theoretical chemistry." Some quantum theoreticians naturally would like to see computational chemistry as a subset of their field (7). However, today the number of scientists employed as computational chemists well exceeds the number employed as theoreticians (8). A recent textbook author (9) views computational chemistry as encompassing "not only quantum mechanics, but also molecular mechanics, [energy] minimization, simulations, conformational analysis, and other computer-based methods for understanding and predicting the behavior of molecular systems."

Computational chemistry includes applications of theoretical chemistry, but theoretical chemistry and computational chemistry are definitely not synonymous. Theoretical chemistry involves development of mathematical expressions that model physical reality; as such, some of theoretical chemistry entails quantum mechanics (QM). Computational chemistry, on the other hand, involves use of computers on which theoretical and many other algorithms have been programmed.

The International Union of Pure and Applied Chemistry (IUPAC, 10) proposed a definition of computational chemistry about 15 years after the term was already well established in the lexicon of chemists: "A discipline using mathematical methods for the calculation of molecular properties or for the simulation of molecular behavior. It also includes, e.g., synthesis planning, database searching, combinatorial library manipulation." The open-ended second part of this statement reflects the disparate opinions of the IUPAC committee and others who contributed comments.

The scope of computational chemistry can be inferred from the methodologies it encompasses. Some of the more common tools include computer graphics, molecular modeling, quantum chemistry, molecular mechanics (MM), statistical analysis of structure–property relationships, and data management (informatics). As with any dynamic field of research, computational chemistry is growing, new methodologies are being developed, and the scope is evolving. For instance, 20 years ago, quantum chemistry was by far the most used approach in computational chemistry, but 10 years later force field (FF) calculations (molecular mechanics and molecular simulations) had grown to be the most used approach (11).

B. Information Resources

Much useful reading material about computational chemistry is available. Some self-help information can be found at various websites. These can be located with any of the common "search engines" (database retrieval systems) that are convenient for finding resources on the World Wide Web. Once an individual is connected to the Internet, the search engines are free. A particularly fast, up-to-date, and comprehensive search engine is at http://www.google.com/. Queries can be in the form of words or

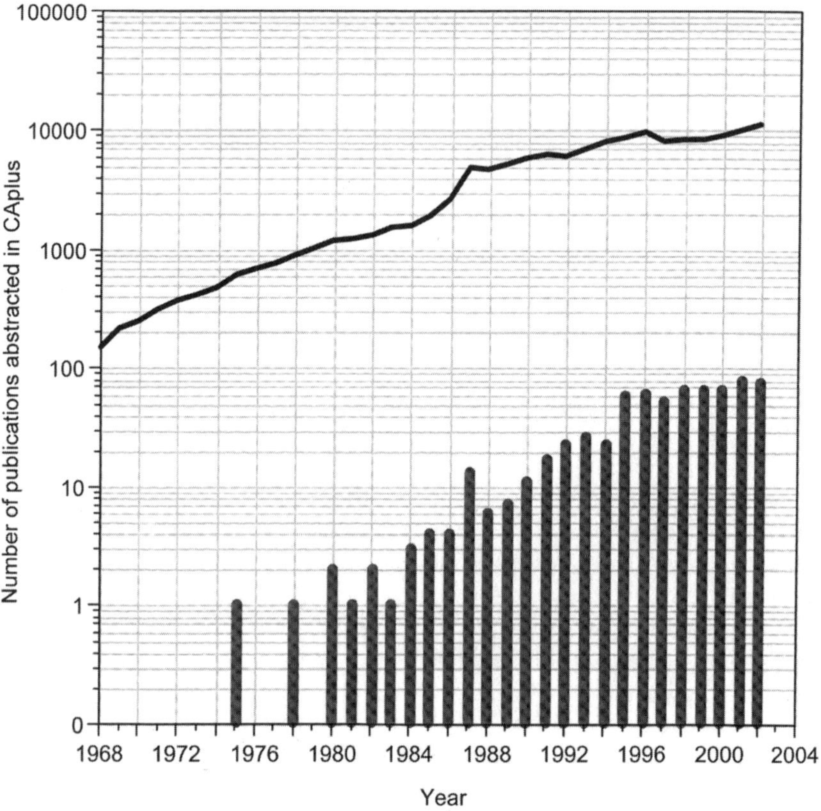

Figure 1 (*Caption on facing page*)

phrases (enclosed in double quotes). Google ranks its hits according to how many other people have previously visited the same hits, thereby showing you the paths to the most frequented websites. Various other search engines, some purporting to specialize in science but which are not as fast as Google, are also available. Also helpful can be the so-called meta search engines; these will send your query to all the popular search engines and then present you with a compilation of the hits from each. A Google search for meta search engines will steer you to some of these.

There are several "lists" (formerly called electronic bulletin boards) available on the Internet where questions about computational chemistry can be asked and information exchanged freely. With the number of subscribers of these lists ranging from a few hundred to several thousand, usually there is someone willing to offer answers, including those from a beginner. The most famous of these lists, and broadest in terms of topics covered, is the Computational Chemistry List (CCL), which is administered by Dr. Jan K. Labanowski (presently at the University of Notre Dame). To post

---

Figure 1 (*Continued from previous page*) Semi-log plot of the annual number of published items (articles, books, reports, etc.) dealing with or using computational chemistry according to CAplus, the main database of the Chemical Abstracts Service (www.cas.org). The number of publications grew rapidly from humble beginnings. The mid-1980s was a period of exceptionally fast growth as chemists in traditional disciplines discovered the amazing utility of the technology. Shown by the bars in the lower part of the plot is the annual number of published items that explicitly use the term "computational chemistry" in their title or abstract. This number is roughly 1% of the total number of publications involving development and applications of computational chemistry. The term "computational chemistry" began to be used in the literature in the 1970s, but did not become prevalent until after 1980 when the *Journal of Computational Chemistry* was founded. As described in Ref. 4, in order to avoid missing relevant papers in CAplus database, special SciFinder search strategies had to be used to obtain the data for this graph. In doing the SciFinder searches, it became apparent that searching on the *concept* "computational chemistry" pulled up many irrelevant hits. Such hits date back to 1910, when obviously the modern concept of computational chemistry was not in use. For purposes of creating the graph in this figure, we performed SciFinder searches of the CAplus database using the terms (not concepts) "computational chemistry," "molecular modeling," "cheminformatics," "computer-aided drug design," "molecular mechanics," "molecular simulations," and "quantitative structure–activity relationships," and then combined the number of hits for each year. Some of these search terms brought up extraneous hits, but it was also apparent that some relevant papers were being missed. Hence, the numbers graphed are approximate, but representative. Owing to the fact that not every paper is fully or accurately catalogued by the staff of CAS, the actual number of publications dealing with computational chemistry is probably larger than illustrated here.

a question on the CCL, anyone can send an e-mail to chemistry@ccl.net. Messages are monitored by human beings to screen out junk e-mails (spam). Also, a vast, rich, searchable archive of previous correspondence is available at http://www.ccl.net/chemistry/. Some questions are asked over and over as new people enter the field. It is possible that an answer to your questions may already be in the database.

A more permanent source of information about the methods used by computational chemists is *Reviews in Computational Chemistry* (12). This book series covers most of the important facets of computational chemistry with some chapters designed for the newcomer and some for the expert. Another excellent source is a five-volume encyclopedia published a few years ago (13). There are also many other relevant books. In fact, a recent tabulation discovered that more than 1600 books have been published on computational chemistry and its closely allied subjects (14). The textbook by Leach (9) is one of the most popular in the field. The book gives a thorough, balanced treatment of quantum chemistry, FF methods, molecular dynamics (MD) simulations, Monte Carlo (MC) simulations, conformational analysis, thermodynamics and statistical mechanics, and molecular design. The textbook by Young (1) broadly introduces many subjects. There is a slew of books on quantum chemistry, ranging from theoretically oriented to more practical; we cite only a tiny sample (15–17). Several books emphasize molecular modeling (18–21). See Ref. 14 for a comprehensive listing of books.

A number of organizations have offered workshops in computational chemistry starting more than 20 years ago. More recently, the American Chemical Society has offered a short course in computational chemistry (see, e.g., www.chemistry.org). Most vendors of software for the chemistry and pharmaceutical industries offer training in the use of their products. An increasing number of universities offer courses on computational chemistry or at least incorporate computational chemistry topics and laboratories in some of the traditional physical, organic, and inorganic courses. Some universities offer advanced degrees in computational chemistry or in cheminformatics. The latter is a relatively new field that combines computational chemistry and data management techniques.

C. Chapter's Scope

In this chapter, we discuss the main tools of computational chemistry in the context of studying the stability and degradation of pharmaceutical compounds. In a single chapter, it is impossible to teach everything there is to know about computational chemistry, of course. The reader is encouraged to pursue further learning and to try out some computational chemistry software, if they have not already done so.

In the next few sections, we give an overview of the main components of computational chemistry methods. Then we discuss the available software and considerations in selecting which to use. We attempt to keep our remarks on how to use the software as general as possible, so as not to be a manual for any one software package. However, we are more familiar with some programs and, for illustrative purposes, describe how they are used. In the next to last section, we take the reader through a typical computational chemistry research scenario. Finally, we give suggestions for the best way to tackle some selected research topics of particular interest to the readers of this book.

II. TIMELY TOOLS OF COMPUTATIONAL CHEMISTRY

A. Computer Graphics

Probably, the most important tool of computational chemistry is computer graphics because this provides the interface between the user and the computer. Molecular structure is the universal language of chemists. Therefore, it was an important advance when a user could enter a molecular structure into the computer by simply drawing lines and pointing and clicking on a building menu.

The simplest graphical depiction of molecules has lines representing bonds connecting points representing atoms. Molecular models can also be shown as balls (atoms) and sticks (covalent bonds) or simply as tubes (covalent bonds). Space-filling models can be produced, representing the modern equivalent of Corey–Pauling–Koltun (CPK) hand-held models. More complex graphics representing molecules as solid objects with colored or translucent surfaces convey not only the shape of the molecule but also electronic properties that pertain to each region of the molecule. An example is shown in Figure 2. The complexity of three-dimensional (3D) molecular models makes high resolution, color, and stereographics highly desirable.

Program options for a calculation can be set up through a GUI, and after a calculation (such as described in the sections below) is complete, the results (output) may be examined visually on the computer screen (22). The quantum chemical and molecular simulations methods (see below) are computationally intense and generate large quantities of data. Computer visualization of the output helps make the data meaningful to chemists. Sometimes, it can be very helpful to the chemist to see the computed results displayed as numbers or properties in or around the molecular structure.

With modern graphical analysis programs, it is possible to plot numerical data in three, four, five, or even six dimensions simultaneously. Such graphs can be useful for showing relationships and finding clusters of data. An example is shown in Figure 3. Complex response surfaces can be color-coded to show how several variables relate to each other (23). Information about a long-standing provider of software for graphical analysis of data can be found at www.sas.com; another is www.spotfire.com.

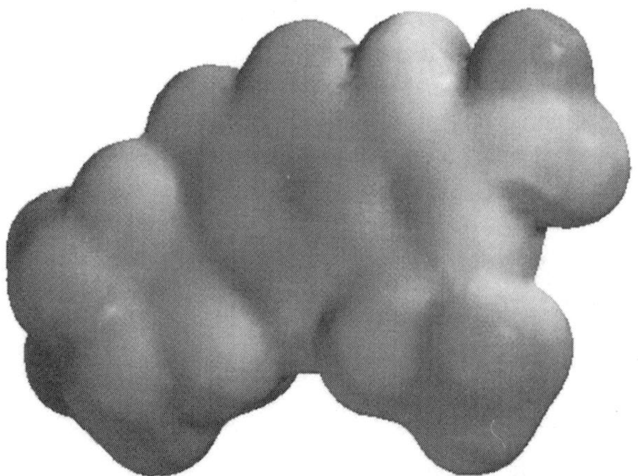

Figure 2 Molecular electrostatic potential energy map of norfloxacin projected onto a molecular surface corresponding approximately to the van der Waals volume of the molecule. Although this figure is not to be reproduced in color in this book, the right-hand side of the molecule is reddish corresponding to the negative charge on the carboxylate group. Hence, this end of the molecule would prefer to interact with a species that is positively charged. The left-hand side is bluish corresponding to a protonated nitrogen in the piperazine ring. The left-hand end would prefer to interact with a species that is negatively charged. The central aromatic region of the molecule is green corresponding to a nearly neutral electrostatic potential.

B. Databases

There are two types of molecular structure database: two-dimensional (2D) and three-dimensional. The 2D type stores atoms (chemical elements) and connectivity information (i.e., which atoms are bonded to which in a molecule). The 3D type stores, in addition, the x, y, z Cartesian co-ordinates of each atom in a molecule.

Most corporate databases of chemical compounds (libraries) are of the 2D type. The databases are managed using software that allows fast registration of new structures, fast retrieval of previously stored compounds, and fast substructure searching. (For more information about chemical database management software, see www.mdl.com or www.daylight.com.)

Whereas 2D databases of compounds play an invaluable role in pharmaceutical discovery research, a computational chemistry calculation on a molecule often requires its 3D structure. An excellent starting point for such a calculation is sometimes one of the molecules in the Cambridge Structural Database (CSD), a 3D database. The CSD (24–26) presently has atomic co-ordinates and other information for over 300,000 small organic and organometallic compounds, most of which have been solved by x-ray crystallography. The number of structures in the database is growing by about 10%

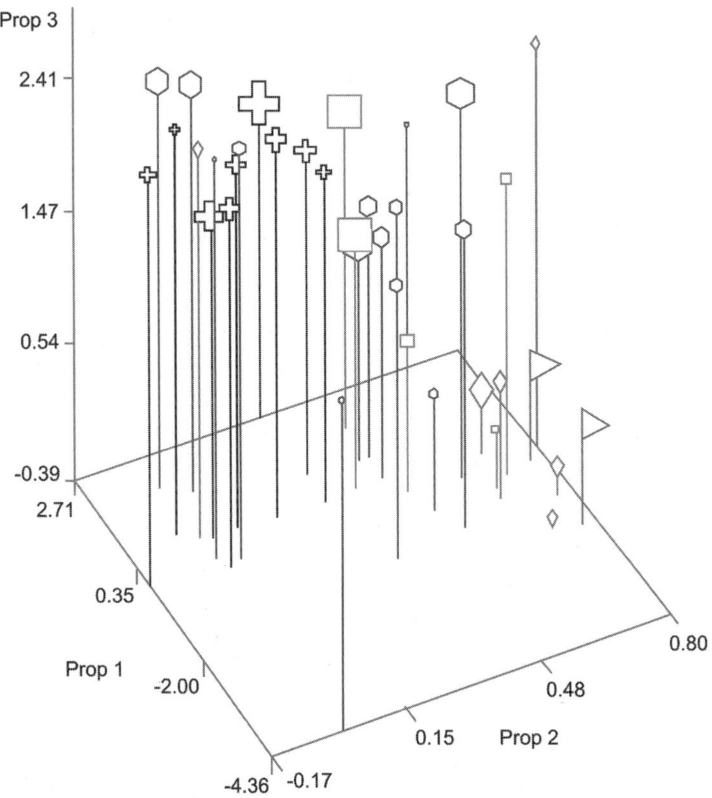

Figure 3 Example of how computer graphics can simultaneously display six dimensions. The example comes from the study of the antibacterial activity of a set of related compounds. Each compound corresponds to one "lollipop" (a shape at the end of a vertical line. Six properties can be plotted for each compound. Three of the dimensions correspond to the axes (labeled Prop 1, Prop *2,* and Prop 3). A fourth dimension is indicated by the kind of shape at the end of the vertical lines. The fifth dimension is indicated by the size of the shapes. A sixth dimension can be indicated by the color of the shapes.

per year. Access to the database requires a subscription (see www.ccdc.cam.ac.uk for further information).

Besides chemical structure databases, both proprietary and public databases contain a wealth of numerical and textual information pertinent to chemistry.

C. Molecular Modeling

Models of molecules have been around for a long time. Chemists have used hand-held molecular models to help them visualize conformation, stereochemistry, and steric accessibility. These models were built of plastic, aluminum, iron, or other materials (wood and cork in the old days). Today, computers perform many of the functions of the hand-held models and can do much more.

A note about terminology: In some situations, chemists use the terms computational chemistry and molecular modeling interchangeably. In other situations, molecular modeling emphasizes in particular that 3D structures of molecules are being viewed (i.e., molecular graphics) and/or studied computationally (27). Both meanings of molecular modeling are used in this chapter.

Modeling involves working with what is usually a simplified description of a system. Despite the simplifications, the model should capture the essence of a particular object, property, or process of interest. The models help scientists sort out complex relationships between many variables. Being able to devise and use good models takes skill and practice. Modeling can be used to estimate and understand molecular properties in cases where experiment is difficult or impossible.

Because of the mathematics involved in computer modeling, proper use requires attention to quantitative details and an appreciation of the underlying theory. State-of-the-art hardware and software make it easy for a novice to display a structure on a computer, but does it mean anything? When a molecule is being generated, manipulated, represented, or depicted in a computer, you should check that the 3D structure is close to experiment, so that any conclusions that are derived from the model are valid. It may not be immediately apparent from just looking at a structure displayed on a computer screen that some bond lengths are too short or too long, for instance.

Energy and shape are two molecular properties by which chemists understand how compounds interact and react. Most molecules are flexible, and at room temperature they are constantly undergoing conformational changes. Sometimes, a chemist will want to know what conformations a molecule can adopt. Some conformations may be more productive for a reaction than others. The most populated conformation is that which gives the lowest free energy. The lowest energy conformation computed by a given method, on the other hand, is called the global minimum energy structure.

1. Not All Energies Are the Same

Different types of calculation will give different types of energy. Depending on the computational chemistry invoked, the program may give an MM (sometimes called "steric") energy, or a quantum mechanical electronic energy and total energy, or a thermodynamical free energy. Most calculations encountered in routine work will yield only one of the first two categories of energy; it requires empirical estimation or lengthy molecular simulations to obtain a free energy. Nevertheless, it is common for chemists to make do with the energies from MM or QM (see below). Not all calculations yield an energy that is directly comparable to an experimental quantity. Some programs will yield a heat of formation, which is an experimentally meaningful number (28). Few if any programs, however, are designed to give directly the enthalpy or entropy of a reaction.

An important point to remember is that any calculated energy is useful only in comparison with other energies that are similarly computed. For this reason, computational chemists like to deal with relative energies. Thus, a fairly accurate conformational energy map can be obtained for many organic and pharmaceutical compounds because it involves relative energies obtained by one method on the same species.

2. The Shape of Things to Come

The process of exploring all the conformations a molecule can adopt is called conformational searching (29). This involves molecular modeling techniques to map out the potential energy surface of a molecule, which describes the energy of the molecule as a function of the spatial location of its atoms. One approach of conformational searching is systematic searching, where, as the name implies, the torsional angles at the rotatable bonds are varied systematically in increments. Another approach is the MC method in which the geometrical variables are varied randomly, and the energy of each random configuration of atoms is calculated (30). (A configuration in this sense is a set of Cartesian co-ordinates of the atoms of the system.) These and other methods for conformational searching tend to be compute-intensive and become prohibitively long for molecules with more than about 10 rotatable bonds. Energy evaluation during a search can done with an FF or quantum chemical method (see below), although the FF methods are preferred because of their much greater speed.

Once the conformations have been determined, then molecular shape comparisons are possible. Overlaying molecules is one of the most common applications of computer-based modeling and is easier and more accurate than trying to manipulate hand-held models of molecules. Molecular modeling offers several ways to superpose molecules. Probably the most common used alignment technique is by least squares fitting of atoms, i.e., minimize the distances between specified pairs of atoms, one from each molecule. An additional advantage of superimposing molecules by computer is that the fit can be quantitated.

D. Quantum Mechanical Modeling

Stress testing involves speeding up the rate at which molecules degrade so the reactions can be conveniently studied in the time frame of pharmaceutical development. Computational chemistry lets us model reactions at the speed of computers. Since bonds are forming, breaking or rearranging during reactions (31), electronic structure calculations are usually better at modeling the system than are FF methods (see, however, Ref. 32).

Theoretical chemistry had its origins in the QM theory developed in the 1920s. The early calculations were done on mechanical adding machines, and it was not till the 1950s that the early (slow) computers became available to research chemists.

Quantum mechanics is embodied in the famous Schrödinger equation from physics,

$$H\Psi = E\Psi \tag{1}$$

where H is a mathematical "operator" called a Hamiltonian and having a kinetic energy term and potential energy terms, Ψ is the wave function describing the positions of particles (electrons and nuclei) in a system, and E is the energy of the system (26). In effect, an operator is a mathematical expression of partial derivatives and distance-dependent terms that when applied to a wave function extracts a property (observable) from the wave function and gives back the wave function unchanged.

In molecular orbital (MO) theory, which is the most common implementation of QM used by chemists, electrons are distributed around the atomic nuclei until they reach a so-called self-consistent field (SCF), that is, until the attractive and repulsive forces between all the particles (electrons and nuclei) are in a steady state, and the energy is at a minimum. An SCF calculation yields the electronic wave function Ψ_e (the electronic motion being separable from nuclear motion thanks to the Born–Oppenheimer approximation). This is the type of wave function usually referred to in the literature and in the rest of this chapter.

1. Minimization/Optimization

By computing the energy of different nuclear configurations, the lowest energy structure can be found. (In the vernacular of computational chemistry, a spatial configuration of the atomic nuclei is called a "molecular geometry" or simply "geometry.") This so-called geometry optimization process is useful because the resulting bond lengths and bond angles, which give the lowest energy, are usually closest to what is observed experimentally. The energy is minimized when the geometry is optimized. Hence, the terms optimization and minimization are used interchangeably in regard to this type of calculation. Other molecular properties are usually computed closer to experiment if an equilibrium (i.e., low energy) molecular geometry is used.

Modern computational chemistry programs usually have various well-tested optimization algorithms for finding the lowest energy (33). Such algorithms have adjustable mathematical parameters that were chosen by the program developer to balance between computer time requirements and completeness of the minimization. It has been pointed out that reliable reproductions of potential energy surfaces of flexible molecules sometimes require more stringent convergence criteria during the optimizations (34).

2. From First Principles and Post Hoc Patching

Popular implementations of MO theory are at the ab initio and semiempirical levels. In the ab initio (from first principles) approach, very few approximations are made (26). The electron density is represented by distributing it among certain standard linear combinations of mathematical functions; today these usually have the form e^{-r^2}, although 40 years ago e^{-r} was preferred because of its better description of electron density close to the nucleus of an atom. (Here r is the distance of the electron from the nucleus.) The former function, called a Gaussian-type basis function, gained favor because the integrals required to solve the Schrödinger equation are much easier to compute. Combinations of the basis functions are called basis sets (15,35). Typically, the basis sets concentrate most of the electron density near the nuclei because this is where the system picks up most of the kinetic and potential energies; then the electron density tapers off toward zero far from the nuclei. Some popular basis sets, in increasing size, have cryptic names like 3-21G, 6-31G, 6-31G*, 6-31G**, double-zeta (DZ), triple-zeta (TZ), etc. These acronyms indicate how many Gaussian-type functions (e^{-r^2}) are used to describe the core, valence, and diffuse electron density on each atom. Generally, the higher the numbers and the longer the acronym, the better the basis set. See e.g., Refs. 15, 29, 35 for details of the notation.

There are different levels of ab initio theory based on the size of the basis set and how much electron correlation is described. The larger the basis set, the more accurately it can describe the electron distribution in an atom or molecule. Electron correlation refers to electrons staying out of each other's way as much as possible. The different levels of ab initio theory are sometimes referred to as "model chemistries."

The basic level of ab initio theory is called Hartree–Fock (HF) or SCF theory. It has been by far the most often used level because it is faster than higher levels and because it is usually adequate for studying geometries, conformations, and hydrogen bonding. The difference between the HF energy and true (experimental) energy of a molecule is called the correlation energy.

Whereas HF theory is good for isolated, gas-phase molecules, some potential problems should be noted. One is the failure of a calculation to reach an SCF. There is no guarantee every SCF run will converge to a stable solution, without which all subsequent analyses of energies, charge distribution, and other molecular properties are precluded. Most calculations run okay, but sometimes electron density will oscillate between the two sides of a molecule, thereby preventing the achievement of an SCF. Techniques are available in many MO programs to damp down on the oscillation if it arises and to otherwise help reach a satisfactory endpoint, i.e., the SCF

(13). Sometimes, a better starting geometry will circumvent an SCF problem.

A second problem is that HF theory does not correctly model the dissociation of a bond. The energy of a dissociating system will rise too high as the separation of the fragments increases. This problem can be ameliorated in cases where you are comparing fragmentation of two molecules that differ only in the substituents remote from the breaking bond. Then the reaction can be compared in terms of relative energies. To better represent the potential energy curve for bond rupture, post-HF methods (see below) must be invoked.

A third problem to be aware of when modeling reaction pathways is the so-called basis set superposition error (BSSE) (37). This effect arises from the fact that when two reactant molecules come in proximity of each other, each molecule can use some of the basis functions on the other molecule to redistribute the electron density and thereby lower the electronic energy. The result is that the approach of two molecules may seem more stabilizing than is real. The BSSE can be reduced by using an adequately large basis set on each separate molecule.

A fourth potential problem is that HF theory does not model van der Waals attractive interactions between nonbonded molecules. Whereas hydrogen bonding is well represented by the HF-SCF model, weak London dispersion attractions are not.

Better (higher) levels of ab initio theory are called post-HF methods (38). These attempt to account for electron correlation and do so with varying degrees of success. Treatment of electron correlation is essential if you are interested in modeling bond breaking or van der Waals interactions, or in obtaining an accurate total energy. There is a veritable alphabet soup of post-HF methods including generalized valence bond (GVB), complete active space self-consistent field (CASSCF), coupled cluster (CC) (39), configuration interaction (CI), Møller–Plesset (MP) many-body perturbation theory (MBPT), and Gaussian-3 (G3). (This last model is not to be confused with the Gaussian function, the Gaussian program (40), or the company Gaussian Inc., although they have some connection.) Møller–Plesset is frequently encountered in the chemical literature; there are different levels: second order (MP2), third order (MP3), and fourth order (MP4). Further complicating the situation is that the different MP levels do not asymptotically approach the true answer, but rather oscillate toward the true answer. However, even the largest basis sets and highest levels of theory yield only close approximations to the true electron density distribution in most nontrivial-sized molecules.

The post-HF methods can be very accurate, but require so much computer time that they are restricted to molecules with less than about 15 atoms. Hence, post-HF methods are generally impractical for studying degradation of pharmaceutically interesting molecules.

3. Semiempirically Speaking

In semiempirical MO calculations (36,41), additional approximations are made, such as treating only the outer-most (i.e., valence) electrons while assuming the core (inner) electrons simply neutralize part of the nuclear charge. Of the remaining integrals, the easier ones are computed exactly and the rest are approximated or treated as parameters chosen such that the output of a calculation will be reasonably close to experimental values of target properties of a selected set of compounds (often small organics). The main advantage of semiempirical calculations is that they are faster than ab initio calculations. The main disadvantage is that the results are generally less accurate than ab initio ones.

Popular implementations of semiempirical methods include MINDO/3 (modified intermediate neglect of differential overlap, third parameterization), MNDO (modified neglect of diatomic differential overlap), AM1 (Austin Model 1), and PM3 (Parametric Method 3) Hamiltonians. MNDO/d has d atomic orbitals added to the second-row atoms and gives improved results for molecules with these elements (42). The PM5 Hamiltonian recently became available in commercial software, and PM7 (or similar name) is in development. Each of these methods is a step toward greater overall agreement with selected experimental properties, primarily heat of formation, ionization potentials, dipole moments, and molecular geometries. Hence, the order of increasing accuracy is: MINDO/3 < MNDO < AM1 < PM3 < PM5 < PM7. However, inevitably with each of these parameterized methods, there are some classes of compounds and some types of properties where there remain deficiencies or where some specific properties were actually handled better by an earlier generation of semiempirical theory than by a subsequent one.

4. A Nobel Winning Topic: Density Functional Theory

A third implementation of QM is density functional theory (DFT) (43–45), and it is useful in both molecular and materials applications. Density functional theory has the advantage of being roughly intermediate in speed and accuracy between ab initio and semiempirical theories. Optimized geometries from DFT can be quite good. For these reasons, use of DFT by chemists is increasing. The 1998 Nobel Prize in Chemistry recognized Professors Walter Kohn and John Pople, proponents of DFT and ab initio theory, respectively.

Just as in the case of solving the Schrödinger equation in HF theory, the total electronic energy in DFT is the sum of the kinetic energy of the electrons, the electron–electron repulsion energy, and the nuclear–electron attraction energy. Analogous to the HF equations, the Kohn–Sham equations are iteratively solved in DFT. A key difference is the appearance of a so-called exchange-correlation functional, which adds some electron correlation. Functionals are cryptically functions of functions. Exchange-correlation functionals go by acronyms like B3LYP (Becke 3 term with Lee, Yang, and Parr exchange), B3PW91 (Perdue and Wang), and BP86. B3LYP is one of the most widely used because of its superior accuracy for properties such as electron ionization energies and electron affinities.

5. Practical Considerations

The decision of which quantum mechanical model to use boils down to what size molecule you want to calculate, how reliable an answer you want, and how much time are you willing to wait for the results. Fortunately, as software and hardware improve, the tipping point of the balance weighing the pros and cons of semiempirical vs. DFT vs. ab initio is shifting such that larger molecules can be handled by the better methods. In special situations, a molecule with a couple of hundred atoms can be treated by an ab initio method (46,47), but the typical molecule of interest to theorists, spectroscopists, and physicists is smaller than what a pharmaceutical chemist usually wants to treat. Large molecular systems are often best left to one of the FF approaches (see next section).

A strategy used by many chemists is to divide the work into manageable steps. In the first step, semiempirical MO or MM (see below) calculations can be done to optimize a starting molecular geometry (e.g., after a 3D structure is constructed by drawing it on a computer screen). Sometimes, an MM geometry is quite accurate and can be used without further refinement. On the other hand, an optimized geometry from semiempirical calculations can be used as input for intermediate level ab initio calculations for more accurate refinement of the 3D structure. Then in the last step, electronic properties can be calculated at a very high but affordable ab initio or DFT level but without further geometry optimization. In the parlance of computational chemistry, a calculation in which the geometry is held fixed is called a "fixed point" calculation. Even in the propitious case when you have a starting geometry from experiment (e.g., X-ray crystallography), the hydrogen positions should be optimized because bond lengths to hydrogen atoms are systematically too short from an X-ray diffraction experiment.)

Another thing to keep in mind is that most quantum chemistry calculations, by default, treat the molecules as gas-phase species in a vacuum. In contrast, most laboratory experiments are done in solvent. Today, fortunately, many of the widely used quantum chemistry programs have a way of approximating the effect of solvent on solute models. The solvent can be treated in two ways. Water is a common solvent, so we will use it as an example. One way is to use the so-called "explicit waters"; in this approach, a few water molecules are sprinkled around the periphery of the solute to mimic the effect of a solvation shell or hydrogen bonding, and the whole ensemble is run in the calculation. The other way is to use "implicit waters" in which an average potential field that would be produced by water molecules is incorporated in the quantum calculations (48); here, the solute is the only species explicitly run in a calculation.

For any kind of quantum mechanical calculation, a caveat to keep in mind is that an experimentalist may be used to writing chemical structures without the hydrogens or in other shorthand notation, but all atoms and electrons in a molecule must be explicitly present in the model structure. Otherwise, the calculations will fail to run or the output, if produced, will be meaningless. The molecular structure run in a calculation must have all valences appropriately filled. Also, in regard to having the correct number of electrons in a molecular model, make sure the formal charge on the species (e.g., –1 for a carboxylic acid in its ionized form or +1 for an ammonium group) is properly set prior to a calculation. The formal charge is used by the program to figure the total number of electrons and the number of filled MOs.

Electronic structure calculations—by any of the three general approaches described above—are suited for predicting a variety of molecular systems (ground states, excited states, and transition states) and properties (equilibrium bond lengths and bond angles, conformational preferences, ionization potentials, electron affinities, charge distributions, conformational energies, reaction pathways, hydrogen bonding, and so on) (49,50).

Although the charge on an atom is not an experimental observable, charge distributions are of great interest to chemists (51–53). The most widely used scheme for dividing up the electron cloud among the atoms in a molecule is the Mulliken population analysis (51,52). The resulting values are called net atomic charges. These have no physical meaning, but can be quite useful for comparisons of a given atom of the same element in a series of related molecules.

From a wave function, one can also calculate the molecular electrostatic potential (MEP), which is an energy of attraction or repulsion experienced by a hypothetical unit charge as it moves in the vicinity of a molecule (54). The MEP gives clues to how one molecule looks to another as they approach. Hence, MEPs can be studied to reveal how two reactants might approach each other.

E. Force Field Modeling

In MM, MD, and MC simulations, an empirical FF describes how the energy of a molecule changes as a function of bond lengths l, bond angles θ, and torsional angles φ. The theory is chemically intuitive, and the energy functions and parameters are set empirically to reproduce experimental molecular geometries and relative energies as closely as possible. Atoms are treated as points in space except for the van der Waals term, which represents the atoms as spheres occupying volumes with soft surfaces. These latter surfaces are attractive at long range and repulsive at distances shorter than the van der Waals radii.

A set of energy terms and associated parameters is called a force field (55). The energy is a combination of bond stretching/compression, bond angle bending, torsional twisting, van der Waals interactions, and electrostatic forces that tend to hold the atoms at their equilibrium positions (56–58). Simpler FFs assume harmonic force constants for stretching and bending movements.

$$E_{\text{total}} = E_{\text{b}} + E_{\theta} + E_{\phi} + E_{\tau} + E_{\text{el}} + E_{\text{vdw}} \tag{2}$$

$$E_{\text{b}} = \sum_{\text{bonds}} k_{\text{b}}(l - l_0)^2 \tag{3}$$

$$E_{\theta} = \sum_{\text{bond angles}} k_{\theta}(\theta - \theta_0)^2 \tag{4}$$

$$E_{\phi} = \sum_{\text{dihedral angles}} k_{\phi}[1 + \cos(n\phi - \delta)] \tag{5}$$

$$E_{\text{electrostatic}} = \sum_{i,\, j>1} \frac{q_i q_j}{4\varepsilon r_{ij}} \tag{6}$$

$$E_{\text{vdw}} = \sum_{i,\, j>1} \frac{A_{ij}}{r_{ij}^{12}} - \frac{B_{ij}}{r_{ij}^{6}} \tag{7}$$

$$E_{\tau} = \sum_{\text{improper angles}} k_{\tau}(\tau - \tau_0)2 \tag{8}$$

Here the force constants are the various parameters k, the "natural" bond lengths (l_0) and angles (θ_0) are indicated by the subscript zero, n controls foldedness of internal rotation around each bond, δ is an angle that controls where the energy minima and maxima occur during rotation around bonds, q is the charge on an atom, ε is the dielectric constant, r here is the interatomic distance between two nonbonded atoms, A and B parameters control where and how deep the energy minima occur in Lennard-Jones interactions, and the "improper" angles τ refer to a mathematically convenient way to keep sp^2 atoms from deviating too far from planarity. The van der Waals and Coulombic interactions are summed between nonbonded atoms, whereas the other FF terms involve atoms covalently bonded to each other. In better FFs, additional terms take into account anharmonicity of bond stretching and angle bending and also special electronic effects. The FF parameters are calibrated to reproduce experimental geometries, relative energies, and sometimes other molecular properties.

In MM, the objective is to compute the energy of a molecular structure and/or to minimize the energy as a function of geometrical degrees of freedom, i.e., the potential energy surface. The computed energy reflects how far the geometrical arrangement of atoms deviates from an idealized bonding situation (such as would be the case when there is no strain in any bond). A better geometry has a lower energy. Well-established optimization methods are again used for energy minimization.

The MM model is conceptually simple, gives very accurate 3D structures for common organic compounds, and provides its information at least an order of magnitude faster than do QM methods. These strengths make MM well suited for treating both small and large molecules. Limitations of MM are that it requires empirical parameters to describe each "spring," and predictions depend on the care with which parameterization has been done. The analogous situation in quantum chemistry is that its predictions depend on the adequacy of the basis set and level of theory.

There are about 10 or so FFs in wide use. Some of these have simpler and/or a minimal number of potential energy terms in order that they can be used to model large biomolecules such as proteins and nucleic acids. Other FFs that would be of more interest to the readers of this chapter are carefully parameterized and have extra terms to reproduce more molecular effects. Examples of the latter are the MM3 (59–61) and MM4 (62–66) methods of Norman Louis Allinger; these are refinements of his MM2 FF (67,68). The Allinger FFs work very well on common kinds of organic molecules. An FF that was designed specifically for pharmaceutically relevant molecules is the Merck molecular force field (MMFF) (69–76). Compared to other FFs, the Allinger and Merck FFs give the best overall results for molecular geometries and conformational energies (77). MM2* and MM3* are close variants of MM2 and MM3 as used in the MacroModel program (marketed by Schrödinger, Inc.; Table 1).

Some of the more approximate or specialized FFs encountered in the literature include CFF, CHEM-X, COSMIC, CVFF, DREIDING, MMX, SHAPES, TRIPOS, VALBOND, and UFF. Well-known FFs for modeling proteins and nucleic acids include AMBER, CHARMM, ECEPP, GROMOS, OPLS and their variants. Some of these latter FFs compromise the quality of reproducing subtle intramolecular electronic effects for the sake of being fast enough to treat biomacromolecules in long molecular simulations.

Molecular simulations are used most often for modeling proteins and nucleic acids. We mention the methods here only because they are methods for computing a free energy directly. However, they are rather complex calculations, so we will keep our comments brief. Molecular dynamics simulations give information about the variation in structure and energy of a molecule over an interval of time (78,79). In MD, each atom moves according to Newton's equations of motion for classical particles:

$$\text{Force} = \text{mass} \times \text{acceleration}, \mathbf{F} = m\mathbf{a} \tag{9}$$

Table 1 Some Commercial Suppliers of Computational Chemistry Software

Vendor	Website (www.*.com)	E-mail	Telephone	Headquarters
Accelrys	accelrys	solutions@accelrys.com	858-799-5000	San Diego, California
CAChe Group of Fujitsu	cachesoftware	info@cachesoftware.com	503-531-3600	Beaverton, Oregon
Gaussian, Inc.	gaussian	info@gaussian.com	412-279-6700	Pittsburgh, Pennsylvania
Hypercube Inc.	hyper	sales@hyper.com	352-371-7744	Gainesville, Florida
Parallel Quantum Solutions	pqs-chem	sales@pqs-chem.com	479-521-5118	Fayetteville, Arkansas
Planaria Software	planaria-software	info@planaria-software.com	—	Seattle, Washington
Schrodinger, Inc.	schrodinger	tnfo@schrodinger.com	503-299-1150	Portland, Oregon
Scientific Computing & Modelling	scm	info@scm.com	31-(0)20-444-7626	Amsterdam, The Netherlands
Semichem	semichem	andy@semichem.com	913-268-3271	Shawnee Mission, Kansas
Tripos, Inc.	tripos	info@tripos.com	314-647-1099	St. Louis, Missouri
Wavefunction, Inc.	wavefun	sales@wavefun.com	949-955-2120	Irvine, California

$$\text{Force} = \text{negative gradient of potential energy}, \mathbf{F} = -\nabla \cdot \mathbf{V} \qquad (10)$$

Thus, at each time step, atoms under the most strain move fastest and farthest. To satisfactorily solve Newton's equations requires extremely short time steps, typically only 1 femtosecond (10^{-15} sec). If the time increment is too long, atoms can come too close in each step, and the energy of interaction from the FF gets so high that the system becomes unstable and erratic in subsequent steps (80).

An important concept for obtaining free energies is the thermodynamic cycle. This cycle is shown in Figure 4. The first law of thermodynamics states that the work done by a system changing between two states is the same for every adiabatic path between the states. Free energy is a state function, so the change in free energy must be the same regardless of how you go around the cycle. Hence,

$$\Delta G_A + \Delta G_C = \Delta G_B + \Delta G_D \qquad (11)$$

There may be situations where it is too difficult to compute the free energy for a reaction or transformation along, for example, route D, whereas it may be relatively easy to compute the free energies for the three routes A, B, and C. Rearranging Eq. (11) gives

$$\Delta G_D = \Delta G_A + \Delta G_C - \Delta G_B \qquad (12)$$

Calculations can thus be set up to run the three steps A, B, and C. Then the results can be combined to yield the free energy change for step D.

Thermodynamic cycles are used in MD simulations for computing accurate relative free energies. Free energy perturbation (FEP) calculations simulate the conversion of one molecule into another similar one (81,82). By

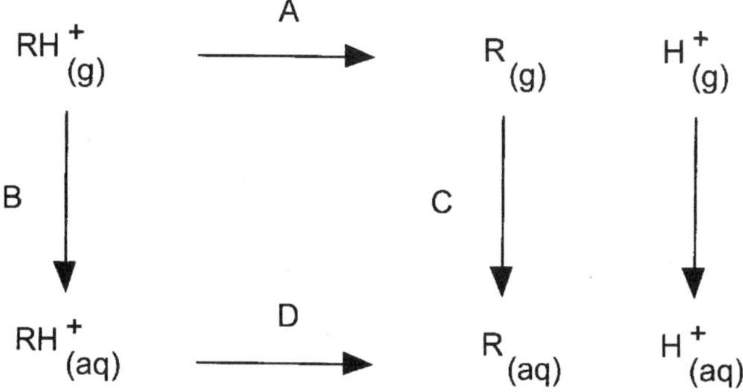

Figure 4 A thermodynamic cycle. The example illustrated here corresponds to a simple ionization, but a similar cycle could be drawn for other reactions. The point of using the cycle is that it is easier to compute the energy changes for the gas phase reaction (step A) and the two hydration processes (steps B and C) than it is to compute the energy for step D (ionization in solution).

changing the FF parameters in tiny increments from those of one chemical structure to those for another similar structure, the change in free energy can be accurately estimated. The incremental changes must be small so that the molecular system stays in equilibrium; in practice, this means the calculations are demanding of computer time and the alchemical transformations must be rather modest (83). Hence, for many industrial applications, FEP calculations are limited (see, however, Ref. 84).

In MD calculations, the molecular system is following along a time course (trajectory). In the second type of molecular simulations, MC, the system follows a random walk through configuration space (85). A huge

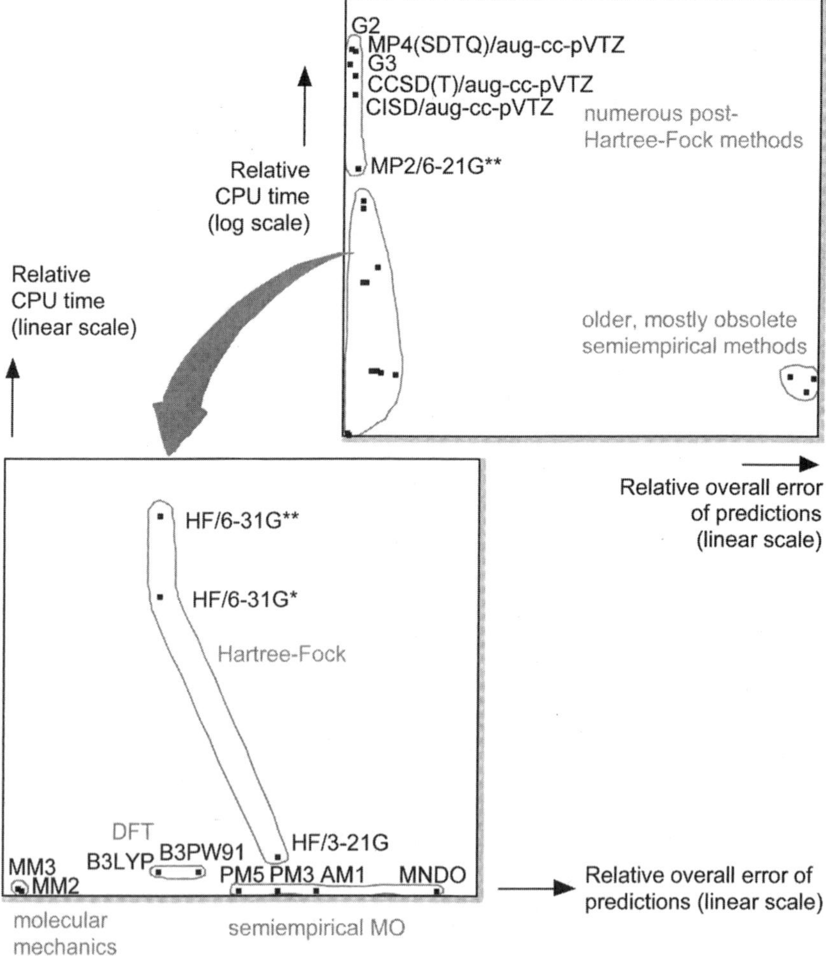

Figure 5 (*Caption on facing page*)

number of more or less randomly chosen configurations are considered. The energy of each is computed. An ensemble average of the computed energies is used to calculate thermodynamic properties via statistical mechanics.

F. Selecting a Computational Chemistry Method

So far, we have introduced a large number of quantum mechanical and FF approaches that have potential utility to chemists interested in stress testing. The perhaps bewildering mosaic of methods from which to choose can be intimidating to the beginner. To help put these methods in perspective and to help the readers of this chapter, we compare the performance of a representative selection of methods in Figure 5. On the abscissa, we plot the relative error of predicted molecular properties obtained by these methods

---

Figure 5 (*Continued from previous page*) Schematic relationship comparing accuracy and computer time requirements of various kinds of computational chemistry methods. In the upper plot, relative central-processor-unit (CPU) time requirements are plotted on a log scale. The other axes in the two plots are on a linear scale. The cluster of points in the lower left-hand corner of the upper plot are enlarged in the lower plot. The lower plot shows the relative performance of refined molecular mechanics methods, semiempirical molecular orbital methods, ab initio molecular orbital (Hartree–Fock) methods, and density functional theory (DFT) methods. The methods with the best balance of accuracy and speed are located closer to the origin of the lower plot. To explain the acronyms in the upper plot, MP4(SDTQ)/aug-cc-pVTZ refers to fourth order Møller–Plesset perturbation theory with single, double, triple, and quadruple excitations of the electrons between the molecular orbitals. Following the slash is a long basis set designation. In the case shown, the basis set is augmented with diffuse functions (e.g., for higher Gaussian basis functions). Further, the basis set is correlation consistent (cc), which means that the basis functions have been selected to work well with post-Hartree–Fock calculations. There are polarization (p) functions on all atoms (i.e., Gaussian basis functions for d orbitals on first-row atoms; Gaussian basis functions for p orbitals on hydrogens). And the basis set is a very large one of triple-zeta (TZ) quality, which means that there are three sets of Gaussian basis functions to represent orbitals occupied by the valence (V) electrons, in addition to a large number of Gaussian basis functions for the core electrons. G2 and G3 are Pople's Gaussian-2 and Gaussian-3 theories which involve elaborate ab initio calculations that are empirically handled to minimize systematic errors stemming from the use of less than complete basis sets and less than perfect account of electron correlation. CCSD(T) is coupled cluster theory with single and double excitations and with triple excitations treated perturbatively. CISD is configuration interaction with single and double excitation of electrons between the molecular orbitals. The 6–31G** is a basis set with ten s Gaussian basis functions, four p Gaussian basis functions, and one d Gaussian basis function on each first-row atom. A single asterisk means the basis set is augmented with a set of d Gaussian basis functions on each first-row atom; two asterisks mean the basis set is further augmented with a set of p Gaussian basis functions on hydrogens.

based on published evaluations (1). The basis for evaluating performance is the agreement between theoretically computed and experimentally observed properties, such as heats of formation, molecular energies, ionization potentials, electron affinities, equilibrium bond lengths and bond angles, of sets of test compounds. (In the case of MM, no electronic properties are computed, so the error of estimation is based on heats of formation and molecular geometries.) On the ordinate, we indicate rough estimates of the relative computer times to run a calculation on a given molecule. Ideally, the scientist will want to use methods that give the best possible accuracy at the least cost in terms of how long it takes to obtain the computational results.

At the horizontal extremities in the figure are older, simple quantum mechanical methods that have mostly fallen to disuse. At the vertical extremities are the post-HF methods. These are used quite frequently, but mostly, for very small molecules. In the lower left corner of the upper right graph are four classes of computational methods. These methods are seen more clearly in the enlargement on the left side of Figure 5. Best in terms of speed and accuracy are the MM methods. However, as we have noted, MM is usually not well suited for studying bond breakage and formation. But use of a good quality FF can yield excellent ground state molecular geometries that can then be used in subsequent quantum chemistry calculations. Of the three quantum mechanical classes of methods in the enlargement, semiempirical MO methods are relatively fast but can be left wanting in terms of accuracy. Each new generation of semiempirical method brings its predictions a little closer on average to ab initio accuracy. (However, ab initio calculations with the very small STO-3G basis set are not any better than semiempirical ones.) Ab initio MO and density functional methods often balance the desires for reliability of the predicted properties and for speed of obtaining results.

In summary, we advise that you begin your research project by exploration with fast, approximate methods, but plan to culminate the project using the best affordable method(s). If you need results immediately, as so often happens in the pharmaceutical industry, then low level ab initio calculations to obtain mainly graphical results might be your most practicable option. Here, a small basis set such as 3–21G is worth trying.

III. SELECTING SOFTWARE

Applicable software has been summarized elsewhere (86), including brief descriptions of each software package, information about developers and vendors, and resources on the Internet and World Wide Web. Ref. 1 presents more recent descriptions of some relevant programs. A variety of free software is available from individual developers, but availability depends on the whims and interests of the programmers. Today most of the computational chemistry software used in industrial, academic, and other laboratories is from commercial sources. Prices on this software range from modest to expensive. Cost depends not only on the capabilities of the program, but also the number of users at a site, the convenience of use, the level of technical support offered to users, and the number of competing software products.

Starting in the 1980s, scores of small companies were created by entrepreneurs to develop and market such software. In the last ten years, there has been much consolidation of this industry, so that now fewer companies serve most of the market. We list some of these companies in Table 1.

There are some programs of particular potential usefulness to the readers of this chapter: SPARTAN (Wavefunction, Inc.), which runs on various current computing platforms (from workstations to personal computers (PCs) and Macintoshes), Jaguar (Schrödinger, Inc.), which runs on workstations, and Gaussian and GaussView (Gaussian, Inc.), which run on various current computing platforms (from workstations to PCs and Macintoshes). SPARTAN is a more general molecular modeling program because it has MM capability, but all three programs have strong and easy-to-use quantum chemistry capabilities. All three have GUIs available, although SPARTAN's is the most integrated and elaborate.

Among other companies listed in Table 1, the largest in the computational chemistry market is Accelrys and has product offerings ranging from chemistry to the life sciences to materials science. Tripos, Inc. is another large company with a broad range of software products and services. New companies pop up on the scene from time to time, so a search of the World Wide Web will likely turn up additional vendors of niche software.

In addition to the commercial programs, there are some quantum chemistry and associated molecular graphics programs that can be obtained (licensed) at no cost. GAMESS (General Atomic and Molecular Electronic Structure System) is a well-established program (87) that can execute ab initio calculations on a variety of current computing platforms (see http://www.msg.ameslab.gov/GAMESS/). The various versions of GAMESS are maintained at the Iowa State University and other academic laboratories. Unlike with most commercial software, the source code is available, so the punctilious user can delve into exactly what the program is doing.

For studying degradation pathways, you need to investigate reaction mechanisms. Hence, at the heart of any software you select should be a robust array of quantum mechanical methods. The software package should include semiempirical MO methods (for treating large molecular systems and for preliminary reconnoitering of reaction pathways), ab initio MO methods with a variety of basis sets, and DFT implementations. Beyond the quantum mechanical core engine, it is very helpful if the software is bundled with MM methods with reliable FFs for geometry optimizations and explorations of conformational space. All these methods should be accessible through an easy-to-use GUI that will allow you to build the model structures on which the calculations are to be done. The GUI should present the program options (methods and parameters) in readily understandable menus. It can also be helpful if the program can easily export output to a spreadsheet program for further analysis.

Most of the established programs are of good quality; they rarely crash. They have been debugged, enhanced, and made to operate as fast as possible thanks to competition in the marketplace of other software. Modern software is user-friendly enough that it can be used without knowing how to program. In fact, most of the commercial programs are designed so that the user cannot alter them.

We strongly recommend that the reader try out software before selecting a product for purchase. Some vendor websites have demonstration packages that can be downloaded to your computer free of charge. These demonstration programs have built-in time limits, so they can be tried out for a period, such as a month, before they automatically quit working. Another opportunity for testing out software, or at least seeing software demonstrated, is at the exhibition of each national meeting of the American Chemical Society. Chemists who have wandered around the exhibition hall of these meetings or other large gatherings of chemists are well aware of the amazing variety of software products being offered. Many vendors proclaim that their software is a "solution" (it sounds better to be selling "solutions" rather than copies of computer programs.) But in order for a program to help you solve your research problems, it must be the appropriate tool and you must use it correctly. Moreover, seeing an expert put a program through its paces is not the same as trying to figure out yourself what to do when trying to run the program back in the privacy of your own office. Most likely, a user will have questions when using the software. When choosing software for purchase, also compare the quality of documentation (manuals) and customer support offered by the vendors.

Fifteen years ago, most of the computational chemistry software was designed to run on expensive mainframes, minicomputers, and workstations. More recently, with the increasing speed and declining price of computer chips, a desktop PC or a laptop computer has become an adequate platform for many calculations. To run software on your machine, you must be aware of which versions of computer operating system (e.g., Microsoft Windows, Apple Mac OS, UNIX, Linux) are compatible with a particular program.

IV. A MODELING SCENARIO

A. Getting Started

Assume now that you have purchased or have access to a suitable program. It is loaded on your PC, Macintosh, or workstation. You would like to take your new technology for a "test drive." We will assume that the software is an integrated package (i.e., with built-in GUI).

Human nature being what it is, the tendency of most scientists is simply to start the program and familiarize themselves with the features of the program by trial and error. Nevertheless, most computational chemistry software comes with documentation in the form of a user's manual and/or a help menu within the program itself. Some software vendors also maintain manuals and/or frequently asked questions (FAQ) on their websites (Table 1). Some programs come with self-guided tutorials that lead the user through examples that illustrate the features of the program; sample data are included with the software.

While not endorsing any particular program, for purposes of this section, we will envision use of a program such as SPARTAN or a similar one. SPARTAN is one of the easiest modeling programs to learn to use. The marketers of SPARTAN have produced several booklets designed to be adjuncts to classroom teaching (88–90).

Running a calculation and obtaining the first beautiful molecular graphics can be a proud accomplishment, but it is not equivalent to being an expert with the program or theory. If being competent with the program is important to you, then further reading of manuals and textbooks will bolster the probability that results you obtain will be meaningful.

B. Building a Model Structure

Once you have launched (started) the software, you will want to construct on the computer a model of the molecule you are interested in. Some programs require that you first use the pull-down menu under "File" and select "New." This tells the program to expect a new molecular structure to be entered. (The program will automatically set up a directory (or folder for a PC) on the hard drive where data can be stored for this model.) One way to enter a structural model is with a "draw" window. Typically, this consists of a "palette" of atom types (C_{sp^3}, C_{sp^2}, N_{amine}, –O–, =O, F, etc.), bond types (single, double, aromatic, etc.), and molecular fragments (preconstructed moieties such as a phenyl ring, amide, carboxylate, etc.). By clicking (with the computer mouse or touch pad) on one of these icons and then clicking on the drawing window, the icon will be placed at the location you indicate. Clicking at the end of a "bond" of your nascent model will cause the new atom or fragment to be attached there. You can continue to pick and place the fragment icons until you have a complete structure. An erase icon lets you use your cursor to change your mind.

There are several things to keep in mind while building a model.

1. Acids and Bases

When you build a model structure, consider the experimental conditions relevant to the system you want to study. If the molecule's environment is acidic and it contains a basic nitrogen, the nitrogen can be protonated and a positive charge must be added to the model. If the molecule's environment is basic and it contains a carboxyl or other ionizable group, then the model can have the acidic hydrogen removed and a negative charge must be added to the model. On the other hand, if you are just interested in the shape of the MOs, then a calculation on a neutral model may be adequate.

2. Leave No Valence Behind

We have already mentioned the necessity of having the hydrogens and formal charges explicitly accounted for in a molecular model prior to calculations. A program will handle a structure with, e.g., $-COO^-$, differently from a structure with $-COOH$. If you attempt to do an MM calculation on an incomplete model, some programs will allow the calculation to proceed, but the results will be substandard.

3. Three-Dimensionality

In some programs such as SPARTAN, the structure-building icons of the drawing window are three-dimensional so that constructing a molecular model is almost like snapping together the pieces of a hand-held molecular modeling kit. In other programs, the structure-building icons of the drawing window are two-dimensional. In the case of a 2D chemical diagram, you will need to "three-dimensionalize" the molecular model before proceeding. This process involves minimizing the energy of your crude starting structure so that such features as the tetrahedral hybridization of C_{sp^3} carbons are introduced. The process of three-dimensionalization is usually done via MM because of its speed and potential for accuracy depending on the FF. The process generates a set of Cartesian (x, y, z) co-ordinates for each atom in the structure.

4. Check and Recheck

After you have a model structure, you should check its reasonableness and completeness. Most programs allow you to use the computer's mouse or touch pad to rotate the model on the computer screen. You should carefully inspect the structure from various orientations and make sure the computer understood what you intended. Some programs do not show double bonds as two lines or do not show aromatic rings with a dotted circle in the center. Hence, you need to make sure the hybridization of the atoms is right, so that phenyl rings are flat, and so on.

Sometimes, if two atoms are too close in the starting structure, severe distortions (obviously bad bond lengths and angles) will be introduced by optimization. The structural defects are often easy for a chemist to spot in the molecular graphics display. In such situations, go back to the drawing menu and try to redraw the distorted parts. Then repeat the optimization.

If your molecule has a stereo center, check that the configuration is what you want. If not, you need to rebuild the atoms at the stereo center(s) and reclean (reoptimize) the model structure. If the substance you want to study is racemic, then you may model either enantiomer because from an MM or QM point of view the results will be the same for either enantiomer. Some programs are equipped with the ability to tell you whether the chiral centers are *R* or *S*, which can be very convenient. For other programs with GUIs, it can be tricky to tell which enantiomer you have on the computer screen by simple visual inspection. You will need to rotate the molecule back and forth on the screen (using the mouse or touch pad). A few programs can display a structure as a stereo pair. So if your eyes are adept at either "relaxed eye" or cross-eyed viewing, you can see the dramatic 3D shape on the screen. Special glasses that help you see stereo can be purchased with some modeling software.

5. Imported Models

Another way to get a structure into the computer is to import (read) a molecule file containing the atomic co-ordinates (and perhaps other atomic and molecular information) into your program. Unfortunately, there is no single standard file format that all programs use. However, some of the commonly encountered formats include those of SYBYL MOL2 files and Protein Data Bank (PDB) files. There are also free programs available for download from the World Wide Web that can interconvert the numerous file formats still in use.

Most chemists today are acquainted with computer programs for creating chemical structure diagrams, which are the 2D depictions of compounds familiar to all chemists (91). ChemDraw from CambridgeSoft Corp. (www.cambridgesoft.com) is one of the most widely used of programs for drawing chemical structures. A companion program from CambridgeSoft is Chem3D, which allows rudimentary molecular modeling. A typical chemist will have many ChemDraw documents stored on a PC. The structure diagrams in these documents can be copied from ChemDraw and pasted into Chem3D, where they can be three-dimensionalized. Chem3D can export the 3D models as PDB files, which can then be imported by other computational chemistry programs for further calculations.

C. Trimming the Fat

It will be to your advantage to keep the model structure as simple as possible. When chemists first sit down at a computer, it is not uncommon for them to think they must build the model on the computer screen to be identical in structure to the compound in the flask. Using the complete structure may be fine if all you plan are a few quick calculations. However, if you plan extensive calculations, either in terms of the range and sophistication of the methods you might want to apply or in terms of the number of compounds to treat in a related series, then it makes sense to keep the models as small as possible. A smaller model will run much faster on the computer and save you time.

In practical terms, simplifying a model means using a hydrogen (or methyl or some other small group) to replace side chains that are remote from a reaction site. Or if you are studying a series of related compounds such that part of the structure is constant, then it might be feasible to replace the invariant part of the molecules with a hydrogen or a small group like methyl. By understanding the chemistry of the compounds, you can simplify your modeling so that you will still extract the essential information but not waste time waiting for overly long calculations to run.

Let us give a few examples of what we mean. Suppose you are interested in the reactions of cephalosporin antibacterial agents (Figure 6). Both chemical and computational studies of these compounds show that the substituent at the 3 position can interact electronically with the β-lactam ring. Hence, if you are interested in modeling a reaction of the β-lactam ring, it suffices to replace the large acylamido side chain at the 7 position and the carboxylate at the 4 position with something smaller, even though these side chains are absolutely required for biological activity. Or suppose you are interested in stress testing the oncolytic gemcitabine (Fig. 6). If you are interested in studying electrophilic substitution on the aromatic ring, then the fluoro-containing side chain may be replaced by a hydrogen.

Just to be absolutely clear, structural simplifications should be done only in cases where the focus is on the electronic properties in a localized part of a molecule. For conformational problems where any or all the side chains may interact sterically or electrostatically, avoid excising your model.

D. Strategic Thinking

At this juncture, the user should consider which methods are going to be applied to shed light on the research questions at hand. You will want to treat all relevant molecules you plan to compare by the same method(s). For instance, the optimized length of some bond in model structure 1 obtained by method A should not be compared to the analogous bond in another model structure 2 optimized by some other method B. As usual, you cannot compare apples and oranges. You need to decide, or at least think about, how much computing you can afford to do and how long you are willing to wait for the calculations to finish. If qualitative pictures of MOs are all that you need, then a semiempirical calculation may suffice. If you want a fairly reliable comparison of the energetics of two competing

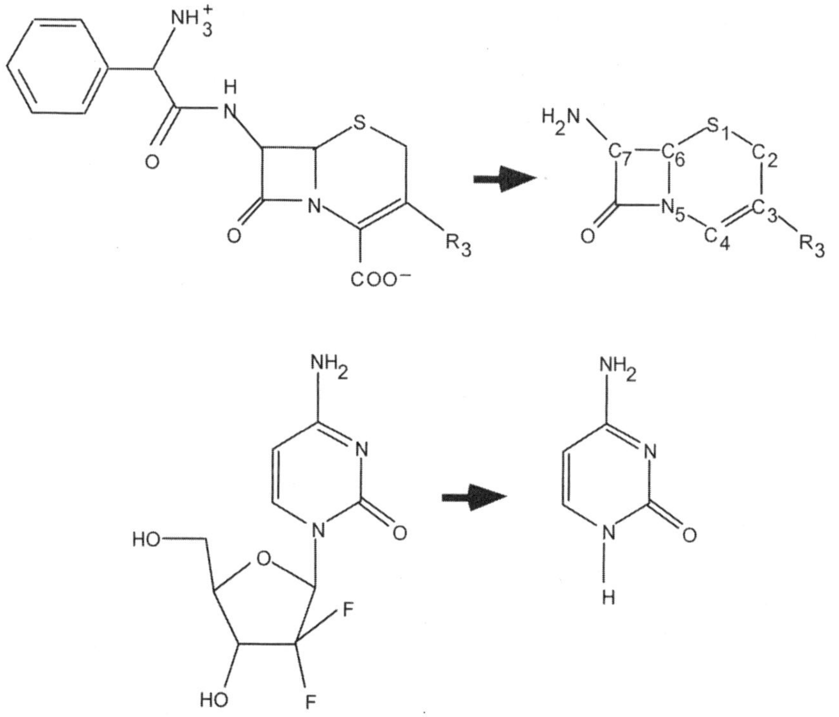

Figure 6 Examples of simplifying molecular structures for the purpose of speeding calculations on the models. The "extraneous" side chains in cephalosporins and gemcitabine are replaced by smaller groups (not all hydrogens are shown explicitly). The point is to retain only those parts of the compounds that deal directly with the electronic questions being studied. Side chains do affect the chemical and biological properties of a compound, but would produce a more or less constant effect on the electronic structure of the model structure retained. In the cephalosporins, the 7-acylamido and 4-carboxylate substituents can be replaced by NH_2 and H, respectively. Substituents at the 3 position of cephalosporins include H, CH_3, Cl, acetoxymethyl, arylthiomethyl, etc.

reaction pathways, then the most sophisticated type of ab initio calculation possible may be in order.

As explained earlier, the more accurate methods take longer to run on a computer than the approximate ones. In fact, the length of your calculation increases exponentially as you try to nail down the last bits of accuracy (Figure 5).

A good strategy is to perform preliminary calculations by a relatively rapid (i.e., approximate) method. Recall, however, that MM methods are generally much, much faster than quantum mechanical ones, and for questions of ground state geometries can be just as accurate. For transition state or excited state geometries, ab initio methods are better. Then after reconnoitering the situation and getting familiar with the molecular geometries and how they may "morph" between reactants and products, repeat the calculations at one—or preferably several—higher levels of theory.

We cannot stress enough the importance of benchmarking your calculated results to experimental data. The experimental data can be in the form of structural, chemical, or other information. However, in real-world research problems, there may be no experimental data for corroborating your calculations on the molecules you want to treat. If possible, test the computational method on a similar molecule for which accurate experimental data are available. Ascertain to your satisfaction that the method is reliable. If even this test is not possible, we recommend aiming to use the best level of theory possible for your problem because you will have no way to detect systematic or other errors. The highest level of theory that is practical has a better chance of agreeing with experiment than a lower one. Lower level quantum methods can sometimes predict molecular properties adequately when comparing similar molecules in which effects of systematic errors are minimized.

E. Conformational Analysis: Down in the Valley

Given some overall strategy of what you hope to accomplish with the calculations, you need to decide which conformation(s) of your reactant(s) to use. A potential energy surface of nontrivial molecules will have many hills and valleys. The deepest valley is called the global minimum, as mentioned earlier. Without some other basis for selecting a conformation, many chemists will want to use the global minimum conformation. However, most pertinent is the conformation a molecule adopts at the time of reaction. This may or may not be the global minimum. You may need to use your chemical intuition to choose the most relevant conformation. Sometimes, you will need to explore several different conformations.

Energy minimization algorithms take the molecule to the vicinity of the lowest point in the valley closest to the starting geometry. Hence, it is important to have a good starting geometry. It is advisable to repeat the geometry optimization two or three times sequentially because movement across a relatively flat valley can be slow. In other words, to check that the structure is fully relaxed, take the optimized geometry from the first run and plug it back into the program as the starting geometry for a second run. Optimization algorithms are generally designed to take longer geometrical steps at the beginning of a run than near the end.

If you are concerned about finding the global minimum structure, you will need to explore conformational space by rotating the structure about single bonds. Conformational search approaches have already been mentioned. For drug-sized molecules, a systematic search method, which varies specified torsional angles through a range of angles in increments, works well. Most programs save all (or all low energy) conformers generated, and then you can select any of these for further calculations.

F. Experimental Design

After the conformation search, you should again energy minimize the most interesting conformer(s) to make sure you are starting the bond lengths and bond angles at equilibrium values according to the theoretical method used. The model is now ready for further calculations.

As an example, consider the problem of trying to decide if some drug-like molecule decomposes through pathway P1 or pathway P2. In designing your computational experiments on these two pathways, you also should use your understanding of the general mechanism(s) involved. Is the reaction nucleophilic substitution, electrophilic substitution, elimination, addition, pericyclic, etc.? Use your basic understanding of these mechanisms to set up the process you want to model on the computer. On the computer, you model the chemistry by varying distances between atoms in the molecule(s) undergoing the reaction or rearrangement. This is where your chemical knowledge and intuition give you a distinct advantage over someone with, say, only a computer science or informatics background.

Every chemist is trained in conceptualizing reactions and rearrangements by "pushing arrows" to track the movement of electrons in the bonds. This is a depiction that chemists have long found useful. Of course, electron pairs do not really move around like this. In the realm of physical reality, interatomic distances lengthen and shorten, and electron density shifts in the course of a reaction, but no electron pairs hop among the bonds and atoms. Quantum mechanics works.

G. Types of Results

One of the simplest ways of examining a molecule is to look at the partial charges on each of its component atoms as obtained from a typical MO calculation. A chemist would expect that an atom with a more positive charge might be more susceptible to nucleophilic attack than some less positive atoms in the molecule. Sometimes, this simple interpretation suffices. But there are other times, however, when one needs to look more closely at the charge distribution. For one thing, an attacking moiety will experience electrostatic interaction not only with the atom being attacked, but also with nearby atoms. The electrostatic field could increase the probability that some other positively charged atom will collide with the reactant.

A more sophisticated way to look at charge distribution is the molecular electrostatic potential energy map of the reactant(s). Programs like SPARTAN can compute and display the MEP of a molecule as part of its quantum mechanical repertoire. In an alternate visualization of the MEP, it is common for such graphics programs to display the electron density contour at 0.02 e/Å^3 as the molecular "surface" (92). This contour roughly coincides with the van der Waals surface and hence is roughly similar in shape to the old-fashioned CPK space-filling models. Onto this electron density surface, the MEP values can be projected in terms of color-coding. The color-coding differentiates negative and positive regions of MEP and shows the magnitude of the MEP values (see Figure 2).

Inspection of the computer graphics can give you a qualitative picture of where an electrophile or nucleophile may prefer to attack. Nucleophiles usually find it easier to attack where the MEP is positive, whereas electrophiles tend to go where the MEP is negative. In fortuitous situations, you might be able to see that one position is more appropriate for reaction than some other position. As you view and rotate the molecular graphics on the computer screen, you can qualitatively compare the steric accessibility of the various possible reactive sites in your molecule. Thus, when comparing two reactive centers in a molecule, you should also look at the regions an approaching reactant would have to traverse.

A relatively easy option in user-friendly software is to look at the frontier MOs. To obtain these, you can simply request (via a pull-down menu or pop-up menu when setting up the calculation) that the MOs be computed. In fact, since you may not know ahead of time what information will prove useful, and since it does not add much overhead (running time) to the calculation, it is good to always ask for the MOs and MEP to be produced. The highest occupied MO (HOMO) and lowest unoccupied (LUMO) are commonly examined, but sometimes the shapes of somewhat lower or somewhat higher MOs also need to be checked.

An electrophile is often likely to attack a position that has more electron density in the HOMO. This is because the electrons in the HOMO are more accessible and more polarizable than are the electrons in the lower energy MOs. Conversely, in the case of a nucleophilic reaction, the attacking agent often prefers to go where the LUMO offers a large, accessible lobe with which the orbitals of the nucleophile can overlap and interact.

Actual energy calculations may be desirable to confirm what the qualitative pictures indicate because the graphics give the picture for a static molecule. As two molecules approach each other, they may change conformation, which in turn can alter the shape of the MEP and MOs. Quantum mechanical energy calculations along the reaction path may therefore be desirable (93). Sometimes, the differences in the MEP or frontier MOs at the two positions may be too subtle to discern or may even indicate contradictory conclusions. In such cases, you can try quantitating the relative difficulty/ease of approaching to position 1 vs. position 2. You can compute the energies along the two (or more) reaction paths by setting up the appropriate computational experiments.

H. The Dry Look (Gas-Phase Reactions)

In searching for the most probable reaction path, the aim would be to find the one with the lowest energy barrier(s) to climb over. However, this brings up another caveat. Theoretically, computed reaction energy surfaces may look entirely different from what is taught in organic chemistry class. This is because those pedagogical examples were for reactions in solution, whereas a "plain vanilla" quantum mechanical calculation is for the gas phase (i.e., vacuum). Hence, where you would expect to see the energy rise as two reactants approach each other, the calculations may show a steady decline in energy as the separation distance decreases. It is only after you include solvation of the reactants that you obtain the expected energy barrier for a reaction. A famous example of computed energy surfaces for an S_N2 reaction (94,95) is depicted in Figure 7.

Some of the more user-friendly, interactive computational chemistry programs are designed based on the assumption that only one molecule will be handled at a time. But to study a reaction you need two molecules at once. Hence, you may need to "trick" the program into thinking that the two reacting molecules are really one molecule. This trick can be done by creating a dummy bond between the two reactants. The dummy bond can be systematically lengthened or shortened, thereby mimicking a reaction pathway. With a program like SPARTAN, setting up a reaction is further complicated because the program was written as if it knew some chemistry; the program will object if you try adding an extra bond between two atoms with all their valence positions already full. Also, the program may automatically reset certain bond lengths based on standard tables of bond lengths stored in the program by the software developers. (A typical set of standard bond lengths can be found in Ref. 96.) This adjustment of bond lengths can undo much work of prior geometry optimization calculations and thus be frustrating. SPARTAN lets you put "constraints" on geometrical variables to hold these near assigned values, but the results are less than precise. It is at this point that convenience of interactive software becomes an impediment.

I. Reaction Pathways: Advanced Treatment

A regrettable fact is that no software package will satisfy all your needs unless they are rather basic. For the general case of computing energies along a reaction pathway between reactant(s) and product(s), you want exact control of the geometrical variables. Some software packages, particularly those that function solely in terms of molecular graphics, do not allow sufficiently precise control of geometry. This is where some other programs, such as Jaguar, MOPAC, Gaussian, or GAMESS, come into play.

In general, a molecular geometry can be represented in terms of a set of atomic co-ordinates or in terms of "internal co-ordinates". The latter

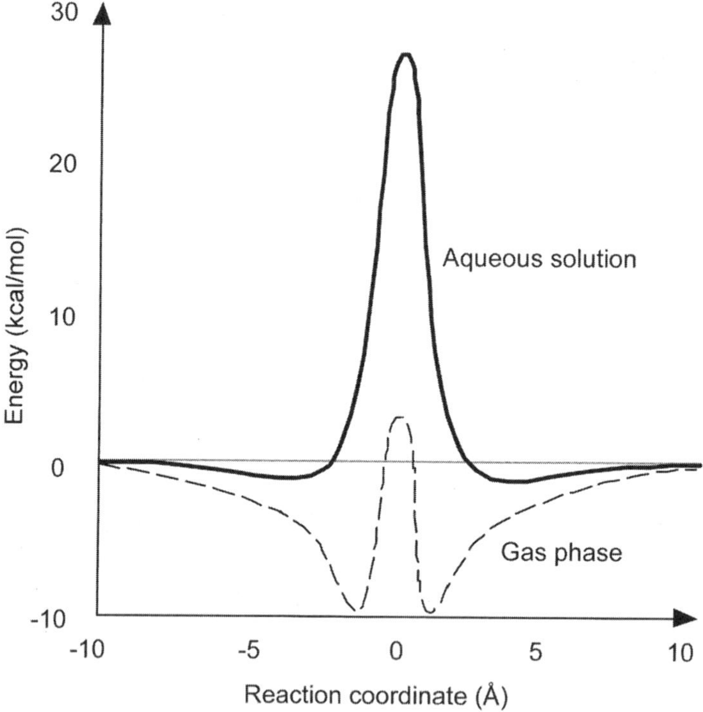

Figure 7 Qualitative depiction of the energy profile along the reaction co-ordinate for the S_N2 reaction: $Cl^- + CH_3Cl \rightarrow ClCH_3 + Cl^-$, which involves nucleophilic substitution of the chloride of methylchloride by a chloride ion. The potential energy curves drop as the two reactants approach until a loose complex is formed. Then the energy rises rapidly to the transition state, which has two equal C–Cl interatomic distances (zero on the abscissa). The energy profile looks quite different in the gas and solution phases. Compared to the reactants (or products), the loose complex and the TS are poorly solvated, so the energies for these are much higher in solution than in a vacuum.

represent the molecule entirely by a set of bond lengths, bond angles, and torsional (dihedral) angles. In the parlance of the field, such a description of a molecular structure is called a Z-matrix.

The situation with internal geometries is depicted schematically in Figure 8. The programs are generally written to place the first atom at the origin. Then the second atom can be positioned with respect to the first by placing it at a bond length away along one of the Cartesian axes, say, x. Then the third atom can be positioned with respect to being a bond length away from the second atom and forming a bond angle in the xy plane with respect to the first atom. Then the fourth atom is placed at a bond length

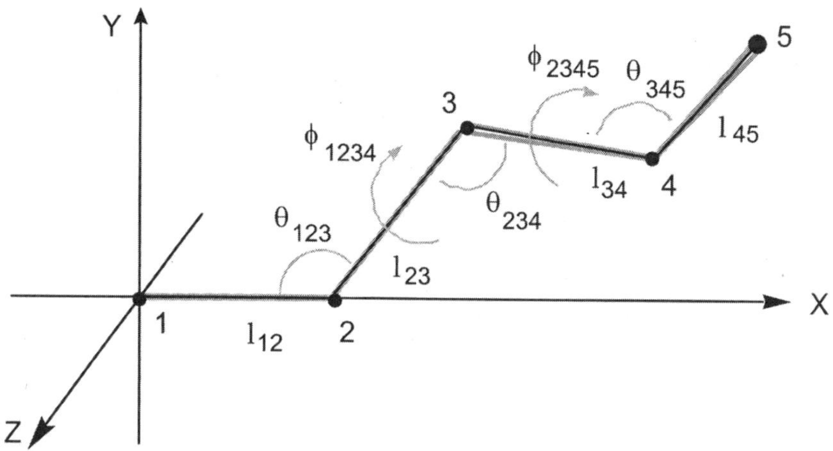

Figure 8 Building a molecular model based on internal geometries (bond lengths *l*, bond angles θ, and torsional angles ϕ). Each subsequent atom is added to the framework with respect to earlier situated atoms. The convention in many programs is that the x Cartesian axis is the horizontal axis on the computer screen, the y axis is vertical, and the z axis comes out of the computer screen toward the user.

away from one of the first three atoms, forming a bond angle with respect to another of the previous atoms, and forming a torsional angle with respect to the remaining previous atom. The other atoms in the molecule can be added in an analogous manner. Each atom is positioned in space with respect to only previously positioned atoms.

The advantage of using internal co-ordinates is that the user has complete control over the relative location of all atoms. With internal geometry, it is very easy to set precisely the distance between two (or more) reactants. You can incrementally vary this separation and thereby model what happens as two molecules "collide" (or, in the reverse reaction, fragment). For instance, you can request a program to optimize all internal co-ordinates except the length of a dummy bond length between two reactant molecules. The length of the dummy bond can be varied in increments over a range. A wide increment of 0.25–0.5 Å can be used in an initial scan of the range. The range should cover from where the molecules first start to "feel" each other's presence (ca. 4.0 Å) to a point closer than that of the new bond being formed (e.g., a typical alkyl C–C bond is 1.54 Å). For plotting the potential energy surface, you will also need the energies of the infinitely separated reactants, which means the energies of each molecule alone. You will also be particularly interested in any dips (corresponding to intermediates) or bumps (corresponding to transition states) in the potential energy surface. Additional points on the reaction co-ordinate curve can be computed to fill in interesting regions.

You can conduct your "reaction experiment" in a solution-like environment. One of the options in the set-up window of a program is to let you to turn on an implicit solvation model (48). Such models attempt to account for the mutual interaction of the dipoles of the water molecules and the electron distribution in the solute molecule, as well as to account for the energy required to create a cavity in the bulk solvent to accommodate the solute. A very dilute solution is assumed, so the solute molecules do not see each other. Several implicit solvation modeling schemes have been proffered in the literature and are incorporated in various quantum mechanical programs.

J. Over the Hill (Transition States)

Some programs provide computational techniques for locating transition states. This capability can be helpful. Finding an energy minimum involves finding a molecular geometry such that a small change of any geometrical variable (e.g., a bond length or a bond angle) raises the molecular energy. However, finding a transition state is trickier because the algorithm must find the "mountain pass" connecting the energy valley of the reactant(s) and the energy valley of the product(s). Algorithms for finding transition states operate by starting with a model structure on either side of the pass, and then the two structures are gradually "morphed" toward some average geometries. The program tries to bring the geometries on each side of the mountain pass closer and closer to the saddle point until a transition state is in hand.

There is a criterion used to judge the stability of an assembly of atoms whose geometry has been optimized by a quantum mechanical method. Some quantum mechanical programs let you compute the normal mode vibrational frequencies of the assemblage. If all these frequencies are positive, the structure is at a minimum on the potential energy surface. If there is one negative vibrational frequency predicted (say, $-100\ \mathrm{cm}^{-1}$), then the structure is a transition state between two stable molecules. If there are two such negative frequencies, that is an indication that the assemblage is at a peak on the potential energy surface; the implication of such a finding is that the structure would spontaneously decompose or rearrange to more stable species.

Once the saddle point on the reaction co-ordinate is found, then there are some other algorithms that can be tried. The dynamic reaction co-ordinate (DRC) computes the path followed by the atoms in a system starting at the saddle point (93). As the system glides down a valley on the potential energy surface, the initially high potential energy is converted to kinetic energy (e.g., more vibration). The intrinsic reaction co-ordinate (IRC) saps off some of the kinetic energy as the system evolves (93). The IRC is also referred to as the minimum energy path. A number of semiempirical and ab initio programs are equipped to handle these algorithms.

K. Reproducibility and Accuracy

One might naively assume that if you ran the same calculations in different programs that you would get identical results. This is sometimes a safe assumption, but not always. Not all programs are created equal. Differing results from different programs arise from several factors: (1) round-off errors due to the number of significant figures stored for each of the millions of numbers handled by the computer in a typical calculation, (2) slightly different implementations of the theoretical methods (obscure details of how some methods were programmed may not have been completely described in the literature), and (3) slightly different parameters controlling such operations as geometry optimizations, SCF iterations, shortcuts in evaluating integrals, and hundreds of other procedures involved in the intricacies of a calculation.

The user should realize that there are a multitude of parameters in every computational chemistry program. The more automated a program, the more likely it is that more of these were preset by the programmer and are thus invisible to the user. Usually, preset parameters were selected by the software developers to give the best possible performance on some particular set of molecules of interest to the developers. Feedback from users of the widely used programs usually stimulates the developers to refine their programs so that the best overall results can be obtained for a variety of research problems. However, before putting too much trust in calculated results, it is prudent to check them carefully.

Sometimes, using more than one program to cross-check the results is advisable. And results should be corroborated with experimental information wherever possible.

Whereas textbook examples show cases where computational chemistry provides an answer conforming to chemical intuition and experiment, real-world research problems may not be as clear-cut.

L. Carried Away by Numbers

The calculations you perform may yield results worthy of publication. We hope so. A common foible for beginners is to report their computed data with too many digits—what could be called "digititis" (inflammation of the digits). Just because a computer program prints out numbers with, for instance, 6 or 8 or more decimal places, that does not mean that all these are significant. Typically, no more than 1–4 decimal places in output should be considered significant. A good rule-of-thumb is never report more than one decimal place beyond what is variable from one computational method to another. Hence, if method A gives 2.47812471 and method B gives 3.01699821 for the same property, report these two values as 2.5 and 3.0.

M. Dealing with Relatives: Avoiding Systematic Error

It is worth reinforcing a caveat alluded to earlier. The absolute value of a quantity like energy may have little meaning by itself. Computational chemistry methods can always provide answers more reliably when the scientist phrases the question in relative terms. Thus, if you calculate the change in energy of molecule A going to intermediate B, the resulting number may not mean much. If possible, you want to set up your computational experiments asking what is the change in energy for molecule A going to B, for molecule A′ going to B′, and for molecule A″ going to B″, where A, A′, and A″ are related and B, B′, and B″ are related, the more closely related the better. Then you will be on safer ground comparing the energy changes for the three transformations.

N. Grasping for Definitiveness

Just as in the case of laboratory experiments, sometimes a computational experiment will not yield a conclusive answer to a research question. For instance, suppose you are comparing the energy landscapes of two reaction pathways. Sometimes, the two landscapes will be predicted to be so similar that no clear preference can be discerned. Or even worse, the calculations may give mutually contradictory results. Charge distributions may predict one answer, whereas the MO shapes may suggest another answer, and the energies suggest still another. Theoretically, the energy landscape should be the definitive answer, but only if the most rigorous methods are used and only if thermodynamic effects on the calculated surfaces can be correctly modeled. Almost always, reaction conditions are greatly simplified in a calculation.

There is thus no guarantee that computational modeling will resolve a research question; such is the nature of research. But as with much of curiosity-driven science, a modeling calculation may be worth investigating and could be very revealing. We have tried to show the opportunities of computational chemistry, but we want the readers to embark on these experiments with their eyes wide open. Your first computer experiments may not work as you hoped, but just as in the case of laboratory experiments, persistence can pay off. If an experimental procedure or technique did not work for you the first time you tried it, you would not shun it forever. Likewise with computational chemistry experiments, if you do not get a satisfactory answer the first time you try it, do not assume the whole field is useless.

The experimentalist has a distinct advantage when turning to computer modeling because of having expertise in the chemistry of the compounds under study. Once you have learned a method, you can apply it to additional research problems in the future.

V. SPECIALIZED APPLICATIONS

In the remaining space we have available for this chapter, we briefly touch upon a number of topics of potential interest to the readers of this book. More in-depth presentations can be found in the textbooks and articles that are cited in this chapter.

A. Prediction of Ultraviolet/Visible Spectra

Electronic transitions in the UV–Vis region are commonly used to detect compounds eluting from a chromatographic system. Suppose you are looking for a particular compound in the eluent. It would help if you knew what its strongest electronic transitions were. Computational chemistry provides a way to estimate transitions in UV–Vis spectra of compounds even before they are isolated and characterized.

An electronic transition involves excitation of an electron from the ground state wave function to one of the excited state wave functions. An adiabatic excitation is one that involves adjustment of the nuclear geometry to minimize the energy of the excited molecular system. A vertical excitation is one that occurs so rapidly that the ground state geometry does not have time to change. This latter type of excitation is usually adequate for modeling UV–Vis spectra.

There are various post-HF methods for obtaining a wave function for an excited state (38). However, a molecule has so many excited states that it may be computationally difficult to determine the wave functions for each of these except when symmetry (i.e., the irreproducible representation in group theory) can be used to distinguish the states.

For drug-sized molecules, an MO calculation is more practical than post-HF methods. Such a calculation will give you a set of filled MOs and a set of unoccupied (so-called virtual) MOs (and, in the case of radicals, one or more singly occupied MOs). Simplistically, electronic excitations can be thought of as promoting an electron from one of the occupied MOs to an unfilled one. In reality, of course, the MOs would adjust to the excitation so that the ground state MOs are only an approximation to the excited state MOs.

A fast approach to predicting spectra is to use a semiempirical MO method specifically parameterized to reproduce experimental electronic transitions. Such a method is INDO/S (intermediate neglect of differential overlap/spectroscopy). The most widely used INDO/S parameterization is that developed by Zerner (41). The name of both the parameterization and program is ZINDO. This semiempirical method does well at predicting spectra of organometallic compounds and organic dyes, such as used for photographic film or hair coloring. However, ZINDO is not good for predicting bond lengths and angles, so it is best to obtain a good geometry by MM or ab initio calculations and then using this geometry for the spectral calculations.

Computing an electronic excitation will give you λ_{max}. Determining the intensity of each peak in a spectrum involves calculation of transition dipole moments. Unfortunately, not all molecular modeling programs have facility to compute these, but some do. Relevant software products (Table 1) include the semiempirical MO programs ZINDO from Accelrys, CAChe and MOPAC from Cache Software/Fujitsu, MOPAC from Schrödinger, AMPAC from Semichem, ArgusLab from Planaria, and HyperChem from Hypercube. Most of these programs run under Windows on a PC. Many ab initio programs can also compute transition dipole moments. To broaden the sharp, calculated excitation lines into the peaks typically seen in an experimental UV spectrum, each line can be replaced by a Gaussian distribution curve and then these curves can be summed.

B. Open-Shell Molecules

By far, most calculations reported in the chemical literature are on closed-shell molecules, i.e., those with the MOs (spatial orbitals) cozily occupied by two electrons each, one of α spin and one of β spin. However, in the case of radicals there is a singly occupied orbital, or in the case of diradicals two singly occupied orbitals. These radicals are referred to as open-shell molecules. Calculations on these are even more challenging than those on closed-shell molecules.

One way to deal with unpaired electrons is to use the unrestricted HF (UHF). Whereas regular ab initio calculations restrict the one-electron spatial orbitals to be identical for α- and β-spin electrons (so-called restricted HF, RHF), in UHF the orbitals are allowed to be different in the SCF processes. Usually, the difference in the spatial orbitals for α and β electrons is only slight. Unfortunately, when applied to a radical, UHF stumbles in a pitfall (97). It is called "spin contamination." Unrestricted HF wave functions cannot be trusted to correspond to pure spin states such as a doublet for radicals or a singlet or triplet for diradicals. Theoretically speaking, the UHF wave function may not be an eigenfunction of the spin operators.

Another way to computationally treat unpaired electrons is to employ restricted open-shell HF (ROHF) theory. Here, we encounter another pitfall. It is an artifact called "symmetry breaking" (97). Whereas ROHF wave functions are pure spin states, the ROHF wave function may not retain the symmetry of the molecule. Suppose a molecule has C_{2v} symmetry. The wave function should have the same symmetry, e.g., the orbital lobes on either side of the symmetry plane should be identical. However, with symmetry breaking, the two sides are not equal. The unsymmetrical ROHF wave function may even give lower energy than a physically correct (symmetrical) wave function. Symmetry breaking occurs because correlation between electrons of opposite spin is insufficient.

What is one left to do? It has been recommended (97) that the most reliable method for treating radicals in general is DFT. With a functional such as B3LYP, unrestricted DFT gives good energies and optimized geometries. Time-dependent DFT is a method seeing increased usage because its results are easy to interpret (98).

C. Photochemistry

As stress chemists are well aware, one of the potential sources of degradative forces on pharmaceutical products is light. Pharmaceutical companies and pharmacists have long known that some biomedical products must be stored in dark bottles. Even bottled soda pop ages faster in the sunlight.

Modeling photochemistry is especially challenging because besides the difficult task of finding the minimum energy pathways from the reactants to the transition state to the various products that can result from degradation, you must also deal with electronic transitions and hence pathways on more than one potential energy surface. The Gordian knot of modeling a photochemical reaction is the funnel region where an excited state reactant or intermediate descends to the ground state potential energy surface. The funnel region is called a "conical intersection" (99).

In practical terms, a post-HF method (38) that is able to reliably optimize ground and excited states must be used. One such method is CASSCF, which is available in ab initio programs such as Gaussian. The drawback of modeling with a post-HF method is that the computer time requirements are heavy. Molecules with 10–15 first-row atoms are about as large as can be handled accurately.

D. Predicting Stability of a Molecule

At one time, measuring the thermochemical properties of compounds was a serious, widespread research area. The old National Bureau of Standards (now the National Institute of Standards and Technology) determined and compiled data of heats of formation for thousands of chemicals. Now such research is less popular, so, if there is a new molecule for which you want the heat of formation, the alternatives are to do the thermochemical experiments or to determine it by computational chemistry. A recently developed collection site for experimental thermodynamic data is at http://trc.nist.gov/.

For a typical reaction involving reactants A and B going to products C and D,

$$a\mathrm{A} + b\mathrm{B} \rightarrow c\mathrm{C} + d\mathrm{D} \tag{13}$$

the standard enthalpy of the reaction can be obtained from the standard enthalpies of formation for each species in the reaction, i.e.,

$$\Delta H_r^\circ = c\Delta H_f^\circ(\mathrm{C}) + \Delta H_f^\circ(\mathrm{D}) - a\Delta H_f^\circ(\mathrm{A}) - b\Delta H_f^\circ(\mathrm{B}) \tag{14}$$

The standard enthalpy of formation of a compound is the change in enthalpy associated with forming the compound from its constitutive elements, each in their standard state, at a given temperature.

There are five computational categories for obtaining the standard enthalpy of formation (28).

1. Post-Hartree–Fock: The Best

The first category consists of the post-HF methods. Unfortunately, the HF model fails to give good enough electronic energies from which heats of formation can be computed. Electron correlation is necessary, and so we must turn to post-HF methods. Two such methods of note are G2 (100) and G3 (101). The latter is more finely tuned than G2. These methods entail lengthy, multistep calculations found empirically to closely approximate reliable experimental data. So-called "chemical accuracy" ($\pm$1 kcal/mol) can often be achieved on small molecules. For 148 such compounds, the average absolute deviation (AAD) between laboratory experiment and computational experiment is 1.56 kcal/mol by G2 and 0.94 by G3. (The set of 148 compounds, referred to in the literature as the "G2 set", consists of molecules with 2–12 atoms.) Quite a few variants of G2 and G3 have been conceived and tested trying to find ways to simplify the calculations and/or give better results, but basically G3 is about as good as has been achieved (28). G3 is available in the Gaussian series of programs.

2. DFT Performance

The second category of method for computing heats of formation is DFT. Benchmarking on a test set of 37 small compounds reveals an AAD from experimental heats of formation as small as 2.34 kcal/mol with the B3LYP functional, whereas for the same test set of compounds, G2 gives 1.46 kcal/mol and G3 gives 0.67 kcal/mol (28). Tests on the G2 test set show that the AAD is smallest when using the B3LYP functional. With other commonly used functionals, AAD increases to 3.49 kcal/mol with B3PW91, 7.11 kcal/mol with BLYP, 7.88 kcal/mol with BPW92, 17.99 with B3P86, 20.22 kcal/mol with BP86, and a horrendous 90.91 kcal/mol for SVWN (28). Generally, the B3LYP predictions of heats of formation perform best for inorganic hydrides and poorest for nonhydrogen-containing compounds. In summary, DFT with B3LYP can give answers faster and can be applied to larger molecules than G3, but at the cost of somewhat less accuracy on average.

3. Semiempirical Performance

In contrast to most other quantum mechanical programs, popular semiempirical MO programs (as well as molecular mechanics programs like MM2 and MM3) are programmed to output directly a calculated heat of formation of molecules. This leads us to the third category: the semiempirical MO methods (36). Here, the AAD values are larger than for the methods mentioned above. MINDO/3, one of the older semiempirical MO methods (dating from 1975), gives AAD at 8.63 kcal/mol for a subset of the G2 set of test compounds (28). The next method from the laboratory of the late Michael J. S. Dewar was MNDO (1977); for it the AAD is 9.15 kcal/mol. Then in 1985 the Dewar group came out with the AM1 method, which gives an AAD of 9.48 kcal/mol. Note that these AADs are getting slightly worse, even though for large test sets of compounds used by Dewar and coworkers the predicted heats of formation got better on average with each newer method (36). Another semiempirical MO method PM3, published by J. J. P. Stewart in 1989 (36), yields an AAD of 7.02 kcal/mol for 140 compounds in the G2 test set (28). The semiempirical MO methods perform best on hydrocarbons, substituted hydrocarbons, and inorganic hydroxides, but give relatively large errors in predicted heats of formation for radicals and nonhydrogen-containing compounds. In summary, semiempirical MO methods can give answers faster than ab initio or DFT, but with generally poorer accuracy. If all you need is a ballpark figure for heats of formation or relative heats of formation of some similar molecules, then semiempirical methods may suffice.

4. Molecular Mechanics Performance

The fourth category of methods to compute heats of formation is MM. For most small organic compounds with experimentally known heats of formation, MM3 is able to predict these well within ± 1 kcal/mol (67,102), i.e., chemical accuracy. Thus, MM can be quite useful for ascertaining the stability of organic molecules, provided they are not too unusual. Allinger has meticulously developed a parade of molecular mechanics methods: MMI, MM2, MM3, and MM4. In general, each advancement improved average agreement with experiment for properties such as molecular geometries and conformational energies. However, because the FF parameters must be developed specifically for each class of compound (hydrocarbons, amines, hydroxyls, acids, etc.), a newer generation may not have been extended to as much of compound space as an earlier one. If MM3 or MM4 can treat the compounds you are interested in, then they are the preferred MM methods.

5. Sum of Parts

The fifth category consists of empirical methods of obtaining heats of formation. These depend on the additive constitutive principle. That is, they assume that the standard heat of formation of a compound depends on the number of atoms of each type or the number of groups present in the compound (28). Another common way to apportion the molecular heat of formation is between the bonds; each bond type (single C–C, double C=C, etc.) contributes a portion of the total heat of formation of the compound. Tables of atomic or bond contributions can be found in the thermochemistry literature (28). These empirical calculations can yield values within a few kilocalories per mole of the experimental values if the molecules consist of well-studied constitutive components and there are no strong strain or conformational effects in play.

E. Applications to Hard–Soft Acid–Base Reactions

Lewis acids are atoms or molecules that accept an electron pair (103). Soft acids have polarizable valence electrons, whereas hard acids do not. Lewis bases are atoms or molecules that are capable of donating an electron pair. Soft bases are polarizable, whereas hard ones are not. Hard acids preferentially interact with hard bases; the interaction is mainly ionic and charge controlled (104). Conversely, soft acids tend to interact (or react) with soft bases; the interaction has covalent character and may be orbital controlled.

The use of DFT to study hardness and softness, as well as chemical principles such as that of maximum hardness (molecules arranging themselves to yield products as hard as possible) has been reviewed recently (105).

There may be an occasion in stress testing when the ideas and associated principles of hard–soft acid–base reactions can come into play. Although molecular modeling programs are not usually designed to tell you the polarizability of a molecule directly, you can vary the charge on a molecule by computing the electron density maps for the neutral, anionic, and cationic forms of the same molecular geometry. Comparing the isodensity maps will give a qualitative idea of how much the spatial extent of the electron density changes. A greater change indicates a softer, more polarizable molecule. A procedure has been described (www.colby.edu/chemistry/PChem/notes/Fukui.pdf) for using SPARTAN to evaluate the hardness and softness of molecules in terms of the Fukui function which is related to polarizability (106).

F. Predicting Acidity and Basicity

Another fundamental molecular property of interest in pharmaceutical stress research as well as in the rest of chemistry is the pK_a of acidic groups (or pK_b of basic groups) in a compound. The pK_a of a compound in hand is more easily—and reliably—determined experimentally than by computational chemistry. In cases where an experiment on a molecule of interest cannot be done for whatever reason, then a reasonable approach for obtaining an approximate pK_a is to look in compilations of pK_a values of known compounds and find some similar ones or at least ones with similar functional groups.

In certain situations, a computational chemistry approach may be useful. The procedure just described for estimating pK_a from similar known compounds has been turned into an algorithm in the program ACD/pK_a DB from Advanced Chemical Development (www.acdlabs.com). The program performs reasonably well (average accuracy of ± 0.2 pK_a units for common organic compounds), and its database can be supplemented with pK_a values of compounds studied in-house.

Alternatively, suppose you want to determine which heteroatom in a molecule is protonated first as pH is lowered. Or conversely, you may want to know which is the most acidic proton in a compound (even if it is a hydrocarbon, for example). In such cases, you can obtain optimized geometries for the parent molecule Z and its conjugate acid ZH^+ (or conjugate base Z^-) for each site of proton attachment or removal. Simply take the differences in total energy (obtained quantum mechanically), $E(ZH^+)$–$E(Z)$ [or $E(Z^-)$–$E(Z)$], and you have a theoretical assessment of the relative gas-phase acidity (basicity). (The electronic energy of a proton is zero because it has no electron.) Of course, these energy differences do not account for solvation, but if the two protonation (or deprotonation) sites are very similar, the vacuum results may suffice. Alternatively, you can turn on implicit (continuum) solvation in your calculation and obtain energies of the simulated solution species.

Some quantum mechanically oriented programs include instructions and routines specifically designed for estimating pK_a values. These programs include Jaguar (with its ab initio and density functional methods) and CAChe (with its semiempirical methods). Jaguar has a "pK_a module" that uses a routine of DFT calculations combined with empirical corrections and the heat of solvation of a proton. For many common functional groups such as carboxylic acids, phenols, amines, and heterocycles, AAD between calculated and experimental pK_a values is 0.5 or better, whereas the deviation is 0.7–0.8 for other functional groups such as alcohols, sulfonamides, and imides.

G. Modeling Hydrolysis

Hydrolysis is one of the most common reactions encountered. Degradation of a pharmaceutical agent can occur if it is stored in aqueous solution or if it is exposed in the solid state to any water vapor during storage, formulation, distribution of the dosage forms, or patient handling. Hydrolysis can be especially problematic for susceptible compounds that are hygroscopic in the solid state.

Hydrolysis reactions have often been modeled with computational chemistry. You can start the computational experiment by modeling the substrate (drug) molecule. Then a nucleophile can be "flown" toward the site of attack, for instance, the carbonyl carbon of an ester or amide linkage (107). The model nucleophile can be a water molecule or a hydroxide ion. A typical computational experiment would be to calculate the quantum mechanical total energy of the substrate and nucleophile fixed at a separation of 4 Å. Then incrementally move the reactant closer in 0.25 Å steps until they are within about 1.25 Å of each other. With gas-phase modeling, the energy will go down until the separation is close to that of a covalent C–O single bond length (i.e., ca. 1.4 Å), and then at still closer distances the energy will start to rise rapidly indicating less stability when the reactants are pushed too close.

The change in total energy between the infinitely separated reactants and the species at the energy minimum of the reaction co-ordinate curve will not be comparable to the heat of reaction (because thermodynamics is neglected in the quantum mechanical model). Nevertheless, the energy change can be quite useful on a relative basis in the case of comparing the hydrolysis of a series of closely related compounds.

Let us give a specific example. Cephalosporins are well-known antibacterial agents. There are tens of cephalosporins on the market and thousands more in the patent literature and in proprietary company archives. A common route of cephalosporin decomposition is via hydrolysis of the β-lactam ring and subsequent rearrangements. The biological mode of action is for the β-lactam ring to pop open when acylating the hydroxyl group of a serine in the active site of bacterial transpeptidases (108). In effect, a nucleophile (–OH) is reacting with the carbonyl carbon of the β-lactam.

One of the sites of substitution differentiating cephalosporins is the 3 position (Fig. 4). Modeling experiments were designed (109) to compare the energy profile for a hydroxide ion attacking the β-lactam carbonyl of a simplified 3-cephem ring system with various substituents at R_3. It was found that the energy change along the reaction pathway correlated with Gram-negative antibacterial potency of the compounds (110). Moreover, these calculated energy changes correlated with experimental base-catalyzed hydrolysis rates, chemical shifts at the Δ^3 double bond, and carbonyl stretching frequencies (111,112). The result was a tidy package where computed properties, physicochemical properties, kinetics, and biological activities tied together in a rational and coherent way. It was not necessary to compute correct heats of formation because the modeling experiments were designed so that relative energies (corresponding to the different R_3) could provide useful answers. In fact, a semiempirical MO method sufficed. The key point is that the computational experiments were set up so that systematic errors would roughly cancel, and results were obtained that could be compared.

H. Reaction Knowledge Bases

With the growing power of computers, chemists began exploring the use of artificial intelligence to help with synthesis planning in the 1970s. The goal was to reduce to simple computer algorithms all the rules, knowledge, and considerations that an experienced synthetic organic chemist would employ in devising the reactions necessary to reach a desired endpoint. Then other chemists could, in principle, use the programs to design synthetic routes as clever as the experts. Among the examples of these efforts were the programs LHASA developed by the Elias J. Corey group at Harvard (113), ORAC by the A. Peter Johnson group in Leeds (114), Munich by the Ivar Ugi group obviously in Munich (115), and CAMEO by the William L. Jorgensen group at Purdue and then Yale (116). While once attracting quite a bit of interest and still receiving some attention, the efforts generally have not panned out to become universally useful. [However, for additional discussion of CAMEO (computer-assisted mechanistic evaluation of organic reactions), see the chapter earlier in this book on drug degradation pathways.]

Instead, computer databases of reactions proved to be of wider interest to chemists. Software companies targeting the chemistry market began compiling reactions from the literature in the 1980s. The databases could be searched in terms of reactants or products, or substructures of these. If hits are found, the user can retrieve the details of the reaction including conditions and reagents as well as the literature reference. One of the earliest such reaction databases and search software that became available commercially was called REACCS (now part of ISIS) (117). Other software products followed, including both specialized databases (to appeal to chemists in specific fields) and comprehensive databases. An example of the latter is the database of the CAS, which has reaction information from the literature dating from 1907 to the present. Chemical Abstracts Service's databases (www.cas.org) can be searched using a program called STN Easy (118) or a program called SciFinder (119). Both software products are ubiquitous at pharmaceutical companies.

The reaction databases let scientists easily and quickly retrieve information about the chemistry of known substances, some of which might be similar to the investigational compounds under study in forced degradation testing. Many of the readers of this book will already be acquainted with these informatics resources on their desktop computers.

I. Atropisomerism

High-performance liquid chromatography can sometimes separate atropisomers, i.e., a compound with highly hindered rotation about a single bond, producing effectively two molecular species.

Addressing conformational questions is the strong suit of computational chemistry and molecular modeling. Both quantum mechanical and

MM work well at predicting relative conformational energies. Quantum mechanics is very reliable at determining barriers to internal rotation. (Molecular mechanics can sometimes give good barriers, although it is primarily parameterized to reproduce the energies and geometries of molecules in their equilibrium states.)

Although conformational searching is usually simple, we take this opportunity to point out a few complications that can arise. Take the case of rotating a molecule about a single bond connecting two relatively bulky, bumpy ends (Figure 9). The standard modeling procedure is to first optimize the geometrical variables including the torsional angle (also called dihedral angle) around the single bond. Then the torsional angle can be varied ("driven" in the parlance of computational chemistry) through 360° in increments. A suitable initial increment to try is 30°. A larger increment would miss some of the hills and valleys of the potential energy surface. An increment smaller than 30° may give more detail about the surface than necessary and would be more time consuming to compute. After initially scanning the potential energy curve at 30° increments, you can always go back and compute the energy for intermediate conformations in regions of particular interest.

There are some pitfalls that can be encountered in driving a torsional angle in a congested molecule. One is a "gearing" effect. If at each increment you optimize the geometrical variables other than the torsional angle being driven and you take as a starting geometry for increment n the geometry optimized at increment $n-1$, the following problem can arise. A bulky side chain (say, R_1) can start rotating as it is driven past a bulky side chain at the other end of the molecule (say R_5). In effect, the two side chains become entangled like the teeth of two gears. What results is that as you drive the torsional angle of interest all the way around 360°, the final conformation at 360° is not the same as your starting conformation at 0° because the rest of the molecule has adopted a different conformation. Hence, as you plot

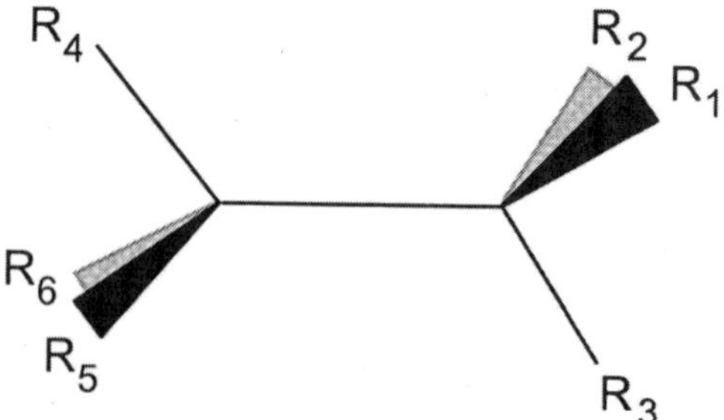

Figure 9 Example of a compound with severely restricted rotation about the single bond because of the bulkiness of the substituents, R_1–R_6.

the energies to see the barriers to internal rotation, the curves will not line up smoothly.

The way to avoid this problem is to start your calculations with an optimized, low energy conformation (e.g., a staggered, rather than eclipsed, conformer). Then use this same starting geometry at every increment of the torsional angle being driven. Hold constant all geometrical variables except the torsional angle being incremented. If you want, you can also optimize the variables at each increment. In effect, you can plot two potential energy curves: one for rigid rotation and one for relaxed rotation. The latter is closer to modeling what the molecule experiences as it rotates.

Another related pitfall can be encountered when the two ends of the molecule are very bulky. As you follow the procedure just recommended above, two large side chains may become hopelessly entangled, i.e., they occupy the same space. No amount of energy minimization will relieve the entanglement. The energy will be very high because of the unfavorable steric clashes. In such situations, it may be impossible to obtain a meaningful energy at that increment. When you plot the potential energy curve, you can simply represent the very high-energy peak by truncating it at the top of the graph. An example is shown in Figure 10.

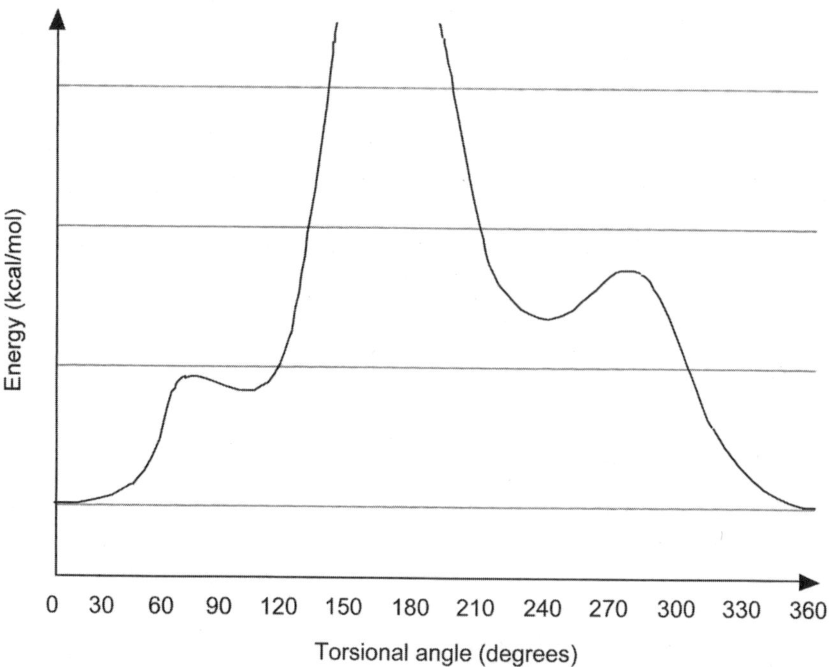

Figure 10 Example of how the potential energy curve can be plotted when the energy becomes too high to calculate at certain conformations.

A final pitfall should be mentioned in regard to modeling conformational changes such as rotation about a single bond or rotation about multiple single bonds as in the case of ring flip between two conformations (e.g., chair and boat). Suppose you have thought about your computational experiment and plan to drive the molecule between the energy minima of two conformational states. Starting at an optimized geometry, you increment the structures along a geometrical variable (a distance or an angle) that should result in the second conformation. When the molecular energies are plotted against the geometrical variable you may notice that the energy rises higher and higher until at some point it drops precipitously before settling out in the valley of the second conformer. Further examination of your results may show that the peak in energy is beyond what chemical intuition tells you should be the transition state between the two conformers. Curious, you may reverse the computational experiment. Start with an optimized geometry of the second conformation and drive it toward the first conformation. What you may find is that the energy again rises until beyond the expected transition state geometry of the first experiment, and then the energy plunges abruptly to the valley of the first conformer.

What is happening is that the strain in the molecule model is building to an excessive state. Then, like a tree branch that snaps back after being pushed out of the way by a passing hiker, potential energy is released suddenly (energy drops) when steric overlap is relieved. Plotting the energies from the two directions, the peaks will not coincide (Figure 11). The true energy barrier is probably located at or between the values of the geometrical variable at the peaks. The true energy barrier height may be slightly lower than the plotted peaks; this lower value of the barrier can arise from minor adjustments in the other geometrical variables during the "driving" process. You can obtain an approximate barrier location and height by estimating them from the graph of the two energy curves. You can also approximate or optimize the conformation near the presumed energy barrier and then drive the structure downhill in each direction in two separate runs.

J. Selected Bibliography

As mentioned at the beginning of this chapter, the number of papers in the literature reporting computational chemistry work on the degradation of pharmaceutical reactions is still not large. One could almost regard this as a virgin area of research compared to some overworked areas of research. Our objective in this section is not to comment on each paper that has appeared, but rather to just cite some papers that are illustrative of the type of computational chemistry experiments that can be brought to bear on research questions facing the chemist doing pharmaceutical stress testing.

Outside the scope of this section are a number of papers that have reported applications of computational chemistry to the degradation of

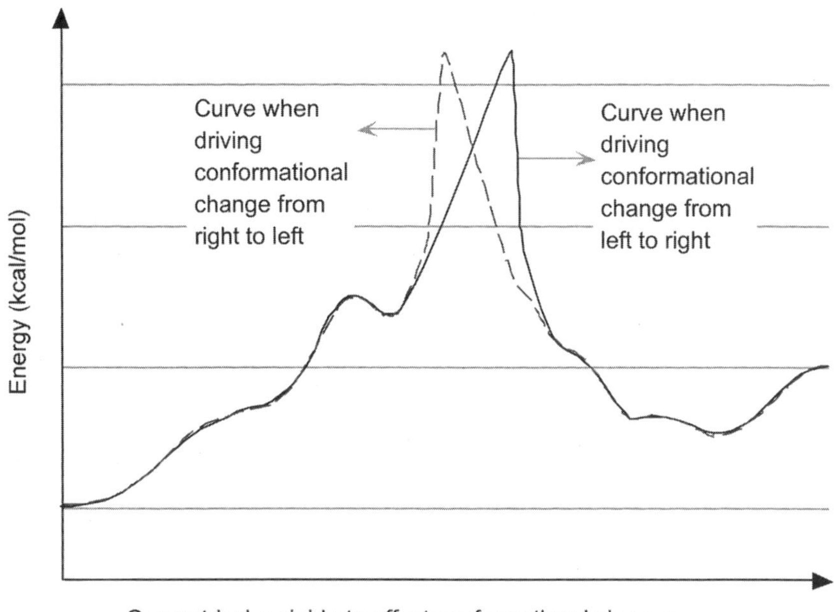

Figure 11 Hypothetical example of how the potential energy curves differ depending on the direction a geometrical variable is driven. In this example, there are two valleys separated by a high barrier. Climbing the energy hill from the left gives a different result compared to climbing the hill from the right. The actual energy barrier is probably between the two peaks because the driving process has forced excess strain into the model structure.

polymers, atmospheric compounds, pesticides, inorganic compounds, and other materials. However, many of the same computational principles that have been presented in this chapter also apply to these other areas. Beyond the scope of this section are the many synthetic reactions that have been investigated by computational chemistry. For instance, the Diels–Alder reaction is an especially favorite one for modeling. Preparative reactions are, in principle, the reverse of degradation, but it would make this chapter too long to cite all the synthetic reactions that have been modeled computationally. We do not include computational studies on the degradation of pharmaceuticals in the presence of enzymes; that is an area involving ligand–protein interactions. Also outside of the scope of this review are studies on chemical kinetics at the macroscopic (rather than atomistic) level, but this is certainly another valid use of computers (see, e.g., Ref. 120).

Cephalosporins, already mentioned in this chapter, have received much attention over the years from computational chemists and other scientists using computational chemistry tools. The treatments have ranged from semiempirical to ab initio; some attempted to model the effects of solvation (121–146). Many of these papers are reviewed in Ref. 107. The β-lactam substructure (azetidinone) of cephalosporins and penicillins has been treated often because it is quite small and has interesting electronic and geometrical factors at play.

The degradations of a variety of other compounds have also been studied computationally (147–152). Some of these computational studies neglected solvation. The studies were generally at the semiempirical level. The articles illustrate that much can be accomplished even without more sophisticated theoretical models. Some of the calculations have been quite advanced and yielded valuable insights and/or predictions. These few studies stand as beacons inviting further applications of computational chemistry to the sort of issues discussed in this book.

VI. CONCLUSIONS

Computational chemistry offers powerful tools for examining research questions arising in stress testing of pharmaceuticals. The methods and software have become very easy to use and more accurate. Whereas they cannot answer many questions faced by the experimentalist, they can give the researcher additional leverage in many research and development situations. The tools can be used for studying a wide range of molecules in regard to reaction pathways, conformations, electronic structure, and other physicochemical properties. Pharmaceutical degradation studies beckon with many novel and unique opportunities for applying computational chemistry. Our basic inquisitiveness as scientists stimulates us to use those tools that elucidate difficult research questions.

As with any scientific tool, computational chemistry software must be used and interpreted with some understanding. The primary purpose of this chapter has been to give a wide-ranging practical tutorial. Gaining experience with the tools will allow the user to phrase research questions in the most effective way.

Looking back at Figure 1, we see that the use of computational chemistry has been growing dramatically. One sure prediction is that use will continue to increase as more scientists discover its value for their particular research problems.

ACKNOWLEDGMENTS

This chapter is dedicated to Richard Bradford Leber and Rebecca Katherine Boyd, who prove that patience pays off. This chapter also honors Edward Lynn Boyd, whose three-quarters of a century has set a good example. The author is grateful to Joanne H. Boyd for assistance with manuscript preparation. Dr. Steven W. Baertschi is to be commended for showing incredible persistence and fortitude in the face of the usual editorial challenges. It has been a pleasure working with such a knowledgeable scientist and seeing his vision for a book move toward reality.

REFERENCES

1. Young DC. Computational Chemistry: A Practical Guide for Applying Techniques to Real-World Problems. New York: Wiley-Interscience, 2001.
2. Boyd DB. Molecular modeling software in use: publication trends. In: Lipkowitz KB, Boyd DB, eds. Reviews in Computational Chemistry. Vol. 6. New York: VCH, 1995:317–354.
3. Lipkowitz KB, Boyd DB, eds. Reviews in Computational Chemistry. Vol. 8. New York: VCH, 1996:v–ix.
4. Lipkowitz KB, Boyd DB, eds. Reviews in Computational Chemistry. Vol. 17. New York: Wiley-VCH, 2001:v–xii.
5. Lipkowitz KB, Boyd DB, eds. Reviews in Computational Chemistry. Vol. 1. New York: VCH, 1990:vii–xii.
6. Hopfinger AJ. Computer-assisted drug design. J Med Chem 1985; 28: 1133–1139.
7. Jensen F. Introduction to Computational Chemistry. Chichester, U.K.: Wiley, 1999.
8. Boyd DB, Lipkowitz KB. Examination of the employment environment for computational chemistry. In: Lipkowitz KB, Boyd DB, eds. Reviews in Computational Chemistry. Vol. 18. New York: Wiley-VCH, 2002:293–319.
9. Leach AR. Molecular Modeling: Principles and Applications. 2nd ed. Harlow, U.K.: Pearson Education, 2001.
10. Van de Waterbeemd H, Carter RE, Grassy G, Kubinyi H, Martin YC, Tute MS, Willett P. Glossary of terms used in computational drug design. Pure Appl Chem 1997; 69:1137–1152.
11. Boyd DB. Evidence that there is a future for semiempirical calculations. J Mol Struct: THEOCHEM 1997; 401:219–225.
12. Lipkowitz KB, Boyd DB, eds. Reviews in Computational Chemistry. Vols. 1–10. New York: VCH, 1990–1997; Vols. 11–18. Hoboken, NJ: Wiley-VCH, 1997–2002. Lipkowitz KB, Larter R, Cundari TR, eds. Reviews in Computational Chemistry. Vols. 19–21. Hoboken, NJ: Wiley-VCH, 2003–2005.
13. Schleyer PvR, Allinger NL, Clark T, Gasteiger J, Kollman P, Schaefer HF III, eds. Encyclopedia of Computational Chemistry. Vols. 1–5. Chichester, U.K.: Wiley, 1998.
14. Lipkowitz KB, Boyd DB. Books published on the topics of computational chemistry. In: Lipkowitz KB, Boyd DB, eds. Reviews in Computational Chemistry. Vol 17. New York: Wiley-VCH, 2001:255–357.
15. Hehre WJ, Radom L, Schleyer PvR, Pople JA. Ab Initio Molecular Orbital Theory. New York: Wiley, 1986.
16. Szabo A, Ostlund NS. Modern Quantum Chemistry: Introduction to Advanced Electronic Structure Theory. New York: McGraw-Hill, 1989.

17. Cramer CJ. Essentials of Computational Chemistry: Theories and Models. New York: Wiley, 2002.
18. Smith WB. Introduction to Theoretical Organic Chemistry and Molecular Modeling. New York: VCH, 1996.
19. Höltje HD, Folkers G. Molecular Modeling—Basic Principles and Applications. Weinheim: VCH, 1996.
20. Schlecht MF. Molecular Modeling on the PC. New York: Wiley-VCH, 1998.
21. Goodman JM. Chemical Applications of Molecular Modelling. Cambridge, U.K.: Royal Society of Chemistry, 1998.
22. Hubbard RE. Molecular graphics and modeling: tools of the trade. In: Cohen NC, ed. Guidebook to Molecular Modeling and Drug Design. San Diego, CA: Academic Press, 1996:19–54.
23. Boyd DB. Application of the hypersurface iterative projection method to bicyclic pyrazolidinone antibacterial agents. J Med Chem 1993; 36:1443–1449.
24. Allen FH, Taylor R. Research applications of the Cambridge Structural Database (CSD). Chem Soc Rev 2004; 33:463–475.
25. Müller K. Molecular modeling and structural data bases in pharmaceutical research. In: Jensen B, Jørgensen FS, Kofod H, eds. Frontiers in Drug Research—Crystallographic and Computational Methods. Alfred Benzon Symposium No. 28, Jun 11–15, 1989, Copenhagen: Munksgaard, 1990: 210–221.
26. Boyd DB. Aspects of molecular modeling. In: Lipkowitz KB, Boyd DB, eds. Reviews in Computational Chemistry. Vol. 1. New York: VCH, 1990:321–354.
27. Boyd DB. Molecular modeling—industrial relevance and applications. In: Ullmann's Encyclopedia of Industrial Chemistry. 6th ed. Weinheim: Wiley-VCH, 1998.
28. Curtiss LA, Redfern PC, Frurip DJ. Theoretical methods for computing enthalpies of formation of gaseous compounds. In: Lipkowitz KB, Boyd DB, eds. Reviews in Computational Chemistry. Vol. 15. New York: Wiley-VCH, 2000:147–211.
29. Leach AR. A survey of methods for searching the conformational space of small and medium-sized molecules. In: Lipkowitz KB, Boyd DB, eds. Reviews in Computational Chemistry. Vol. 2. New York: VCH, 1991:1–55.
30. Saunders M, Houk KN, Wu YD, Still WC, Lipton M, Chang G, Guida WC. Conformations of cycloheptadecane. A comparison of methods for conformational searching. J Am Chem Soc 1990; 112:1419–1427.
31. Pross A. Theoretical and Physical Principles of Organic Reactivity. New York: Wiley-Interscience, 1995.
32. Lipkowitz KB, Peterson MA. Molecular mechanics in organic synthesis. Chem Rev 1993; 93:2463–2486.
33. Schlick T. Optimization methods in computational chemistry. In: Lipkowitz KB, Boyd DB, eds. Reviews in Computational Chemistry. Vol. 3. New York: VCH, 1992:1–71.
34. Boyd DB, Smith DW, Stewart JJP, Wimmer E. Numerical sensitivity of trajectories across conformational energy hypersurfaces from geometry optimized molecular orbital calculations: AM1, MNDO, and MINDO/3. J Comput Chem 1988; 9:387–398.

35. Feller D, Davidson ER. Basis sets for ab initio molecular orbital calculations and intermolecular interactions. In: Lipkowitz KB, Boyd DB, eds. Reviews in Computational Chemistry. Vol. 1. New York: VCH, 1990:1–43.
36. Stewart JJP. Semiempirical molecular orbital methods. In: Lipkowitz KB, Boyd DB, eds. Reviews in Computational Chemistry. Vol. 1. New York: VCH, 1990:45–81.
37. Kestner NR, Combariza JE. Basis set superposition errors: theory and practice. In: Lipkowitz KB, Boyd DB, eds. Reviews in Computational Chemistry. Vol. 13. New York: Wiley-VCH, 1999:99–132.
38. Bartlett RJ, Stanton JF. Applications of post-Hartree–Fock methods: a tutorial. In: Lipkowitz KB, Boyd DB, eds. Reviews in Computational Chemistry. Vol. 5. New York: VCH, 1994:65–169.
39. Crawford TD, Schaefer HF III. An introduction to coupled cluster theory for computational chemists. In: Lipkowitz KB, Boyd DB, eds. Reviews in Computational Chemistry. Vol. 14. New York: Wiley-VCH, 2000:33–136.
40. Frisch MJ, Trucks GW, Schlegel HB, Scuseria GE, Robb MA, Cheeseman JR, Montgomery JA Jr, Vreven T, Kudin KN, Burant JC, Millam JM, Iyengar SS, Tomasi J, Barone V, Mennucci B, Cossi M, Scalmani G, Rega N, Petersson GA, Nakatsuji H, Hada M, Ehara M, Toyota K, Fukuda R, Hasegawa J, Ishida M, Nakajima T, Honda Y, Kitao O, Nakai H, Klene M, Li X, Knox JE, Hratchian HP, Cross JB, Adamo C, Jaramillo J, Gomperts R, Stratmann RE, Yazyev O, Austin AJ, Cammi R, Pomelli C, Ochterski JW, Ayala PY, Morokuma K, Voth GA, Salvador P, Dannenberg JJ, Zakrzewski VG, Dapprich S, Daniels AD, Strain MC, Farkas O, Malick DK, Rabuck AD, Raghavachari K, Foresman JB, Ortiz JV, Cui Q, Baboul AG, Clifford S, Cioslowski J, Stefanov BB, Liu G, Liashenko A, Piskorz P, Komaromi I, Martin RL, Fox DJ, Keith T, Al-Laham MA, Peng CY, Nanayakkara A, Challacombe M, Gill PMW, Johnson B, Chen W, Wong MW, Gonzalez C, Pople JA. Gaussian 03. Pittsburgh, PA: Gaussian, Inc., 2003.
41. Zerner MC. Semiempirical molecular orbital methods. In: Lipkowitz KB, Boyd DB, eds. Reviews in Computational Chemistry. Vol. 2. New York: VCH, 1991:313–365.
42. Thiel W, Voityuk AA. Extension of MNDO to d orbitals: parameters and results for the second-row elements and for the zinc group. J Phys Chem 1996; 100:616–626.
43. Bartolotti LJ, Flurchick K. An introduction to density functional theory. In: Lipkowitz KB, Boyd DB, eds. Reviews in Computational Chemistry. Vol. 7. New York: VCH, 1995:187–216.
44. St-Amant A. Density functional methods in biomolecular modeling. In: Lipkowitz KB, Boyd DB, eds. Reviews in Computational Chemistry. Vol. 7. New York: VCH, 1995:217–259.
45. Bickelhaupt FM, Baerends EJ. Kohn–Sham density functional theory: predicting and understanding chemistry. In: Lipkowitz KB, Boyd DB, eds. Reviews in Computational Chemistry. Vol. 15. New York: Wiley-VCH, 2000:1–86.

46. Davidson ER. Perspectives on ab initio calculations. In: Lipkowitz KB, Boyd DB, eds. Reviews in Computational Chemistry. Vol. 1. New York: VCH, 1990:373–382.
47. Cioslowski J. Ab initio calculations on large molecules: methodology and applications. In: Lipkowitz KB, Boyd DB, eds. Reviews in Computational Chemistry. Vol. 4. New York: VCH, 1993:1–33.
48. Cramer CJ, Truhlar DG. Continuum solvation models: classical and quantum mechanical implementations. In: Lipkowitz KB, Boyd DB, eds. Reviews in Computational Chemistry. Vol. 6. New York: VCH, 1995:1–72.
49. Scheiner S. Calculating the properties of hydrogen bonds by ab initio methods. In: Lipkowitz KB, Boyd DB, eds. Reviews in Computational Chemistry. Vol. 2. New York: VCH, 1991:165–218.
50. Dykstra CE, Augspurger JD, Kirtman B, Malik DJ. Properties of molecules by direct calculation. In: Lipkowitz KB, Boyd DB, eds. Reviews in Computational Chemistry. Vol. 1. New York: VCH, 1990:83–118.
51. Williams DE. Net atomic charge and multipole models for the ab initio molecular electric potential. In: Lipkowitz KB, Boyd DB, eds. Reviews in Computational Chemistry. Vol. 2. New York: VCH, 1991:219–271.
52. Bachrach SM. Population analysis and electron densities from quantum mechanics. In: Lipkowitz KB, Boyd DB, eds. Reviews in Computational Chemistry. Vol. 5. New York: VCH, 1994:171–227.
53. Francl MM, Chirlian LE. The pluses and minuses of mapping atomic charges to electrostatic potentials. In: Lipkowitz KB, Boyd DB, eds. Reviews in Computational Chemistry. Vol. 14. New York: Wiley-VCH, 2000:1–31.
54. Politzer P, Murray JS. Molecular electrostatic potentials and chemical reactivity. In: Lipkowitz KB, Boyd DB, eds. Reviews in Computational Chemistry. Vol. 2. New York: VCH, 1991:273–312.
55. Boyd DB, Lipkowitz KB. Molecular mechanics. The method and its underlying philosophy. J Chem Educ 1982; 59:269–274.
56. Dinur U, Hagler AT. New approaches to empirical force fields. In: Lipkowitz KB, Boyd DB, eds. Reviews in Computational Chemistry. Vol. 2. New York: VCH, 1991:99–164.
57. DeKock RL, Madura JD, Rioux F, Casanova J. Computational chemistry in the undergraduate curriculum. In: Lipkowitz KB, Boyd DB, eds. Reviews in Computational Chemistry. Vol. 4. New York: VCH, 1993:149–228.
58. Landis CR, Root DM, Cleveland T. Molecular mechanics force fields for modeling inorganic and organometallic compounds. In: Lipkowitz KB, Boyd DB, eds. Reviews in Computational Chemistry. Vol. 6. New York: VCH, 1995:73–148.
59. Allinger NL, Yuh YH, Lii JH. Molecular mechanics. The MM3 force field for hydrocarbons. 1. J Am Chem Soc 1989; 111:8551–8566.
60. Lii JH, Allinger NL. Molecular mechanics. The MM3 force field for hydrocarbons. 2. Vibrational frequencies and thermodynamics. J Am Chem Soc 1989; 111:8566–8575.
61. Lii JH, Allinger NL. Molecular mechanics. The MM3 force field for hydrocarbons. 3. The van der Waals' potentials and crystal data for aliphatic and aromatic hydrocarbons. J Am Chem Soc 1989; 111:8576–8582.

62. Allinger NL, Chen K, Lii JH. An improved force field (MM4) for saturated hydrocarbons. J Comput Chem 1996; 17:642–668.
63. Nevins N, Chen K, Allinger NL. Molecular mechanics (MM4) calculations on alkenes. J Comput Chem 1996; 17:669–694.
64. Nevins N, Lii JH, Allinger NL. Molecular mechanics (MM4) calculations on conjugated hydrocarbons. J Comput Chem 1996; 17:695–729.
65. Nevins N, Allinger NL. Molecular mechanics (MM4) vibrational frequency calculations for alkenes and conjugated hydrocarbons. J Comput Chem 1996; 17:730–746.
66. Allinger NL, Chen K, Katzenellenbogen JA, Wilson SR, Anstead GM. Hyperconjugative effects on carbon–carbon bond lengths in molecular mechanics (MM4). J Comput Chem 1996; 17:747–755.
67. Burkert U, Allinger NL. Molecular Mechanics. In: ACS Monograph 177. Washington, DC: American Chemical Society, 1982.
68. Bowen JP, Allinger NL. Molecular mechanics: the art and science of parameterization. In: Lipkowitz KB, Boyd DB, eds. Reviews in Computational Chemistry. Vol. 2. New York: VCH, 1991:81–97.
69. Halgren TA. The representation of van der Waals (vdW) interactions in molecular mechanics force fields: potential form, combination rules, and vdW parameters. J Am Chem Soc 1992; 114:7827–7843.
70. Halgren TA. Merck molecular force field. I. Basis, form, scope, parameterization, and performance of MMFF94. J Comput Chem 1996; 17:490–519.
71. Halgren TA. Merck molecular force field. II. MMFF94 van der Waals and electrostatic parameters for intermolecular interactions. J Comput Chem 1996; 17:520–552.
72. Halgren TA. Merck molecular force field. III. Molecular geometries and vibrational frequencies for MMFF94. J Comput Chem 1996; 17:553–586.
73. Halgren TA, Nachbar RB. Merck molecular force field. IV. Conformational energies and geometries for MMFF94. J Comput Chem 1996; 17:587–615.
74. Halgren TA. Merck molecular force field. V. Extension of MMFF94 using experimental data, additional computational data, and empirical rules. J Comput Chem 1996; 17:616–641.
75. Halgren TA. MMFF. VI. MMFF94s option for energy minimization studies. J Comput Chem 1999; 20:720–729.
76. Halgren TA. MMFF. VII. Characterization of MMFF94, MMFF94s, and other widely available force fields for conformational energies and for intermolecular-interaction energies and geometries. J Comput Chem 1999; 20:730–748.
77. Pettersson I, Liljefors T. Molecular mechanics calculated conformational energies of organic molecules: a comparison of force fields. In: Lipkowitz KB, Boyd DB, eds. Reviews in Computational Chemistry. Vol. 9. New York: VCH, 1996:167–189. Liljefors T, Gundertofte K, Norrby PO, Pettersson I. Molecular mechanics and comparsion of force fields. In: Bultinck P, Winter HD, Langenaeker W, Tollenaere JP, eds. Computational Medicinal Chemistry for Drug Discovery. New York: Marcel Dekker, 2004:1–28.

78. van Gunsteren WF, Berendsen HJC. Computer simulation of molecular dynamics: methodology, applications and perspectives in chemistry. Angew Chem Int Ed Engl 1990; 29:992–1023.
79. Gubbins KE, Quirke N. Molecular Simulation and Industrial Applications: Methods, Example and Prospects. Amsterdam: Gordon & Breach, 1996.
80. Boyd DB. Computer-aided molecular design. In: Kent A, Williams JG, eds. Encyclopedia of Computer Science and Technology. Vol. 33. New York: Marcel Dekker, Suppl 18, 1995:41–71.
81. Lybrand TP. Computer simulation of biomolecular systems using molecular dynamics and free energy perturbation methods. In: Lipkowitz KB, Boyd DB, eds. Reviews in Computational Chemistry. Vol. 1. New York: VCH, 1990:295–320.
82. Meirovitch H. Calculation of the free energy and the entropy of macromolecular systems by computer simulation. In: Lipkowitz KB, Boyd DB, eds. Reviews in Computational Chemistry. Vol. 12. New York: Wiley-VCH, 1998:1–74.
83. Balbes LM, Mascarella SW, Boyd DB. A perspective of modern methods in computer-aided drug design. In: Lipkowitz KB, Boyd DB, eds. Reviews in Computational Chemistry. Vol. 5. New York: VCH, 1994:337–379.
84. Reddy MR, Erion MD, Agarwal A. Free energy calculations: use and limitations in predicting ligand binding affinities. In: Lipkowitz KB, Boyd DB, eds. Reviews in Computational Chemistry. Vol. 16. New York: Wiley-VCH, 2000: 217–304.
85. Woods RJ. The application of molecular modeling techniques to the determination of oligosaccharide solution conformations. In: Lipkowitz KB, Boyd DB, eds. Reviews in Computational Chemistry. Vol. 9. New York: VCH, 1996:129–165.
86. Boyd DB. Compendium of software and Internet tools for computational chemistry. In: Lipkowitz KB, Boyd DB, eds. Reviews in Computational Chemistry. Vol. 11. New York: Wiley-VCH, 1997:373–399.
87. Schmidt MW, Baldridge KK, Boatz JA, Elbert ST, Gordon MS, Jensen JH, Koseki S, Matsunaga N, Nguyen KA, Su S, Windus TL, Dupuis M, Montgomery JA. General atomic and molecular electronic-structure system. J Comput Chem 1993; 14:1347–1363.
88. Hehre WJ, Burke LD, Shusterman AJ. A Spartan Tutorial. Irvine, CA: Wavefunction, Inc., 1993.
89. Hehre WJ, Nelson JE. Introducing Molecular Modeling into the Undergraduate Chemistry Curriculum. Irvine, CA: Wavefunction, Inc., 1997.
90. Hehre WJ, Shusterman AJ, Nelson JE. The Molecular Modeling Workbook for Organic Chemistry. Irvine, CA: Wavefunction, Inc., 1998.
91. Helson HE. Structure diagram generation. In: Lipkowitz KB, Boyd DB, eds. Reviews in Computational Chemistry. Vol. 13. New York: Wiley-VCH, 1999:313–398.
92. Mezey PG. Molecular surfaces. In: Lipkowitz KB, Boyd DB, eds. Reviews in Computational Chemistry. Vol. 1. New York: VCH, 1990:265–294.

93. McKee ML, Page M. Computing reaction pathways on molecular potential energy surfaces. In: Lipkowitz KB, Boyd DB, eds. Reviews in Computational Chemistry. Vol. 4. New York: VCH, 1993:35–65.
94. Chandrasekhar J, Jorgensen WL. Energy profile for a nonconcerted SN2 reaction in solution. J Am Chem Soc 1985; 107:2974–2975.
95. Whitnell RM, Wilson KR. Computational molecular dynamics of chemical reactions in solution. In: Lipkowitz KB, Boyd DB, eds. Reviews in Computational Chemistry. Vol. 4. New York: VCH, 1993:67–148.
96. Lide DR. CRC Handbook of Chemistry and Physics. 84th ed. Boca Raton, FL: CRC Press, 2003.
97. Bally T, Borden WT. Calculations on open-shell molecules: a beginner's guide. In: Lipkowitz KB, Boyd DB, eds. Reviews in Computational Chemistry. Vol. 13. New York: Wiley-VCH, 1999:1–97.
98. Te Velde G, Bickelhaupt FM, Baerends EJ, Fonseca Guerra C, Van Gisbergen SJA, Snijders JG, Ziegler T. Chemistry with ADF. J Comput Chem 2001; 22:931–967.
99. Robb MA, Garavelli M, Olivucci M, Bernardi F. A computational strategy for organic photochemistry. In: Lipkowitz KB, Boyd DB, eds. Reviews in Computational Chemistry. Vol. 15. New York: Wiley-VCH, 2000:87–146.
100. Curtiss LA, Raghavachari K, Trucks GW, Pople JA. Gaussian-2 theory for molecular energies of first- and second-row compounds. J Chem Phys 1991; 94:7221–7230.
101. Curtiss LA, Raghavachari K, Redfern PC, Rassolov V, Pople JA. Gaussian-3 (G3) theory for molecules containing first and second-row atoms. J Chem Phys 1998; 109:7764–7776.
102. Allinger NL. Heats of formation by density functional theory calculations. Energetics of Stable Molecules and Reactive Intermediates. NATO Science Series, Series C: Mathematical and Physical Sciences. Vol. 535. 1999:417–430.
103. Pearson RG. Hard and soft acids and bases. J Am Chem Soc 1963; 85: 3533–3539.
104. Pearson RG, Songsted J. Application of the principle of hard and soft acids and bases to organic chemistry. J Am Chem Soc 1967; 89:1827–1836.
105. Geerlings P, De Proft F, Langenaeker W. Conceptual density functional theory. Chem Rev 2003; 103:1793–1873.
106. Mendez F, Gazquez JL. Chemical reactivity of enolate ions: the local hard and soft acids and bases principle viewpoint. J Am Chem Soc 1994; 116:9298–9301.
107. Boyd DB. β-Lactam antibacterial agents: computational chemistry investigations. In: Greenberg A, Breneman CM, Liebman JF, eds. The Amide Linkage: Structural Significance in Chemistry, Biochemistry, and Materials Science. New York: Wiley, 2000:337–375.
108. Boyd DB. Theoretical and physicochemical studies on β-lactam antibiotics. In: Morin RB, Gorman M, eds. β-Lactam Antibiotics: Chemistry and Biology. Vol. 1. New York: Academic Press, 1982:437–545.
109. Boyd DB, Hermann RB, Presti DE, Marsh MM. Electronic structures of cephalosporins and penicillins. 4. Modeling acylation by the β-lactam ring. J Med Chem 1975; 18:408–417.

110. Boyd DB, Herron DK, Lunn WHW, Spitzer WA. Parabolic relationships between antibacterial activity of cephalosporins and β-lactam reactivity predicted from molecular orbital calculations. J Am Chem Soc 1980; 102: 1812–1814.
111. Boyd DB. Substituent effects in cephalosporins as assessed by molecular orbital calculations, nuclear magnetic resonance, and kinetics. J Med Chem 1983; 26:1010–1013.
112. Boyd DB. Electronic structure of cephalosporins and penicillins. 15. Inductive effect of the 3-position side chain in cephalosporins. J Med Chem 1984; 27: 63–66.
113. Corey EJ, Long AK, Greene TW, Miller JW. Computer-assisted synthetic analysis. Selection of protective groups for multistep organic syntheses. J Org Chem 1985; 50:1920–1927.
114. Johnson AP. Computer aids to synthesis planning. Chem Brit 1985; 21:59, 62–64, 66–67.
115. Ugi I, Bauer J, Bley K, Dengler A, Dietz A, Fontain E, Gruber B, Knauer M, Reitsam K, Stein N. Computer-supported chemical calculating, thinking, and inventing. LaborPraxis (Lab 2000) 1992:170–172, 174, 176–178.
116. Jorgensen WL, Laird ER, Gushurst AJ, Fleischer JM, Gothe SA, Helson HE, Paderes GD, Sinclair S. CAMEO: a program for the logical prediction of the products of organic reactions. Pure Appl Chem 1990; 62:1921–1932.
117. Chen L, Nourse JG, Christie BD, Leland BA, Grier DL. Over 20 years of reaction access systems from MDL: a novel reaction substructure search algorithm. J Chem Inf Comput Sci 2002; 42:1296–1310.
118. Ridley DD. Online Searching: A Scientist's Perspective. A Guide for the Chemical and Life Sciences. New York: Wiley, 1996.
119. Ridley DD. Information Retrieval: SciFinder and SciFinder Scholar. New York: Wiley-VCH, 2002.
120. Marin U. Prediction of drug stability from analytical data obtained in stress testing. Intell Instrum Comput 1986; 4:28–36.
121. Petrongolo C, Ranghino G, Scordamaglia R. Ab initio study of β-lactam antibiotics. I. Potential energy surface for the amidic carbon–nitrogen bond breaking in the β-lactam+hydroxide ion reaction. Chem Phys 1980; 45:279–290.
122. Petrongolo C, Pescatori E, Ranghino G, Scordamaglia R. Ab initio study of β-lactam antibiotics. II. Potential energy surface for the amidic carbon–nitrogen bond breaking in the 3-cephem+hydroxide ion reaction and comparison with the β-lactam+hydroxide ion reaction. Chem Phys 1980; 45:291–304.
123. Miyauchi M, Kurihara H, Fujimoto K, Kawamoto I, Ide J, Nakao H. Studies on orally active cephalosporin esters. III. Effect of the 3-substituent on the chemical stability of pivaloyloxymethyl esters in phosphate buffer solution. Chem Pharm Bull 1989; 37:2375–2378.
124. Frau J, Coll M, Donoso J, Munoz F, Garcia Blanco F. Theoretical calculations of β-lactam antibiotics. Part 1. AM1, MNDO and MINDO/3 calculations of some penicillins. J Mol Struct: THEOCHEM 1991; 77:109–124.
125. Frau J, Donoso J, Munoz F, Garcia Blanco F. Theoretical calculations of β-lactam antibiotics. Part 2. AM1, MNDO and MINDO/3 calculations of some cephalosporins. J Mol Struct: THEOCHEM 1991; 83:205–218.

126. Vilanova B, Munoz F, Donoso J, Garcia Blanco F. Analysis of the UV absorption band of cephalosporins. Appl Spectrosc 1992; 46:44–48.
127. Frau J, Donoso J, Munoz F, Garcia Blanco F. Theoretical calculations of β-lactam antibiotics. III. AM1, MNDO, and MINDO/3 calculations of hydrolysis of β-lactam compound (azetidin-2-one ring). J Comput Chem 1992; 13:681–692.
128. Chen G, Fu X, Tang A. Ab initio studies on the thermolysis of azetidine. Chin J Chem 1992; 10:193–199.
129. Frau J, Donoso J, Vilanova B, Munoz F, Garcia Blanco F. Theoretical calculations of β-lactam antibiotics. Part 4. AM1, MNDO, and MINDO/3 calculations of hydrolysis of bicyclic system of penicillins. Theor Chim Acta 1993; 86:229–239.
130. Frau J, Donoso J, Munoz F, Garcia Blanco F. Theoretical calculations of β-lactam antibiotics. V. AM1 calculations of hydrolysis of cephalothin in gaseous phase and influence of the solvent. J Comput Chem 1993; 14:1545–1552.
131. Vilanova B, Munoz F, Donoso J, Frau J, Garcia Blanco F. Alkaline hydrolysis of cefotaxime. An HPLC and proton NMR study. J Pharm Sci 1994; 83:322–327.
132. Burks JE Jr, Chelius EC, Johnson RA. Kinetic differences in the chlorination of cephalosporin versus carbacephalosporin enols: evidence of sulfur neighboring group participation. J Org Chem 1994; 59:5724–5728.
133. Wolfe S, Kim CK, Yang K. Ab initio molecular orbital calculations on the neutral hydrolysis and methanolysis of azetidinones, including catalysis by water. Relationship to the mechanism of action of β-lactam antibiotics. Can J Chem 1994; 72:1033–1034.
134. Wolfe S, Hoz T. A semiempirical molecular orbital study of the methanolysis of complex azetidinones. A combined MM and QM analysis of the interaction Δ^2- and Δ^3-cephems with the penicillin receptor. Can J Chem 1994; 72: 1044–1050.
135. Frau J, Donoso J, Munoz F, Garcia Blanco F. Theoretical calculations of β-lactam antibiotics. Part VI. AM1 calculations of alkaline hydrolysis of clavulanic acid. Helv Chim Acta 1994; 77:1557–1569.
136. Frau J, Donoso J, Munoz F, Garcia Blanco F. Theoretical calculations on β-lactam antibiotics. Part VII. Influence of the solvent on the basic hydrolysis of the β-lactam ring. Helv Chim Acta 1997; 79:353–362.
137. Frau J, Donoso J, Munoz F, Garcia Blanco F. Semiempirical and ab initio calculations on the alkaline hydrolysis of the β-lactam ring. Influence of the solvent. J Mol Struct: THEOCHEM 1997; 390:247–254.
138. Frau J, Donoso J, Munoz F, Garcia Blanco F. Semiempirical calculations of the hydrolysis of penicillin G. J Mol Struct: THEOCHEM 1997; 390:255–263.
139. Frau J, Donoso J, Munoz F, Vilanova B, Garcia Blanco F. Study on the alkaline hydrolysis of the azetidin-2-one ring by ab initio methods. Influence of the solvent. Helv Chim Acta 1997; 80:739–747.
140. Frau J, Donoso J, Munoz F, Vilanova B, Garcia Blanco F. Alkaline hydrolysis of *N*-methylazetidin-2-one. Hydration effects. J Mol Struct: THEOCHEM 1998; 426:313–321.

141. Coll M, Frau J, Donoso J, Munoz F. Ab initio study of β-lactam compounds: acidic hydrolysis. J Mol Struct: THEOCHEM 1998; 426:323–329.
142. Coll M, Frau J, Munoz F, Donoso J. Ab initio study of the basic hydrolysis of the pyrazolidinone ring. J Phys Chem A 1998; 102:5915–5922.
143. Coll M, Frau J, Vilanova B, Donoso J, Munoz F, Garcia Blanco F. Theoretical study of the alkaline hydrolysis of an oxo-β-lactam structure. J Phys Chem A 1999; 103:8879–8884.
144. Coll M, Frau J, Donoso J, Munoz F. PM3 study of reactivity of non-classical β-lactam structures. J Mol Struct: THEOCHEM 1999; 493:287–299.
145. Coll M, Frau J, Vilanova B, Donoso J, Munoz F. Ab initio study of the alkaline hydrolysis of a thio-β-lactam structure. Chem Phys Lett 2000; 326: 304–310.
146. Coll M, Frau J, Vilanova B, Donoso J, Munoz F, Garcia Blanco F. Theoretical study of the alkaline hydrolysis of a bicyclic aza-β-lactam. J Phys Chem B 2000; 104:11389–11394.
147. Holder AJ, Upadrashta SM. A semiempirical computational investigation of the antipsoriatic drug anthralin. J Pharm Sci 1992; 81:1074–1078.
148. Nicholls AW, Akira K, Lindon JC, Farrant RD, Wilson ID, Harding J, Killick DA, Nicholson JK. NMR spectroscopic and theoretical chemistry studies on the internal acyl migration reactions of the 1-*O*-acyl-b-D-glucopyranuronate conjugates of 2-, 3-, and 4-(trifluoromethyl)benzoic acids. Chem Res Toxicol 1996; 9:1414–1424.
149. Williams CI, Whitehead MA, Jean-Claude BJ. A semiempirical PM3 treatment of benzotetrazepine decomposition in acid media. J Org Chem 1997; 62:7006–7014.
150. Schnurpfeil G, Sobbi AK, Spiller W, Kliesch H, Wohrle D. Photooxidative stability and its correlation with semi-empirical MO calculations of various tetraazaporphyrin derivatives in solution. J Porphyrins Phthalocyanines 1997; 1:159–167.
151. Hoffner J, Schottelius MJ, Feichtinger D, Chen P. Chemistry of the 2,5-didehydropyridine biradical: computational, kinetic, and trapping studies toward drug design. J Am Chem Soc 1998; 120:376–385.
152. Reid DL, Calvitt CJ, Zell MT, Miller KG, Kingsmill CA. Early prediction of pharmaceutical oxidation pathways by computational chemistry and forced degradation. Pharmaceut Res 2004; 21:1708–1717.

13

Solid-State Excipient Compatibility Testing

Amy S. Antipas and Margaret S. Landis
Pfizer Global Research & Development, Groton, Connecticut, U.S.A.

The choice of the best excipients for the formulation of remedies is of vital importance in ensuring the stability and efficacy of the resulting preparations (1). As formulation scientists, it is imperative that the products we develop have acceptable chemical and physical stability during the period of their distribution and storage. It is not uncommon that an active pharmaceutical ingredient (API) will be stable as bulk drug but unstable when blended with the excipients required for formulation of dosage forms. Understanding the reactivity of the API in the solid state when mixed with excipients is critical to commercial formulation development. Because the gathering of real-time stability and compatibility data is impractical in the early stages of development, we must rely on stress testing and accelerated stability methods for predicting ambient condition interactions and rates of degradation. Often such studies will require innovative approaches to minimize the amount of compound used and to maximize the detection of small quantities of degradation products. This chapter will focus on summarizing approaches to designing, measuring, and interpreting solid-state excipient compatibility data.

I. DESIGNS OF TRADITIONAL EXCIPIENT COMPATIBILITY EXPERIMENTS

A. Attributes of API: Pre-formulation Profiles

Prior to the initiation of any solid-state excipient compatibility testing of a potential drug candidate, it is best to generate a pre-formulation profile of the API (2,3). This profile should include pH-solubility profiles, pH-stability profiles, p*K*a estimation and log *P* information, as well as knowledge about degradants formed from forced degradation studies in the solution state under acid, base, and oxidative conditions. Analysis of this pre-formulation data in relation to the chemical structure, whereby nucleophilic, electrophilic, hydrogen-bond donating, and hydrogen-bond accepting sites are highlighted, gives the solid dosage formulator insight into the areas of molecular reactivity of the API and its potential to interact with excipients during formulation studies. On this note, it is always worthwhile to review the metabolites associated with *in vivo* degradation of the API, as it can sometimes yield important information on reactive areas of the molecular scaffold. Additional information on predicted reactivity may be provided by computer models (4).

Although solution state property and stability data are important, it is the data and characteristics of the solid state of the API that are of most value to the formulator. Therefore, it is recommended that further experimental information on the solid-state form of the API be gathered prior to initiation of the compatibility studies. Relevant solid-state parameters of the API that could be investigated for further information include (but are not limited to):

- Thermal and thermal/humidity stability
- Hygroscopicity
- Thermal behavior
- Single crystal or crystal packing information
- Particle size distribution and surface area
- Crystal habit descriptions
- Hot-stage polarized light microscopy data
- Photostability
- Effects of mechanical aggravation

Minimally, one should have a brief foreknowledge of the thermal and thermal/humidity solid-state stability of the API prior to initiation of excipient compatibility studies. These protocols should include investigation of stability at various temperature and humidity conditions and should always include information about both chemical stability and physical-form integrity of the API. Thermal and thermal moisture-induced solid-state chemical reactions are well known (5), with hydrolysis and oxidation being the most prevalent mechanisms of decay. Changes in physical form with thermal and moisture stress are also common and well described in the literature (6). Published reviews (7) describe many standard spectroscopic techniques used to characterize physical-form changes of the bulk API.

An important parameter of the API to investigate prior to excipient studies is the ability of the compound to gain and/or lose water when exposed to environments having variable humidity because it is known that water will equilibrate and redistribute in solid-state mixtures. Additionally, solid-state photochemical assessment should be considered as it can be dramatically different than solution-state photoreactivity (8). These brief studies will provide early warnings on preparation, storage, and subdivision precautions.

Thermal analysis, i.e., differential scanning calorimetry (DSC), data can provide much information about the solid-state API for consideration during excipient compatibility testing. Melting point and heat of fusion data provide an understanding of the bonding strengths within the crystal lattice. Additionally, thermal transitions associated with the API form can be observed, such as thermal polymorphic interconversion, loss of waters of hydration, and decomposition temperatures. Knowledge of temperature-related behavior of the API could guide the storage and evaluation methods of the excipient compatibility study and circumvent the use of incompatible storage and testing conditions.

There are a number of crystal aspects of the API that should be briefly examined. Knowledge of crystal habit, particle size distribution, surface area, and optical properties are important because these characteristics will affect the stability of all solid dosage forms in excipient compatibility testing (9,10). Although single crystal data may not be available at early formulation stages, predicted data may be available, based on powder x-ray diffraction (PXRD) studies, and should be considered (11).

A cursory evaluation of mechanical grinding, milling, or compaction on the API can provide valuable insight into the types and extent of degradation noted in the excipient compatibility studies. During tablet production, the API will be subjected to high mechanical stress from processes like high-shear blending, mechanical granulation, and compaction (12). Assessment of the effects of mechanical aggravation on the API and the use of grinding and compaction in excipient compatibility studies will provide a more realistic view of stability observed in larger-scale production in later stages of development. Crystalline to amorphous transformations and polymorphic transitions (13) are the most common changes in physical form associated with mechanical aggravation. Several examples of changes in chemical stability due to mechanical activation are known. It has been shown (14) that increased amorphous content can be correlated to increased chemical reactivity of the API. Waltersson and Lundgren (15) investigated the increase in hydrolytic stability of model compounds, salicylic acid, and procaine, following ball milling and attributed the increased reactivity to the increase in surface activity and number of defect sites. The tendency of an API to experience this type of activation is only recently beginning to be predictable (16). Thus, actual assessment of the propensity for mechanically induced changes should be evaluated prior to or concomitant with excipient compatibility studies. A variety of auxiliary methods have been described to assess these changes, such as changes in thermal calorimetry profiles (17), changes in vapor sorption (18), sensitive solution calorimetry (19), PXRD (20,21), and optical microscopy solubility/dissolution characteristics (22).

It is important to note that the overall purity of the material should be considered prior to investigation of excipient compatibility, such as starting impurity levels, levels of residual water content and residual solvents, as well as the presence and levels of heavy metal impurities. A consideration of the enantiomeric and diastereomeric purities of the materials should be given and may be correlated to instability noted in compatibility studies.

In general, if an API form has stability problems in the bulk form, it is best to solve these issues via salt and form selection studies designed to discover and identify more thermodynamically stable forms prior to any excipient compatibility evaluation. It is known that different polymorphic forms and hydrated/solvated forms can have dramatically different stability profiles (23–26).

B. Attributes of Excipients

Information about excipients is useful in the initial planning and interpretation of the excipient compatibility results. Important factors to consider for excipients include their physical–chemical properties. *The Handbook of Pharmaceutical Excipients* lists important information on structure, moisture content, melting point, pH, solubility, and equilibrium moisture at variable relative humidity for individual excipients (27). An example of relevant physical–chemical parameters for some select excipients is detailed in Table 1. A spectroscopic review of excipients (28) has been completed, and extensive reviews of some of the most common types of excipients (i.e., carbohydrate based) are published (29).

Two parameters of excipients that are important to the compatibility formulator are (i) the ability of the excipients to absorb water at variable humidity and (ii) the pH that the excipient will impart in the solid-state environment. Knowledge of water sorption of excipients is well documented (27) and is used to estimate the amount of water the excipients will introduce into a solid-formulation mixture (30). The percentage of water and the dispensation of water, whether bound or variably adsorbed, was shown to have a dramatic effect on the hydrolytic stability of aspirin (31). It is well known that water will redistribute within solid pharmaceutical systems and this redistribution has been modeled and studied extensively (18). The pH influence that an excipient imparts to the formulation matrix can be directly related to

Table 1 Relevant Physical–Chemical Properties of Selected Common Excipients

Excipient (common use)	Moisture content	Melting point	pH	Solubility	% Equilibrium moisture at 75% RH
Microcrystalline cellulose (diluent)	Typically < 5% w/w	260–270°C (decomp.)	5.0–7.0	Practically insoluble in water	6% w/w gain
Lactose monohydrate (diluent)	4.5–5.5% w/w (5% as monohydrate water)	201–202°C	5.0–7.0	Soluble	1% w/w gain
Calcium phosphate dibasic dihydrate (diluent)	21% w/w as dihydrate water	Decomposes below 100°C with loss of water	7.4	Practically insoluble in water	19% w/w
Sodium starch glycolate (disintegrant)	as much as 10% w/w	200°C (decomp.)	5.5–7.5	Practically insoluble in water	23% w/w gain
Ascorbic acid (antioxidant)	0.1% w/w	190°C (decomp.)	2.1–2.6	Soluble	—

chemical stability. For example, the degradation of a fluoropyridinyl drug in a capsule formulation was correlated with the pH of the excipients and not with the amount of moisture present (32). Because many excipients are generally insoluble in water, a standard method to assess excipient pH is the measurement of the pH of a 5–20% w/w slurry of the excipient in water. Other spectroscopic techniques using pH indictors in the solid state are also known (33).

Some additional solid-state experimental information that may be useful to gather on the excipients includes:

- Known incompatibilities of excipients
- Known stabilization effects of excipients
- Reactive impurities in excipients
- Mechanical properties of the excipients

One should consider known incompatibilities of excipients with specific classes of API and other excipients. Known incompatibilities are detailed and well documented in standard references (27). The most well-known example of incompatibility is reducing cellulosic excipients with primary and secondary amine containing drugs resulting in Maillard type degradation (34,35). Based solely on initial examination of the chemical structure of the API, many carbohydrate excipients can be immediately ruled out of testing protocols. Similarly, if the API is known to be hydrolytically labile, the choice of excipients with low moisture contents and limited moisture uptakes may be better suited for evaluation in compatibility studies. Lastly, if pre-formulation studies have determined that pH plays a major role in degradation of an API, excipients with compatible pH profiles can be selected, i.e., acid labile drugs should not be formulated in the presence of acidic polymers such as hydroxypropyl methylcellulose acetate succinate (HPMCAS) and hydroxypropyl methylcellulose phthalate (HPMCP).

On the other hand, many excipients can act to chemically stabilize an API in the solid state and in solid dosage forms. The most common class of stabilizing excipients is cyclodextrins (36). Cyclodextrins can envelop the API in their hydrophobic cavities and shield it from common degradation reactions such as hydrolysis, oxidation, or photodegradation. Some excipients or additives may also act as complexing agents that provide hydrolytic (37) and oxidative (38) stabilization. Many excipients, such as cyclodextrins, dyes, and colored additives, are capable of providing extensive photostabilization in the solid state (39–41).

A brief review of the excipient synthesis and isolation can give vital clues about the presence of potential reactive impurities in excipients remaining from processing and derivatization reactions. Examples include the known residual presence of sodium glycolate in sodium starch glycolate, a common tablet disintegrant that can play a role in chemical stability of API components. Known impurities of enteric polymers have been identified as sources of degradation of Duloxetine in solid dosage formulations (42). The presence of peroxide impurities in polymeric polyvinylpyrrolidone (PVP) -based excipients is well known and documented (43).

Review of the mechanical properties of the excipients is important when initiating excipient compatibility studies. These parameters are well studied and their importance in solid dosage form design and compatibility is extensively reviewed (44,45). If excipient compatibility studies will involve processing and compacting samples, knowledge of these parameters is very useful. Compaction pressures may affect excipient studies with regard to stability and degree of interaction of materials present in the mixtures. The grade of excipient material used in the compatibility studies should be similar to that used in later stage solid dosage form development for accurate prediction of compatibility.

Any and all preliminary information on the solid-state form of the API and the excipients will enable the scientist to (i) design the best experimental layout for excipient compatibility studies that focuses on the relevant aspects of the API and excipients, (ii) have a better understanding of appropriate stress conditions and timeframes over which to conduct the studies, and (iii) provide a more complete basis for which to interpret the final results of the excipient compatibility testing.

C. Initiation of Excipient Compatibility: Design of Experiments

According to Monkhouse (46), there are four major attributes of a drug–excipient compatibility study: (i) sample preparation, (ii) statistical design, (iii) storage conditions, and (iv) method of analysis. Traditionally, a one factor at a time approach employing the preparation of binary blends of the API with excipients has been used in compatibility screening. Many different ratios of API to excipient have been reported, but one should attempt to reflect the relative amounts in a tablet in order to obtain the most meaningful data. Blends can be prepared by dry mixing the components in a vial using a vortex. However, be aware that the homogeneity of the blend will be important in ensuring that all of the API is in contact with the excipient and is especially critical if you are not sampling the entire vial.

It has been reported that the chemical stability of a drug substance in a binary drug substance–excipient mixture may differ completely from a multi-component drug substance–excipient mixture because of the potential for interactions to occur among the excipients as well as between the drug and excipients (47). A well-conceived statistical design could easily reveal these additional interactions. According to the proponents of statistical designs, more information can be obtained with less work, iteration time, and cost vs. the one factor at a time approach. Some examples of statistical designs can be found in what follows.

El-Banna et al. (48) described the use of a Box–Wilson type fractional factorial design. They explored six factors which included filler, lubricant, binder, disintegrant, light, and humidity. For the full factorial design ($N = 2^6$), six factors at two levels, 64 experiments must be performed. A more practical fractional factorial design ($N = 2^{6-3}$) containing eight experiments can still elucidate the main effects, as well as some of the interactive effects, as seen in the design in Table 2.

Durig and Fassihi (49) utilized a Plackett–Burman saturated factorial design that allows accurate investigation of multiple factors simultaneously without having to investigate all possible combinations. Taken to the extreme, this type of design can be used to evaluate up to N–1 factors from only N experiments. One disadvantage of this approach is that there is no estimation of the inherent experimental error or measurement of the significance of observed effects because of the absence of replicates. In addition, only the main effects are detected and not the interactions between two or more factors. As a result, the scientist must balance the significance and utility of the data vs. the need to incorporate additional experiments. In examining the stability of pyridoxal HC1, Durig and Fassihi employed a Plackett–Burman design consisting of 13 variables at two levels. As seen

Table 2 Box–Wilson Type Fractional Factorial Design

Trial no.	Factors						
	X_1	X_2	X_3	X_4 (X_1X_2)	X_5 (X_1X_3)	X_6 ($X_1X_2X_3$)	X_2X_3
1	−	−	−	+	+	−	+
2	+	−	−	−	−	+	+
3	−	+	−	−	+	+	−
4	+	+	−	+	−	−	−
5	−	−	+	+	−	+	−
6	+	−	+	−	+	−	−
7	−	+	+	−	−	−	+
8	+	+	+	+	+	+	+

Note: X_1 lactose (−) or mannitol (+); X_2 stearic acid (−) or magnesium stearate (+); X_3 PVP (−) or gelatin (+); X_4 maize starch (−) or Avicel (+); X_5 presence (+) or absense (−) of light; X_6 0% (−) or 3% (+) humidity.

in Table 3, 24 experiments were used to examine the 13 variables with the addition of pseudo-variables to aid in determining the system error. Using the average effects of the pseudo-variables, the standard deviation of the variable effect was calculated in order to provide estimations for the minimum significant variable effects at the 90% and 60% confidence levels. In this design, it was possible to observe both stabilizing and destabilizing effects of excipients.

II. APPROPRIATE STRESS CONDITIONS

A. Thermal

Elevated thermal conditions are often used to accelerate the degradation processes that occur at ambient room temperature with the assumption that the kinetics of the reactions follow linear Arrhenius behavior. In order to minimize the time required for the experiment, the temperature is often maximized. Care must be taken when using this method of acceleration because raising the temperature above 70–80°C may cause the energy of the system to exceed the activation energies of alternative degradation mechanisms thus resulting in unrepresentative data. Sims et al. (50) studied the compatibility of SB-243213-A in excipient mixtures to explore conditions, which would have predicted the degradation that was seen with the clinical formulation after 3 months of storage at 50°C. As seen in Figure 1 when 100°C was used as the stress condition, the desired degradants (Imp A and B) are formed but the additional peaks early in the chromatogram indicate a shift in the primary degradation processes. When the temperature is lowered to 60°C

Table 3 Plackett–Burman Design for Pyridoxal HCL Compatibility Studies

Trial	Variable													Pseudo-variable									
no.	A	B	C	D	E	F	G	H	I	J	K	L	M	N	O	P	Q	R	S	T	U	V	W
1	+	+	+	+	+	−	+	−	+	+	−	−	+	+	−	−	+	−	+	−	−	−	−
2	−	+	+	+	+	+	−	+	−	+	+	−	−	+	+	−	−	+	−	+	−	−	−
3	−	−	+	+	+	+	+	−	+	−	+	+	−	−	+	+	−	−	+	−	+	−	−
4	−	−	−	+	+	+	+	+	−	+	−	+	+	−	−	+	+	−	−	+	−	+	−
5	−	−	−	−	+	+	+	+	+	−	+	−	+	+	−	−	+	+	−	−	+	−	+
6	+	−	−	−	−	+	+	+	+	+	−	+	−	+	+	−	−	+	+	−	−	+	−
7	−	+	−	−	−	−	+	+	+	+	+	−	+	−	+	+	−	−	+	+	−	−	+
8	+	−	+	−	−	−	−	+	+	+	+	+	−	+	−	+	+	−	−	+	+	−	−
9	−	+	−	+	−	−	−	−	+	+	+	+	+	−	+	−	+	+	−	−	+	+	−
10	−	−	+	−	+	−	−	−	−	+	+	+	+	+	−	+	−	+	+	−	−	+	+
11	+	−	−	+	−	+	−	−	−	−	+	+	+	+	+	−	+	−	+	+	−	−	+
12	+	+	−	−	+	−	+	−	−	−	−	+	+	+	+	+	−	+	−	+	+	−	−
13	−	+	+	−	−	+	−	+	−	−	−	−	+	+	+	+	+	−	+	−	+	+	−
14	−	−	+	+	−	−	+	−	+	−	−	−	−	+	+	+	+	+	−	+	−	+	+
15	+	−	−	+	+	−	−	+	−	+	−	−	−	−	+	+	+	+	+	−	+	−	+
16	+	+	−	−	+	+	−	−	+	−	+	−	−	−	−	+	+	+	+	+	−	+	−
17	−	+	+	−	−	+	+	−	−	+	−	+	−	−	−	−	+	+	+	+	+	−	+
18	+	−	+	+	−	−	+	+	−	−	+	−	+	−	−	−	−	+	+	+	+	+	−
19	−	+	−	+	+	−	−	+	+	−	−	+	−	−	−	−	−	−	+	+	+	+	+
20	+	−	+	−	+	+	−	−	+	+	−	−	+	+	+	−	−	−	−	+	+	+	+
21	+	+	−	+	−	+	+	−	−	+	+	−	−	−	−	+	−	−	−	−	+	+	+
22	+	+	+	−	+	−	+	+	−	−	+	+	−	−	+	−	+	−	−	−	−	+	+
23	+	+	+	+	−	+	−	+	+	−	−	+	+	+	−	+	−	+	−	−	−	−	+
24	+	+	+	+	+	−	+	−	+	+	−	−	+	+	−	−	+	−	+	−	−	−	−

Note: A, stearic acid; B, magnesium stearate; C, AEROSIL 380; D, lactose; E, LUDIPRESS; F, corn starch; G, AVICEL PH101; H, methylcellulose; I, ethylcellulose; J, EUDRAGIT RSPM; K, mannitol; L, relative humidity; M, temperature; N–W, pseudo variables. (+) is high level and (−) is low level.

and 80°C, the degradation profile is similar to what was expected based on the clinical tablet experience.

B. Mechanical Stress

Mechanical stress may be introduced into the system in several ways. Some of the most common include grinding, milling, or co-milling the drug or blend. By adding mechanical stress using these methods, it is hypothesized that amorphous pockets of drug are formed or crystal defects are induced such that the rate of degradation will increase. In studying the effects of mechanical comminution on the stability of procaine penicillin G, Waltersson and Lundgren (15) found that the rate of solid-state degradation nearly

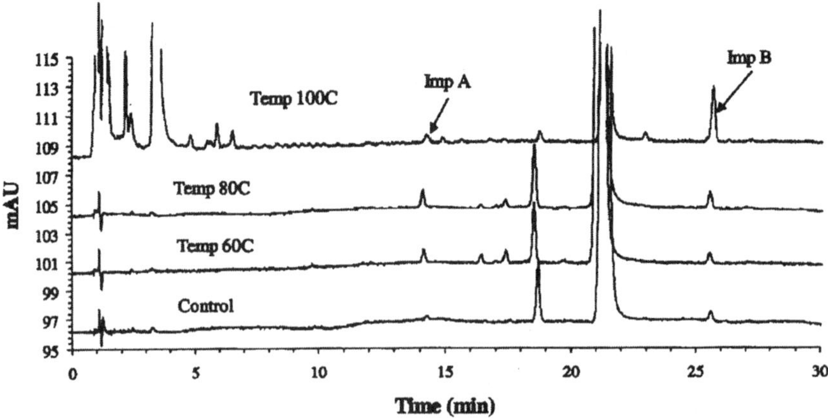

Figure 1 Degradation of SB-243213-A at different temperatures.

doubled after the drug was ball milled for 20 hr, Table 4. This trend continued when the drug was blended with Avicel® or Emcompress®.

Mechanical stress may also be added to the system through the use of compaction. Some possible reasons for differences in reactivity after compaction include:

1. More intimate interactions of the drug with the excipients or impurities
2. Mechanically induced chemical reactions
3. Changes in physical form, i.e., induction of amorphous defects, changes to partially amorphous or other physical forms
4. Different surface area of contact, i.e., changes in surface area to volume ratio

Table 4 Observed Rate Constant for the Solid-state Degradation of Procaine Penicillin G Stored at 55°C and 67% RH

	Rate constant, k_0 (mg/day) (Mean ± SD)
Pure drug, unmilled	0.240 ± 0.005
Pure drug, milled 20 hr	0.434 ± 0.011
Avicel + unmilled drug	0.473 ± 0.012
Avicel + milled drug	1.018 ± 0.008
Emcompress + unmilled drug	0.428 + 0.009
Emcompress + milled drug	0.708 ± 0.013

Source: Excerpted from Table 3 in Waltersson and Lundgren Ref. 15.

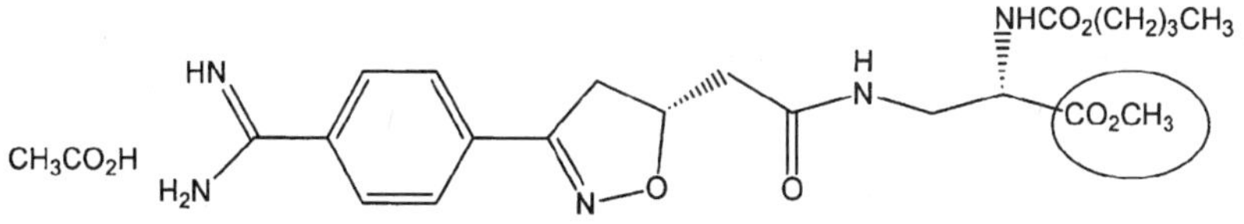

Figure 2 Structure of DMP-754. Area of ester hydrolysis is highlighted.

In trying to formulate DMP-754, Badway et al. (51) investigated binary blends as well as compacts of DMP-754 (Fig. 2) with anhydrous lactose and concluded that compaction of the blends resulted in an increase in the amount of hydrolysis seen (Table 5). Badway et al. postulated that this result was due to an increase in the number of contact points between the drug and the lactose resulting in an increased rate of moisture transfer leading to degradation.

Guo et al. (52) studied the relationship between the solid-state chemical instability of quinapril hydrochloride (QHC1) (Fig. 3) and its physical characteristics. QHC1 degrades via an intramolecular cyclization resulting in aminolysis and production of a diketopiperazine (DKP) compound. Crystalline QHC1 exists as an acetonitrile solvate, which is loosely incorporated into the lattice channels. As seen in Figure 4a and b, loss of the acetonitrile occurs with minimal mechanical force and results in loss of crystallinity, which could result in an increase in the amount of degradation because the activation energy for the cyclization reaction is significantly lower in the amorphous state than in the crystalline state (Table 6) (53,54). Compression of samples on a Carver press also resulted in partial loss of crystallinity (Fig. 5) leading us to extrapolate that the compression force used in tableting could result in the formation of some amorphous character, which would decrease stability.

Compaction may also decrease the reaction rate of compounds that degrade via a mechanism that produces a gaseous product, as the compression will inhibit its escape. For example, in the QHCl case, the degradation produces two gaseous products, HC1 and water (52). Experiments exploring the effect of sample size indicate that the degradation rate is decreased when the sample size is large (Fig. 6). The results indicate that the restriction of

Table 5 Ester Hydrolysis of DMP-754 in Lactose Blends and Compacts After 1 Month at 40° C/75% RH

	% Hydrolysis
Blend	1.75
Compact	6

Source: Values extracted from Figure 3 in Ref. 51.

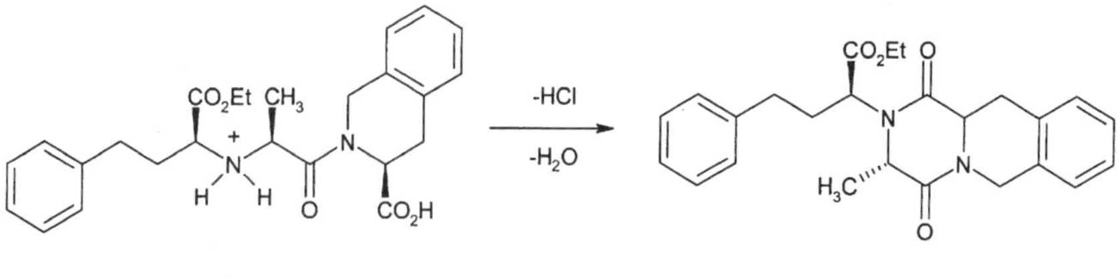

Figure 3 Structure of QHCl and degradation to DKP.

gases to escape from the reaction matrix tends to slow down the reaction significantly. Compaction of the samples would be expected to have similar effects as larger samples. The reaction rate is also increased when the gas removal is facilitated by applying a vacuum (inset in Fig. 6).

C. Water

Water is often added into excipient compatibility designs because hydrolysis is one of the most common routes of drug degradation. Most excipients contain an appreciable level of free water or are able to absorb water from the environment (see Section I.B). Water can be added into the system through several methods: (i) the formation of a slurry or suspension, (ii) the addition of a certain percentage of water into a closed system, or (iii) exposure of the system to controlled humidity. The suspension technique can be used to rapidly assess whether chemical or physical stability problems exist; however, the presence of such an excess of water may cause a shift in degradation mechanisms from that seen in the solid state where the amount of water present depends on the properties of the drug and the excipients (55). Serajuddin et al. studied the degradation of multi-component blends with various drugs after the addition of 20% water into a closed system (56). A specified amount of water was added into the system because their experience with humidity chambers was that the excipient interactions at high humidity depended on the amount of free moisture present and on the relative hygroscopicities of the drug substance and/or the excipients thus leading to variability in the data. In developing methods for on-line stress testing using a STEM block reactor, Sims et al. (50) discovered that having a controlled and humid atmosphere produced more predictive results than having the sample in direct contact with the moisture. More traditional methods of excipient compatibility testing have employed the use of exposure to controlled humidity using saturated salt solutions or humidity chambers. The conditions used (−15° C, 5°C/ambient humidity, 25° C/60% RH, 30° C/60% RH and 40°C/75% RH), are often based on the guidance from the Food and Drug Administration (FDA) entitled "Stability Testing of Drug Substances and Drug Products" (57).

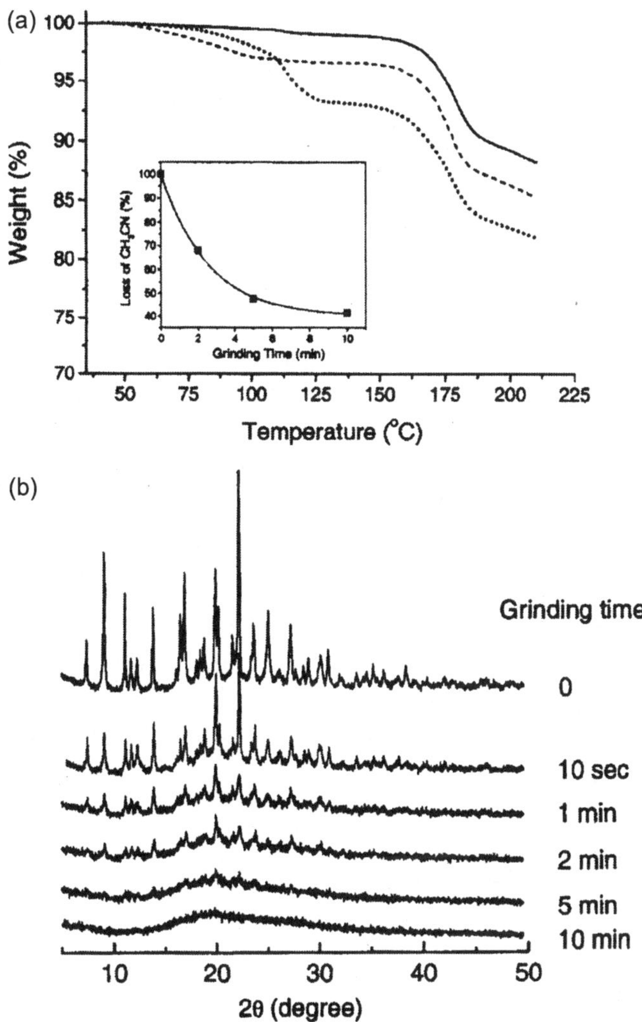

Figure 4 (a) TGA analysis of QHC1–CH_3CN describing weight loss (%) with increasing temperature and the loss of acetonitrile in QHCl–CH_3CN vs. grinding time (see inset). (b) PXRD patterns of samples obtained after grinding crystalline QHCl–CH_3CN for different time intervals.

D. Oxidation

Oxidative instability is the second most common cause of chemical degradation of API in pharmaceutical formulations. If prior knowledge and/or preformulation stability experiments have predicted reactivity toward oxidative degradation, additional oxidative stress conditions can be included into excipient compatibility protocols in several ways.

Table 6 Comparison of Reactivity for the Cyclization Reaction of QHCl

	E_a (Kcal/mol)
Crystalline[a]	−60
Amorphous	30–35
In solution[b]	20

[a]Activation energy for a similar cyclization reaction as crystaline solid (53).
[b]Activation energy for a similar cyclization reaction as solution (54).

One of the most common ways to investigate the oxidative reactivity of compounds is to store the excipient blends in an environment having a pure oxygen headspace. It is generally accepted that acceleration of oxidation via this method may require high temperature and humidity (58). For these stress configurations to be accomplished, hermetically sealed containers, such as sealed glass septum vials or heat sealed foil packs and blisters, are highly recommended (59).

Harsher conditions may employ pressurized oxygen headspaces, for which Parr® type apparatus are employed. Incorporation of added metal impurities (commonly copper and iron salts) in conjunction with oxygen headspace has been reported (60). One research group utilized high temperatures (80°C), copper (II) salts, and oxygen gas headspace to study the

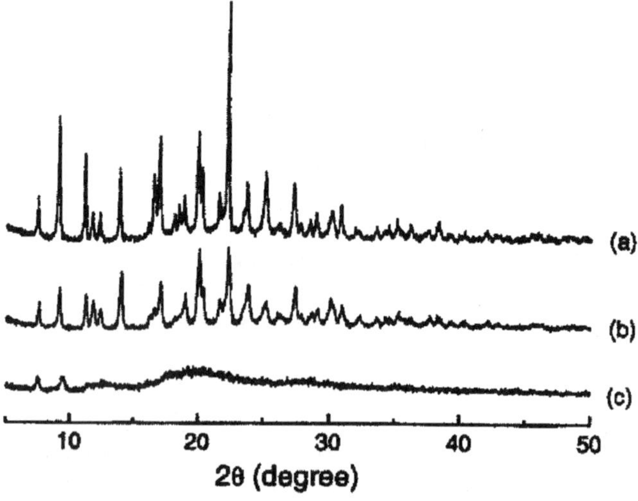

Figure 5 PXRD of crystalline QHC1–CH_3CN (a), after compression using a Carver press (~10^4 lb/cm^2) (b), and sample after desolvation under vacuum at 45°C for 24 hr (c).

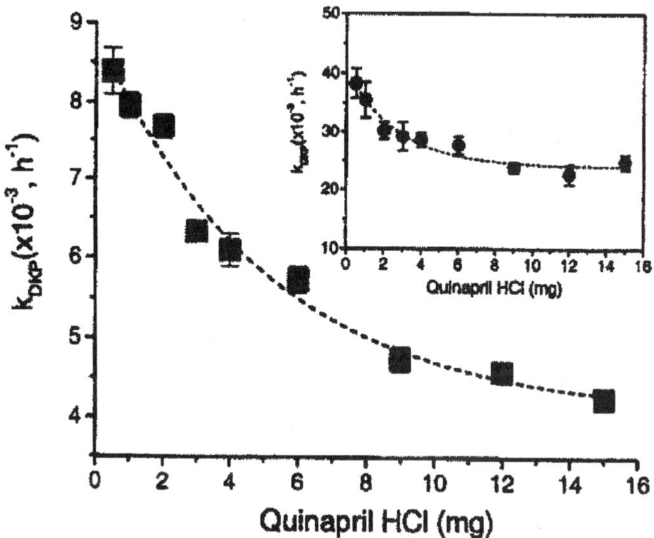

Figure 6 Effect of sample mass on the cyclization reaction rate constant of amorphous QHCl at 80°C. Inset shows results of same experiment but conducted under vacuum.

decomposition of sulpyrine, noting that the oxidative decomposition depended heavily on water content (61). Not as common, but potentially still useful, is the use of radical initiators incorporated into solid dosage forms that can be stressed at increased temperature with oxygen headspaces (60).

For any gaseous headspace stress condition, particle size and surface area may play a major role. Thus, blends and compacts may show widely different results, with compacted material being the most realistic scenario for oxidation in solid dosage forms. Negative controls for this type of oxidative stress may involve the use of nitrogen (60) or argon headspaces. For further investigation into the mechanism and stabilization of solid formulations toward oxidation, the formulator could use some of the newly emerging technologies such as oxygen scavengers included in packaging configurations, oxygen impermeable capsule shells and tablet film coatings having limited gas permeability.

Another common source of oxidation in solid dosage forms is linked to excipient-related peroxide impurities. PVP and high molecular weight polyethylene glycols (PEGs) are known to contain peroxide impurities that can increase with age and storage conditions. Because the excipient storage and handling history can be related to the levels of these impurities, variation in the amount of oxidative degradation can be noted in excipient compatibility studies and early solid dosage form evaluations.

Table 7 N-Oxide Levels for Drug Excipient Mixtures After 31 days Storage at 125°C

Drug–excipient mixture	Degradant amount ($n = 1$)
R–HCl/lactose anhydrous	0.01
R–HCl/lactose monohydrate	0.01
R–HCl/povidone	0.26
R–HCl/crospovidone	0.26
R–HCl/magnesium stearate	0.01
R–HCl/polysorbate 80	0.03

Note: N-Oxide Expressed as % w/w of Raloxifene–HCl.

Following observations of oxidative degradation of Raloxifene hydrochloride (R-HCL) in tablets and direct mixtures containing povidone and crospovidone excipients, Hartanuer et al. (62) proposed that peroxide impurities in the povidone and crospovidone were directly responsible for the degradation observed. Accelerated binary studies of the API with all the individual tablet components revealed that povidone and crospovidone were the most likely cause of the oxidative instability (Table 7). To further elaborate on this degradation, studies involving the addition of hydrogen peroxide directly to tablet formulation matrices of Raloxifene prior to granulation and compaction were examined.

Stability results again supported the indictment of peroxide impurities in the povidone and crospovidone excipients used in the core tablet formulation (Fig. 7) as being responsible for oxidation of Raloxifene to the N-oxide degradant. Increasing amounts of added peroxide led directly to increasing amounts of the N-oxide degradant being formed in the tablet formulations. These peroxide spiking experiments aided in the full identification of the N-oxide degradant and provided valuable data for a realistic control strategy that would impose limits on the impurities allowed in designated excipients for manufacture of the final dosage form product.

E. Packaging Aspects

If the aim of excipient compatibility is to be predictive of the degradation expected with clinical or commercial dosage forms, then the packaging configuration should be representative of what will be used in that setting. Factors that could influence stability measurements include container headspace and permeability of oxygen and water vapor through the walls and cap (if a bottle) of the container.

Table 8 lists the water vapor transmission through common types of packaging materials (63). As indicated by Waterman et al., the amount of

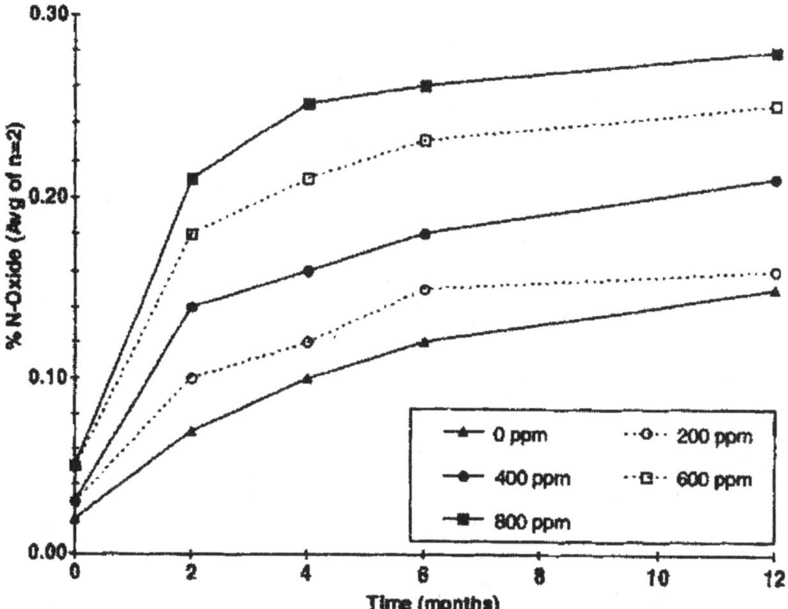

Figure 7 Influence of peroxide impurities on Raloxifene chemical stability.

water vapor permeating a typical HDPE bottle can be calculated using the following equation:

$$\text{Amount of water} = \frac{(\text{transmission})(\text{surface area of container})(\text{time})}{(\text{thickness of barrier})}$$

If hydrolysis is expected to be an issue, desiccants can be a valuable addition to the packaging scheme. The rate and capacity for water adsorption of desiccants will vary depending on the type of adsorbent and the configuration (i.e., canister vs. sachet). Table 9 summarizes various desiccant options for use with pharmaceutical products (63).

Understanding oxygen transmission through commonly used pharmaceutical packaging materials (Table 10) will aid in the proper choice for stabilizing oxygen sensitive formulations (60). It should be noted that oxygen permeability of material often increases with temperature. The amount of oxygen permeating a typical HDPE bottle can be calculated in a similar manner to the method used for water vapor permeation.

$$\text{Volume of } O_2 = \frac{(\text{transmission})(\text{surface area of container})(\text{time})}{(O_2 \text{ pressure})(\text{thickness of barrier})}$$

A foil/foil blister sealed under a nitrogen atmosphere would provide the most protective packaging, although this type of configuration can be

Table 8 Water Vapor Transmission Rates for Common Packaging Materials

Material	Water vapor transmission[a] [g mm/(m^2 day)]
PVC	1.8
Polypropylene	0.54
HDPE	0.12
Aclar UltRx	0.006
Aclar 22A	0.011
Nylon 6	7.5–7.9
Oriented PET	0.39–0.51
Cold-formed foil blister	<0.005

[a]At 38°C and 90% RH.

expensive. An alternative would be the use of oxygen scavenging packets, which could be added to a bottle like traditional desiccant canisters. A packet of size 20 is able to scavenge up to 20 mL of O_2 or the equivalent of 100 mL of air (64). These oxygen scavengers are useful in stabilization of the product and in diagnosis of the issue.

III. ANALYSIS

The initial analysis of excipient compatibility samples usually involves visual inspection of the samples for changes in color, tablet integrity, and deliquescence. Initial observations of this type can be a sign of instability of the API and excipients and should be noted and considered when assessing compatibility. Several subjective systems exist to quantify the changes in color following compatibility and stress testing of solid dosage forms (65). More recently, electronic systems are used to record, evaluate, and track the changes in tablet color (66,67) to avoid human subjectivity in assessments.

Table 9 Desiccant Options for Use with Pharmaceutical Products

Desiccant type	H_2O (g) adsorbed/ adsorbent (g) (25°C/ 75% RH)	H_2O (g) adsorbed/ adsorbent (g) (25°C/ 20% RH)	H_2O (g) adsorbed/ adsorbent (g) (25°C/ 10% RH)	Hours to $\frac{1}{2}$ capacity (25°C/75% RH)	Approx. % RH reached
Silica gel	0.33	0.12	0.05	1.2	10–20
Clay	0.26	0.11	0.08	1.5	10–20
Molecular sieves	0.22	0.18	0.15	0.5	2–10
$CaSO_4$	0.10	0.05	0.03	1.2	15–30
CaO	0.28	0.28	0.27	27	1–25

Table 10 Oxygen Permeability (Transmission Rate) for Packaging Materials

Material	Oxygen transmission [cm^3 mm/(m^2 day atm)]
Low-density polyethylene	241
High-density polyethylene	102 (26.3 at 0°C)
Polypropylene	89
Polystyrene	127
Polyvinylchloride	4
Polycarbonate	114
Unoriented polyethylene terephthalate (PET)	2.5
Oriented PET	2

A. Measurement of Chemical Instability

1. High Performance Liquid Chromatography

One of the most widely used methods for detecting the formation of degradants after stability challenges in the face of excipients is the use of HPLC. Although the use of this technique requires sample preparation to extract the API and its degradants from the excipient matrix, it remains a valuable tool because it has the ability to discriminate between decay products based on polarity. The ability to use various types of detectors (UV, MS, light scattering, electrochemical, fluorescence, chemiluminescence) imparts the flexibility and sensitivity to the technique. One essential requirement in the use of HPLC for the detection of degradants is that the analytical method used must be stability indicating. In other words, the method must be capable of discriminating between the API and any decomposition products formed as well as be sufficiently sensitive to detect and quantify the degradation products (68). Because the identities of the degradation products are typically unknown at the time of early excipient compatibility studies, degradation is measured by comparing the relative peak areas of compounds eluting at specific retention times over some specified study duration. As mentioned by Olsen et al. (69), it is important to use highly discriminating investigational methods capable of resolving and detecting degradation products so that mass balance can be assessed.

The combination of solid-phase extraction (SPE) with HPLC analysis or preparative HPLC can be a valuable tool in concentrating and identifying degradation products. SPE can be a useful technique for the isolation and concentration of analytes from a complex mixture. Selection of the appropriate column depends on the properties of the API and the suspected degradants (70,71). Mixed mode columns having both non-polar and ion exchange character can be useful when the identities of the degradants are unknown.

Preparative HPLC is another convenient method for isolating degradants from excipient compatibility matrices (72,73). The peaks from stressed samples can be collected, the solvent removed with a rotary evaporator, and the remaining solution lyophilized to obtain purified compounds. The samples can then be analyzed by other methods such as mass spectrometry and nuclear magnetic resonance (NMR) in order to identify the molecular composition.

2. Isothermal Microcalorimetry

Isothermal microcalorimetry has been used in the assessment of excipient compatibility in the solution and the solid state (19,74–76). As discussed by Buckton in Chapter 11, the basis for evaluation of chemical interactions using this method is the measurement of minute amounts of evolved or absorbed heat after establishing a baseline at a constant temperature. The advantage of using this technique in the evaluation of excipient compatibility is that the data can be generated in the timeframe of several hours to a week as opposed to the traditional accelerated temperature methods that can require 6 to 12 weeks. In addition, the sensitivity of the method may allow one to monitor the reaction at ambient temperatures rather than at highly elevated temperatures. One disadvantage of the technique is the non-specificity of the measurement. The evolution or absorption of heat could be a result of other physical processes occurring such as dissolution, evaporation, phase transitions, or crystallization (77). As a result, it is necessary to investigate the origins of the observed measurement using more specific assays. For example, as the technique is non-destructive, the sample could be analyzed by HPLC once the measurement is completed.

Experimental procedures for running excipient compatibility studies using isothermal microcalorimetry include the collection of power–time curves for each component of the mixture alone, as well as in combinations (Fig. 8). The separate drug and excipient curves can then be used to construct a theoretical "non-interaction" curve for the blend, which then is subtracted from the actual blend curves in order to define the interaction between the components.

Variables that the investigator must keep in mind are the effects of sample particle size, the influence of different mixing methods, temperature, and the effect of moisture (added either as aliquots of water or as controlled humidity in the chamber). Selzer et al. (78,79) has investigated the compatibility of a model drug in binary excipient mixtures (studied as powders, granules, and tablets). The data indicates that granulation or compaction of the powder results in a significantly higher heat flow when compared with the blend itself and is likely caused by the additional processing. This could

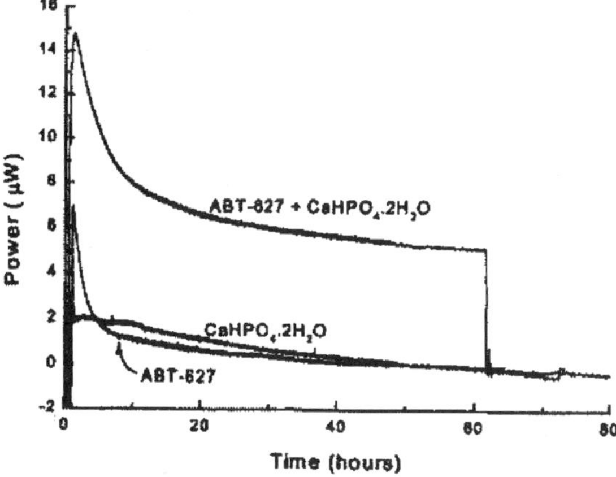

Figure 8 Typical raw power–time curves used for an excipient compatibility study.

be a result of increased association of the drug with the excipients or of physical processes occurring after compaction, such as relaxation.

Phipps and Mackin (80) and Schmitt et al. (77) have advocated using isothermal microcalorimetry as a screening tool to assign relative risk and eliminate highly unstable excipients from subsequent model formulations. As seen in Table 11, Schmitt found that the results of an excipient screen with ABT-627 using isothermal microcalorimetry at 50°C qualitatively

Table 11 ABT-627 Excipient Compatibility Comparison Using Isothermal Microcalorimetry or HPLC Analysis of Binary Mixtures at 50°C

		Area Percent Impurities by HPLC		
Excipient	Microcalorimetry interaction power (μW)	Initial	After 3 weeks	After 5.2 weeks
Dibasic calcium phosphate	5.23	0	0.06	0.22
Microcrystalline cellulose	2.92	0	0.056	0.108
Lactose monohydrate	−0.345	0	0.051	0.076
Pre-gelatinized starch	−1.31	0.05	0.048	0.102
Magnesium stearate	6.51	0.546	1.25	2.04
Stearic acid	0.512	0	0.05	0.03
Sodium starch glycolate	7.12	0	0.21	0.51
Povidone K30	2.59	0.059	0.10	0.54
Crospovidone	2.37	0.052	0.25	0.39

agreed with the results obtained after the same blends were analyzed by HPLC after sitting in a 50°C oven for 3 to 6 weeks. The time to complete the excipient screening using microcalorimetry took only 3 days, whereas the conventional method took 6 weeks.

3. High-Sensitivity DSC

High Sensitivity DSC (HSDSC) can be used as a screening tool to identify gross incompatibilities with excipients. As with traditional DSC, a power differential is measured between a reference and the sample as a function of temperature. Changes in the melting behavior of the components in a mixture, after comparison to those that occur with the individual components under the identical stress conditions, may be used as an indication of a chemical incompatibility that occurs when the components are mixed. As indicated by Wissing et al. (81), the use of HSDSC is controversial because melting differences may arise due to reasons other than chemical incompatibility. In addition, initial studies from Mroso et al. (82) proclaiming the utility of this method, were run using a system where the incompatibility was linked to the melting behavior. It is debatable whether incompatibility between components of systems where the reaction is not linked to melting behavior could be detected.

Wissing et al. (81) and McDaid et al. (83), however, promote the use of HSDSC with stepwise isothermal ramping methods. Using ramping methods alone, the technique would have inferior sensitivity to microcalorimetry, and using isothermal methods alone at room temperature may result in inferior sensitivity if the degradation mechanism is energetically weak. McDaid compared binary blends and compacts containing 5% API with 95% magnesium stearate or lactose using HSDSC to traditional accelerated methods where the samples were held for 6 weeks at 5°C/50% RH, 40°C/20% RH, and 40°C/75% RH. HSDSC samples were tested as the dry powder or compacts or as a 2:1 slurry of water with solid. The temperature ramps ran from 30° to 90°C with the temperature held constant for 1–2 hr every 5°C (Figs. 9 and 10). The results from the conventional excipient compatibility studies indicated an incompatibility of the API with magnesium stearate only at conditions of 40°C/75% RH. HSDSC results indicated no incompatibilities in the dry state; however, an incompatibility with magnesium stearate was seen in the slurry. It was postulated that the thermal event at 35°C was due to dissolution of the drug into the aqueous phase of the slurry. This deviation was reduced when the sample was given sufficient time to dissolve before the experiment was initiated. It was concluded that in order to better compare the data to the conventional methods, the experiment might be repeated using a saturated salt solution to maintain the humidity in the cell rather than to slurry the components.

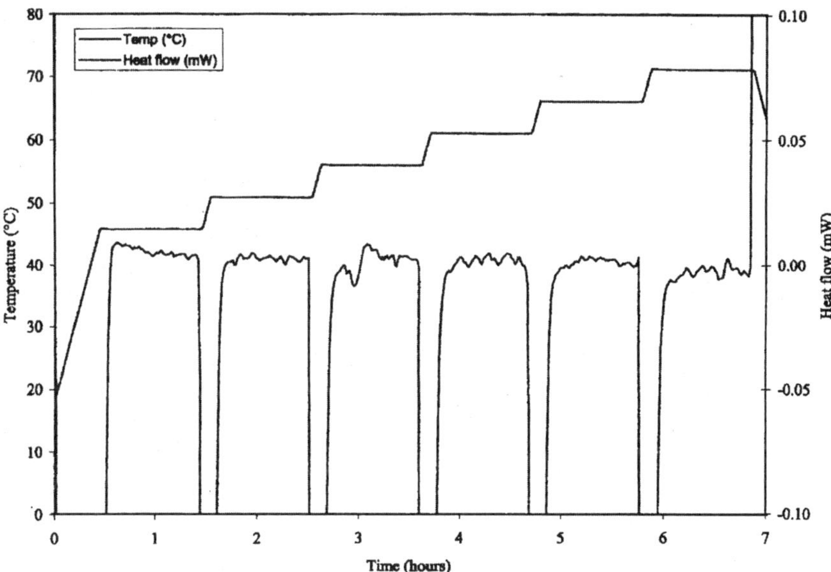

Figure 9 HSDSC profiles for dry compacts of drug A and magnesium stearate (50/50, w/w) held for 1 hr every 5°C, total sample size ~75 mg.

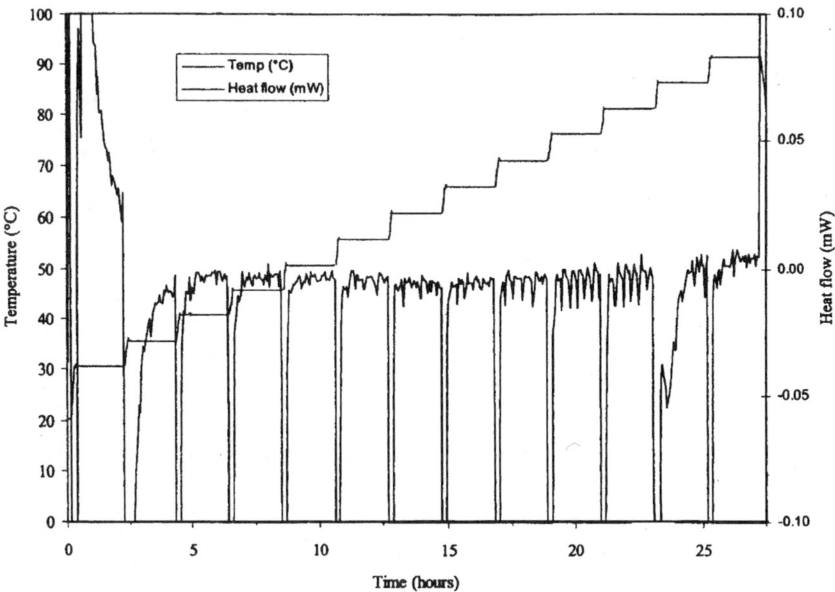

Figure 10 HSDSC profiles for drug A–magnesium stearate–water slurries (16.7:16.7:66.6%, w/w), total sample size ~120 mg, showing thermal events at 35°C and 85°C (held for 2 hr every 5°C).

B. Physical-Form Stability and Assessment

In the process of stressing API in the presence of excipients, one should take into account the potential for physical change of the API to occur in the formulation mixtures being evaluated. Depending on the stage of development and the depth of excipient compatibility studies, physical form assessment may be cursory or more extensive, but should be considered at some level.

Physical-form changes such as crystallization of amorphous API, polymorphic conversions, conversions of API to hydrate or solvate forms, and conversion of crystalline forms to amorphous forms are some common phase transitions that may occur under the conditions of excipient compatibility and accelerated testing. Assessment of physical-form changes should be directly linked to chemical stability data to obtain the best overall view of compatibility. If tracking decomposition kinetics in early formulation studies, knowledge of physical-form integrity is essential before kinetic analysis can be applied. It is always advantageous to begin to track physical-form integrity in the early excipient compatibility studies to avoid significant problems occurring in later development stages (84,85).

In the case studies examined in this section, a combination of several analytical methods is utilized to fully characterize physical-form changes of API in excipient mixtures following preparation and accelerated stress testing. Some common solid-state methods used to study the physical forms of API in solid dosage formulation matrices include Raman spectroscopy (86), PXRD (87), reflectance FT-IR spectroscopy (88), thermal analysis (89), solid-state NMR, (90) and chemical imaging (7). It is recommended that these methods be used in combination with each other to describe physical changes of the API during excipient compatibility testing and accelerated stress conditions. The results of these techniques are often correlated with auxiliary analytical methods such as light microscopy/hot stage microscopy, scanning electron microscopy, and dissolution and solubility assessments.

Following complete characterization of the physical-form stability of the API alone, Serajuddin et al. (6) traced the physical-form changes of SQ-33600 disodium salt through the solid dosage formulation process. Using PXRD studies, it was revealed that the API turned amorphous upon initial wet granulation (Fig. 11, curve A). This finding led to a dry granulation process being utilized for initial processing of SQ-33600. Thermal-humidity challenges of prototype capsules and tablets of both wet and dry granulated materials were completed and powder x-ray analysis again detailed changes in the crystal form. The amorphous material was shown to convert to crystalline hydrate on further exposure to several high relative humidity stress conditions, such as 52% RH and 75% RH. Figure 11 shows the PXRD analysis of the prepared granules following humidity challenge (Fig. 11, curves B and C). This example shows the necessity of tracking changes in the physical form of the API through initial formulation processes and following

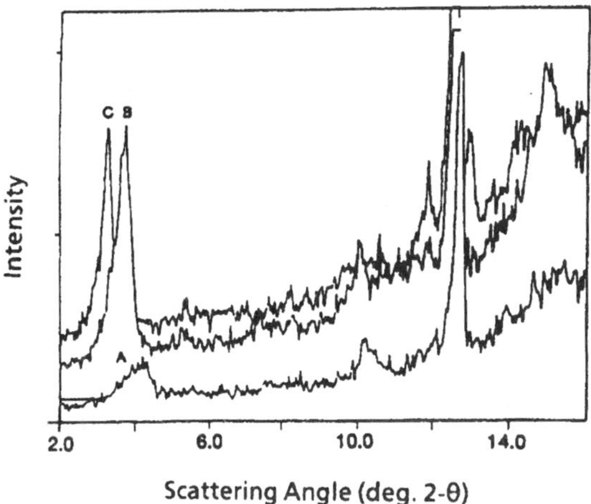

Figure 11 Physical changes occurring to SQ-33600 disodium salt during solid-formulation processes as described using PXRD analysis. Sample A represents the initial wet-granulated amorphous material. Samples B and C represent samples following storage at 52% RH and 75% RH, respectively.

accelerated stability challenges. Supporting dissolution studies were effectively utilized to determine that the physical-form change was expected to have limited impact on the performance of the proposed final dosage form.

More recently, Markovich et al. (91) utilized a combination of solid-state infra-red (IR) and NMR methods to study the amorphous to crystalline API transition of SCH 48461 in solid dispersion capsule formulations. In this illustrative study, dissolution testing initially revealed inter-and intralot variations of capsules stored under accelerated stability conditions (25°C/60% RH, 30°C/60% RH, and 40°C/80% RH). PXRD analysis could not explain the dissolution data being collected on lots stored at accelerated conditions and revealed no differences from original diffraction patterns. Two additional analytical techniques, attenuated total reflectance IR (ATR-IR) spectroscopy and solid-state ^{13}C NMR spectroscopy, were employed to study the physical form in the actual solid dispersion formulations.

Because amorphous and crystalline solid-state forms contain non-equivalent spatial relationships at the molecular level, they often display differences in functional group vibrational modes that can be measured by IR spectroscopy. Total attenuated reflectance IR spectroscopy is utilized because it is non-destructive and can be used to directly measure actual tablet and capsule samples. Similarly, solid-state NMR spectroscopy is another non-destructive direct analytical method that can detect and measure differences in nuclear resonance frequencies and relaxations, such as those displayed by amorphous and crystalline material. Cross-polarization magic angle spinning (CP-MAS) variations enhance the power of solid-state NMR and involve (i) strong proton decoupling, which eliminates coupling to neighboring proton nuclei, thereby simplifying the acquired spectra, (ii) utilizing rapid magic angle spinning to remove random orientation effects, and (iii) utilizing nuclear cross-polarization techniques to provide stronger signal-to-noise ratios and faster acquisition times.

ATR-IR analysis of the relative intensities of the strong carbonyl band of SCH 48461 (1740 cm^{-1}) and the intense ether band of the PEG 8000 excipient (1100 cm^{-1}) were utilized to track differences in lots of formulated capsule cores (Fig. 12a and b). The ratio of the intensity of these vibrations

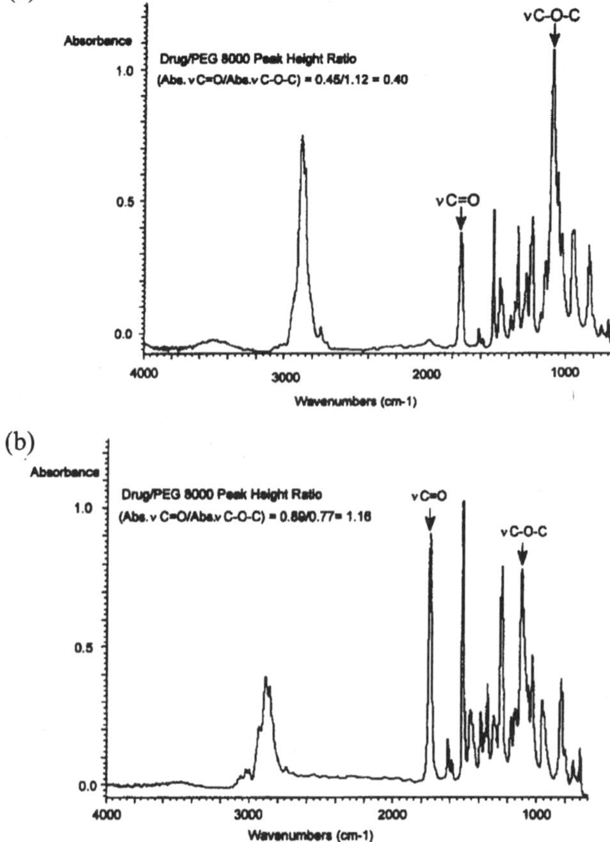

Figure 12 Comparison of the ATR-IR carbonyl and ether band intensities of initially prepared SCH 48461 capsule cores of (a) a rapidly dissolving capsule lot (Lot A) and (b) slower dissolving capsule lot (Lot C).

revealed large differences in two formulated lots of material, thereby effectively explaining the dissolution results previously obtained.

Solid-state CPMAS ^{13}C NMR analysis of the samples was used to confirm the data generated using the ATR-IR technique. Solid-state NMR spectra of SCH 48461 capsule cores following storage for 6 months at room temperature and after 18 month storage at 30°C/60% RH are shown in Figure 13, spectra A and B. These spectra show typically broad signals associated with amorphous material. The obvious change in line width of the sample stored for 24 months at room temperature immediately suggests that a physical-form change may have occurred, as narrow line-widths are more closely associated with crystalline materials (Fig. 13, spectra C). In a series of further cross-depolarization and interrupted-decoupling

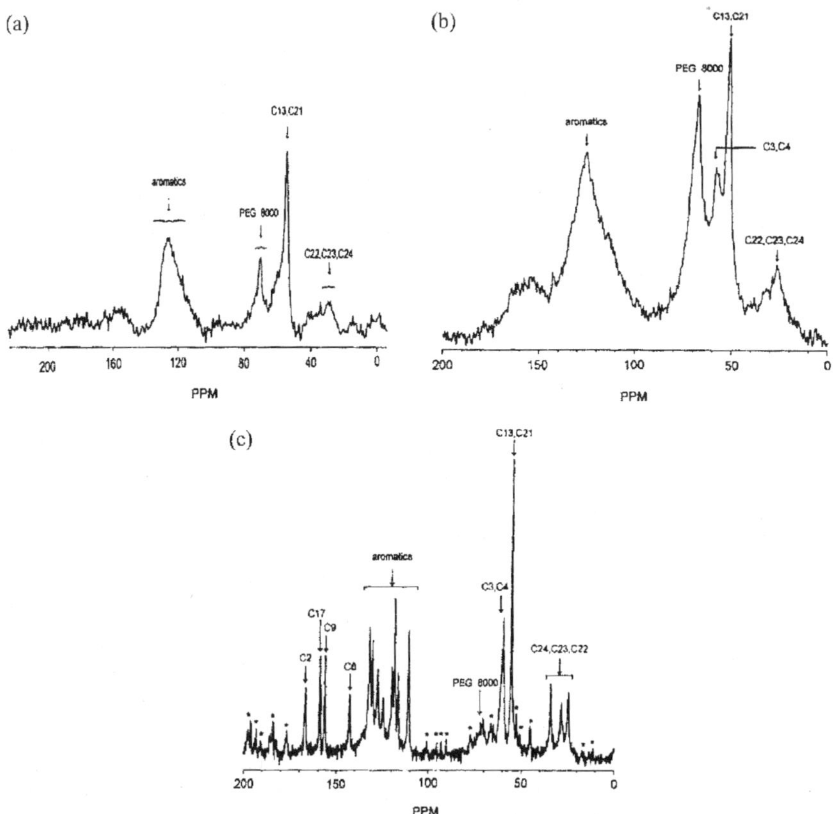

Figure 13 Solid-state CP-MAS ^{13}C NMR spectra of intact capsule cores of SCH 48461 formulations (a) after storage for 6 months at room temperature (b) after storage at 30°C/60% RH for 18 months, and (c) after storage for 24 months at room temperature.

experiments, the presence of crystalline material in several lots of SCH 48461–PEG 8000 solid dispersion formulation preparations was confirmed.

The combination of solid-state ATR-IR and solid-state NMR data supported the conclusion that the presence of crystalline material was responsible for changes in the dissolution profiles of the different lots. The results appear consistent with historical examples of changes in API physical form of solid, high molecular weight, polyethylene glycol dispersion formulations of amorphous indomethacin and griseofulvin (92–95).

In the foregoing examples, many techniques were utilized to obtain the fullest picture of the changes and interactions of the API in the formulation mixtures. Very often, these changes and interactions are linked to changes in chemical stability or performance of the dosage form such that some initial monitoring of these physical changes and interactions should be considered and incorporated in excipient compatibility testing when applicable.

IV. KINETICS AND PREDICTIONS BASED ON EXCIPIENT COMPATIBILITY DATA

Kinetic information on the chemical changes of excipient compatibility samples is a direct outcome of most formulation compatibility studies. Because accelerated conditions of thermal and thermal humidity stress are employed, degradation will often occur at these conditions. A brief kinetic evaluation of the data can address the behavior and extent of decay such that degradation data can effectively be utilized to determine levels and conditions of compatibility (96). It is not the aim of this section to recommend full kinetic treatment of decay; rather it is to describe simple concepts and exercises that will help the excipient compatibility formulator utilize their data most effectively. Several experimental factors can be included in the initial experimental design of excipient compatibility studies to make kinetic analysis more powerful, and even with small studies having a limited amount of samples for analysis, a brief kinetic treatment of the data is recommended.

Overall, for any kinetic analysis, the more distinct data points acquired, the better characterization of the decay. This factor must be weighed against the resources available for the study, but the maximum number of data points should be collected whenever possible. It is recommended that multiple samples be analyzed per data point to rule out spurious results. An assessment of uniformity of prepared samples should be strongly considered. It is recommended that over the timeframes of the study, the number of samples and data points be rationally prescribed (59), such that for harsher conditions analysis of many early data points may be the most beneficial. Whenever possible, a variety of temperatures (more than three) with identical, controlled humidity levels (generally moderate to high, 40–75% RH) may be able to contribute to the estimation of valuable kinetic parameters. It should also be noted that on the basis of review of related literature (50) harsh temperatures of >70°C may not provide realistic and relevant degradation data for simple kinetic analyses. Rigorous kinetic consideration of largely degraded samples (>50–60% decay) should be avoided, as secondary degradation reactions and involvement of decay products in further decay reactions can convolute analysis. For highest quality kinetic data, all samples should be analyzed immediately after sampling, using validated analytical methodology.

Often, changes in decay kinetics are observed in bulk API stability and excipient compatibility studies because the system converts from a homogeneous solid mixture to a heterogeneous, multi-component mixture involving gas, liquid, and solid phases (97). For initial consideration, total loss of API, loss of API via a specific major degradation mechanism, or growth of a major, significant degradant with time can be investigated kinetically. For emphasis, it should be restated that prior to kinetic analysis, confirmation of API physical-form integrity in the excipient samples is recommended. Modeling of chemical API decay may be severely convoluted by the kinetics of physical-form transformations.

The brief kinetic data treatment may begin with a plot of potency or growth of a major degradation product with respect to time, for a given set of temperature and humidity conditions. If the data is best fit by a simple linear plot of these separate parameters with time, the degradation in the excipient mixture is likely following zero-order kinetics. An example is detailed in Figure 14 and illustrates the kinetics of formation of free salicylic acid from the decomposition of aspirin in the solid state. Analysis reveals that at three separate temperatures, the formation of the degradation product is linear with respect to time, with the slope of the line being the temperature-dependant rate constant of the reaction. Zero-order reactions are common in the solid state and effectively model degradation occurring in saturated adsorbed moisture layers of the drug or excipient.

Another common decay pattern of drug substances in the presence of excipients is exemplified by the example of thiamine hydrochloride in microcrystalline cellulose as described by Carstensen et al. (98) and detailed in Figure 15. Here, the degradation profile shows initial rapid decay followed by a decline and leveling to a pseudo-equilibrium level. It should be noted that the rapid initial decay is described by many distinct samplings and the number of later samplings are helpful in determining the level at which decay slows, so that in general, more distinct samples are very helpful in kinetic analysis.

Carstensen directly relates the level at which degradation slows to the amount of water present in the matrix and utilizes this equilibrium level, denoted A_∞, in further kinetic analysis. Kinetic treatment of the data reveals a first order decay character to the degradation, with a linear slope of the log of the thiamine hydrochloride concentration at a specific point (A) in relation to the observed equilibrium level (A_∞), with respect to time in days.

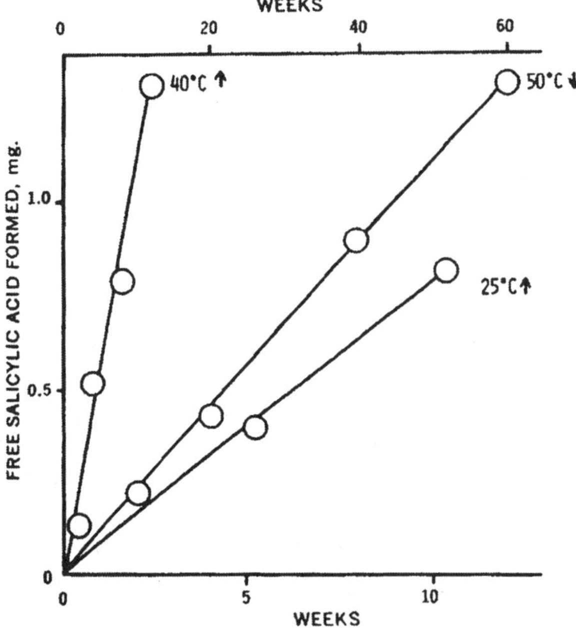

Figure 14 The kinetics of formation of salicylic acid from the decomposition of aspirin in the solid state at varying temperature.

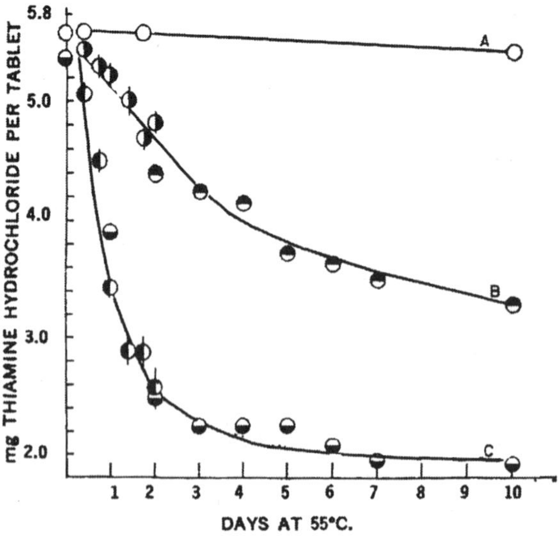

Figure 15 Stability of thiamine hydrochloride in a cellulose-magnesium stearate tablet containing various amounts of moisture following storage at 55°C.

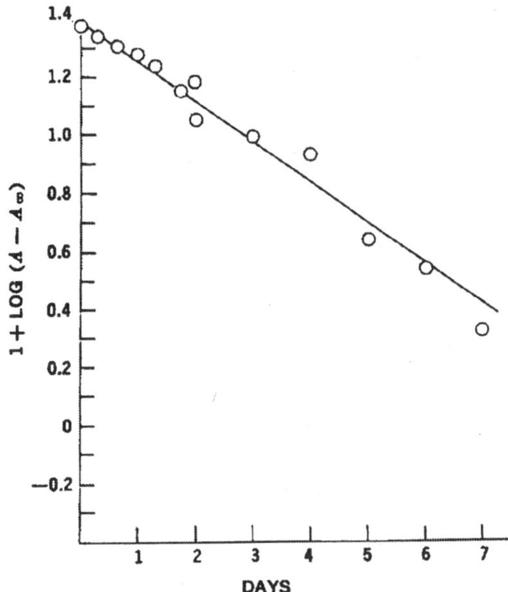

Figure 16 Plot of the logarithm of thiamine hydrochloride content after the subtraction of equilibrium content ($A-A_{\infty}$) as a function of time at 55°C with addition of 4% moisture.

This plot of [$A-A_{\infty}$] with time is shown in Figure 16 and illustrates the usefulness of using basic kinetic observations (i.e., pseudo-equilibrium levels) to explain compatibility data sets.

First-order degradation that is characterized by initial rapid decay with subsequent slowing or halt of degradation is also observed when reactive impurities are responsible for decay. In the specific case of reactive impurities, the level at which degradation slows for all samples of the same composition will be similar or identical, whereas the rate at which they achieve that level will vary with temperature. This is an example where brief kinetic analysis of the data reveals a valuable clue about the decay that is occurring in the system and can lead directly to a statement about compatibility of certain lots of excipients. There are additional scenarios for which first-order decay may be observed. Direct solid–solid chemical reaction decay routes also exhibit first-order decay kinetics, with the decay being limited by the growth of the impurities at the surfaces of the reacting solids. In this specific case, the decay level may closely relate to the surface area of the API and/or reactive excipient. Similarly, a first-order decay profile might be anticipated when a small but significant amount of reactive amorphous material or reactive defects are initially generated in the excipient compatibility preparation

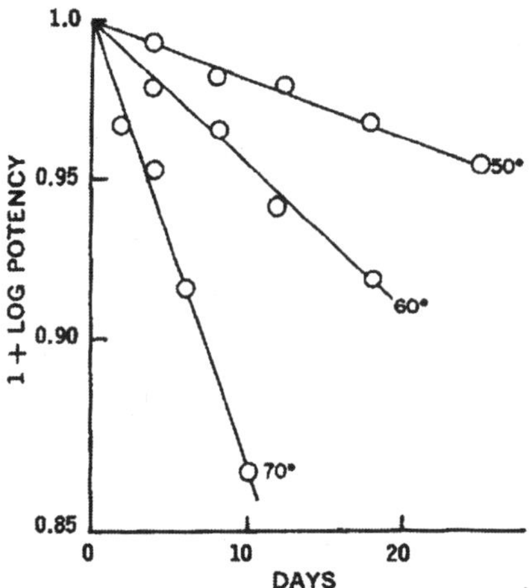

Figure 17 Pseudo-first-order plot of thermal degradation of ascorbic acid (vitamin C) in a solid dosage form.

process. Rapid decay reactions are observed until the amount of amorphous material or defects are depleted.

When several temperature-dependent rate constants have been determined or at least estimated, the adherence of the decay in the system to Arrhenius behavior can be easily determined. If a plot of these rate constants vs. reciprocal temperature ($1/T$) produces a linear correlation, the system is adhering to the well-studied Arrhenius kinetic model and some prediction of the rate of decay at any temperature can be made. As detailed in Figure 17, Carstensen's adaptation of data, originally described by Tardif (99), demonstrates the pseudo-first-order decay behavior of the decomposition of ascorbic acid in solid dosage forms at temperatures of 50°C, 60°C, and 70°C (100). Further analysis of the data confirmed that the system adhered closely to Arrhenius behavior as the plot of the rate constants with respect to reciprocal temperature ($1/T$) showed linearity (Fig. 18). Carstensen suggests that it is not always necessary to determine the mechanism of decay if some relevant property of the degradation can be explained as a function of time, and therefore logically quantified and rationally predicted.

Review of compatibility data in this manner is important and useful in many cases. If Arrhenius treatment fits the decay observed in the compatibility samples, data obtained under relatively short-term accelerated stress conditions can efficiently be used to extrapolate the amount of decay expected at realistic long-term storage conditions. The adherence of decay to Arrhenius kinetics provides the formulator with a powerful tool for prediction and understanding of degradation. This decay model is the basis for the International Committee on Harmonization (ICH) quality guidelines

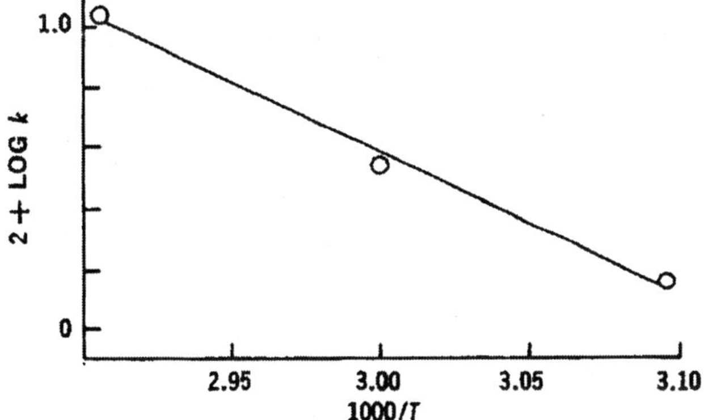

Figure 18 Arrhenius plots of the temperature-dependant rate constants derived from Figure 17.

describing stability testing for new drug substances and products, followed by the FDA and the entire pharmaceutical industry (57). If the API decay in excipient systems can be described by Arrhenius behavior, there are detailed nomographs (101) that can be referenced to determine extent of decay projected for the sample under any combination of time and temperature conditions, making compatibility judgments the most quantitative and realistic.

Lastly, through the kinetic exercises described herein, it may be discovered that there are conditions of temperature and humidity stress where the system more closely follows Arrhenius behavior and those conditions where the decay behavior will deviate greatly from the model. In this case, the kinetic analysis will serve to define the stress conditions under which Arrhenius behavior is valid, thereby directing and focusing further studies to limited stress conditions so that more powerful, predictive data can be generated under closely prescribed conditions.

Excipient compatibility testing can become a complicated and extensive series of experiments. It has been questioned by Monkhouse and Maderich (102) if these studies, in any form, are predictive enough to be worthy of the experimental expense. Several groups are working toward the automation of excipient compatibility testing while others are considering high throughput approaches (103), Effective utilization of these more modern approaches will lead to several advantages including the efficient analysis of many more distinct data points so that kinetic analysis will be fully empowered, and the ability to evaluate and test many more experimental parameters to provide greater overview of compatibility and to evaluate many more processing parameters at earlier stages, leading to the identification of optimal process without large-scale investigations.

Because a large degree of resources are involved in generating of data, it is highly recommended that compatibility data be compiled and referenced in complete databases. Databases will prove useful in later stages of development as a valuable reference to formulators looking to switch or exchange excipients in commercial formulations and for early-stage formulators who may be examining compatibility of similar classes of compounds and molecule scaffolds. Although this concept of rigorous mining of excipient compatibility data is not exceedingly novel, there are only limited references to these types of database systems in the literature (104).

Overall, the concepts presented in this summary suggest that (i) an initial understanding of the properties of the API and excipients should be utilized to design excipient compatibility studies, (ii) the understanding of the role of water in the interactions of excipients with API should be considered for all designs of compatibility testing, and (iii) the physical form and its involvement in the solid state needs to be considered when interpreting the data.

REFERENCES

1. Whittet T. Decomposition of medicaments due to excipients and containers and its prevention. Pharm Acta Helv 1959; 34:489–520.
2. Stahl VPH. Dir characterisierung und aufbereitung des wirkstoffs bein der Entwircklungfester Arneiformen. Pharm Ind 1989; 51(4):425–439.
3. Dudinkski J, Lachman L, Shami E, Tingstad J. Preformulation studies I: molindone hydrochloride. J Pharm Sci 1973; 62:622–624.
4. Jorgensen WL, Laired ER, Gushurst AJ, Fleischer JM, Goethe SA, Helson HE, Paderes GD, Sinclair S. CAMEO: a program for the logical prediction of the products of organic reactions. Pure Appl Chem 1990; 62(10):1921–1932.
5. Paul IC, Curtin DY. Thermally induced organic reactions in the solid state. Acc Chem Res 1973; 6(7):217–225.
6. Serajuddin ATM, Morris KR, Newman AW, Bugay DE, Ranadive SA, Singh AK, Szyper M, Varia SA, Brittain HG. Characterization of humidity-dependent changes in crystal properties of a new HMG-CoA reductase inhibitor in support of its dosage form development. Int J Pharm 1994; 108:195–206.
7. Bugay DE. Characterization of the solid-state: spectroscopic techniques. Adv Drug Delivery Rev 2001; 48:43–65.
8. Food and Drug Administration. QIB: Stability Testing: Photostability Testing of New Drug Substances and Products. Federal Register, 1996:1–8.
9. York P. Solid-state properties of powders in the formulation and processing of solid dosage forms. Int J Pharm 1983; 17:1–28.
10. Teraoka R, Otsuka M, Matsuda Y. Evaluation of photostability of solid state dimethyl 1,4-dihydro-2,6-dimethyl-4-(2-nitro-phenyl)-3,5-pyridinecarboxylate by Fourier-transformed reflection–absorption infrared spectroscopy. Int J Pharm 1999; 184:35–43.
11. Harris KDM. New opportunities for structure determination of molecular materials directly from powder diffraction data. Crys Growth Des 2003; 3(6):887–895.

12. Wray PE. The physics of tablet compaction revisited. Drug Dev Ind Pharm 1992; 18(6&7):627–658.
13. Lefebvre C, Guyot-Hermann AM. Polymorphic transitions of carbemazepine during grinding and compression. Drug Dev Ind Pharm 1986; 12(11–13): 1913–1927.
14. Pikal MJ, Lukes AL, Lang JE. Thermal decomposition of amorphous beta-lactam antibacterials. J Pharm Sci 1977; 66:1312–1316.
15. Waltersson J, Lundgren P. The effect of mechanical comminution on drug stability. Acta Pharm Suec 1985; 22:291–300.
16. Morris KR, Griesser UJ, Eckhardt CJ, Stowell JG. Theoretical approaches to physical transformations of active pharmaceutical ingredients during manufacturing processes. Adv Drug Deliv Rev 2001; 48:91–114.
17. Chiou KL, Kyle LE. Differential thermal, solubility and aging studies on various sources ofdigoxin and digitoxin powder: biopharmaceutical inplications. J Pharm Sci 1979; 68(10):1224–1229.
18. Konty MJ. Distrubution of water in solid pharmaceutical systems. Drug Dev Ind Pharm 1988; 14(14):1991–2027.
19. Pikal M, Dellerman K. Stability testing of pharmaceuticals by high-sensitivity isothermal calorimetry at 25°C: cephalosporins in the solid and aqueous solution states. Int J Pharm 1989; 50(3):233–252.
20. Brittain HG. X-ray diffraction. III. Pharmaceutical application of x-ray powder diffraction. Pharm Tech North Am 2001; 25(3):142–150.
21. Suryanarayanan R. X-ray powder diffractometry. Drug Pharm Sci 1995; 70: 187–221.
22. Florence AT, Salole EG. Changes in crystallinity and solubility on comminution of digoxin and observations on spironolactone and oestradiol. J Pharm Pharmacol 1976; 28:637–642.
23. Byrn SR, Lin C. The effect of crystal packing and defects on desolvation of hydrate crystals of caffeine and L-(−)-l,4-cyclohexadien-l-alanine. J Am Chem Soc 1976; 98:4004–4005.
24. Clay RJ, Knevel AM, Byrn SR. The desolvation and oxidation of crystals of dialuric acid monohydrate. J Pharm Sci 1982; 71:1289–1291.
25. Halebilian J, McCrone W. Pharmaceutical application of polymorphism. J Pharm Sci 1969; 58(8):911–929.
26. Aruga M, Awazu A, Hanano M. Kinetic studies on decomposition of glutathione. I. Decomposition in the solid state. Chem Pharm Bull 1978; 26(7): 2081–2091.
27. Kibbe AH, ed. Handbook of Pharmaceutical Excipients. 3rd ed. Washington, DC: American Pharmaceutical Association, 2000:665.
28. Bugay DE, Findlay WP, eds. Pharmaceutical excipients: characterization by IR, raman and NMR spectroscopy. In: Drugs and the Pharmaceutical Science. Vol. 94. New York, NY: Marcel Dekker, 1999:669.
29. Hancock BC, Shamblin SL. Water vapour sorption by pharmaceutical sugars. Pharm Sci Tech Today 1998; 1(8):345–351.
30. Lundgren P.a.A., C, Methods for the evaluation of solid state stability and compatibility between drug and excipient. Acta Pharm Suecica 1985; 22(6):305–314.

31. Patel NK, Patel IJ, Cutie AJ, Wadke DA, Monkhouse DC, Reier GE. The effect of selected direct compression excipients on the stability of aspirin as a model hydrolyzable drug. Drug Dev Ind Pharm 1988; 14(1):77–98.
32. Chen J-G, Markovitz DA, Yang AY, Rabel SR, Pang J, Dolinksky D, Wu L-S, Alessandro M. Degradation of a fluoropyridinyl drug in capsule formulation: degradant identification, proposed degradation mechanism and formulation optimization. Pharm Dev Tech 2000; 5(4):561–570.
33. Walling C. The acid strengths of surfaces. J Am Chem Soc 1950; 72: 1164–1168.
34. Castello RA, Mattocks AM. Discoloration of tablets containing amines and lactose. J Pharm Sci 1962; 51:106–108.
35. Wirth DD, Baertschi SW, Johnson RA, Maple SR, Miller MS, Hallenbeck DK, Gregg SM. Maillard reaction of lactose and fluoxetine hydrochloride, a secondary amine. J Pharm Sci 1998; 87(1):31–39.
36. Brewster ME, Loftson T. The use of chemically modified cyclodextrins in the development of formulations for chemical delivery systems. Pharmazie 2002; 57:94–101.
37. Higuchi T, Lachman L. Inhibition of hydrolysis of esters in solution by formation of complexes I. J Am Pharm Assoc Sci Ed 1955; XLIV(9):521–526.
38. Bhattacharya S. Influence of intact and hydrolyzable protein in solid state. J Inst Chem Calcutta 1969; 41:147–153.
39. Crowley PJ. Excipients as stabilizers. Pharm Sci Tech Today 1999; 2(6): 237–243.
40. Bayomi B, Abanumay KA, Al-Angary AA. Effect of inclusion complexation with cyclodextrins on photostability of Nifedipine in solid state. Int J Pharm 2002; 243:107–117.
41. Thoma K, Klimek R. Photostabilization of drugs in dosage forms without protection from packaging materials. Int J Pharm 1991; 67:169–175.
42. Jansen PJ, Kemp CA, Maple SR, Baertschi SW. Characterization of Impurities found by interaction of Duloxetine HCl with enteric polymers hydroxypropyl methyl cellulose acetate succinate and hydroxypropyl methylcellulose phthalaie. J Pharm Sci 1998; 87(1):81–85.
43. Waterman K, Adami R, Hong J. Impurities in Drug Products in, Handbook of Isolation and Characterization of Impurities in Pharmaceuticals, Ahuja, SA, San Diego: Academic Press, 2003:75–88
44. Brittain HG, Bogdanowich SJ, Bugay DE, DeVincentis J, Lewen G, Newman AW. Physical characterization of pharmaceutical solids. Pharm Res 1991; 8(8):963–973.
45. Jones TM. The physico technical properties of starting materials used in tablet formulation. Int J Pharm Tech Prod Mfr 1981; 2(2):17–24.
46. Monkhouse D. Excipient compatibility possibilities and limitations in stability prediction. Paperback APV, 1993. 32 (Stability Testing in the EC, Japan and the USA):67–74.
47. Leuenberger H, Becher W. A factorial design for compatibility studies in preformulation work. Pharm Acta Helv 1975; 50(4):88–91.

48. El-Banna HM, Ismail AA, Gadalla MAF. Factorial design of experiment for stability studies in the development of a tablet formulation. Pharmazie 1984; 39:163–165.
49. Dung T, Fassihi AR. Identification of stabilizing and destabilizing effects of excipient–drug interactions in solid dosage form design. Int J Pharm 1993; 97:161–170.
50. Sims J, Carreira J, Carrier D, Crabtree S, Easton L, Hancock S, Simcox C. A new approach to accelerated drug–excipient compatibility testing. Pharm Dev Tech 2003; 8(2):119–126.
51. Badway S, Williams R, Gilbert D. Chemical stability of an ester prodrug of a glycoprotein IIb/IIIa receptor antagonist in solid dosage forms. J Pharm Sci 1999; 88(4):428–433.
52. Guo Y, Byrn S, Zografi G. Physical characteristics and chemical degradation of amorphous quinapril hydrochloride. J Pharm Sci 2000; 89(1):128–143.
53. Leung SS, Grant DW. Solid state stability studies of model dipeptides: aspartame and aspartylphenylalanine. J Pharm Sci 1997; 86(1):64–71.
54. Gu L, Strickley RG. Diketopiperazine formation, hydrolysis, and epimerization of the new dipeptide angiotensin-converting enzyme inhibitor RS-10085. Pharm Res 1987; 4(5):392–397.
55. Ahlneck C, Lundgren P. Methods for the evaluation of solid state stability and compatibility between drug and excipient. Acta Pharm Suec 1986; 22(6): 305–314.
56. Serajuddin A, Thakur A, Ghoshal R, Fakes M, Ranadive S, Morris K, Varia S. Selection of solid dosage form composition through drug–excipient Compatibility Testing. J Pharm Sci 1999; 88(7):696–704.
57. Food and Drug Administration. Q1A(R2) Stability Testing of New Drug Substances and Products. Federal Register, 2003:65717–65718.
58. Eyjolfsson R. Diclofenac sodium: oxidative degradation in solution and solid state. Drug Dev Ind Pharm 2000; 26(4):451–453.
59. Carstensen JT. Stability of solid dosage forms. In: Timoney DA, ed. Progress in the Quality Control of Medicines. Chapter 5 Elsevier Biomedical Press, 1981:97–112.
60. Waterman K, Adami R, Alsante K, Hong J, Landis M, Lombardo F, Roberts C. Stabilization of pharmaceuticals to oxidative degradation. Pharm Dev Tech 2002; 7(1):1–32.
61. Yoshioka S, Ogata H, Shibazaki T, Ejima A. Stability of sulpyrine. V. Oxidation with molecular oxygen in the solid state. Chem Pharm Bull 1979; 27(10): 2363–2371.
62. Hartanuer KJ, Arbuthnot GN, Baertschi SW, Johnson RA, Luke WD, Pearson NG, Rickard EC, Tingle CA, Tsang PKS, Wiens RE. Influence of peroxide impurities in povidone and crospovidone on the stability of raloxifene hydrochloride in tablets: identification and control of an oxidative degradation product. Pharm Dev Tech 2000; 5(3):303–310.
63. Waterman K, Adami R, Alsante K, Antipas A, Arenson D, Carrier R, Hong J, Landis M, Lombardo F, Shah J, Shalaev E, Smith S, Wang H. Hydrolysis in pharmaceutical formulations. Pharm Dev Tech 2002; 7(2):113–146.

64. Anonymons. Ageless oxygen absorber presenting product purity, integrity and freshness. Mitsubishi Gas Chemical company of Japan, Tokyo, 1994.
65. Carstensen JT, Johnson JB, Valentine W, Vance JJ. Extrapolation of appearence of tablets and Powders from Accelerated Storage Tests. J Pharm Sci 1964; 53(9):1050–1054.
66. Wirth M. Instrumental color measurement: a method for judging the appearance of tablets. J Pharm Sci 1991; 80(12):1177–1179.
67. Stark G, Fawcett JP, Tucker IG, Weatherall IL. Instrumental evaluation of color of solid dosage forms during stability testing. Int J Pharm 1996; 143(1):93–100.
68. Hong D, Shah M. Development and Validation of HPLC Stability-Indicating Assay. In: Drugs and the Pharmaceutical Sciences. New York: Marcel Dekker, 2000:329–384.
69. Olsen B, Baertschi S, Riggin R. Multidimensional evaluation of impurity profiles for generic cephalexin and cefaclor antibiotics. J Chromatogr 1993; 648: 165–173.
70. Kuiken J, Mitchell T, Mann T, Burke M. SPE method improves drug analysis. Drug Discov Dev 2000; Nov/Dec:75–78.
71. Moreno P, Salvado V. Determination of eight water- and fat-soluble vitamins in multi-vitamin pharmaceutical formulations by high-performance liquid chromatography. J Chromatogr A 2000; 870:207–215.
72. Dorman D, Lorenz L, Occolowitz J, Spangle L, Collins M, Bashore F, Baertschi S. Isolation and structure elucidation of the major degradation products of cefaclor in the solid state. J Pharm Sci 1997; 86(5):540–549.
73. Dubost D, Kaufman M, Zimmerman J, Bogusky M, Coddington A, Pitzenberger S. Characterization of a solid state reaction product from a lyophilized formulation of a cyclic heptapeptide. A novel example of an excipient-induced oxidation. Pharm Res 1996; 13(12):1811–1814.
74. Angberg M, Nystroem C, Castensson S. Evaluation of heat-conduction microcalorimetry in pharmaceutical stability studies. VII. Oxidation of ascorbic acid in aqueous solution. Int J Pharm 1993; 90(1):19–33.
75. Oliyai R, Lindenbaum S. Stability testing of pharmaceuticals by isothermal heat conduction calorimetry: ampicillin in aqueous solution. Int J Pharm 1991; 73(1):33–36.
76. Tan X, Meltzer N, Lindenbaum S. Solid-state stability studies of 13-*cis*-retinoic acid and all-*trans*-retinoic acid using microcalorimetry and HPLC analysis. Pharm Res 1992; 9(9):1203–1208.
77. Schmitt E, Peck K, Sun Y, Geoffroy J. Rapid, practical and predictive excipient compatibility screening using isothermal microcalorimetry. Thermochim Acta 2001; 380:175–183.
78. Selzer T, Radau M, Kreuter J. Use of isothermal heat conduction microcalorimetry to evaluate stability and excipient compatibility of a solid drug. Int J Pharm 1998; 171:227–241.
79. Selzer T, Radau M, Kreuter J. The use of isothermal heat conduction microcalorimetry to evaluate drug stability in tablets. Int J Pharm 1999; 184: 199–206.

80. Phipps M, Mackin L. Application of isothermal microcalorimetry in solid state drug development. Pharm Sci Technol Today 2000; 3(1):9–17.
81. Wissing S, Craig D, Barker S, Moore W. An investigation into the use of stepwise isothermal high sensitivity DSC as a means of detecting drug-excipient incompatibility. Int J Pharm 2000; 199:141–150.
82. Mroso P, Li Wan Po A, Irwin W. Solid-state stability of aspirin in the presence of excipients: kinetic interpretation modeling and prediction. J Pharm Sci 1982; 71(10):1096–1101.
83. McDaid F, Barker S, Fitzpatrick S, Petts, C, Craig D. Further investigations into the use of high sensitivity differential scanning calorimetry as a means of predicting drug–excipient interactions. Int J Pharm 2003; 252:235–240.
84. Morissette SL, Soukasene S, Levinson D, Cima MJ, Almarsson O. Elucidation of crystal form diversity of the HIV protease inhibitor ritonavir by high-throughput crystallization. Proc Natl Acad Sci 2003; 100(5):2180–2184.
85. Bauer J, Spanton S, Henry R, Quick J, Dziki W, Porter W, Morris J. Ritonavir: an extraordinary example of conformational polymorphism. Pharm Res 2001; 18(6):859–866.
86. Taylor LS, Langkilde EW. Evaluation of solid-state forms present in tablets by Raman spectroscopy. J Pharm Sci 2000; 89(10):1342–1353.
87. Suryanarayanan R, Herman CS. Quantitative analysis of the active ingredient in a multi-component tablet formulation by powder x-ray diffraction. Int J Pharm 1991; 77:287–295.
88. Lach JL, Bornstein M. Diffuse reflectance studies of solid–solid interactions. J Pharm Sci 1965; 54(12):1730–1736.
89. Weslowski M. Thermal methods of analysis in solid dosage technology. Drug Dev Ind Pharm 1985; 11(2 and 3):493–521.
90. Byrn SE, Bugay DE, Tishmack PA. Solid state nuclear magnetic resonance spectroscopy—pharmaceutical applications. J Pharm Sci 2003; 92(3):441–474.
91. Markovich RJ, Anderson Evans C, Coscolluela CB, Zibas SA, Rosen J. Spectroscopic identification of an amorphous-to-crystalline drug transition in a solid dispersion SCH-48461 capsule formulation. J Pharm Biomed Anal 1997; 19:661–673.
92. Chiou W, Riegleman S. Pharmaceutical applications of solid dispersion systems. J Pharm Sci 1971; 60:1281–1302.
93. Chiou W. Pharmaceutical applications of solid dispersion systems: x-ray diffraction and aqueous solubility studies on griseofulvin–polyethylene glycol 6000 systems. J Pharm Sci 1977; 66:989–991.
94. Ford J, Rubinsten M. Ageing of indomethacin–polyethylene glycol 6000 solid dispersion. Pharm Acta Helv 1979; 54(12):353–358.
95. Ford J. The Current status of solid dispersion. Pharm Acta Helv 1986; 61(3):69–88.
96. Waterman KC, Adami RC. Accelerated aging: prediction of chemical stability in pharmaceuticals. Int J Pharm 2005; **293** (1-2):101–125.
97. Tingstad J, Dudzinski J. Preformulations studies II: stability of drug substances in solid pharmaceutical systems. J Pharm Sci 1973; 62(11):1856–1860.
98. Carstensen JT, Osadca M, Rubin S. Degradation mechanisms for water-soluble drugs in solid dosage forms. J Pharm Sci 1969; 58:549–553.

99. Tardif R. Reliability of accelerated storage tests to predict stability of vitalimes (A, B1, C) in tablets. J Pharm Sci 1965; 54:281–284.
100. Carstensen JT, Rhodes C. Stability of solids and solid dosage forms. J Pharm Sci 1974; 63(1):1–14.
101. Scott MW, Lordi NG. Design and application of accelerated stability testing of pharmaceuticals. J Pharm Sci 1965; 54(4):531–537.
102. Monkhouse DC, Maderich A. Whither compatibility testing? Drug Dev Ind Pharm 1989; 15(13):2115–2130
103. Henry CM. New wrinkles in drug discovery In: Baum RM, Chemical and Engineering News. Washington, DC: American Chemical Society, 2004; 37–42.
104. Zimmer A. CompaSys: informations sytem fur galenische vertraglichkeit. Pharmazie 1990; 135(39):56–58.

14

Stress Testing: Frequently Asked Questions

Steven W. Baertschi
Eli Lilly and Company, Lilly Research Laboratories, Lilly Corporate Center, Indianapolis, Indiana, U.S.A.

Karen M. Alsante
Pfizer Global Research & Development, Analytical Research & Development, Groton, Connecticut, U.S.A.

There are many potential problems and questions that the scientific researcher may encounter when attempting to design and carry out a stress-testing study for a pharmaceutical compound. This chapter is intended to address some of the more frequently encountered problems or questions. Since many of the questions are dealt with in more detail in other parts of the book, the reader may be referred to other chapters or publications for further information.

1. Are stress-testing studies, the data from which may be included in the regulatory submission for a new drug entity, considered GMP studies?

This is an important question that deserves some discussion. The stages at which stress-testing studies are carried out are generally prior to the establishment of "quality standards". Stress-testing studies are designed to provide the groundwork for establishment of such standards. Thus, stress-testing studies should not be considered GMP studies. Instead, the focus should be on the thoroughness of the scientific investigation, the soundness of design, the quality of documentation, the "defendability" of the conclusions, and the retrievability of data.

2. Are protocols or SOPs required for carrying out stress-testing studies?

A survey of 20 major pharmaceutical companies indicated that 70% of the companies follow some kind of standard operating procedure and 50% require a protocol for stress-testing studies (1). There is, however, no regulatory requirement that mandates the use of protocols or SOPs.

3. How much validation of the analytical methods used for stress-testing studies is appropriate?

It should be remembered that stress-testing studies are investigational and the validation should demonstrate that the studies are "suitable for its intended purpose" (2). The "intended purpose" of a stress-testing method is to help understand the degradation chemistry of the drug and to provide separation and detection of as many degradation products as possible. The specificity of these methods cannot be fully validated since all the degradation products are not yet known. Validation for an investigational stress-testing method will therefore be much more limited than for official control methods. See Chapter 4 for additional discussion.

4. If the salt form or the physical characteristics of the drug substance change, do new stress-testing studies need to be performed?

If either the salt form or the physical characteristics (e.g., particle size, polymorphic form, surface area, etc.) change, all solid-state stress-testing studies should be repeated, since such changes could affect degradation rates and even degradation pathways.

5. How "hard" should a drug substance be stressed?

This is one of the most frequently asked questions related to stress-testing studies, probably because there are no official regulatory guidances that deal with such specifics. The primary question is whether the drug must be forced to degrade (regardless of how harsh the conditions or how long the exposure) or simply exposed to conditions of "reasonable harshness" with the understanding that if the drug does not degrade under this set of conditions then it can be regarded as "stable" to the particular stress condition. We assert that there should be realistic limits to stress-testing studies, and these limits are discussed in detail in Chapter 2. Additional guidance and discussion can be found in the PhRMA "Available Guidance and Best Practices" article (3), in Chapter 1, and elsewhere (4). As discussed in the PhRMA article, the target of stress testing is the "lesser of 10% degradation of the active ingredient or exposure to energy in slight excess of accelerated storage...". The approach discussed in the PhRMA article acknowledges that a compound may not degrade under a given stress condition after a reasonable amount of time, and that no further stressing is advised in these cases. Increasing stress conditions to force degradation (without regard to whether or not the stressing is excessive) can lead to degradation pathways that are not representative of "real world" degradation. Such degradation will cause unnecessary method development for separation of components that will never be observed under realistic conditions, e.g., upon storage according to ICH guidelines (4) or under reasonable shipping or distribution excursions or patient use.

6. If a compound has aqueous solubility problems, should co-solvents be employed to facilitate dissolution for aqueous acid/base degradation studies? If so, what co-solvents are recommended?

It is appropriate to employ a co-solvent when the solubility of the drug is limited under a given condition. The two most common co-solvents used are acetonitrile and methanol (1). It should be noted that dissolution facilitated by a co-solvent may not always increase the degradation rate, as there are many factors involved. For further discussion of this topic see "Hydrolytic" section of Chapter 2.

Special attention should be given to the drug substance structure when choosing the appropriate co-solvent. One should carefully investigate the chemical composition of the drug substance and take care not to use a co-solvent that may react with it. For example, methanol and other alcohols are avoided for acidic conditions if the compound contains a carboxylic acid, ester, amide, aryl amine, or hydroxyl group. This prevents significant experimental artifact components involving reaction with methanol and other alcohols.

Also, 1 N NaOH and acetonitrile are miscible only for solutions containing 20% acetonitrile or less. Reducing the base strength to 0.1 N NaOH allows for higher levels of acetonitrile as a co-solvent. Acetonitrile is the most commonly used co-solvent (1).

7. How do you choose which lot of a drug substance should be used in stress-testing studies? How many lots should be used for stress testing?

The lot of drug substance chosen for stress testing is ideally representative of the manufactured or marketed form, although this is not always possible with the solid form in the early phases of development. If the solid form changes, the solid-state stress testing should be repeated. Changes in the solid-state characteristics or polymorphic form should not require new solution studies to be performed. One lot is normally sufficient for stress-testing purposes. From the *ICH Stability Guideline*: "stress testing is likely to be carried out on a single batch of material (5)."

8. Are there guidances or guidelines available for designing and carrying out stress-testing studies?

The *ICH Stability Guideline* (Q1A) defines stress testing and provides a few paragraphs to describe the kinds of conditions (i.e., heat, humidity, acid/base, oxidative, and light) that should be employed during stress testing. The PhRMA has published an "Available Guidance and Best Practices" article on stress testing as an outcome of a workshop on the topic (3). Alsante et al. have published a useful guide for "purposeful degradation studies" (i.e., stress testing) (4). Singh (12) and Klick et al. (13) have also published approaches to stress testing/forced degradation. A benchmarking study that describes common stress-testing practices of 20 major pharmaceutical companies has been published (1). For further discussion of this topic see Chapter 1, Section IV.

9. Do degradation products that arise during stress-testing studies need to be structurally characterized if they do not form at significant levels during long-term stability or accelerated stability studies in either the drug substance or product?

There is no clear, definitive requirement in the ICH guidances or in FDA guidelines that degradation products that form only in stress-testing studies must be identified structurally. It is difficult to envision, however, how an understanding of the "intrinsic stability characteristics" of a drug compound can be developed unless some information about the structures of degradation products along with the conditions that lead to their formation is developed. This question is discussed thoroughly in Chapter 2, under the section of "Intrinsic Stability: Structures of the major degradation products."

From the stress-testing benchmarking study (1), 14 companies generally identify major degradation products observed during stress testing on the drug substance even if the degradation products are not observed during formal stability studies (e.g., 25°C/60% RH, 30°C/60% RH, 40°C/75% RH). Of the 14 companies, 10 companies identify all major degradation products that form in stress testing, and 2 companies generally identify only those approaching ICH thresholds (i.e., the degradation products that are formed during formal stability that approach ICH thresholds).

10. How do you choose what wavelength to monitor when performing stress-testing studies using RP-HPLC with UV detection as the analytical separation technique?

Since both the loss of the parent drug and the increasing levels of degradation products need to be monitored, two different methods can be utilized, if desired, to analyze stressed samples, although the use of one method to monitor both has some advantages as is discussed in Chapter 4. For monitoring of the parent drug, it is common to monitor the λ_{max} of the parent. For monitoring of unknown degradation products, the goal is to maximize detectability and to minimize the differences in response factors. Monitoring at low wavelengths (e.g., 205–220 nm) is therefore recommended. For further discussion see Chapter 4.

11. What is a good alternate separation method to employ if RP-HPLC is the primary separation method?

Ideally, one wants an "orthogonal" (nonoverlapping) separation technique for the alternate method. In this respect, CE is a good first choice. Other choices include TLC, NP-HPLC, and RP-HPLC using different columns, different pH conditions, and different mobile phases. Peak purity evaluations using photodiode array (PDA) UV analysis (to evaluate UV-homogeneity) as well as LC-MS analyses are recommended. The ICH supports this approach in suggesting, "Peak purity tests may be useful to show that the analyte chromatographic peak is not attributable to more than one component (e.g., using diode array or mass spectrometry) (6)." For more discussion of this topic see Chapters 2 and 4.

12. How does one know whether or not all the major degradation products formed under a given stress condition are being detected with the analytical method? How do you know what the response factors of the unknown degradation product are? How should mass balance concerns be addressed during stress testing?

These questions are critical and difficult questions, and more discussion is warranted than will be provided here. These questions are discussed in detail in Chapter 2 (Section XI), in Chapter 6, and by Clarke & Norris (7). Briefly, it is nearly impossible to know whether or not all the major degradation products under a given condition are being detected until the structures of the detected products are known and the pathways of degradation can be proposed. When using UV detection, the response factors are nearly impossible to know unless purified standards are available. Mass balance concerns will always be present when using separation techniques that cannot ensure elution and resolution of all unknown products and detectors that are not universal and do not respond on the basis of mass. Whenever mass balance concerns are present, additional analysis should be performed using an orthogonal separation and/or detection scheme. The use of a detector such as a chemiluminescent nitrogen detector (which responds on the basis of the mass of nitrogen present in an eluted compound) can provide reliable response factors of unknown compounds as long as the compound contains nitrogen and the molecular formula is known. A recently introduced detector known as a "charged aerosol detector" has shown promise as a universal detector that responds to non-volatile compounds on the basis of the amount of mass eluting off the column (14). When using UV detection, it is prudent to use PDA detection to examine the UV spectra of the parent peak and degradation products. Any degradants with UV spectra significantly different than the parent will likely have different molar absorptivity, and hence different UV response factors. The use of low wavelengths (e.g., 205–210 nm) is recommended to increase the universality of UV detection and to minimize differences in response factors.

13. How sensitive should the analytical method be? What limit of detection is needed for routine stress-testing purposes?

While there is not an absolute requirement for sensitivity, we advocate that a limit of detection of 0.1% is appropriate for routine stress-testing purposes.

14. At what concentration of the parent drug should acid/base aqueous stress-testing studies be carried out?

While there are no specific requirements, most companies use a concentration between 0.1 and 1 mg/mL (1). Some companies use multiple concentrations, but most (14 out of 20 surveyed) use one concentration.

15. Should samples be analyzed in duplicate, or triplicate?

While there are no requirements for duplicate or triplicate analysis of stress-testing samples, we recommend that samples be analyzed in duplicate (or triplicate, if deemed appropriate), especially for studies that are intended to provide results for regulatory submissions.

16. When should stress-testing studies be performed in the development timeline: for drug substance and drug product?

This question may have several answers, as indicated by the different practices of major pharmaceutical companies. Certainly, stress testing needs to occur in order to develop and validate a stability-indicating analytical method. Because of this, some stress-testing studies need to occur at the very beginning of the development process, in the pre-clinical phase. Since the stability requirements for the clinical trial period are much less than what is needed for the market, stress-testing studies can be minimal in scope, with the goal of providing enough stability information to ensure the stability of the drug substance and product throughout the early clinical trials. Many companies perform additional stress-testing studies as the compound progresses through the clinical trial period to more thoroughly understand the intrinsic stability and to prepare for the needs of various formulations and of a marketed product. Determination of the structures of the major degradation products usually occurs later in the development cycle (e.g., Phase II to Phase III) because of the significant costs associated with isolation and structure elucidation coupled with the high fallout rate of new drugs from pre-clinical to the market. For additional discussion of this topic see Ref. 1 and Chapter 5.

17. How much material is needed for a stress-testing study of a drug substance powder?

The amount of material needed for a stress-testing study can vary greatly depending on the number of conditions being evaluated and the concentrations needed for the analytical evaluation. For a thorough stress-testing set up like that described in Chapter 4, 200 mg to 1 g may be required, although if the drug substance availability is limited, adjustments can be made to the protocols. For follow-up isolation and identification work, an additional 1–5 g may be needed to allow for generation of larger amounts of degradation products suitable for purification and structure elucidation. Alsante et al. have recommended that at least 300 mg of drug substance are needed at the early stage of development (when there are limited quantities of material) for experimental purposes while 10–15 g may be required during late stage development for thorough characterization. In terms of the amount of drug product required, early stage work requires approximately 25 tablets (solid) or 50 mL (solution) (see Ref. 4, p. 112.).

18. How do you decide which degradation products to characterize?

While there are no official "rules", we recommend characterization of the major degradation products formed under each stress condition that the drug degrades. A "rule-of-thumb" is to limit characterization to those products that are formed at levels greater than 10% of the total amount of degradation. Thus, if the drug degrades 10% and the individual degradation product is detected at 3% relative to the parent, this represents 30% of the total degradation and this product would be targeted for characterization. Alternatively, if the drug degrades 10% and the individual degradation product is present at 0.8% relative to the parent, this would represent only 8% of the total degradation and the product would not be targeted for characterization. See the PhRMA "Available Guidance and Best Practices" article (3) and Alsante et al. (4) page 115, for additional references.

19. How do you achieve buffered solutions across a pH range? (i.e., should one use the same buffer at ALL pH levels . . .)

Different companies use different approaches to address this problem. The use of different buffer systems that are true buffers at specific pH conditions provides for the best pH control, but the effects of the buffer on degradation rate (i.e., buffer-catalysis) can complicate the interpretation of kinetic data. The use of a single buffer" system (e.g., phosphate) is possible, as long as it is recognized that not all pH ranges will be truly buffered, and the pH can therefore change upon addition of the drug substance or during the degradation process. Measuring the pH after addition of the drug substance and at the specific time points of analysis is important to ensure that the pH is maintained. For additional discussion on this topic, see Alsante et al. (1) and Waterman et al. (8).

20. How much time and material are required to identify degradation products?

From Alsante et al., Ref. 4, page 126: Isolation of low-level degradants can be cumbersome and time consuming. Consider a 0.1% level degradant present in a drug substance bulk lot. Based on traditional NMR experiments, 5 mg of the impurity would be needed to obtain structural confirmation. To isolate 5 mg of the impurity from the bulk, a minimum of 5 g of bulk drug substance would be needed, assuming 100% recovery. Because actual recoveries are generally closer to 50% for low-level (0.1% range) isolations, 10 g of bulk drug substance would generally be requested.

In addition to requiring significant bulk material, the timeframe to complete the isolation is considerable. If the maximum analytical load for a 4.6 mm × 150 mm column has been determined to be 5 mg, assuming the isolation will be performed using semi-preparative chromatography (20 mm × 300 mm column), approximately 190 mg of sample can be loaded onto the preparative column. For a 0.1% level unknown, this translates to 190 μg of unknown injected onto the preparative column. Therefore, a total of 27 injections are required. If the assay time were estimated to be 1 hr, it would take at least 27 hr to perform the injections needed to obtain 5 mg (once again assuming 100% recovery). This timeframe does not include the time needed for method scale-up development, concentration and solubility experiments, and mass spectrometry and NMR experimentation. On the other hand, if a sample was available from stress-testing studies that contained 10% of the unknown, only 1 g of bulk would be needed and the estimated timeframe of the isolation would be drastically reduced. In the example above, 19 mg of unknown can be injected onto the preparative column (assuming the maximum analytical load does not change and resolution is retained with the higher level impurity). Therefore, only one injection would be needed to obtain the amount necessary for an NMR analysis, reducing the time to 1 hr.

21. What degradation information is requested in a regulatory submission?

From the PhRMA "Available Guidance and Best Practices" article on forced degradation studies (3), the following information should be supplied:

For marketing applications, current FDA and ICH guidance recommends inclusion of the results, including chromatograms of stressed samples, demonstration of the stability-indicating nature of the analytical procedures, and the degradation pathways of the drug substance in solution, solid state, and drug product. The structures of significant degradation products and the associated procedures for their isolation and/or characterization also are expected to be included in the filing.

Federal regulations require more from the pharmaceutical industry than just reporting that impurities and degradation products may exist. The 1987 FDA Stability Guideline gives guidance on the procedure to follow when degradation products are detected (9):

The following information about them should be submitted when available:

- Identity and chemical structure.
- Cross-reference to any available information about biological effect and significance at the concentrations likely to be encountered.
- Procedure for isolation and purification.
- Mechanism of formation, including order of reaction.
- Physical and chemical properties.
- Specification and directions for testing for their presence at the levels or concentrations expected to be present.
- Indication of pharmacological action or inaction.

More specific guidance for reporting of stress testing was found in FDA draft guidance documents dealing with stability and method validation (10). According to the documents, the applicant should provide:

- Degradation pathways of the drug substance, alone and in drug product.

- A discussion of the possible formation of polymorphic and enantiomeric substances; the possible formation of any stereoisomers is implied.
- Data showing that neither the freshly prepared nor the degraded placebo interferes with the quantitation of the active ingredient.
- Data from stress studies of the drug substance and drug product demonstrating the specificity of the assay and analytical procedures for degradation products. These data may take the form of representative instrument output (e.g., chromatograms) and/or degradation information obtained from stress studies (e.g., results of the peak purity experiments performed on degraded samples).

22. What degradation conditions should be performed for drug substance? Are there differences for drug product?

Table 1 shows a general outline for degradation studies of new drug substances and drug products that was endorsed at the PhRMA Acceptable Analytical Practices for Forced Degradation workshop (3).

Stress-testing studies of the drug substance include appropriate solution and solid-state conditions (e.g., acid/base hydrolysis, heat, humidity, oxidation, and light exposure, in accordance with regulatory guidelines) (5,9). Drug product degradation cannot be predicted from the stress-testing studies of the drug substance in the solution and solid state alone. The non-active pharmaceutical ingredients (excipients) can also react with the drug substance or catalyze degradation reactions. Stress-testing studies of the drug product depend on the chemical composition of the drug product formulation. For drug product formulations, heat, light, and humidity are often used (5). Stress-testing experiments will vary depending on whether the formulation is a solution or solid drug product. For solid drug product,

Table 1 General Protocol for Forced Degradation Studies (Stress Testing) of Drug Substance and Drug Products

	Drug substance		Drug product	
Condition	Solid	Solution/ suspension	Solid (tablets, capsules, blends)	Solution (IV, oral suspension)
Acid/base		✓		X
Oxidative	X	✓	✓	✓
Photostability	✓	X	✓	✓
Thermal	✓		✓	✓
Thermal/humidity	✓		✓	

✓—recommended; X—optional, suggested for some compounds.

key experiments are thermal, humidity, photostability and oxidation, if applicable. The most common type of interaction in solid dosage forms is between water and the drug substance; therefore, thermal/humidity challenges are critical (11). For more detailed discussion on drug substance and drug product degradation, see Alsante (4) and Singh (12).

ACKNOWLEDGMENTS

The assistance of W. Kimmer Smith and Patrick J. Jansen in reviewing this chapter is gratefully acknowledged.

REFERENCES

1. Alsante KM, Baertschi SW, Martin L. A Stress testing benchmarking study. Pharm Technol 2003; 27:2, February: 60–72.
2. International Conference on Harmonisation, Guideline on Validation of Analytical Procedures, Q2A, Code of Federal Register, Vol 60, no. 40, p. 11260, March (1995).
3. Reynolds DW, Facchine KL, Mullaney JF, Alsante KM, Hatajik TD, Motto MG. Available guidance and best practices for conducting forced degradation studies. Pharm Technol 2002; 26(2):48–54.
4. Alsante KM, Friedmann RC, Hatajik TD, Lohr LL, Sharp TR, Snyder KD, Szczesny EJ. Degradation and impurity analysis for pharmaceutical drug candidates (Chapter 4). In: Ahuja S, Scypinski S, eds. Handbook of Modern Pharmaceutical Analysis. Boston: Academic Press, 2001.
5. International Conference on Harmonisation, "Stability Testing of New Drug Substances and Products", Q1A(R2), February 2003.
6. International Conference on Harmonisation, "Validation of Analytical Procedures: Methodology", Q2B, November 1996.
7. Clarke HJ, Norris KJ. Sample selection for analytical method development (Chapter 7). In: Ahuja S, Alsante KM, eds. Handbook of Isolation and Characterization of Impurities in Pharmaceuticals. San Diego: Elsevier Science, 2003.
8. Waterman KC, Adami RC, Alsante KM, Antipas AS, Arenson DR, Carrier R, Hong J, Landis MS, Lombardo F, Shah JC, Shalaev E, Smith SW, Wang H. Hydrolysis in pharmaceutical formulations. Pharm Dev Tech 2002; 7(2): 113–146.
9. US Food and Drug Administration. Drug Stability Guidelines, February 1987.
10. FDA, International Conference on Harmonization: Guidance on Q6A Specifications: Test Procedures and Acceptance Criteria for New Drug Substances and New Drug Products: Chemical Substances. Federal Register (Notices) 65 (251), December 29, 2000: 83041–83063.
11. Cartensen JT. Drug Stability Principles and Practices. Vol. 68. 2nd ed. New York: Marcel Dekker, 1995.
12. Singh S, Bakshi M. Guidance on conduct of stress tests to determine inherent stability of drugs. Pharm Technol On-Line 2000; 24:1–14.

13. Silke K, Muijselaar PG, Waterval J, Eichinger T, Korn C, Gerding TK, Debets AJ, Sänger-van de Griend C, van den Beld C, Somsen GW, Desong GJ, "Toward a generic approach for stress testing of drug substances and drug products", Pharmaceutical Technology Feb 2005; 48–66.
14. Dixon RW, "Development and testing of a detection method for liquid chromatography based on aerosol charging", Analytical Chemistry 2002; 74: 2930–2937.

Index